NUTRITIONAL PHYSIOLOGY OF FARM ANIMALS

NUTRITIONAL PHYSIOLOGY OF FARM ANIMALS

J. A. F. ROOK
Agricultural Research Council, London, England
P. C. THOMAS
Hannah Research Institute, Ayr, Scotland

Longman *London and New York*

Longman Group Limited
Longman House
Burnt Mill, Harlow, Essex, UK

*Published in the United States of America
by Longman Inc., New York*

First published 1983

British Library Cataloguing in Publication Data
Nutritional physiology of farm animals.
  1. Animal nutrition
  I. Rook, J. A. F.   II. Thomas, P. C.
  636.08'4   SF95
ISBN 0-582-45587-1

Library of Congress Cataloging in Publication Data
Nutritional physiology of farm animals.
  Bibliography: p.
  Includes index.
  1. Animal nutrition.   2. Veterinary physiology.
I. Rook, J. A. F. (John Allan Fynes), 1926–
II. Thomas, P. C. (Phillip Charles), 1942–
SF768.N87   636.089'2   82-243
ISBN 0-582-45587-1   AACR2

Printed in Singapore by
Kyodo Shing Loong Printing Industries Pte Ltd.

CONTENTS

PREFACE

Historically, the study of animal nutrition was concerned with the identification of essential nutrients, the determination of nutrient requirements under defined conditions of activity, environment and productive state, and the clinical, physiological and biochemical consequences of failing to meet those requirements. As the subject has evolved, however, a more dynamic aspect has emerged. The supply of nutrients is now recognized to be a major determinant of the nature and rate of metabolic reactions within the body, of the overall balance between the synthetic and degradative processes, and of the efficiency and characteristics of animal production.

This book is designed to present this newer approach to the study of animal nutrition, where possible in terms of the underlying physiology and biochemistry. An elementary appreciation of these subjects has been assumed as has a more detailed knowledge of food composition and of the processes of digestion in both simple-stomached and ruminant animals. The first chapter proceeds from this basis, with a brief review of the mechanisms for digestion and absorption of the food constituents that have a central role in the supply of nutrients to the body tissues. The second chapter considers in principle the physiological mechanisms that are fundamental to an understanding of the transfer and metabolism of materials within the body. There is then, in Chapter 3, a detailed consideration of the transport of major nutrients and the part played by the various tissues of the body in the regulation of metabolism. Following this are the two main sections of the book. The first of these sections deals with the regulation of food intake, the relationship between nutrient supply and metabolism under various physiological conditions, the consequences of nutrient imbalances and the unique role of the trace nutrients. This is followed by a section dealing with the relationship between diet and the yield and quality of animal products, and with the ways in which nutritional responses in animal performance are modified by environment and gastrointestinal disease. Each chapter is presented as a self-contained essay but the arrangement of the chapters is designed to give a continuity to the theme of the book and to allow the reader to appreciate the extent to which the different subject areas in animal nutrition are presently conceived in physiological and biochemical terms.

We are grateful to our colleagues for their helpful comments during the planning and preparation of this book but we are especially indebted to Dr P. D. Wilson and Miss Marilyn Beatson for their direct and invaluable assistance.

J. A. F. Rook
P. C. Thomas

CONTRIBUTORS

Campling, R. C., MSc, PhD, MIBiol
Reader in Animal Production, Wye College, University of London

Faulkner, Anne, BSc, PhD
Principal Scientific Officer, Department of Lactational Physiology and Biochemistry, Hannah Research Institute, Ayr

Fisher, C., BSc, PhD
Senior Principal Scientific Officer and Head of the Department of Nutritional and Environmental Studies, ARC Poultry Research Centre, Roslin, Midlothian

Forbes, J. M., BSc, PhD
Senior Lecturer, Department of Animal Physiology, University of Leeds

Gilbert, A. B., BSc, PhD
Principal Scientific Officer, Department of Reproductive Physiology, ARC Poultry Research Centre, Roslin, Midlothian

Hill, K. J., DVSc, MRCVS
Principal Scientist, Nutrition and Agriculture Division, Unilever Research, Colworth Laboratory, Colworth House, Sharnbrook and Special Professor in Animal Physiology, School of Agriculture, University of Nottingham

Lean, I. J., BSc, PhD, MIBiol
Lecturer in Animal Production, Wye College, University of London

Lindsay, D. B., BSc, MA, DPhil
Principal Scientific Officer, Department of Biochemistry, ARC Institute of Animal Physiology, Cambridge; Special Professor in Animal Physiology, School of Agriculture, University of Nottingham

Lewis, D., MSc, PhD, DSc, FRSC
Professor of Applied Biochemistry and Head of the Department of Applied Biochemistry and Food Science, University of Nottingham

Lister, D., BSc, PhD, FIBiol
    Senior Principal Scientific Officer and Head of the Animal
    Physiology Division and of the Applied Physiology Section,
    Meat Research Institute, Langford; Research Fellow in Animal
    Physiology, University of Bristol
Peaker M., BSc, PhD, FIBiol
    Director, Hannah Research Institute, Ayr and Professor of Dairy
    Science, University of Glasgow
Pearson, R. Anne, BSc, PhD
    Principal Scientific Officer, Department of Nutrition, ARC
    Poultry Research Centre, Roslin, Midlothian
Perry, B. N., BSc, PhD
    Principal Scientific Officer, Applied Physiology Section, ARC
    Meat Research Institute, Langford; Research Fellow in Animal
    Physiology, University of Bristol
Suttle, N. F., BSc, PhD
    Principal Scientific Officer, Biochemistry Department, More-
    dun Research Institute, Edinburgh
Rook, J. A. F., PhD, DSc, FRSC, FIBiol, FRSE
    Second Secretary, Agricultural Research Council, London;
    Visiting Professor in Animal Nutrition, Wye College, Univer-
    sity of London; formerly Director, Hannah Research Institute,
    Ayr and Professor of Animal Nutrition, University of Glasgow
Thomas, P. C., BSc, PhD, MIBiol
    Senior Principal Scientific Officer and Head of the Department
    of Animal Nutrition and Production, Hannah Research Insti-
    tute, Ayr; Honorary Lecturer in Animal Nutrition, University
    of Glasgow
Topps, J. H., BSc, PhD, FRCS
    Head of the Department of Agricultural Chemistry and Bio-
    chemistry, School of Agriculture, Aberdeen
Vernon, R. G., BSc, PhD
    Principal Scientific Officer and Head of the Department of
    Lactational Physiology and Biochemistry, Hannah Research
    Institute, Ayr
Webster, A. J. F., MA, VetMB, PhD, MRCVS
    Professor of Animal Husbandry, University of Bristol; formerly
    Principal Scientific Officer and Head of the Calorimetry Section,
    Rowett Research Institute, Aberdeen
Wood, J. D., BSc, PhD
    Principal Scientific Officer and Head of the Growth Section,
    Deputy Head of the Animal Physiology Division, ARC Meat
    Research Institute, Langford; Research Fellow in Animal Phy-
    siology, University of Bristol

ABBREVIATIONS

ACTH	Adrenocorticotrophic hormone (adrenocorticotropin)
ADP	Adenosine diphosphate
AMP	Adenosine monophosphate
ATP	Adenosine triphosphate
ATPase	Adenosine triphosphatase
CDP	Cytidine diphosphate
CNS	Central nervous system
CoA	Coenzyme A
CP	Crude protein
CTP	Cytidine triphosphate
DE	Digestible energy
DM	Dry matter
DNA	Deoxyribonucleic acid
FAD	Flavin adenine dinucleotide
FADH$_2$	Reduced flavin adenine dinucleotide
FFA	Free fatty acid(s)
FMN	Flavin mononucleotide
FSH	Follicle stimulating hormone
GDP	Guanosine diphosphate
GMP	Guanosine monophosphate
GTP	Guanosine triphosphate
K_i	Inhibitor constant
K_m	Michaelis–Menten constant
LH	Luteinizing hormone
ME	Metabolizable energy
mRNA	Messenger ribonucleic acid
NAD	Nicotinamide adenine dinucleotide
NADH	Reduced nicotinamide adenine dinucleotide
NADP	Nicotinamide adenine dinucleotide phosphate
NADPH	Reduced nicotinamide adenine dinucleotide phosphate
NPN	Non-protein nitrogen

P	Probability
Pi	Inorganic phosphate
PPi	Inorganic pyrophosphate
RNA	Ribonucleic acid
RNase	Ribonuclease
rRNA	Ribosomal ribonucleic acid
T_3	Tri–iodothyronine
T_4	Thyroxine (tetraiodothyronine)
tRNA	Transfer ribonucleic acid
TSH	Thyroid stimulating hormone (thyrotropin)
UDP	Uridine diphosphate
UMP	Uridine monophosphate
UTP	Uridine triphosphate
VFA	Volatile fatty acid(s)
V_{max}	Maximum velocity

INTRODUCTION

Section 1

INTRODUCTION

1 THE PROVISION OF NUTRIENTS

D. Lewis and K. J. Hill

Most foodstuffs contain a mixture of nutrients – proteins, fats, carbohydrates, minerals, vitamins and water – and, as few of these can be absorbed directly by the animal, they must be prepared or modified to make them available. This is accomplished by the process of digestion in which foodstuffs are converted to diffusible or assimilatable substances by enzymes secreted in the digestive tract or, especially in herbivores, by the action of microorganisms living in symbiotic association with the animal.

Apart from the intracellular enzymes present in the epithelial cells of the small intestine, the animal's digestive enzymes are produced by the salivary, gastric, and pancreatic glands and, along with other products of glandular activity, comprise the secretions which enter the digestive tract. Enzyme provision is therefore a function of the secretory activity of the digestive glands, whilst the duration of enzyme action is dependent on the rate at which food material passes along the tract. These two are coordinated by a series of nervous and hormonal mechanisms which ensure the different phases of digestion occur in orderly sequence, commencing with the breakdown of food into small pieces by the teeth, its transport along the oesophagus to the stomach, and the production by the gastric contractions of a semi-solid mixture of food and digestive secretions. Subsequent movement of the ingesta and its admixture with pancreatic, biliary and intestinal secretions is dependent on the activities of the small intestine.

Secretory activity (of the salivary glands) at the cranial end of the tract is controlled only by neural mechanisms, and subsequently there is a progessive change through mixed nervous and hormonal control of the gastric glands to predominantly hormonal control of the pancreatic and biliary secretions. Nervous stimulation of secretory activity ensures a rapid response to the ingestion of food, whilst hormonal stimulation results in a more gradual, but sustained, level of secretory activity. Optimal conditions for digestion are therefore achieved by close integration of substrate presentation, secretory (enzymic) activity and capacity for absorption.

THE DIGESTIVE TRACT

The higher animals are dependent on plants and other animals for their nutrients and it is conventional to classify them on the basis of their eating habits in the natural state, though under domestication their diets may be considerably different from those eaten under natural conditions. Carnivores obtain most of their food by eating other animals, and in these species digestion is mainly enzymic in nature and microbial digestion is minimal. In the herbivores, however, microbial digestion is of great significance and allows utilization of plant materials that are not broken down by the enzymes present in the digestive secretions.

The domesticated herbivores fall into two groups: those possessing a rumen (cow, sheep, goat), in which there is extensive microbial fermentation of the vegetable diet in a specialized region of the digestive tract, prior to its digestion by the alimentary enzymes; and those with simple stomachs (horse, pig), in which fermentation takes place in the posterior part of the digestive tract. The relative sizes of the main regions of the digestive tract in the different species illustrates these adaptations to different modes of digestion (Table 1.1) and, although the basic characteristics of the digestive process are similar in all higher animals, the presence of a rumen, in particular, has resulted in numerous modifications to secretory and digestive activity which optimize the microbial contribution to digestion.

THE DIGESTIVE SECRETIONS

There is, in most animals, anticipatory secretion of saliva, gastric juice and pancreatic juice at the sight or smell of food or at its presence in the mouth. This anticipatory response is readily conditioned so that, even in the absence of food, the noise or disturbance associated with food preparation will provoke secretory activity. Experimental work on the secretory responses to different stimuli therefore has to be carefully controlled to avoid spurious results arising from conditioned responses.

Saliva

When food enters the mouth there is secretion of saliva attributable to reflex stimulation of the salivary glands by means of buccal receptors

Table 1.1 Relative volume of the different regions of the digestive tract
(Colin, 1886)

Species	Total volume of digestive tract (l)	Fraction of total volume		
		Stomach	Small intestine	Large intestine
Dog	7	0.63	0.23	0.14
Pig	27	0.29	0.33	0.38
Horse	210	0.09	0.30	0.61
Cow	360	0.71	0.18	0.11

sensitive to tactile and taste stimulation, activation of sensory centres in the brain-stem and impulse discharge along the efferent cranial nerves. The volume and composition of saliva secreted in response to different substances are, however, markedly different, e.g. moist edible substances produce a saliva rich in mucin which facilitates swallowing, whereas dry, fibrous or alkaline materials provoke a copious watery secretion. These variations are produced, to some extent, by admixture of secretions from the different salivary glands, but it is apparent that mechanisms exist which permit analysis of food texture and composition and give rise to an integrated signal for the release of a salivary secretion of appropriate volume and composition.

Gustatory signals are probably the major component of this system, since different tastes are associated with different characteristics of the secretory response and the magnitude of taste nerve activity, i.e. taste receptor discharge, has been shown to be related to the volume of saliva produced (Kawamura and Yamamoto, 1978). However, as most of the taste fibres respond to more than one kind of taste stimulus, differences in secretory activity by the salivary glands are not attributable only to taste nerve activity. Central activity is likely to be involved, and it is probable that it is the activation of different response patterns in the medulla that gives rise to qualitative differences in efferent nerve activity to the salivary glands and hence to differences in secretory activity (Erickson, 1963).

The characteristics of the receptor patterns in the brain-stem and the mechanisms by which different patterns influence the volume and composition of the saliva have not been resolved, but are fundamental to further understanding of food selection and taste, and of control of salivary enzyme secretion.

Saliva assists in the mechanical disintegration of food during mastication and lubricates, by its mucin content, the passage of food along the oesophagus. The water-soluble components of foods are dissolved in the saliva in the mouth and are then able to activate the taste buds which initiate further secretory activity. Mixed saliva collected from the mouth is a colourless, slightly opalescent fluid, consisting mainly of water and small amounts of electrolytes. The carbohydrate-splitting enzyme, α-amylase, is present in the saliva of a number of species (man, ape, pig, rat, rabbit) but is absent, or present only in very low concentrations, in others (dog, cat, horse, sheep, cow, goat) (Chauncy, Henriques and Tanzer, 1963.)

Numerous other enzymes are present in saliva, e.g. lipase, maltase, phosphatase and peroxidase, but it is probable that these originate from the oral bacteria and unlikely that they play any important rôle in the digestive process. A lipase (pre-gastric esterase), active against milk fat glycerides containing short-chain fatty acids (especially butyric acid), is secreted by buccal glands in a number of species, particularly the calf. It is trapped in association with milk fat globules in the milk clot in the stomach, and is responsible for the release of considerable amounts of free fatty acids (Nelson, Jensen and Pitas, 1977).

In contrast to simple-stomached species the saliva of ruminants is markedly alkaline, due to the presence of considerable amounts of sodium bicarbonate and phosphate, which are important in maintaining the well-buffered fluid conditions necessary to provide a suitable environment for the rumen microorganisms (Bailey and Balch, 1961). The buffering effect is maintained by the continuous nature of parotid salivary secretions, partly brought about by the wider distribution of reflex salivary pathways in the ruminant. Thus, mechanical and chemical stimulation of parts of the oesophagus and reticulo-rumen are as effective in provoking secretion as oral stimulation. Ruminant saliva also contains appreciable quantities of urea produced by the liver from ammonia absorbed from the rumen, and subsequently extracted from the blood by the salivary glands.

Gastric juice

In simple-stomached species the stomach is both a temporary storage organ and a digestive chamber and, within it, foods of different composition and consistency are acted upon by the saliva and the gastric enzymes, and transformed by contractions of the pyloric region to a semi-liquid mass which is released at intervals into the duodenum. Gastric juice is acidic and powerfully proteolytic, but the degree and rate of proteolysis in the stomach are related to the extent to which food becomes impregnated with the juice.

Although the juice comprises the total secretion from the surface epithelial cells, and from the cardiac, peptic and pyloric glands, it is derived primarily from the peptic glands and consists of a mixture of hydrochloric acid (parietal cell secretion) and a non-parietal alkaline secretion containing pepsin, mucin and electrolytes. Pure gastric juice may have a pH of 1.0 or slightly less. Pepsins are the main proteolytic enzymes secreted by the stomach and they are synthesized in the peptic cells as inactive precursors, pepsinogens. Pepsinogen granules accummulate during fasting and are released when secretion occurs.

The initial secretion of enzyme-rich gastric juice occurs from the anticipation of food ingestion, and the presence of food in the mouth, and is due to passage of impulses from the vagal nerve centres to the stomach. The major secretory response occurs when food reaches the stomach and consists essentially of acid secretion. It results from several integrated mechanisms:

1. the release of the hormone, gastrin, by the action of peptic digests on gastrin-producing cells in the pyloric region of the stomach;
2. activation, by gastric distension, of cholinergic reflexes which lead to release of gastrin; and
3. the stimulation of the acid-producing cells by the products of protein digestion.

Meals containing different amounts of protein, and/or proteins of different composition, tend to provoke secretory responses which differ in acidity and volume of juice produced (Saint-Hilaire, Lavers, Kennedy and Code, 1960).

The total secretory response to a meal is, however, the result not only of stimulation of gastric secretion but also of its inhibition, which may be of nervous or humoral origin. Accummulation of acid in the stomach will inhibit further acid secretion because gastrin release from the pyloric region is inhibited when the pH falls below 2.5. Inhibitory effects on acid secretion are also obtained from the duodenum when acid, hyptonic solutions or fat are introduced into the lumen, and these effects are also probably due to release of hormones (cholecystokinin-secretin).

The pattern of gastric digestive activity shows some variation with species. Thus in the pig, because the large cardiac zone acts as a food storage area, the secretion of gastric juice tends to be continuous. It is, however, greater during the day-time when food is being consumed (see Kidder and Manners, 1978). The gastric juice is of high acidity and rapidly reduces the pH of the contents of the body of the stomach to a level appropriate for peptic proteolysis. The pH in the cardiac region does tend, however, to remain higher because of mucus and bicarbonate secretion which may relate to its function as a fermentation chamber.

The frequent feeding of the ruminant and the reservoir function of the rumen ensure that there is a regular flow of digesta into the abomasum. Its composition is modified by the removal of water and electrolytes by the omasum but, normally, material entering the abomasum is a finely divided suspension of bacterial bodies, non-fermented food residues and residual fermentation products. Largely because of the flow of this material the secretion of gastric juice is continuous and the abomasal contents therefore remain at a pH which is low enough for optimal peptic proteolysis (Hill, 1968).

Secretion in the small intestine

The digesta leaving the stomach meet the pancreatic juice and the bile in the lumen of the duodenum and the enzymes of the intestinal cells at the brush-border interface. The enzymes involved reduce many of the food components to their absorbable form and collectively accomplish digestion in the intestine.

Pancreatic juice

Pancreatic juice contains bicarbonate as its main anion and this is the major factor responsible for reducing the acidity of the stomach contents when they enter the duodenum. Its major component, however, is a range of enzymes active against most of the dietary ingredients.

In fasting animals basal pancreatic secretion is maintained at a low rate and enzyme synthesis and secretion are greatly reduced. As with saliva and gastric juice, there is anticipatory secretion resulting from the activation of central neural mechanisms in response to the sight, smell, ingestion and mastication of food, and this secretion ensures that digestion in the duodenum of newly arrived stomach contents proceeds rapidly. Subsequently secretion is stimulated mainly by hormones, particularly secretin and cholecystokinin–pancreozymin (CCK–PZ) which are liberated from the duodenal mucosa by contact with the acidic stomach contents.

Secretin is released by a low pH in the duodenum and has been believed generally to be responsible only for bicarbonate secretion whilst CCK–PZ, released mainly by amino acids and fatty acids, stimulates only enzyme secretion. Recent findings indicate that secretin also stimulates enzyme secretion and that CCK–PZ not only stimulates some bicarbonate secretion but greatly potentiates secretin effects on bicarbonate secretion (Singh and Webster, 1978).

Hormone-induced enzyme secretion from the pancreatic cells is mediated by intracellular control mechanisms which couple signals received through receptors at the base of the acinar cells with events inside the cells and result in the extrusion of zymogen granules from the apical portions of the cells. The receptors are genetically determined macromolecules which carry specific recognition sites for exogenous or endogenous ligands. Receptor-ligand interaction results in a series of intracelluar changes mediated by cyclic GMP and cyclic AMP and these result in enzyme synthesis and extrusion (Rosselin, Fromageot and Bonfils, 1979).

The enzymes secreted by the pancreas are synthesized and stored in the pancreatic cells as inactive zymogen granules and it is generally held that the enzyme content of these granules is mixed. Secretion of the digestive enzymes in response to stimulation should therefore result in parallel discharge of the various enzymes contained within the zymogen granules under all conditions of glandular activity, and there is evidence from several species that this is indeed the case (Steer and Glazer, 1976). The basic concept underlying this view of pancreatic secretion is that there is mass transport of newly synthesized digestive enzymes through a series of intracellular, but extracytoplasmic, compartments in the pancreatic acinar cells, each of which contains a mixture of proteins. Proportional representation of each enzyme within this mixture remains constant while the entire mixture migrates as a single wave from the points of synthesis towards the cell surface. Thus, in response to stimulation, there should be a rise in the concentration of digestive enzymes in the juice and a rise in the output of enzymes, although the ratio of these enzymes should remain constant. Because parallel secretion of enzymes has not been observed consistently an alternative concept, the membrane transport hypothesis, has been developed, which proposes that enzymes are secreted as the result of their variable and differential release from the storage pools into the cytoplasm. Their subsequent transport out of the cell across the luminal plasma membrane is governed by independent equilibria for each enzyme. Concentrations of individual enzymes in the pancreatic juice may then vary independently.

Bile

Bile is produced by the liver and, apart from the bile pigments (which are excretory products), it contains an electrolyte mixture similar to that of pancreatic juice, the salts of the bile acids, and phospholipids (mainly lecithin).

The bile salts are cyclopentano–phenanthrene compounds closely related to, and derived from cholesterol. The primary acids in most species are cholic, deoxycholic, chenodeoxycholic and lithocholic acids, and the acid side chains of their sodium salts are conjugated either with taurine or glycine to form taurocholic or glycocholic acids.

There is a distinct relationship between dietary habits and the type of bile salts found in the bile; carnivorous species have bile salts with three or four hydroxyl groups as taurine conjugates; while herbivores, with the exception of bovines, tend to have dihydroxy acids sometimes conjugated almost entirely with glycine. Omnivorous animals have both types of acids and conjugates.

There is continuous formation of bile by the liver, but in most animals there is only an intermittent need for bile as a digestive secretion and consequently bile is stored in the gall-bladder. The walls of the gall-bladder secrete mucin and absorb water from the bile so that gall-bladder bile is more concentrated than hepatic bile. The concentrated bile is discharged into the duodenum when the gall-bladder contracts during the digestion of a meal – contraction following the liberation of CCK-PZ by the acid stomach contents in the duodenum.

The extent to which hepatic bile is concentrated in the gall-bladder varies in different animals. In ruminants and the pig only slight absorption of water takes place and this probably relates to the need for a continuous flow of bile into the duodenum.

The bile salts are intimately involved in the micelle stage of lipid absorption but thereafter pass along the small intestine where some 95% of the total bile salts are absorbed from the ileum. The remainder are deconjugated and pass to the caecum and colon from where, after further breakdown by the bacterial flora, they are excreted in the faeces.

The small intestine is the major absorptive site of the digestive tract and, as such, its mucosa is exposed to digesta of widely varying composition. Possibly because of this and because relatively small changes in the magnitude of bidirectional fluxes of water and ions can convert absorption to secretion, the intestine may at times behave as a secretory rather than as an absorptive organ. Fluid and electrolytes may therefore pass from the mucosal cells to the lumen of the gut.

Enzyme activity appears, however, to be confined to the intestine-lumen interface and the end products of gastric and pancreatic digestion are either hydrolysed on the surface of the intestinal mucosal cells by brush-border enzymes, or hydrolysed within the cytoplasm of the mucosal cells after transport from the lumen to the mucosa has occurred. Enzymes present in the intestinal secretion are therefore probably derived from desquamated cells and not from active secretion. Adaptative changes in the intestinal mucosal enzymes in response to alterations in, for example, dietary carbohydrate content may result from the intimate contact between substrate and the enzyme-producing cells of the gut mucosa.

Secretions in the large intestine

The large intestine comprises the caecum and the colon and is the final region of the tract through which the digesta pass before they are voided as the faeces. The caecum is a simple tubular structure with a blind end and is of considerable size in the non-ruminant herbivores to allow for the extensive microbial fermentation which takes place in these species.

The colon is a major site for water, electrolyte and VFA absorption from the ileal and caecal contents which pass into it, and in the ruminant and the pig is both extensive and much coiled to provide the necessary surface area. It is lined with mucus-secretory cells which assist the passage of the progressively more dehydrated digesta.

THE BIOCHEMISTRY OF DIGESTION

Until comparatively recently the processes of digestion and absorption were regarded as relatively discrete entities. Digestion occurred as a result of the luminal breakdown of macromolecules by enzymes from the digestive secretions whilst absorption was a process of relatively simple transfer through the mucosal surfaces, mainly of the small intestine. It is now recognized that there is, in addition, a more complex process of mucosal breakdown and absorption.

Carbohydrate digestion

Saliva contains significant quantities of only one enzyme, α-amylase, and like pancreatic amylase this enzyme initiates the breakdown of starch into a mixture of maltose, maltotriose and various dextrins. It is active over a pH range of 4.0 to 9.0 with an optimum, in the presence of chloride, of 7.0. Amylose, a linear polymer of glucose units linked by α-1,4 bonds, can be broken down at each link other than the two terminal ones. In the case of branched-chain polysaccharides such as amylopectin and glycogen the 1,6 branch links are resistant to α-amylase action and their products of digestion therefore contain certain dextrins because hydrolysis has stopped at a 1,6 link.

As the food enters the stomach and the pH falls salivary α-amylase activity is steadily reduced but, in the duodenum, following its admixture with pancreatic and duodenal secretions and bile, the pH rises and conditions become suitable for the action of pancreatic amylase which continues the breakdown of starch and intermediates.

The mucosal cells of the small intestine also produce a number of carbohydrases which are located on the brush border of the mature cells and these include lactase, trehalase and several maltases. Lactase has been shown to hydrolyse lactose, cellobiose and gentiobiose and is, therefore, both a β-galactosidase and a β-glucosidase. Trehalase appears to have limited activity but the maltases hydrolyse substrates other than maltose. Thus maltase Ia (isomaltase) attacks dextrins containing α-1,6 bonds, maltase Ib (sucrase) attacks sucrose, and maltase II (glucoamylase) and maltase III (heat stable glucoamylase) attack maltodextrins and starch.

Most of the dietary carbohydrate is absorbed as monosaccharide although the rate of absorption varies with different sugars, glucose and galactose being absorbed most rapidly, fructose more slowly and all other sugars at a much slower rate. This is probably due to the fact that they are absorbed partly by diffusion, but mainly by processes that are specific and are 'active' or 'energy demanding'. The intestinal absorption of glucose has been most studied in this context and, although it is generally accepted that the absorption of glucose from the lumen of the gut into the blood stream depends upon the activity of an energy-coupled specific translocation process which is located in the brush border pole of the epithelial cells of the gut mucosa, the intimate detail of the process has not been fully resolved.

Protein digestion

The enzymes concerned with protein breakdown are divided primarily into proteases (or endopeptidases) and peptidases (or exopeptidases). The exopeptidases act upon peptide linkages adjacent to free polar groups: the carboxypeptidases require an adjacent free carboxyl group whilst the aminopeptidases require a free amino group adjacent to the bond that is to be split. The specificity of the exopeptidases appears to be variable: pancreatic carboxypeptidase, for example, attacks a wide range of substrates whereas leucine amino peptidase is highly specific.

The endopeptidases hydrolyse internal peptide bonds of proteins, and the free polar groups adjacent to the bond split are usually inhibitory. The characteristics of endopeptidases have been studied by using synthetic peptides in which a substituent has been placed on either a free carboxyl group or an amino group respectively, e.g. conversion to an amide or the introduction of a carbobenzoxy derivative. It has been concluded that pepsin preferentially attacks peptide bonds that involve the amino group of an aromatic acid (especially phenylalanine or tyrosine), that trypsin has a preferential activity towards peptide bonds involving the carboxyl group of dibasic amino acids and that chymotrypsin is most active towards peptide bonds involving the carboxyl group of aromatic amino acids (complementary to pepsin).

This characteristic of preferential attack can be illustrated by reference to carbobenzoxyglutamyltyrosylglycineamide, which has bonds appropriate for attack by chymotrypsin and pepsin. However, chymotrypsin is inhibited by the exposure of the carboxyl group of glycine whilst pepsin is inhibited by exposure of the amino group of glutamic acid. Thus:

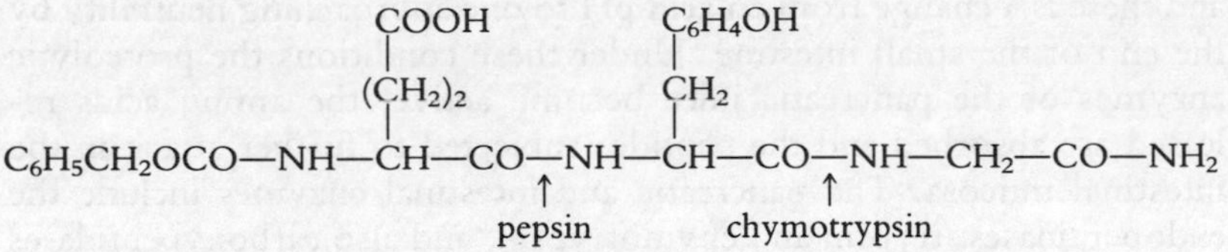

$$COOH \qquad\qquad C_6H_4OH$$
$$| \qquad\qquad\qquad |$$
$$(CH_2)_2 \qquad\qquad CH_2$$
$$| \qquad\qquad\qquad |$$
$$C_6H_5CH_2OCO—NH—CH—CO—NH—CH—CO—NH—CH_2—CO—NH_2$$

pepsin $\qquad$ chymotrypsin

Carbobenzoxyglutamyltyrosylglycineamide

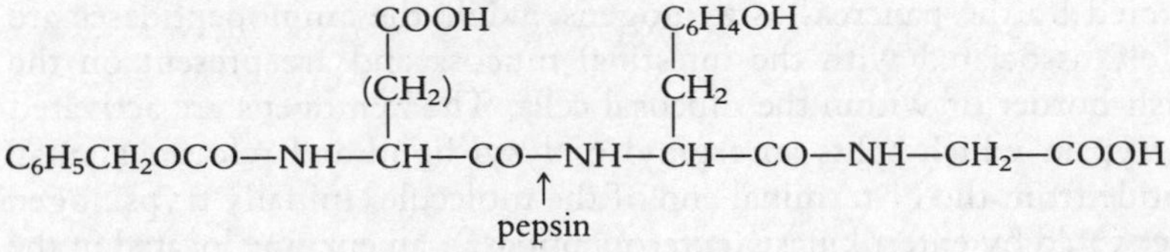

$$COOH \qquad\qquad C_6H_4OH$$
$$| \qquad\qquad\qquad |$$
$$(CH_2) \qquad\qquad CH_2$$
$$| \qquad\qquad\qquad |$$
$$C_6H_5CH_2OCO—NH—CH—CO—NH—CH—CO—NH—CH_2—COOH$$

pepsin

Carbobenzoxyglutamyltyrosylglycine (not attacked by chymotrypsin)

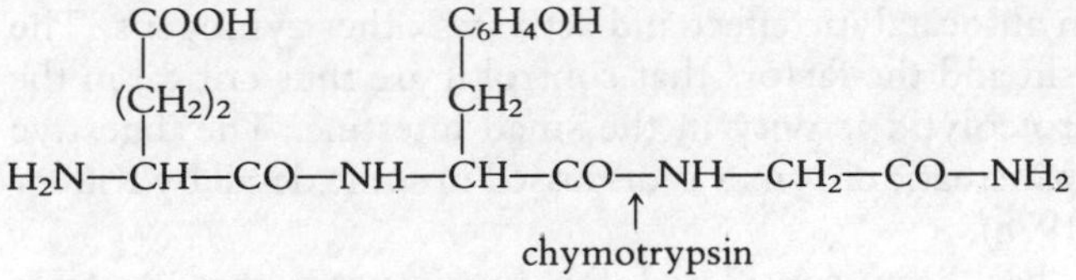

$$COOH \qquad\qquad C_6H_4OH$$
$$| \qquad\qquad\qquad |$$
$$(CH_2)_2 \qquad\qquad CH_2$$
$$| \qquad\qquad\qquad |$$
$$H_2N—CH—CO—NH—CH—CO—NH—CH_2—CO—NH_2$$

chymotrypsin

Glutamyltyrosylglycineamide (not attacked by pepsin)

The endopeptidases have also been classified into broad categories based on bonding to other substances, e.g. serine proteases, metalloproteases or sulphydryl proteases.

Despite the particular attention given in recent years to the concept of integrated digestion and absorption at the mucosal surface, activity within the lumen of the alimentary tract is of major significance. Digestion of protein starts in the stomach following exposure to the pepsins of the gastric juice and these, in common with other proteolytic enzymes, are secreted as inactive precursors (pepsinogens in particular, zymogens in general) which are activated by hydrolytic removal of a peptide from the N-terminal end of the molecule. This process occurs under the acid conditions in the stomach and is autocatalytic since pepsin itself catalyses the activation. The nature of the intramolecular activation involves a split between amino acid residues 44 and 45 (Sanny, Hartsuck and Tang, 1975), whilst the autocatalytic process is due to hydrolysis of a glutamyl-isoleucyl bond with the release of a 41 amino acid peptide (which can be inhibitory of pepsin action at low concentration). This is probably a protective device to inhibit premature activation of the enzyme within the secretory gland.

As the contents of the stomach pass along the duodenum there is an entry of three fluids: duodenal secretion, pancreatic secretion and bile; and there is a change from an acid pH to one approaching neutrality by the end of the small intestine. Under these conditions the proteolytic enzymes of the pancreatic juice become active, the amino acids released are absorbed and the peptides subjected to further attack in the intestinal mucosa. The pancreatic and intestinal enzymes include the endopeptidases, trypsin and chymotrypsin, and also carboxypeptidases and aminopeptidases. The endopeptidases and carboxypeptidases are secreted by the pancreas as zymogens, while the aminopeptidases are largely associated with the intestinal mucosa and are present on the brush-border or within the mucosal cells. The zymogens are activated by trypsin which splits an arginyl or lysyl bond and releases a small peptide from the N-terminal end of the molecule. Initially trypsinogen is activated by enterokinase (enteropeptidase), an enzyme located in the brush-border of the duodenal mucosa, and the trypsin that is then produced has an autocatalytic effect and activates other zymogens. The activity of trypsin and the factors that control it are thus critical in the regulation of proteolytic activity in the small intestine. The digestive function of the pancreatic enzymes is discussed in some detail by Kidder and Manners (1978).

Although it has been considered for many years that proteins undergo complete hydrolysis to free amino acids within the small intestine, it has become apparent recently that there is also uptake by the mucosa of small peptides which is followed by their hydrolysis within the absorptive cells. This process has been shown to be important in the absorption of protein digestion products (see Matthews and Achibi, 1976) and is not dependent upon the carriers responsible for the uptake of free amino acids.

It is still believed, however, that protein digestion products enter the portal blood in the form of free amino acids, indicating that the peptides which enter the mucosa are degraded by intestinal-cell exopeptidases. It has also been shown that there is some competition for mucosal uptake between peptides and that they can share within a group the same mucosal peptide uptake system.

During the passage of food through the alimentary tract, considerable quantities of endogenous protein are added in the form of digestive secretions and desquamated mucosal cells. The precise magnitude of this contribution has not been ascertained. Nasset (1965), for example, suggested that it was several times greater than the protein content of the diet but more recent data (e.g. Corring, 1975) indicate that the amounts may be considerably smaller. The endogenous protein is itself partly digested and absorbed, and this complicates the assessment of dietary protein effects. The residue, which is not digested and absorbed, constitutes a major component of metabolic faecal nitrogen. Because of the difficulty in obtaining reliable figures for such endogenous nitrogen, most digestibility measurements are termed apparent digestibility and are based on the net decrease in nitrogen content during passage of food through the gut.

Lipid digestion

Dietary fats consists mainly of triglycerides with some phospholipids, sterols and sterol esters. Endogenous phospholipids also enter the gut contents mainly in the bile. There is a recognized gastric lipase but its activity against triglycerides containing long-chain fatty acids is rather low. The major enzymes with lipolytic activity are found in duodenal contents and originate from the pancreas. The classical lipolytic enzyme of pancreatic juice is a glycerol-ester hydrolase but this term is misleading as the enzyme is rather unspecific and will split the carboxylic-acid esters of many substrates. One common factor is that the substrate must be present in a dispersed phase. A second lipolytic activity of pancreatic juice is that of a carboxylic-acid ester hydrolase which splits many esters including cholestrol esters. A third pancreatic enzyme is phospholipase A, present in its zymogen form, which hydrolyses fatty acids in the α-position of glycerophospholipids.

True pancreatic lipase has been purified and characterized and has a molecular weight of approximately 40 000. It has an absolute requirement for Ca^{2+} and is only active against water-insoluble substrates; its activity is proportional to the surface area of the substrate. Lipase of pancreatic origin has a high specificity for the primary ester bonds of triglyceride, the products being 1,2 diglyceride and 2 monoglyceride. The chain length of the fatty acid in the triglyceride molecule is of minor importance for the rate of hydrolysis.

The equilibrium of the reaction catalysed by lipase with long-chain glycerides as substrate is dependent on the pH of the medium. At alkaline pH, 2-monoglyceride and fatty acid are the main products whereas in slightly acidic conditions di- and triglycerides are found in the equilibrium mixture. Pancreatic lipase can be described as a hydrophobic acyl transferase and the positional specificity of the enzyme is of considerable biological significance.

The interaction of bile salt with the lipase–substrate system is also of importance and it has been suggested that the bile salts act by promoting the binding of lipase to its substrate. A weakly acidic medium, as in the duodenum, can act to stabilize such a system. Thus a rôle for the lipase-catalysed hydrolysis in the lumen of the small intestine is to lead to the formation of monoglyceride and fatty acids, which in the presence of the bile salts form a mixed micellar phase. The phospholipase of pancreatic juice, which has an absolute requirement for bile salts, is specific for the fatty acid in the 2-position of phosphatidylcholine.

Thus the luminal phase of fat digestion involves entry of lipids into the duodenum, and with the addition of bile and pancreatic juice extensive changes in physical and chemical form occur resulting in an emulsion which equilibrates with an initial micellar phase and is subjected to the action of pancreatic lipase. Different triglyceride fractions enter into the dual emulsion–micellar complex in different ways, which may relate to variations in their overall digestion and absorption. It is widely considered that the mixed bile salt–fatty acid–monoglyceride micelles have a rôle in the transport of less polar lipids from the oil phase to the acceptor system, and in this way the mixed micelles serve as vehicles for other lipids including sterols and fat-soluble vitamins.

These considerations must be borne in mind in considering the uptake of lipids by intestinal cells, but there is some controversy as to whether or not the intact micelles enter as such or are disrupted at the mucosal surface. There is also some lack of clarity in explaining differences in the entry rates of various fatty acid components initially of dietary origin.

When considering the digestion and absorption of specific fatty acids it is necessary to be aware of the position of the fatty acids in the glyceride, especially when it is recognized that in most vegetable fats the saturated fatty acids are largely restricted to the 1-position whereas in animal fats (especially lard) they are mainly in the 2-position. The differences in absorption of saturated and unsaturated fatty acids must be examined in these terms.

Long-chain unsaturated fatty acids are almost completely absorbed from the intestinal tract into the lymphatic system and the absorption of corresponding saturated fatty acids is similar although more limited. Medium- and short-chain acids are also well absorbed. The shorter-chain acids (less than 10 carbon atoms) are taken up into the portal blood whereas the longer-chain acids pass into the lymphatic system; fatty acids of intermediate length are transported by both routes. The chemical form of transport is also different – mainly as triglycerides in the lymphatic system and as unesterified acids in the portal system.

In summary it can be stated that for practical nutritional purposes unsaturated fatty acids are digested better than saturated ones, the digestibility decreasing with increasing chain length; glycerides are better used than free fatty acids and fatty acids located in the 2-position arc bcttcr uscd than those in the 1-position.

Microbial digestion

As indicated earlier, the site of microbial fermentative activity in the digestive tract varies from species to species. Because of its obvious significance and ready accessibility very extensive studies have been carried out on the rumen, and our knowledge of its fermentative activity and metabolic implications far exceeds that available on sites of microbial activity in non-ruminant herbivores. Detailed comparisons of the significance of microbial digestive activity are not therefore possible but it is clear from studies on fibre digestibility (Table 1.2) that the microbial contribution to the digestive process is likely to be less in the non-ruminant.

Table 1.2 Comparison of hemicellulose and cellulose digestibility coefficients in ruminants and non-ruminants fed alfalfa, brome grass and orchard grass (Keys, Van Soest and Young, 1969)

	Digestibility		
	Sheep	Pig	Rat
Alfalfa			
Hemicellulose	0.49	0.42	0.46
Cellulose	0.53	0.38	0.23
Brome grass			
Hemicellulose	0.76	0.46	0.11
Cellulose	0.72	0.38	0.04
Orchard grass			
Hemicellulose	0.76	0.46	0.08
Cellulose	0.68	0.42	0.04

Qualitative information is available on, for example, the VFA concentration in different regions of the alimentary tract (Table 1.3) and the proportions of individual fatty acids at the sites of major microbial activity in some non-ruminant herbivores (Table 1.4), but it must be recognized that the concentration of the acid within the digesta is not an indication of the amount produced but represents the difference between that produced and that absorbed. The amount metabolized by the gut wall and by bacteria must also be taken into account. Similarly,

Table 1.3   VFA concentrations (mmol/kg) in digesta from
            different parts of the digestive tracts of the fowl
            (Annison, Hill and Kenworthy, 1968), pig
            (Friend, Nicholson and Cunningham, 1964) and
            the sheep (Annison, 1954; Ward, Richardson and
            Tsieh, 1961)

	Fowl	Pig	Sheep
Rumen	—	—	119
Stomach, gizzard or abomasum	5	55	13
Small intestine	10	3	19
Caecum	107	182	60
Colon	51	190	7

Table 1.4   VFA proportions (mmol/mol total VFA) within
            the sites of major microbial activity in the fowl
            (Annison *et al.*, 1968), pig (Friend *et al.*, 1964) and
            the sheep (Annison, 1954)

	Fowl caecum	Pig caecum	Sheep rumen
Acetic acid	610	550	540
Propionic acid	270	370	250
Butyric acid	110	60	170
Longer-chain acids	10	20	40

the proportions in which organic acids are found in the digesta do not
necessarily indicate their relative rates of production, as it is possible
that the different acids are absorbed or metabolized at different rates.
Thus such data indicate qualitatively the sites of major microbial
activity but cannot supply quantitative information concerning the
contribution of fermentation products to the nutrition of the animal.

Microbial digestion in the ruminant

A variety of organisms occurs in the rumen, the composition of
the population being largely determined by an equilibrium established
in relation to the diet, and there is considerable information about the
substrates attacked, about the products formed and about the nutritional requirements of the organisms for growth (Tables 1.5 and 1.6).
It is of particular interest that many organisms require strictly anaerobic growth conditions, which implies a nutritional requirement that
is specific for carbon dioxide, ammonia, and certain vitamins. The
microflora modify the food consumed by the animal prior to its arrival

Table 1.5 Substrates and fermentation products of some bacteria of the rumen (after Hungate, 1966)

Organism	Substrates	Products
Bacteroides succinogenes	Cellulose, cellobiose, glucose, CO_2	Succinate, acetate, formate
Ruminococcus	Cellulose, cellobiose, xylan, CO_2	Succinate, lactate, acetate, formate, ethanol, H_2
Butyrivibrio	10–20 C carbohydrates, varying among strains	Butyrate, lactate, ethanol, formate, CO_2, and sometimes acetate and propionate
Bacteroides ruminicola	Many sugars, CO_2	Succinate, acetate, formate
Bacteroides amylophilus	Starch, maltose, CO_2	Succinate, acetate, lactate, ethanol
Succinimonas amylolytica	Starch, maltose, CO_2	Succinate, acetate, propionate
Succinivibrio dextrinosolvens	Dextrin, maltose, xylose, pectin, CO_2	Acetate, succinate, lactate
Lachnospira multiparus	Pectin, esculin, salicin, cellobiose, glucose, fructose	Formate, acetate, lactate, ethanol, CO_2, H_2
Peptostreptococcus elsdenii	Lactate, glucose, fructose, maltose, mannitol, sorbitol	2–6 C fatty acids, H_2, CO_2
Selenomonas ruminantium	7–13 C carbohydrates, esculin, sometimes salicin, glycerol, mannitol	Acetate, propionate, CO_2 and often formate, butyrate, lactate, succinate
Streptococcus bovis	10–14 C sugars, starch, esculin salicin	Lactate
Eubacterium	Glucose, cellobiose and other 4–6 C sugars	Formate, lactate, acetate, butyrate, CO_2, H_2
Methanobacterium	CO_2, H_2, formate	CH_4 and H_2O

Table 1.6 Nutritional requirements of some bacteria of the rumen (after Hungate, 1966)

	CO$_2$	One or more VFA	NH$_3$	Vitamins
Bacteroides succinogenes	E†	E	E	Biotin (E), p-aminobenzoic acid (PAB) (+ to −)
Ruminococcus	E	E	E	Biotin (E), folic acid or PAB (E), pyridoxamine (E, + to −), thiamine (+ to −), riboflavin (+ to −)
Butyrivibrio	+ to −	E to −	E to −	Biotin (E), PAB (E), pyridoxal (E)
Bacteroides ruminicola	E	E to −	+ to −	Some B vitamins (E)
Bacteroides amylophilus	E	−	E	None required
Succinimonas amylolytica	E	E	E	
Succinivibrio dextrinosolvens	+	−	+	
Lachnospira multiparus		Acetate +	−	
Peptostreptococcus elsdenii	−	Acetate +	−	
Selenomonas ruminantium	+ to −	E to −	+ to −	
Streptococcus bovis	+	+ to −	E	Biotin (E), thiamine (+), pantothenic acid (+ to −)
Eubacterium	E	E to −	E	
Methanobacterium	E	E	E	B$_{12}$ (E), unknown factor (E)

† E: essential for growth; + : growth stimulation; − : not stimulatory.

at the conventional sites of digestion and absorption, and possess an ability to digest cellulose and hemicellulose, which releases products of nutritional value from otherwise indigestible material. They ferment polysaccharides to VFA and convert some of the dietary protein to bacterial protein with release of low-molecular weight nitrogenous compounds. The microorganisms also contribute to the animal's vitamin supply, especially of B vitamins.

Carbohydrates

In the rumen, carbohydrate and other substrates are fermented and there is a simultaneous production of microbial cells and microbial products, and a concurrent evolution of heat; as far as the host animal is concerned most of the microbial waste products and the microbial cell material contribute to its nutrient supply. It is relatively straightforward to identify the metabolic routes whereby the VFA and the waste product methane are formed, and also to describe the pathways whereby microbial cellular material is synthesized; but it is very difficult to derive a reliable quantitative appraisal of the impact of these reactions on the nutrition and metabolism of the host animal. The biochemical pathways for the formation of methane and VFA are shown in Fig. 1.1 and, although not all the steps involved are included, it does serve to demonstrate the biochemical complexity of events in the rumen. From the point of view of the whole animal there is little virtue in identifying which microorganisms carry out particular processes, or in elucidating the mechanisms whereby certain of the intermediates and other metabolites are used for microbial synthetic reactions. It is more profitable to assess the quantitative significance to the animal of these reactions as a whole.

The extensive conversion of dietary carbohydrate to acetic, propionic and butyric acids has a major effect on glucose supply to the ruminant and accentuates the importance of gluconeogenesis (the formation of glucose from materials other than sugars). The short-chain fatty acids probably represent two-thirds of the energy supply of the animal and are utilized in many ways that spare or form glucose. It was shown by Leng, Steele and Luick (1967) that approximately half of the glucose in the ruminant is formed from propionate. Of the propionic acid formed in the rumen approximately one-fifth is converted to lactic acid during passage through the rumen wall and enters a gluconeogenic pathway in the liver via phosphoenolpyruvate. The remainder of the propionic acid passes unchanged to the liver where it can be converted to phosphoenolpyruvate via methylmalonyl-CoA, succinate and oxaloacetate. Acetic and butyric acids, on the other hand, do not give rise to glucose. Glucose is vital for certain living processes and the substantial degradation of hexoses in the rumen results in a precarious carbohydrate economy: changes either in the diet or in the

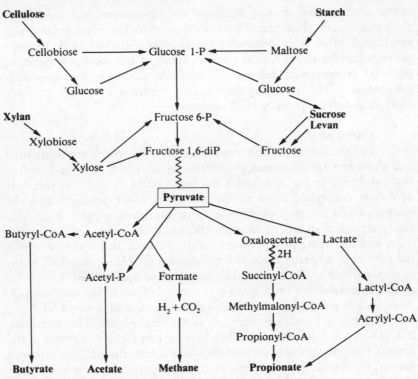

Fig. 1.1.   Metabolic pathways for the production of VFA.

animal's demands for carbohydrate are liable to alter the carbohydrate balance from the normal to the pathological (e.g. ketosis). It is thus especially important to recognize the special rôle of the propionic acid component of the VFA produced in the rumen and also to be aware of the significance of the net passage of starchy carbohydrate material out of the rumen (undergraded dietary plus microbially synthesized material).

It has often been assumed that, since there is very rapid fermentation of starch and related products in the rumen, very little passes in undegraded form to the duodenum. During recent years this assumption has been questioned and several workers have reported that perhaps 100 to 200 g/kg of dietary starch escapes microbial breakdown. In assessing these reports it is important to ensure that satisfactory procedures have been employed for the determination of α-linked glucose polymers and for the collection of suitable duodenal samples, and to recognize the importance of overall digestibility. Selected data given in Table 1.7 indicate the digestibility of starch when different diets were given and provide values for the proportion of starch that has been degraded in the rumen, i.e. prior to passage to the intestines. In the case of hay the overall digestibility was low but some 180 g/kg of

Table 1.7 Extent and sites of digestion of starch in the ruminant (see Armstrong and Beever, 1969)

	Proportions in diet (g/kg)	Digestibility of starch	Proportion of digested starch disappearing before small intestine (g/kg)
Ground maize	200 ⎱	0.96	750
Ground lucerne hay	760 ⎰		
Ground maize	800 ⎱	0.98	690
Ground lucerne hay	100 ⎰		
Hay, milled and pelleted	1000	0.76	820
Barley	850 ⎱	0.99	940
Soya bean	100 ⎰		
Hay	750 ⎱	0.97	900
Dairy cubes	250 ⎰		
Hay	200 ⎱		
Dairy cubes	180 ⎬	0.99	950
Flaked maize	620 ⎰		
Hay	670 ⎱	1.00	910
Rolled barley	330 ⎰		
Hay	330 ⎱	1.00	930
Rolled barley	670 ⎰		
Hay	330 ⎱	1.00	900
Flaked maize	670 ⎰		
Rolled barley	1000	1.00	920

that digested left the rumen intact: this was not of much quantitative importance, however, since the starch content of the food was low. With most of the other diets less than 100 g/kg of the digested starch left the rumen intact. There was, however, a significant difference with those diets containing ground maize, when some 300 g/kg of the starch escaped ruminal breakdown (see Table 1.8). Many of the data on ground maize refer to cattle whereas those for the other cereals relate to sheep. The quantity of glucose that becomes available to the animal can be calculated from these data, and for those diets which contained ground maize it seems that the glucose requirement was likely to be met by that absorbed from the small intestine. Where the glucose supply is in any way precarious it would seem that the inclusion of ground maize in the diet might constitute a useful precaution.

There are numerous observations showing that VFA production representations half to three-quarters of the effective digestible energy

Table 1.8   The effect of the type of cereal in the diet on the extent and sites of digestion of starch in the ruminant (see Armstrong and Beever, 1969)

	Digestibility coefficient of starch	Proportion of digested starch disappearing before small intestine (g/kg)
Diets containing barley or flaked maize	0.99	920
Diets containing ground maize	0.98	680

value of the diet. The significance of these acids to the economy of the animal can also be evaluated in other ways, e.g. by measuring the rate at which a particular metabolite enters the blood stream of the animal from the alimentary tract (entry rate). This particular approach has been evaluated by Annison, Brown, Leng, Lindsay and West (1967), who made a comparison between the effective entry of glucose, acetate, 3-hydroxybutyrate and long-chain fatty acids (see Table 1.9).

The particular significance of acetate can readily be recognized. Propionate was not included in this evaluation since its fate is inextricably associated with that of glucose and, in fact, its contribution is covered essentially by glucose. An alternative form of VFA evaluation is to partition the CO_2 output (Annison *et al.*, 1967). In this procedure the fraction of the CO_2 output derived from a substance represents the ratio of the terminal value of the specific activity of the respired CO_2 to that of the traced substance, and is an effective measure of the contribution made by particular nutrients to the overall energy supply of the animal. This technique also reveals the particular significance of

Table 1.9   Entry rates and oxidation of metabolites serving as sources of energy in sheep fed 24 meals per day at 1-h intervals or fasted for a period of 24 h (Annison *et al.*, 1967)

Metabolite	Entry rate (mg/min per kg$^{0.75}$)		CO_2 output (g/kg of total CO_2)	
	Fed	Fasted	Fed	Fasted
Glucose	5.0	3.8	91	112
Acetate	10.8	5.8	316	221
3-hydroxybutyrate	1.4	1.5	104	48
Palmitate	—	1.0	—	47
Oleate	—	0.9	—	40
Stearate	—	0.9	—	44

acetate and also of the longer-chain fatty acids, which are mobilized from depot lipids, after a fasting period (Table 1.9).

Proteins

It has been recognized for some 30 years that there is a rather complex form of nitrogen cycle in the ruminant (Fig. 1.2). Protein that enters the rumen is hydrolysed by the microorganisms to yield peptides, amino acids and ammonia. NPN consumed can also produce amino acids and ammonia whilst any urea that re-enters the rumen from the blood or via saliva leads to further ammonia production. Simultaneously with these breakdown reactions there is synthesis of microbial protein from the NPN compounds in the rumen. The

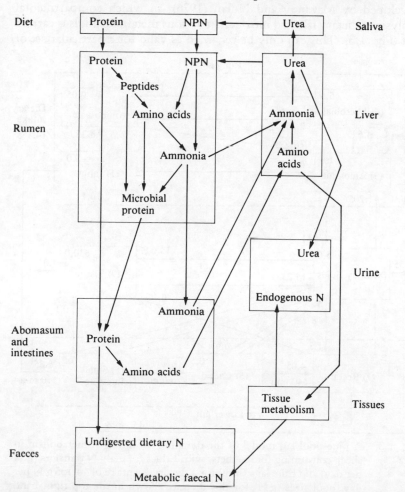

Fig. 1.2.   A schematic representation of nitrogen metabolism in the ruminant.

relative rapidity of the breakdown and synthetic reactions exerts a controlling effect upon the nutritive value of the proteins given. Two of the major factors that regulate this balance are the solubility of the ingested protein and the amount and type of carbohydrate present. There is continuous passage along the alimentary tract of some unchanged dietary protein, a proportion of microbial protein and some NPN. It is usually assumed from this point the digestive processes are essentially the same as in non-ruminants. The significance of the rumen action therefore lies essentially in the extent to which food protein is converted into microbial protein, and thus upon the relative nutritive values of the ingested dietary protein and that synthesized in the rumen. A recent quantitative approach to this metabolic pattern has been developed by Mazanov and Nolan (1976), in which compartmental analysis of dietary labelled nitrogen in various metabolic pools is carried out (Fig. 1.3). This can only be regarded as valid for a particular set of

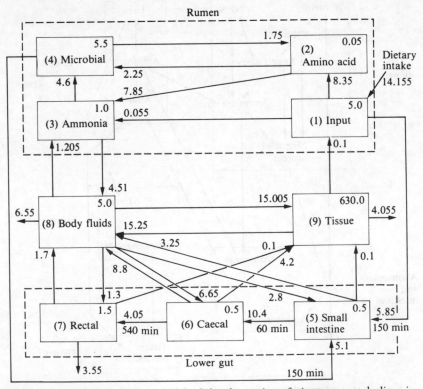

Fig. 1.3.   A nine-pool lag model of the dynamics of nitrogen metabolism in sheep consuming forage diets, with values for dialy N transfers (g N per day) and time lags (min) for a dietary N intake of 14.155 g N per day; pool sizes (g N) for this diet are shown in the top right-hand corner of each box. (After Mazanov and Nolan, 1976.)

defined conditions but represents a useful approach to quantitative metabolic studies. A particularly important development in the quantitative study of ruminant protein nutrition followed from the observations of Bauchop and Elsden (1960) that for a series of anaerobic bacteria some 10.5 g of cellular dry matter was produced per mol of ATP generated by substrate fermentation (the so-called Y_{ATP} value). Although recent studies have indicated that this value is not constant, it has led to alternative forms of expression in which the quantity of microbial protein produced per kg of organic matter apparently digested in the rumen is used; a mean value of approximately 200 g/kg has been suggested (Buttery, 1977).

In order to devise optimum conditions for the production of microbial protein it is first of all necessary to attempt to ensure a constant and optimum rumen ammonia level. Below such a level uncoupled fermentation of organic matter occurs, whilst if the level is exceeded there is wastage, or even toxic effects, of ammonia. There is, however, controversy regarding the rumen ammonia level that allows optimum microbial protein synthesis to occur. Miller (1973) suggested that there is fixation of rumen ammonia at concentrations in excess of 1 mmol/l whilst Okorie, Buttery and Lewis (1977) claimed that maximum protein synthesis occurs at levels of not more than 1 mmol/l.

Lipids

Ruminant diets may contain up to 100 g of lipid per kg, present mainly in the form of triglycerides and galactolipids, with small amounts of phospholipid. Forages can have comparatively high proportions of mono- and digalactosyldiglycerides but cereal lipids are largely triglyceride. The fatty acid composition can vary widely, depending on the dietary components, but in forage lipids there may be a high proportion of linolenic acid and in cereal lipids of linoleic acid.

In the rumen there is a rapid hydrolysis of lipids by microbial (mainly bacterial) lipases with the release of free fatty acids and sugar components, followed by biohydrogenation of unsaturated fatty acids. The mechanism of hydrogenation is incompletely understood but the process is facilitated by absorption of released unsaturated fatty acids onto food particles: in the hydrogenation of linoleic acid the main product is stearic acid but conjugated diene and a *trans*-monoene acids are present as intermediates. These compounds, and other geometrical isomers, can be detected in ruminant tissues, in comparatively high concentrations with low-fibre diets that give poor reducing conditions in rumen liquor. Oleic acid is reduced more rapidly than other 18:1 acids and ruminal organisms involved in hydrogenation may be highly specific in their action.

Ruminal microorganisms also synthesize long-chain fatty acids and bacterial lipids are characterized by comparatively high proportions of odd-numbered chain acids (derived from propionic acid) and branched-chain acids (derived from isobutyric and isovaleric acids, for example) that are esterified to phospholipids. The bacterial lipids may be hydrolysed following lysis in the rumen, or under the action of pancreatic lipases in the small intestine. Because of the extensive hydrolysis of lipids within the rumen, monoglycerides may not be available to form the mixed micelles required for absorption of long-chain fatty acids in the simple-stomached animal. There is, however, a partial hydrolysis to lysophospholipids of biliary and bacterial phospholipids under the action of pancreatic phospholipases, and these facilitate the dispersion and absorption of the longer-chain fatty acids.

MINERALS AND VITAMINS

Minerals

Until 1960 it was concluded that there were 16 essential mineral elements for animals: calcium, phosphorus, potassium, sodium, chlorine, sulphur and magnesium as major elements; and iron, iodine, copper, manganese, zinc, cobalt, molybdenum, selenium and chromium as trace elements. Since that time there have been tentative suggestions that bromine, barium, tin and tungsten may also be essential. Some of the necessary elements, when included in the diet at too high a level, may be toxic, e.g. copper, selenium and molybdenum.

Digestion requires release from the foodstuff but does not usually involve substantial change of the mineral component, although the form of its combination may be altered and there may be a need to release the element from a binding agent. The inclusion in the diet of an alternative binding agent, e.g. chelating agents such as ethylenediaminetetra-acetate (EDTA), has been found on occasion, to facilitate the absorption of certain elements. There is a variety of interactions between pairs or groups of minerals such that absorption or need for one is limited by others.

Absorption may be by simple diffusion or may involve a specific transport mechanism but the exact mechanism has not been determined for all minerals, and the details of the mechanisms that have been identified have not been worked out in all instances. As an example, calcium is absorbed by an active transport process occurring mainly in the upper small intestine. The process is regulated by 1,25-dihydroxycholecalciferol, a metabolite of vitamin D that is produced in the kidney in response to low plasma calcium concentration. Low alimentary pH favours calcium absorption but it is inhibited by a number of dietary factors including phytates, oxalates and phosphates.

The regulation of iron absorption is largely carried out by the intestinal epithelial cells although the exact mechanism is not clear. There has for some time been a mucosal-block theory in which it is considered that the amount of an iron-binding protein, apoferritin, is the controlling factor. Ferrous ion appears more readily to evade entering this binding form. It has also been stated that a diet high in phosphate causes a decrease in the absorption of iron whereas a diet very low in phosphate markedly increases iron absorption. Recent observations make it unlikely that ferritin regulates absorption but suggest that iron is taken into the mucosal cells bound to one or more specific carriers. There is further information on transfer mechanisms into blood plasma and other fluids, involving a specific iron-binding protein.

For potassium, sodium and chlorine, which play a major rôle in the regulation of the osmotic properties of body fluids, absorption is not a specific process. The movement of these elements across the gut epithelia, which encompassess absorption from and secretion into the gut, is dependent on general transport mechanisms and is sensitive to the balance between intra- and extracellular ions within the body tissues.

Vitamins

In any consideration of the vitamins it is important to recognize their complex functional rôle (Ch. 10). Most of the vitamins are, however, readily absorbed from the intestine (e.g. thiamine and pantothenic acid) and are not usually stored in the body to a significant degree. Although there is ready absorption, there are conditions where there is competitive inhibition or metabolic antagonism that may limit uptake, e.g. aminopterin or methotrexate inhibit absorption of folic acid. On the other hand, vitamin B_{12} is absorbed by a complex transport system from the ileum but its absorption is dependent on an earlier combination, in the presence of hydrochloric acid, with a constituent of normal gastric juice designated the intrinsic factor, which is a mucopolysaccharide secreted by the parietal cells of the gastric mucosa.

Vitamins in the diet are vulnerable in that they can be readily destroyed by heat, storage in light or exposure to oxidative conditions: a particular example of this is vitamin C (ascorbic acid). However, it should be equally recognized that some vitamins can be produced in the alimentary tract by the microorganisms present (e.g. in the rumen). Probably the only original source of vitamin B_{12} is microbial synthesis.

PRACTICAL ASPECTS OF NUTRIENT PROVISION

It is apparent from the foregoing brief review that the overall pattern of nutrient digestion is well established although numerous aspects of detail remain to be elucidated. Under practical conditions, however, nutrient provision to the animal is the end result of a complex interplay of physical, chemical and microbial factors in which synergistic and antagonistic reactions occur. The ability to minimize the less productive processes and exploit the more beneficial ones, both in terms of the animal itself and of diet manufacture, lies at the heart of effective ration formulation. Some examples of the subtleties involved are discussed below.

Added fats in rations

Although most individual raw materials contain lipids as an integral part of their structure, the total amount present in a simple mixed ration is well below the digestive capabilities of most animals and it is therefore often highly economic to include additional fat in compound rations. The case for the inclusion of added fats depends upon two general arguments: fats serve as rich sources of energy-yielding nutrients, and they improve the physical condition of the final ration. The energy contribution of fat is determined by its digestible or metabolizable energy value but there are, in addition, two further advantages which are difficult to express in quantitative economic terms: fats supply essential fatty acids, and fat utilization involves a lower heat increment or specific dynamic action than that associated with proteins and carbohydrates (see Carew and Hill, 1958, for poultry). This latter point implies that a unit of digestible or metabolizable energy derived from fat is of greater net value to an animal than an equivalent amount derived from protein or carbohydrate. It is possible therefore that a 5 to 10% increment must be added when ascribing the energy-yielding value of fat as compared with other energy sources. Quantitative values for their contribution to essential fatty acid requirements are not possible at this time.

The benefits in physical characteristics of including added fat in the ration of a farm animal are well recognized but again difficult to express in quantitative terms. It is known that rations containing added fats are more palatable and they generally lead to greater intake in terms of energy per unit of time. Fats also assist in the formation of a stable pellet (e.g. for poultry), which results in less crumbling and a less dusty product. Inclusion of a fat in rations that pass through various stages in a feed mill also results in less wear and tear on the processing machinery.

There are considerable variations in the nutritional value of different fats and the factors responsible for this are reasonably well recognized. Thus there is a reduction in the digestibility of saturated fatty acids as the chain length is increased (Table 1.10), and unsaturated fatty acids are better utilized than saturated ones (Table 1.11).

Table 1.10 Effect of chain length upon the corrected apparent digestibility coefficients of fatty acids

Fatty acid	Lard (1)[†]	Tallow (1)	Triglycerides (2)	Maize oil (3)	Lard (3)	Tallow (3)
12:0	–	–	0.90	–	–	–
14:0	0.85	0.79	0.67	1.00	0.95	0.99
16:0	0.74	0.40	0.46	0.88	0.84	0.88
18:0	0.55	0.28	0.40	[‡]	0.52	0.67
20:0	–	–	–	0.93	[‡]	[‡]

[†] References:
1. Davis and Lewis, 1969;
2. Flanzy, Rerat and Francois, 1968;
3. Carlson and Bayley, 1968.
[‡] Values observed were negative.

Table 1.11 Effects of degree of saturation on the corrected apparent digestibility coefficients of fatty acids

Fatty acid	Lard (1)[†]	Tallow (1)	Triglyceride (2)	Maize oil (3)	Lard (3)	Tallow (3)
16:0	0.74	0.40	0.46	0.88	0.84	0.88
16:1	0.94	0.92	[‡]	[‡]	[‡]	[‡]
18:0	0.55	0.28	0.40	[§]	0.52	0.67
18:1	0.91	0.90	0.90	0.96	0.95	0.98
18:2	0.94	0.97	0.95	1.00	1.00	[‡]

[†] References:
1. Davis and Lewis, 1969;
2. Flanzy et al., 1968;
3. Carlson and Bayley, 1968.
[‡] Values observed were > 1.00.
[§] Values observed were negative.

A further factor that is of importance in the degree of digestibility of a particular fatty acid is its position within the triglyceride. There is considerable information to indicate that fatty acids in the β- or 2-position in the triglyceride are better digested than those in the α- or 1-position; this probably relates to their rôle in establishing the micellar structure associated with the lymphatic pathway of absorption (see Freeman, 1969). Davis and Lewis (1969) showed the high digestibility of palmitic acid in lard (largely in the β- or 2-position) as compared with its value in interesterified lard when its location had been randomized (Table 1.12). A similar result was obtained by Flanzy *et al.* (1968).

Table 1.12   The effect of the position of the fatty acid within the triglyceride upon the corrected apparent digestibility coefficients of fatty acids (Davis and Lewis, 1969)

Fatty acid	Lard	Interesterified lard	Tallow
14:0	0.85	0.80	0.79
16:0	0.74	0.56	0.40
18:0	0.55	0.35	0.28
16:1	0.94	0.94	0.92
18:1	0.91	0.95	0.90
18:2	0.94	0.98	0.97

It is also recognized that the free fatty acid content of a fat influences digestibility (Renner and Hill, 1961). The data available have been summarized by Freeman (1976), who suggested that there was a reduction of digestibility coefficient in some 0.15 with a change from 0 to 1000 g free fatty acid per kg. This was probably accounted for by the availability of mono- and diglycerides for the establishment of a micellar form. It would appear, however, from an appraisal of the data available that there is no significant fall in digestibility until the free fatty acid content rises above 500 g/kg.

The age of the animal also appears to have an effect upon fat digestibility although there may be species differences. The data collected by Freeman (1976) suggest that for poultry the full potential for utilization is not achieved until 2 weeks of age. The observations are, however, rather variable and difficult to present in a quantitative form.

A factor recognized as important in establishing the value of an added dietary fat is the synergistic effect of a proportion of unsaturated fatty acids within a fat, which results in a more than arithmetically proportional benefit in terms of overall digestibility (see Sibbald, Slinger and Ashton, 1960; Renner and Hill, 1961). This effect can be seen where the progressive inclusion of increments of soya bean oil into beef tallow leads to a disproportionate advantage in terms of overall digestibility (Table 1.13).

The implications of these effects of synergism upon digestibility are considerable. The value of a saturated (or hard) fat can be improved by including within it a relatively small proportion of an unsaturated (or soft) fat. The actual value of an added fat may well depend substantially

Table 1.13   The corrected apparent digestibility coefficient of
beef tallow as influenced by the presence of soya
bean oil (Payne and Lewis, 1966)

	Digestibility	Metabolizable energy (MJ/kg)
Beef tallow	0.75	29.50
Beef tallow + 50 g soya bean oil per kg	0.86	33.81
Beef tallow + 100 g soya bean oil per kg	0.93	36.56
Beef tallow + 200 g soya bean oil per kg	0.94	36.99

upon the nature of the basal ration to which it is added. The concept can
also have an effect upon the value ascribed to a fat based upon an
experimentally determined metabolizable energy value, since it will be
influenced by the basal ration used. This effect is highlighted in the
findings of Leeson and Summers (1976), who express the metabolizable
energy value as a proportion of the gross energy value (Table 1.14).
It may be desirable to determine metabolizable energy values using a fat-free basal ration but, if so, a premium must be added for
synergistic advantage under particular conditions (see Leeson and
Summers, 1976).

Table 1.14   Relationships between metabolizable and gross
energy values for different fats (Leeson and
Summers, 1976)

	Metabolizable energy (ME) (MJ/kg)	Gross energy (GE) (MJ/kg)	ME/GE
Maize oil	42.68	39.30	1.09
Fish oil	40.71	39.30	1.04
Tallow	33.23	39.30	0.85

Many of the basic factors that govern the nutritive value of an added
fat have been identified in studies with poultry but there is no reason to
believe that similar factors are not important in other simple-stomached
species. It is clear that there are many benefits of including a fat in a
ration but most of these, beyond a value in terms of energy-yielding
nutrients, are difficult to express in quantitative terms. A selection of
published values as energy-yielding sources for different fats is given in
Table 1.15 (the value for maize oil is unexpectedly low).

Table 1.15   Digestible and metabolizable energy values (MJ/kg) for various fats used in pig rations

	Digestible energy	Metabolizable energy	Metabolizable energy (N)[†]	Reference[‡]
Tallow	34.02	33.05	32.76	1
Lard	32.47	32.22	31.55	1
Maize oil	31.88	30.71	30.54	1
Coconut oil	41.00	—	—	2
Beef tallow	33.22	—	—	3
Soya bean oil	35.27	—	—	3
Hydrogenated edible fat[§]	32.97	—	—	4

[†] The metabolizable energy (N) is corrected for zero nitrogen retention by subtracting 28.33 MJ/kg nitrogen retained during the collection period.
[‡] References:
1. Diggs, Becker, Jensen and Norton, 1965;
2. Creswell and Brooks, 1971;
3. Bayley and Lewis, 1963;
4. D. Lewis, unpublished results.
[§] From Proctor and Gamble, Newcastle upon Tyne.

Lipid digestion in ruminants is a more complex process than in simple-stomached herbivores because of interactions with the rumen flora before the digesta arrive at the conventional sites of fat digestion. Not only is the dietary fat itself modified but there may be overall alteration of fermentation pathways with effects, for example, on fibre digestibility. High levels of fat may lead to escape of unchanged dietary fat from the rumen and hence modification of the composition of body or milk fat (see Devendra and Lewis, 1976).

Modification of carbohydrate fermentation in ruminants

Optimization of roughage digestion by the development of a microbial fermentation chamber at the anterior end of the digestive tract has been accompanied, inevitably, by loss of efficiency in other aspects of metabolic function. Thus there is loss of energy-yielding nutrients such as methane and recycling of energy sources via propionate to maintain the glucose supply.

Elimination or reduction of such activities is an obvious approach to increase digestive efficiency and there has been considerable interest in, for example, the development of inhibitors of methane production particularly for use in highly fermentable diets. Unsaturated fatty acids (e.g. linolenic acid) and saturated acids in the series C_{10} to C_{18} all reduce methane production to less than half of the normal level with slight depression of cellulose digestion, whilst other compounds, notably the sulphated fatty alcohols, have more striking effects in depressing methane production but these affect cellulose digestion appreciably. The limitation of methane wastage is clearly an area worthy of attention but no fully satisfactory approach has yet been devised.

Theoretical consideration of the loss of reducing potential during rumen fermentation shows that acetate and CO_2 production yield energy whereas propionate, butyrate and methane production are energy demanding (see Fig. 1.1). The fatty acids are of net value whereas the methane constitutes a net loss. It is difficult to differentiate the benefit of propionate production from the loss of methane formation since the two are inescapably related. The reactions are amenable to physico-chemical analysis in redox terms, but, as a complex biological system with various inputs and outputs, rumen fermentation cannot yet be satisfactorily analysed in stoichiometric terms and probably requires the application of compartmental analysis techniques.

It has been observed, and it can be predicted from knowledge of the metabolic processes, that the loss of energy as heat during the digestion process with ruminants is much greater than with other species. In the latter, loss as heat during digestion rarely exceeds $0.01 J/J$ gross energy in the food whereas the complex of activities in the rumen leads to a corresponding value of approximately 0.06. Although under certain circumstances the process may help to maintain body heat and hence have a sparing effect on oxidative metabolism, it represents considerable energy loss which appears to be difficult to control.

In this context it is also necessary to consider the extent to which the VFA absorbed are available as a source of free-energy for the animal. An evaluation of the efficiency of utilization of fatty acids (see Blaxter, 1967) can be carried out by estimating the magnitude of the heat increment, i.e. that portion of the total potential energy supply that is effectively wasted during utilization. It is known that in the case of the ruminant the heat increment is generally some two or three times its magnitude for other classes of animals, and that the heat increment is also greater for VFA than for glucose. Although results for individual fatty acids are available it is only those for the type of mixtures that might be encountered in the rumen that have physiological significance, and for those there is a rather constant heat increment of approximately $0.16 J/J$ (i.e. efficiency of utilization of $0.84 J/J$) during maintenance feeding, as opposed to a value of $0.06 J/J$ for glucose (Table 1.16). This stage of utilization therefore appears to add a penalty of approximately $0.10 J/J$ to the ruminant for the possession of the microbiota in the rumen.

A great deal of attention has been given to the importance of rumen VFA ratios, especially minimal propionic levels in relation to the efficiency of diet utilization, and there is some evidence from feeding trials that an increased proportion of propionic acid is advantageous.

Table 1.16   The efficiency of utilization for maintenance in the sheep of the metabolizable energy of various mixtures of VFA given as intraruminal infusions, and of glucose given as an intra-abomasal infusion (Blaxter, 1967)

Substrates infused	Composition of the mixture mmol/mol total VFA			Efficiency of utilization for maintenance J/J
	Acetic	Propionic	Butyric	
Volatile fatty acids	250	450	300	0.87
	500	300	200	0.83
	750	150	100	0.86
	900	600	40	0.85
	1000	0	0	0.59
	0	1000	0	0.86
	0	0	1000	0.76
Glucose				0.94

Thus in experiments with cattle and sheep given rations containing different proportions of hay to flaked maize the efficiency of utilization of metabolizable energy increased from 0.30 to 0.60 J/J as the flaked maize replaced the hay. The proportion of acetate in the VFA rumen declined at the same time from approximately 600/400 mmol/mol, with a compensatory increase mainly in propionic acid. Corresponding effects on efficiency associated with changes in rumen fermentation pattern have often been reported but they are not invariably observed because it is difficult to eliminate from dietary comparisons other variables such as effects on food intake, flow through the alimentary tract, digestibility and composition of body gain, and in this situation it may be profitable to consider the theoretical basis of the rôle of propionate.

In the rumen a six-carbon hexose is first degraded to a triose which can either be oxidatively decarboxylated to acetate or reduced to propionate. In the formation of acetate an equivalent amount of CO_2 is released: this is fully-oxidized material and therefore does not represent any residual free-energy that can be rendered available. The reduction of CO_2 to methane does, however, constitute a loss, and whether to ascribe the loss to methane or to acetate formation becomes merely an exercise in tautology. In the same way the formation of propionate involves a reductive phase, but this again can either be allocated to propionate or even acetate since the reducing potential is probably only available in parallel with the oxidative production of acetate. It might be concluded therefore that the advantage of propionate rests in the fact that its production might well have diverted a reducing potential from the wasteful route of CO_2 conversion to methane, i.e. there may be an inverse relationship between propionate proportion and methane formation. It can be noted that for a predominantly flaked maize diet, methane production represented some 0.03J/J of food energy (Blaxter and Wainman, 1964), whereas for a ration based on a concentrate added to a fibrous basal component loss as methane was within a range of 0.07 to 0.09J/J (see Blaxter, 1967).

Modification of rumen protein digestion

Techniques of manipulating nitrogen metabolism in the rumen have been concerned, historically, with the addition of NPN sources (urea) to the diet as an inexpensive source of ammonia for microbial growth. At normal dietary protein levels, however, the additional ammonia is not utilized efficiently and, as it tends to be released rapidly from added urea, the ruminal concentrations reached may be toxic to the animal. Numerous attempts have been made, therefore, to produce compounds, either of urea or other substances, which are broken down only slowly in the rumen and provide a continuous slow release of ammonia. Commercially viable techniques have not yet been evolved.

In recent years the emphasis has changed to that of prevention of protein breakdown in the rumen by a variety of chemical and physical treatments of dietary protein, and marked alterations in the amount and composition of the protein materials which enter the small intestine have been produced by these processes. Although full exploitation of this approach is dependent on further data on, for example, amino acid requirements, the emphasis given to studies on protein metabolism in the rumen has led to reassessment of the extent of protein degradation of individual raw materials and the effects of conventional processing procedures on degradation.

Ideas about protein digestion and on formulation concepts to meet specific protein needs are therefore changing and proposals which incorporate current thinking have recently been put forward by the Agricultural Research Council (1980). The concepts can be expressed in simple terms, but there are many assumptions involved and many areas where the necessary data are not yet available. Briefly, an initial assessment is made of the microbial protein that can be synthesized within the rumen based upon the quantity produced for a particular input of digestible organic matter. A maximum microbial protein synthesis is assumed in relation to the rumen ammonia concentration which may arise from rumen–degraded protein (RDP), although it is important to recognize the numerous factors that can influence this component. Recognition is made of endogenous urinary nitrogen and it is then assumed that the remainder of the needs of the ruminant must be met by undegraded dietary protein (UDP), a component which is again influenced by a variety of factors. The system at present lacks data on the degree of degradation of dietary protein and the factors influencing it, and has yet to be refined to encompass amino acid data and numerous other factors. Nevertheles, there is a progressive move towards more precise definition of protein requirements and provision which should lead to increased productive efficiency.

REFERENCES

Agricultural Research Council, 1980. *The Nutrient Requirements of Ruminant Livestock*, pp. 121–68. Commonwealth Agricultural Bureaux, Slough.

Annison, E. F., 1954. Studies on the volatile fatty acids of sheep blood with special reference to formic acid, *Biochem. J.* **58**: 670–80.

Annison, E. F., Brown, R. E., Leng, R. A., Lindsay, D. B. and West, C. E., 1967. Rates of entry and oxidation of acetate, glucose, D(-)-β-hydroxybutyrate, palmitate, oleate and stearate, and rates of production and oxidation of propionate and butyrate in fed and starved sheep, *Biochem, J.* **104**: 135–47.

Annison, E. F., Hill, K. J. and Kenworthy, R., 1968. Volatile fatty acids in the digestive tract of the fowl, *Br. J. Nutr.* **22**: 207–16.

Armstrong, D. G. and Beever, D. E., 1969. Post-abomasal digestion of carbohydrate in the adult ruminant, *Proc. Nutr. Soc.* **28**: 121–31

Bailey, C. B. and Balch, C. C., 1961. Saliva secretion and its relation to feeding in cattle. 2. The composition and rate of secretion of mixed saliva in the cow during rest, *Br. J. Nutr.* **15**: 383–402.

Bauchop, T. and Elsden, S. F., 1960. The growth of micro–organisms in relation to their energy supply, *J. gen. Microbiol.* **23**: 457–69.

Bayley, H. S. and Lewis, D., 1963. The use of fats in pig rations, *J. agric. Sci., Camb.* **61**: 121–5.

Blaxter, K. L., 1967. *The Energy Metabolism of Ruminants*. 2nd edn. Hutchinson, London.

Blaxter, K. L. and Wainman, F. W., 1964. The utilisation of the energy of different rations by sheep and cattle for maintenance and for fattening, *J. agric. Sci., Camb.* **63**: 113–28.

Buttery, P. J., 1977. Aspects of the biochemistry of rumen fermentation and their implication in ruminant productivity. In *Recent Advances in Animal Nutrition – 1977* (ed. W. Haresign and D. Lewis), pp. 8–24. Butterworth, London.

Carew, L. B. and Hill, F. W., 1958. Studies of the effect of fat on metabolic efficiency of energy utilisation, *Poult. Sci.* **37**: 1191 (Abstr.).

Carlson, W. E. and Bayley, H. S., 1968. Utilisation of fat by young pigs: fatty acid composition of ingesta in different regions of the digestive tract and apparent and corrected digestibilities of corn oil, lard and tallow, *Can J. Anim. Sci.* **48**: 315–22.

Chauncy, H. H., Henriques, B. L. and Tanzer, J. M., 1963. Comparative enzyme activity of saliva from the sheep, hog, dog, rat and human, *Archs. oral Biol.* **8**: 615–27.

Colin, G. C., 1886. *Traite de Physiologie Comparee des Animaux*. Ballière et Fils, Paris.

Corring, T. 1975. Apport de proteines d'origine endogene par la secretion du pancreas exocrine chez le porc, *Annls. Biol. anim. Biochim. Biophys.* **15**: 115–8.

Cresswell, D. C. and Brooks, C. C., 1971. Composition, apparent digestibility and energy evaluation of coconut oil and coconut meal, *J. Anim. Sci.* **33**: 366–9.

Davis, R. H. and Lewis, D., 1969. The digestibility of fats differing in glyceride structure and their effects on growth, performance and carcass composition of bacon pigs, *J. agric. Sci., Camb.* **72**: 217–22.

Devendra, C. and Lewis, D., 1976. Fat in the ruminant diet: a review, *Indian J. Anim. Sci.* **44**: 917–38.

Diggs, B. G., Becker, D. E., Jensen, A. H. and Norton, H. W., 1965. Energy value of various feeds for the young pig, *J. Anim. Sci.* **24**: 555–8.

Erickson, R. P., 1963. Sensory neural patterns and gustation. In *Olfaction and Taste*, Vol. 1 (ed. Y. Zotterman), pp. 205–13. Pergamon Press, New York.

Flanzy, J., Rerat, A. and Francosi, A. C., 1968. Étude de l'utilisation digestive des acides gras chez le porc, *Annls. Biol. anim. Biochim. Biophys.* **8**: 537–48.

Freeman, C. P., 1969. Properties of fatty acids in dispersions of emulsified lipid and bile salt and the significance of these properties in fat absorption in the pig and the sheep, *Br. J. Nutr.* **23**: 249–63.

Freeman, C. P., 1976. Digestion and absorption of fat. In *Digestion in the Fowl* (ed. K. N. Boorman and B. M. Freeman), pp. 117–42. British Poultry Science, Edinburgh.

Friend, D. W., Nicholson, J. W. G. and Cunningham, H. M., 1964. Volatile fatty acid and lactic acid content of pig blood, *Can J. Anim. Sci.* **44**: 303–8.

Hill, K. J., 1968. Abomasal function. In *Handbook of Physiology*, Sect. 6. Vol. V (ed. C. F. Code and W. Heidel), pp. 2747–59. American Physiological Society, Washington, DC.

Hungate, R. E., 1966. *The Rumen and its Microbes*. Academic Press, New York.

Kawamura, Y. and Yamamoto, T., 1978. Studies on the neural mechanisms of the gustatory-salivary reflex in rabbits, *J. Physiol., Lond.* **285**: 35–47.

Keys, J. E., Van Soest, P. J. and Young, E. P., 1969. Comparative study of the digestibility of forage cellulose and hemicellulose in ruminants and nonruminants, *J. Anim. Sci.* **29**: 11–5.

Kidder, D. E. and Manners, M. J., 1978. *Digestion in the Pig*. Scientechnia, Bristol.

Leeson, S. and Summers, J. D., 1976. Fat ME values: the effect of fatty acid saturation, *Feedstuffs, Lond.* **48** (46): 26.

Leng, R. A., Steele, J. W. and Luick, J. R., 1967. Contribution of propionate to glucose synthesis in sheep, *Biochem. J.* **103**: 785–90.

Matthews, D. M. and Achibi, S. A., 1976. Peptide absorption, *Prog. Gastroenterol.* **71**: 151–61.

Mazanov, A. and Nolan, J. V., 1976. Simulation of the dynamics of nitrogen metabolism in sheep, *Br. J. Nutr.* **35**: 149–74.

Miller, E. L., 1973. Evaluation of foods as sources of nitrogen and amino acids, *Proc. Nutr. Soc.* **32**: 79–84.

Nasset, E. S., 1965. The role of the digestive system in protein metabolism, *Fedn Proc. Fedn Am. Socs exp. Biol.* **24**: 953–8

Nelson, J. H., Jenson, R. G. and Pitas, R. E., 1977. Pregastric esterase and other oral lipases – a review, *J. Dairy Sci.* **60**: 327–62.

Okorie, A. V., Buttery, P. J. and Lewis, D., 1977. Ammonia concentration and protein synthesis in the rumen, *Proc. Nutr. Soc.* **36**: 38A (Abstr.).

Payne, C. G. and Lewis, D., 1966. Fats and amino acids in broiler rations, *Br. Poult. Sci.* **7**: 199–207.

Renner, R. and Hill, F. W., 1961. Factors affecting the absorbability of saturated fatty acids in the chick, *J. Nutr.* **74**: 254–8.

Rosselin, G., Fromageot, P. and Bonfils, F., 1979. *Hormone Receptors in Digestion and Nutrition. Proc. 2nd int. Symp. Horm. Receptors Digestivve Tract Physiol.* Elsevier/North Holland Biomedical Press, Amsterdam.

Saint-Hilaire, Suzanne, Lavers, Majorie K., Kennedy, J. and Code, C. F., 1960. Gastric acid secretory values of different foods, *Gastroenterology* **39**: 1–11.

Sanny, C. G., Hartsuck, Jean A. and Tang, J., 1975. Conversion of pepsinogen to pepsin. Further evidence for intramolecular and pepsin-catalyzed activation, *J. biol. Chem.* **250**: 2635–9.

Sibbald, I. R., Slinger, S. J. and Ashton, G. C., 1960. Factors affecting the metabolizable energy content of poultry feeds, *Poult. Sci.* **40**: 303–8.

Singh, M. and Webster, P. D., 1978. Neurohumoral control of pancreatic secretion, *Gastroenterology* **74**: 294–309.

Steer, M. L. and Glazer, G., 1976. Parallel secretion of digestive enzymes by the *in vitro* rabbit pancreas, *Am. J. Physiol.* **231**: 1860–5.

Ward, J. K., Richardson, D., and Tsien, W. S., 1961. Volatile fatty acid concentrations and proportions in the gastrointestinal tract of full-fed beef heifers, *J. Anim. Sci.* **20**: 830–2.

2 THE REGULATION OF NUTRIENT UTILIZATION: BASIC PRINCIPLES AND MECHANISMS

R. G. Vernon and M. Peaker

Metabolism is concerned with the total chemical changes occurring in the cell or in the body. The processes involved can be classified into synthetic mechanisms, or *anabolism*, and degradative mechanisms, or *catabolism*. Complex anabolic and catabolic processes are taking place continuously and, at the biochemical level, overall catabolic processes may involve anabolic steps, and *vice versa*. Moreover, the catabolism of one substance may lead to anabolism of another with the transfer of chemical energy. Therefore, there is the tendency to use the term metabolism whatever the type of process involved and to restrict its constituent terms of anabolism and catabolism to the overall direction, or outcome, of a series of biochemical reactions in the body. Thus growth is an anabolic process: the breakdown of fats in adipose tissue, a catabolic process.

The control of metabolism has two facets: first, the maintenance of homeostasis, by which the body controls the concentrations of nutrients within the internal environment of the body at optimal levels for the maintenance of essential bodily functions; secondly the diversion of metabolic substrates for the anabolic processes of growth, reproduction (for example, egg production in birds, foetal growth and lactation in mammals) and, in times of dietary plenty, for fattening. The underlying mechanisms controlling the latter are of particular importance in agriculture since the efficiency of growth and fattening (for meat), reproduction (young animals and eggs) and lactation (milk) determine the social and economic value of raising animals for food.

Although the control of metabolism can be divided in this way and related to the nutritional concept of animals being fed for *maintenance* (i.e. of essential functions) and *production*, the maintenance and production processes are completely integrated within the body and are controlled or modulated according to the state of the external environment (of which diet is a part) and the reproductive state of the animal.

THE CONCEPT OF PARTITIONING

Some organs or processes take precedence over others for the supply of available nutrients in the body. In other words, substrate supply is partitioned. This partitioning is not constant but is being continually modified. The dairy cow provides a good example. In early lactation substrate supply is directed towards milk secretion and fat deposits are mobilized. In late lactation, however, milk yield falls and, with the same dietary intake, partitioning changes and the animal deposits fat in adipose tissue. In growing animals, muscle is laid down in preference to fat.

Partitioning can be extremely complex, particularly under modern agricultural systems. Thus the dairy cow may be pregnant, lactating and, if she has not reached her fully adult size, growing – all at the same time. It is not surprising therefore that problems of metabolic control in the partitioning of nutrient supply are being studied by those interested in the underlying biological principles as well as by those with a direct interest in improving agricultural productivity.

Changes in partitioning can occur, and can occur very rapidly, if changes in the external environment cause the animal to take corrective action to preserve homeostasis. Thus in lactating animals exposed to a cold environment, substrate supply is re-partitioned towards providing energy for heat production (e.g. shivering) and the maintenance of body temperature, and milk production falls. Similarly, in starvation milk production is very quickly reduced and the available substrate supply diverted to processes vital for the animal's own life.

In general, animals re-partition their metabolic substrate supply in the face of stresses which, if partitioning were to continue as before, could lead to the loss of constancy of the internal environment – the *milieu intérieur* of Claude Bernard as contained in his famous dictum: 'La fixité du milieu intérieur est la condition de la vie libre, indépendante'. It is as well to remember that in the mnemonic for the definition of stress – Situations That Require Emergency Signals for Survival – emergency signals can over-ride those controlling the overall strategic pattern of metabolism.

Partitioning does not always favour the individual animal, however. Reproduction is often a severe metabolic strain on the mother. During lactation, which must be viewed as a part of reproduction, body reserves may almost entirely be lost and the mother's 'condition' may suffer. Therefore, the lactating animal's metabolism is adjusted towards an altruistic rôle to favour development of her young. In evolutionary terms, and provided that the losses sustained by the mother are not so great as to cause an immediate danger to the mother's (and thereby to her unweaned offspring's) life, it is clear that reproduction operates to perpetuate, in the concept of the 'selfish gene', the mother's genes and not the maternal organism *per se*.

In dairy animals, the strong drive to partition in favour of milk production can have pathological consequences. Selective breeding has produced animals with very large mammary glands and it seems that, to supply substrates for milk synthesis, many cows teeter on the brink of metabolic disaster and do indeed suffer clinical and subclinical conditions associated with high levels of production. It appears that a number of these production diseases are the result of exacerbation of normal strategies of metabolism by artificial selection for superficially-good characters. There seems little doubt that future selection must be based on the ability to cope metabolically with the demands made by additional production.

Levels of control

In creatures possessing different organs with specific functions, partitioning of nutrients can be determined initially by directing nutrients to particular organs. This can be achieved primarily by controlling the blood flow to the organs, and hence the proportion of a nutrient reaching a given organ, and by regulating the permeability of the plasma (outer) membrane of cells, which will determine the ability of the cell to take up a specific nutrient. Both mechanisms are extensively used by mammals.

Once within a cell, a nutrient can be used for several different purposes. A variety of mechanisms exist within the cell which influence the fate of nutrients. Cells produce 'signals' which reflect their metabolic status, and coordinate their metabolism, so ensuring that essential needs are met.

Events within the cells of individual organs and in the body as a whole are coordinated by hormones and nerves which are sensitive to the overall metabolic status of the animal. Hormone concentrations and nervous activity are sensitive to the external environment of the animal and also to changing physiological states (such as pregnancy and lactation), and so they can modulate metabolism to meet novel demands on the animal.

All these aspects are considered in more detail in the following sections.

Complex interactions

As already indicated, the partitioning of nutrients can be affected by:

1. diet – amount and composition;
2. external environment;
3. developmental or reproductive state.

However, none of these factors can be viewed as being completely in isolation since not only can reproduction influence partitioning but signals can clearly be generated which, should dietary intake be inadequate, can prevent growth and reproduction from taking place. Similarly, metabolic demand can itself influence food intake and there is evidence that reproductive hormones can also affect appetite. In addition, in many animals the external environment controls the timing of reproductive cycles to optimize appearance of the young with the availability of food supplies. Some of these interrelationships are illustrated in Fig. 2.1.

It should always be borne in mind that the integration of functions is so extensive that it is impossible to separate fully control of one system in the body from that of another.

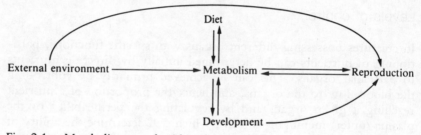

Fig. 2.1.   Metabolic control within the animal; arrows represent positive or negative influences.

PARTITION OF NUTRIENTS BETWEEN CELLS

The rôles of blood flow and capillary permeability

Uptake mechanisms

The rate of uptake of a substance by a cell depends upon the concentration of that substance in the extracellular fluid. For simple diffusion the rate will depend on the concentration gradient across the plasma membrane, and for facilitated and active transport on the concentration of the substance and the affinity of the transport process.

For carrier-mediated systems the effect of alterations in the external concentration will depend on the starting concentration. If the external concentration lies on the plateau of concentration v. rate (i.e. the system is saturated and uptake is at V_{max}) then small changes will have no effect on uptake or on cellular metabolism. If, however, the starting concentration lies on the rising part of the curve, major changes in uptake and in metabolism may occur with relatively small changes in concentration (Fig. 2.2). In the body, the control of uptake is not as simple because the interstitial fluid bathing most of the cells forms a compartment between

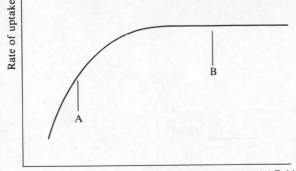

Concentration in interstitial fluid

Fig. 2.2. A diagram to illustrate the effect of varying the concentration of a substance in extracellular fluid on uptake by a cell via a saturable, carrier-mediated process. If the initial concentration is A then increases or decreases will have a marked effect on uptake. Similar changes will have no effect if the initial concentration is B.

the blood capillaries and the cells, separated from blood on one side by the capillary wall and from intracellular fluid on the other by the plasma membrane (Fig. 2.3). Therefore, the concentration in interstitial fluid will depend on the relative rates of uptake by the cell and replenishment from blood.

Events in the capillary

For many substances, passage across the capillary wall follows Fick's law of diffusion, i.e. it depends on the concentration gradient. Assuming that the surface area of the capillary walls remains constant and that the concentration in interstitial fluid is held constant by cellular uptake, the net rate of transport out of the capillary will depend on the concentration of the substance in capillary blood and on capillary permeability (capillary permeability is a measure of the ability of a substance to permeate the wall and is largely dependent on molecular size). Since the capillary blood will be depleted by passage of the substance into interstitial fluid and into the cell, the rate of transport

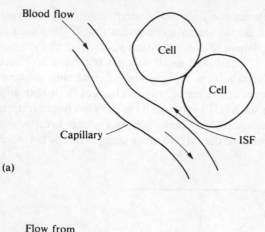

(a)

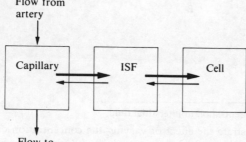

(b)

Fig. 2.3   (a) The morphological arrangement of the capillary, interstitial and
cellular compartments for movements of substances between
plasma and the cell.

(b). The same drawn as diagrammatic compartments with exchanges between compartments shown by arrows; the broad
arrows show the direction of net flux for a substance taken up
and metabolized by a cell.
ISF: interstitial fluid.

will depend on the concentration in the capillary being kept high by
fresh blood flowing into the capillary, i.e. the rate of blood flow. Hence
the rate of blood flow through a tissue is of major importance in
determining the availability of a substance to the cell (Fig. 2.3).

A simple equation relating these terms to the kinetics of diffusion has
been derived:

$$\frac{A \cdot P}{Q} = \log_e \frac{1}{1 - E}$$

where A is the surface area of the capillary wall; P is the permeability
coefficient; Q is the rate of blood flow; and E is the extraction ratio.

The extraction ratio is defined as the proportion of the amount of a substance presented to the tissue in blood which passes into the interstitial fluid and is, for the present purposes, taken up by the cells, i.e.

$$(C_a - C_v)\, Q/(C_a Q),\ \text{which simplifies to}\ (C_a - C_v)/C_a$$

where C_a and C_v are the concentration of a substance in arterial and venous blood respectively. Thus when $E = 1$, all the substance would be removed, and if the uptake mechanism by the cells were not saturated then uptake would be said to be rate-limited by availability. Of course, effective rate limitations could occur with lower values of E since the affinity of the cellular uptake mechanisms might not permit uptake at very low concentrations.

The effects of varying blood flow (Q) on extraction ratio (E) for two substances with different permeability coefficients (P) are shown in Fig. 2.4. It can be seen that, as blood flow is reduced, E approaches 1.0, and with a high permeability coefficient $E = 1$ is approached sooner. Therefore, both blood flow and the permeability coefficient can limit the rate of supply of a substrate to a tissue. For substances with high permeability coefficients, the rate of transport into interstitial fluid

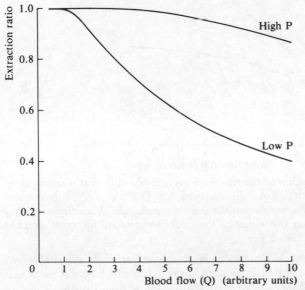

Fig. 2.4. An illustration of the effects of varying blood flow (Q) on extraction ratio (E) from the equation $(A \cdot P)/Q = \log_e 1\, (1 - E)$ (see text). Two curves are shown for different permeability coefficients (P) – high is four times that of low – and correspond to differences in permeability coefficient between sodium ions (high) and glucose (low). Larger molecules have lower coefficients.

can be limited by blood flow; at high blood flows and a low permeability coefficient, transport can be diffusion-limited. These limitations to transport are illustrated by the following equation which was derived from that above by applying diffusion kinetics to fluid flowing through a tube:

$$C = Q(1 - \exp^{-PA/Q})$$

In this case C is capillary clearance – the imaginary volume of blood from which the substance is completely removed – and is analogous to renal clearance, an equally imaginary concept which is a useful means of expressing functional abilities. The effects of varying blood flow (Q) on clearance (C) are shown in Fig. 2.5. At low blood flows, or with a high permeability coefficient, blood flow is rate-limiting since changes in

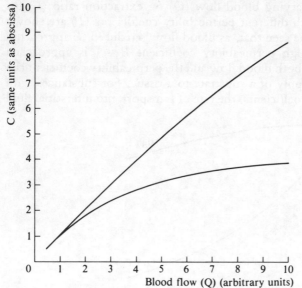

Fig. 2.5.   An illustration of the effects of varying blood flow (Q) on capillary clearance (C) from the equation $C = Q(1 - \exp^{-PA/Q})$ (see text). Two curves are shown for different permeability coefficients (P) – high is four times that of low. All the units are the same as those shown in Fig. 2.4.

flow lead to changes in clearance. With a low permeability coefficient (one quarter that of the high in the example shown) blood flow is not rate-limiting at higher rates of flow – diffusion is then limiting the rate of transport and increase in flow lead to little change in clearance.

All of these considerations are highly simplified because the topic of capillary permeability is a complex one. The question is: how important are these limitations in substrate supply to the metabolism and function of the cell?

Substrate availability

The *concentration* of a substance in interstitial fluid has been related to the *amount* supplied to the tissue (i.e. $C_a \cdot Q$) and to capillary permeability. Changes in supply brought about by changes in the concentration in arterial blood (C_a) or in blood flow (Q) may have marked effects, or virtually no effect, on uptake by the cell. Whether there is such an effect will depend on the nature of the uptake mechanism and on capillary permeability, as well as on the starting point of the changes. There are many possible combinations of circumstances but three examples are selected and other combinations should be apparent.

1. At the starting point, the cellular uptake mechanism is not saturated and diffusion out of the capillary is not rate-limiting. Thus an increase in blood flow will increase uptake.
2. At the start, the cellular uptake mechanism is saturated and, therefore, neither blood flow nor diffusion out of the capillary are rate-limiting. An increase in blood flow will have no effect on cellular uptake; a decrease will have no effect until the concentration in the interstitial fluid falls from the plateau for V_{max}.
3. At the start, the cellular uptake mechanism is not saturated, and diffusion out of the capillary is rate-limiting. An increase in blood flow will have little or no effect on uptake. An increase in arterial concentration will, however, increase uptake since the concentration gradient is increased.

In some circumstances and in some tissues, supply can normally be rate-limiting. For example, in muscle during intense exercise, the availability of oxygen is insufficient to support oxidative phosphorylation despite an increase in blood flow, and the tissue obtains its energy from glycolysis. It has also been suggested that supply is rate-limiting in highly-active tissues. For example, the mammary gland of ruminants extracts about 85% of certain amino acids from the blood (i.e. $E = 0.85$) and it has been argued that function may be limited by supply. However, attempts to demonstrate this by increasing availability (raising the concentration in arterial blood) have not been convincing. It is possible that, although extraction is high, the transport mechanism(s) is still saturated (i.e. at V_{max}) under normal circumstances. Blood flow has been shown to be very important in controlling gluconeogenesis in ruminant liver. The metabolic apparatus (enzyme activities) for maximal rates of gluconeogenesis is present in liver cells, but the actual rate depends on the supply of precursors in the hepatic portal vein. Since the capillaries in liver appear to be extremely permeable (see below) changes in blood flow are probably a major mechanism controlling glucose production.

Reductions in tissue blood flow can have marked effects on metabolism within a tissue. For example, during stress, the discharge of noradrenalin from sympathetic nerve endings and of adrenalin from the adrenal medulla cause marked constriction of the arterioles in the mammary gland. Blood flow is reduced, and the availability of substrates for milk synthesis falls to a level such that cellular uptake and milk production decrease. This illustrates one mechanism by which rapid changes in the partitioning of nutrient supply can be effected in an emergency.

Control of blood flow

In many tissues there is a direct relationship between function and blood flow: when the rate of metabolism changes so does the rate of blood flow (Fig. 2.6). Changes in blood flow are generally believed to

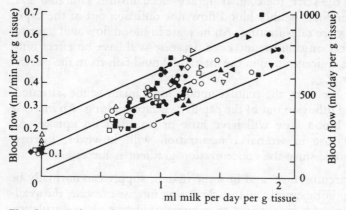

Fig. 2.6. Relation between milk production and mammary-gland blood flow in goats. (After Linzell, 1971.)

be mediated by local chemical products of metabolism or function, which are released by cells and diffuse through the interstitial fluid to cause dilatation of the arterioles. Although the identity of such dilator agents is still uncertain, the following have been suggested as being involved in various organs and tissues: carbon dioxide (or the related change in pH), adenosine, adenine nucleotides, and kinins. In addition, the reduced oxygen tension in interstitial fluid has also been suggested as a factor in dilatation.

Nerves may also play a rôle in inducing vasodilatation, particularly in exocrine glands which switch on very quickly (e.g. the salivary glands). Generally, however, nerves act to reduce blood flow as part of the normal process of continuous adjustment for homeostatsis within the vascular system or during times of stress.

It should be pointed out that the liver, an organ of major interest in metabolism, appears to have little control of its own blood flow. Only a small proportion of the total blood flow is derived from the hepatic artery and the liver receives blood 'second-hand' from the gut in the hepatic portal vein. Therefore, the blood supply to the liver is largely determined by gut blood flow.

Capillary permeability – regional differences

The capillary walls can be viewed as having water-filled pores, and the movements of many substances can be explained on this basis. However, for small lipid-soluble molecules, passage may also occur through the cell membranes of the capillary endothelium. The special case of lipoprotein lipase (see below), which is located on the endothelium to hydrolyse lipoproteins and release free fatty acids and glycerol, should be noted; in this case the question of substrate supply is related as much to the kinetics of the enzyme as it is to diffusion through the capillary wall.

Although a number of studies have been made on capillary permeability in several tissues, information is largely lacking on tissues of central metabolic interest. Nevertheless, the capillaries of some organs are more permeable to large molecules than those of others; liver capillaries are more permeable than others studied, which may be related to the rôle of the liver in breakdown and synthesis of relatively large plasma proteins.

Implications for the partitioning of substrate supply

Blood flow varies markedly between tissues (Table 2.1). Therefore, substrate supply within the body is partitioned according to blood flow and tissue weight. If an organ grows allometrically (i.e. out of proportion to the rest of the body) its share of the substrate supply will change. If a new function begins or the rate of a process accelerates (e.g. milk secretion by the mammary gland, egg formation in chickens), blood flow rises and substrate supply is increased.

Of course, differences in blood flow reflect the substrate supply, not substrate use by the tissue. For instance, the adult brain will take up little of the amino acids with which, by virtue of its high blood flow to support energy metabolism, it is liberally supplied. Therefore, actual partition need not necessarily match the potential partition as indicated by the different rates of blood flow in various tissues, although high blood flows do indicate that a tissue has a high rate of metabolism.

Although substrate supply is dependent on blood flow, there are mechanisms by which the supply may be utilized to a greater extent by a particular tissue. Unfortunately, little is known of this important aspect of metabolic control but the following mechanisms have to be

Table 2.1   Rates of blood flow through some tissues and organs of
            sheep and goats

	Blood flow (ml/min per 100 g tissue)
Skeletal muscle	5
Skin	5–20
Mammary gland (non-lactating)	10
(lactating)	25–50
Large intestine	65
Rumen	68
Brain	70
Small intestine	130
Heart (coronary circulation)	150
Liver	320
Kidney	550

considered. The first is by increasing the amount of carrier proteins for
uptake. The second is by increasing the affinity of the uptake mechanism in the case of facilitated diffusion or active transport. Thus a tissue
with a low K_m for the uptake of a particular substrate will be able to
extract more of that substrate than a tissue with a higher K_m. The third
is by keeping the intracellular concentration of a substrate low and
thereby maintaining a large concentration gradient across the plasma
membrane. The fourth is by changing capillary permeability, and the
fifth is the special case of lipoprotein referred to above. These mechanisms may be under control by hormonal and sometimes neuronal
factors, and in terms of the partitioning of substrate supply they are the
means by which partitioning within the body is thought to be achieved.

The translocation of substances across membranes

Structure of biological membranes

The membrane which bounds the cell and other, intracellular,
membranes contain approximately 400 g lipid (mainly phospholipid)
and 600 g protein per kg. These components are thought to be arranged
as shown in Fig. 2.7 (the *fluid-mosaic* model of membrane structure as
postulated by S. J. Singer and G. L. Nicholson in 1972). Essentially,
the phospholipids are thought to form a bilayer with a hydrophobic
hydrocarbon centre; this accounts for the high electrical resistance and
low permeability to highly polar molecules. The proteins are thought
to be embedded in the lipid bilayer (hence the term *mosaic*) with some

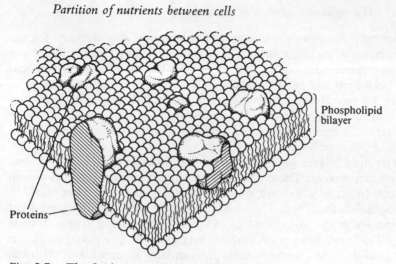

Fig. 2.7. The fluid-mosaic model of membrane structure. (From Singer and Nicholson, 1972.)

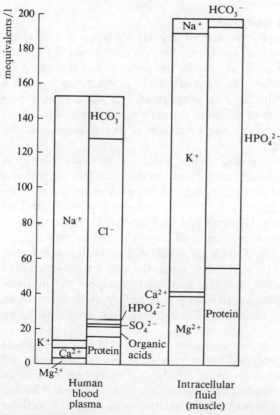

Fig. 2.8. The ionic composition of human blood plasma and intracellular fluid. (From Lehninger, 1975.)

completely spanning the bilayer and others not; this accounts for the asymmetry of membranes both in terms of chemical characteristics and the directional nature of transport systems. The lipid bilayer is not rigid and both lipid and protein molecules are thought to diffuse laterally in the membrane, hence its fluidity and flexibility. These latter properties are influenced by the fatty acid composition of the liquid bilayer: the greater the degree of unsaturation of the fatty acids, the more fluid and flexible the membrane.

The lipid bilayer greatly restricts the diffusion of polar substances across membranes. Therefore, the concentrations of substances within the cell (most of which are ionised) can differ markedly from those of extracellular fluid (see Fig. 2.8). Similarly, the concentrations of substances in the mitochondria and other intracellular compartments can differ from those of the surrounding cytosol. The passage of polar compounds across membranes is thus usually accomplished with the aid of special membrane proteins termed *translocases* or *carrier proteins*.

Non-mediated transport

The non-mediated transport of substances into the cell is by simple diffusion. The substance is neither chemically modified nor associated with another molecule during the process, and moves down the concentration gradient. The rate of uptake is described by Fick's first law of diffusion, that is it is proportional to the concentration gradient. Also, in the case of diffusion through a membrane, the rate of passage will be influenced by the solubility of the substance in the membrane components.

Passage of substances in and out of cells via the lipid bilayer is thought to occur by non-mediated transport but whether such transport occurs through the protein regions of the membrane is not clear. Certainly the process appears to be important for only neutral or slightly polar compounds. Glycerol and undissociated weak acids such as long-chain fatty acids may enter and leave the cell by this means. Similarly, monocarboxylic acids such as acetic, propionic, acetoacetic, hydroxybutyric and lactic acids may enter the cell by non-mediated transport, though systems for the mediated transport of all these substances may yet be discovered. The passage of pyruvic acid through the mitochondrial inner membrane has recently been shown to be by mediated transport.

A major deficiency of non-mediated transport is that the rate of uptake is effectively determined by the concentration gradient only and is not susceptible to other forms of regulation, except perhaps long-term changes in the chemical composition of the membrane. Also the direction of flow is determined by the relative intra- and extracellular concentrations of the substances.

Mediated (facilitated) transport

Mediated transport of substances across membranes involves membrane proteins known as translocases or carrier proteins. The translocases have properties similar to those of enzymes. Thus the transport of a substance will show saturation kinetics, that is the rate of transport will reach a plateau at high concentrations of substrate, unlike non-mediated transport (Fig. 2.9). The K_m (substrate concentration required for half-maximal rate of uptake) of a translocase can therefore

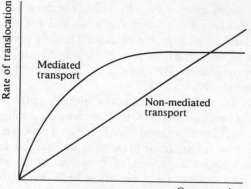

Fig. 2.9. The rate of passage through a membrane of a substance as a function of its concentration.

be determined. For example, the translocase of the human erythrocyte has a K_m for D-glucose of 6.2 mmol, for D-mannose of 18.5 mmol and for D-fructose of >200 mmol. These figures show that, again like enzymes, translocases show a marked substrate specificity with, for example, the human erythrocyte having a much greater affinity for D-glucose than for D-fructose or L-glucose. Similarly, amino acid translocases of animal membranes have a much greater affinity for L-amino acids than for D-amino acids.

Being proteins, the translocases can be subjected to the various types of regulatory mechanisms that are applied to enzymes. Hence mediated transport is open to much more refined regulation than non-mediated transport.

The uptake of ionized substances (e.g. amino acids and many organic anions) and some weakly polar substances (e.g. glucose) is by mediated transport. Mediated transport systems can be divided into passive and active types. Passive transport mechanisms in some respects resemble non-mediated transport in that the system can operate in either direction with the substrate moving down the concentration gradient. Also there is no energy requirement. The sugar translocases and some amino acid translocases are examples of such a system.

Active transport systems permit the uptake of substances against a concentration gradient and, in the case of ionized substances, against an electrochemical gradient. They are unidirectional and require energy, that is they require ultimately a supply of ATP. The major active transport system of mammalian cells is the Na^+/K^+ pump.

As shown in Fig. 2.8, the intra- and extracellular concentrations of Na^+ and K^+ are markedly different. The high K^+ and low Na^+ concentrations in cells are maintained by an ATP-dependent translocase which exchanges intracellular Na^+ for extracellular K^+ to counteract the non-mediated loss of K^+ and gain of Na^+ by cells. The high K^+ concentration of cells is important for protein synthesis and for the activity of several enzymes, and its leakage out of the cell largely gives rise to the membrane potential. In some cells (e.g. kidney and brain) it has been calculated that approximately 70% of the ATP produced is used for the purpose of pumping Na^+ and K^+.

Glucose and amino acids are transported into the blood against a concentration gradient during absorption from the intestine and during reabsorption from the glomerular filtrate in the kidney. There are different amino acid translocases for small neutral, large neutral, basic and acidic amino acids, and also for proline. The active transport systems for both glucose and amino acids are stimulated by high extracellular Na^+ concentrations and it is thought that the energy inherent in the Na^+ gradient across the membrane provides the driving force for the uptake of glucose and amino acids against a concentration gradient. Ultimately, therefore, the energy for the uptake of these substances comes from ATP hydrolysis by the Na^+/K^+ pump. The uptake of amino acids by tissues involves Na^+-dependent, active as well as passive translocases.

Both active and passive transport systems are subject to hormonal control.

Pinocytosis and exocytosis

Pinocytosis is the process of engulfment of solid or liquid material by the cell membrane. The membrane forms vesicles which then move into the cell to be lysed with the release of their contents. Most cell types of the mammalian body do not have this capacity to any marked extent. The liver, however, is the site of breakdown of blood protein and absorption of these proteins may well occur by a pinocytotic mechanism.

The reverse process, usually called exocytosis, is responsible in a number of tissues, particularly glands, for the export of manufactured materials. For example, in the mammary gland milk proteins and lactose, which are synthesized in the secretory cell, are packaged by the Golgi apparatus into vesicles which then release their contents into the lumen of the gland by fusing with the cell membrane.

Lipoprotein lipase

Most of the lipids in blood plasma occur as lipoprotein complexes (see Ch. 3). Lipids such as triacylglycerols do not cross plasma membranes, probably because of their very low solubility in water, and they have to be hydrolysed before their fatty acids are available to tissues. Tissues like adipose, muscle and mammary gland which utilize triacylglycerol fatty acids secrete the enzyme lipoprotein lipase. This enzyme migrates to the endothelial wall of the blood capillaries of the tissue where it hydrolyses the triacylglycerols of chylomicrons and very-low-density lipoproteins (see Ch. 3). The fatty acids and glycerol thus released can then cross the capillary wall and be taken up by the cell. The rate of lipoprotein lipase production is regulated by hormones and provides an effective means for regulating the uptake of lipid by cells.

Activating enzymes

Many nutrients require activation before they can be metabolized. Some of the enzymes which catalyse these reactions are restricted to specific tissues, hence only these tissues can utilize the substance. For example, glycerol kinase is primarily located in the liver and kidney and to a lesser extent in mammary gland and intestinal mucosal cells. So despite the fact that cell membranes are freely permeable to glycerol, it is metabolized by only a few tissues (this is really a special case of control by transcription). Most activating enzymes are widely distributed (e.g. hexokinase, fatty acid acyl–CoA synthetase).

Relative rôle of blood flow and membrane transport in the regulation of nutrient utilization

Both blood flow (and hence rate of nutrient supply) and membrane transport processes (and hence rate of nutrient uptake) have crucial rôles in the regulation of nutrient utilization. Both are subject to nervous and hormonal control. The ability to regulate the blood flow to an organ provides a very rapid and effective way of directing nutrients to specific parts of the body but changes in blood flow change the rate of supply of all nutrients to a tissue. This is ideal for the mammary gland, for example, which requires many different nutrients during lactation, but is not sufficiently selective for some organs. During peak lactation the animal usually needs to release fatty acids from adipose tissue for use elsewhere in the body while suppressing the uptake of nutrients by adipose tissue. This objective cannot be achieved by varying the blood flow to adipose tissue, but is accomplished by reducing the rate of uptake of nutrients, by changing membrane permeability and by reducing lipoprotein lipase activity. Similarly, muscle will use glucose when it is available or fatty acids and ketones when glucose is in short supply (e.g. during fasting). The utilization of glucose by muscle is largely regulated by altering the permeability of the cell membrane to the sugar (under the control of the hormone insulin).

Blood flow and membrane permeability, then, provide powerful complementary mechanisms for regulating the fate of nutrients.

PARTITION OF NUTRIENTS IN THE CELL

Intracellular compartmentation

The cell contains a number of membrane-bound compartments – the nucleus, mitochondria, Golgi apparatus, endoplasmic reticulum, etc. – in which various enzyme systems are localized (Fig. 2.10). The membranes of these compartments are similar in structure and have the same general characteristics as the membrane (the plasma membrane) around the cell.

The mitochondrial compartment has a key rôle in intermediary metabolism. It is the site of oxidative phosphorylation and as such produces most of the ATP requirements of the cell; it also contains several other important enzyme systems (Fig. 2.10). Mitochondria are surrounded by a double membrane; the outer one is apparently permeable to a variety of metabolites but passage of most substances through the inner membrane requires specific translocases. The inner mitochondrial membrane differs from the plasma membrane of the cell in that it contains approximately 800 g protein and only 200 g lipid per kg. Many of these proteins are either translocases or membrane-bound enzymes. Some of the mitochondrial translocases are shown in Fig. 2.11; they are all examples of passive, mediated transport and all appear to catalyse exchange reactions. Exchange of ADP for ATP (there is no net transport of adenine nucleotide from the mitochondria) is crucial for the supply of ATP to the remainder of the cell. Other translocases have important rôles in intermediary metabolism.

Certain groups of substances cannot cross the mitochondrial membrane. These include the nicotinamide adenine dinucleotides (NAD, NADH; NADP, NADPH); therefore there are distinct pools of these dinucleotides in the mitochondria and cytosol. Derivatives of CoA, acetyl-CoA or long-chain fatty acyl-CoA for example, cannot cross the membrane. Translocation of acetyl-CoA is necessary for fatty acid synthesis from glucose in the cytosol and is achieved indirectly –

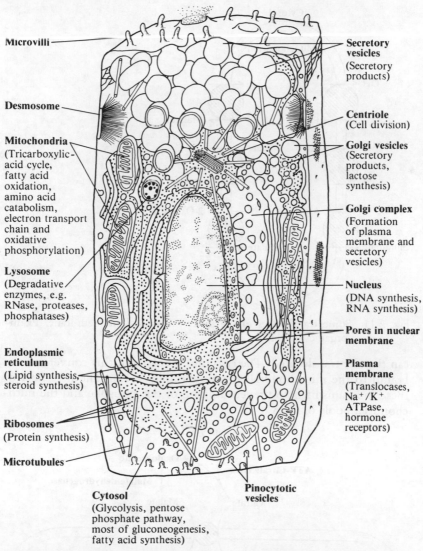

Microvilli

Secretory vesicles
(Secretory products)

Desmosome

Centriole
(Cell division)

Mitochondria
(Tricarboxylic-acid cycle, fatty acid oxidation, amino acid catabolism, electron transport chain and oxidative phosphorylation)

Golgi vesicles
(Secretory products, lactose synthesis)

Golgi complex
(Formation of plasma membrane and secretory vesicles)

Lysosome
(Degradative enzymes, e.g. RNase, proteases, phosphatases)

Nucleus
(DNA synthesis, RNA synthesis)

Pores in nuclear membrane

Endoplasmic reticulum
(Lipid synthesis, steroid synthesis)

Plasma membrane
(Translocases, Na^+/K^+ ATPase, hormone receptors)

Ribosomes
(Protein synthesis)

Microtubules

Cytosol
(Glycolysis, pentose phosphate pathway, most of gluconeogenesis, fatty acid synthesis)

Pinocytotic vesicles

Fig. 2.10. Intracellular structures and localization of some important enzyme systems in a secretory epithelial cell (theoretical magnification × 7500). (From Krstić, 1979.)

by conversion of acetyl-CoA to citrate and its translocation in this form (Fig. 2.12). The citrate translocase, actually a tricarboxylic acid translocase, is inhibited by palmityl-CoA; this may be of importance in the regulation of fatty acid synthesis from glucose in some species.

The uptake of long-chain fatty acyl-CoA for subsequent oxidation in the mitochondria requires its prior conversion to acylcarnitine which

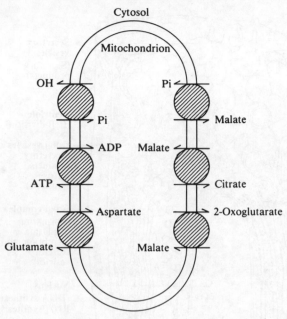

Fig. 2.11   Some translocases of the inner mitochondrial membrane. Pi: inorganic phosphate.

can then be translocated. The enzymes involved in this conversion are
bound to the mitochondrial membrane (Fig. 2.13). The net effect of
these mechanisms is to prevent mixing of the cytosolic and the mitochondrial pools of CoA.

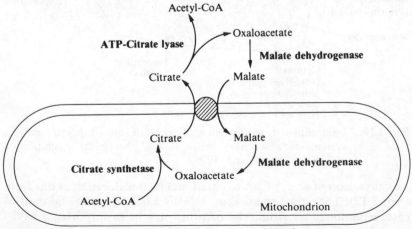

Fig. 2.12.   Translocation of acetyl-CoA across the inner mitochondrial membrane.

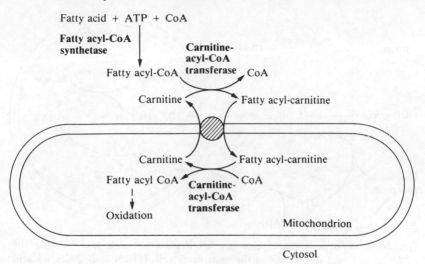

Fig. 2.13. Translocation of long-chain fatty acids across the inner mitochondrial membrane.

Mitochondria also accumulate ions, especially Ca^{2+} for which there is an active transport system coupled to electron transport. This is thought to have a rôle in regulating the Ca^{2+} concentration in the cytosol, which in turn probably influences the activity of a variety of enzymes.

Apart from the mitochondria, translocases have been demonstrated in other membrane-bound compartments. For example, there is a system for the active transport of Ca^{2+} into the sarcoplasmic reticulum of muscle cells. This involves an ATPase (Ca^{2+}-dependent ATPase) and the process is thought to be responsible for the relaxation of muscle. Another example is the Golgi apparatus of the mammary gland. This is the site of lactose synthesis, and there is evidence that translocases are responsible for the uptake of glucose and UDP-galactose from the cytosol, and for the transport of UMP formed by lactose synthesis back into the cytosol (Fig. 2.14).

This latter example exemplifies processes that occur in secretory tissues – the exocrine and endocrine glands. In these tissues, the secretory products synthesized within the cell are often sequestered in or actually synthesized within a membrane-bound intracellular compartment before release into the lumen of the exocrine gland, or the blood of an endocrine gland, by exocytosis of vesicles. The Golgi apparatus is often the site of this process. The importance of sequestration is two-fold. First, it may prevent the inhibition of a synthetic process by accumulation of product at the site of synthesis. Secondly, it removes the product from participation in 'turnover' and therefore saves energy being used for resynthesis to replace that which is broken down; this

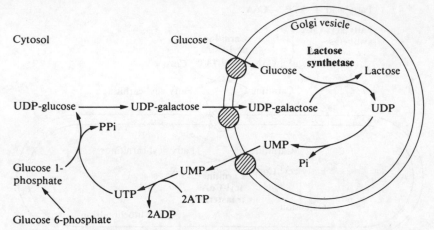

Fig. 2.14. Translocation of glucose, UDP-galactose and UMP across the
Golgi membrane in the mammary cell. (From Kuhn, Carrick and
Wilde, 1980, with modification.)

may be a reason why 'secretory' processes (e.g. egg laying and milk
secretion) are relatively more 'efficient' than 'growth' processes in
which synthesized products are subject to 'turnover'.

Apart from physically-discernible compartments there is evidence
for other types of pools or compartments within the cell. Specific
proteins which bind substances (e.g. fatty acids and Ca^{2+}) have been
demonstrated. The effect of these is to create two pools, albeit in
equilibrium, of the substance (i.e. free and bound). Such binding
proteins can modify the concentration of the 'free' substance, and
therefore the rate of its metabolism and effects on other systems. Fatty
acids, for example, are detergents and can inactivate a number of
enzymes, thus it is to the cell's advantage to keep 'free fatty acid' concentration as low as possible. The release of Ca^{2+} bound to membranes appears to be an important step in the action of some hormones.

There is evidence for two pools of glucose-6-phosphate in the
cytosol of the hepatocyte. Glucose-6-phosphate produced by gluconeogenesis does not appear to be available to glucose-6-phosphatase
for hydrolysis to glucose, but first appears to be incorporated into
glycogen. G6P produced by glycogenolysis, however, can be hydrolysed by glucose-6-phosphatase to glucose (Fig. 2.15). A physical
explanation for this phenomenon is lacking.

The presence of intracellular compartments means that the concentration of a substance may vary in different parts of the cell. As the
concentration of a substance influences its own metabolic fate and, in
some cases, the metabolism of other substances, intracellular compartmentation plays an important rôle in the regulation of metabolism.
Also, the rate of translocation of a substance from one pool or

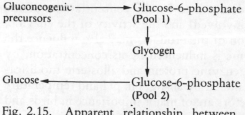

Fig. 2.15. Apparent relationship between separate pools of glucose-6-phosphate in the cytosol of liver cells.

compartment to another provides a further step whereby metabolism can be regulated.

Regulation of enzyme activity

Enzymes are unique proteins that catalyse biochemical reactions and as such have a crucial rôle in the regulation of metabolism. Metabolism involves the synthesis and degradation of covalent bonds which are usually stable at physiological temperatures. As shown in Fig. 2.16, a chemical reaction involves the formation of an activated intermediate and it is the free energy of activation, $\Delta G^{\ddagger}$, which determines the rate of reaction (the greater $\Delta G^{\ddagger}$ the less likely the reaction will occur). The net free energy change of the reaction, ΔG, determines the thermodynamic feasibility of the reaction and the equilibrium constant. The effect of enzymes is to reduce the free energy of activation ($\Delta G^{\ddagger}$) and thus they can increase the rate of reaction by 10^{8}- to 10^{12}-fold. Enzymes are remarkable catalysts: they operate under very mild conditions of temperature, pressure and pH; they exhibit great specificity (most accept only one or a few substrates); the yield of the reactions they promote is 100%, hence there is no accumulation of side-products within the cell.

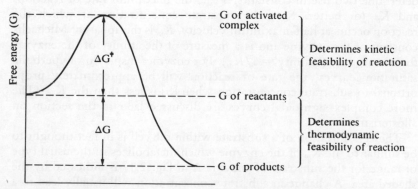

Fig. 2.16. Changes in free energy (G) during the course of a reaction.

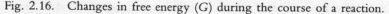

The rate of a reaction is determined by the concentrations of the substrate(s) and cofactors (if involved) and the activity of the enzyme; in some cases the concentration of the products may also influence the rate. The activity of an enzyme is influenced by its concentration, by covalent modification of the enzyme protein and allosteric modification. Enzyme activity is also altered by changes in pH and temperature but it is unlikely that these factors are of major importance in birds and mammals.

Substrate concentration
An enzyme-catalysed reaction comprises several stages:

1. the enzyme (E) binds the substrate at a specific binding site (the active site), forming the enzyme-substrate complex $(E\text{-}S)$;
2. activation of the enzyme-substrate complex occurs and results in the formation of an enzyme-product complex $(E\text{-}P)$;
3. the product (P) is released resulting in the regeneration of the free enzyme.

These stages can be represented by:

$$E + S \rightleftharpoons E\text{-}S \rightleftharpoons E\text{-}P \rightleftharpoons E + P.$$

This is a simplification, of course; several intermediate stages may occur between E-S and E-P and in many reactions there is more than one substrate. The critical step of the sequence is thought to be the formation of the enzyme-substrate complex. As is evident from the above equation, the rate of formation of E-S will be influenced by the concentrations of S and E.

Plots of the rate of reaction (V) as a function of substrate concentration ($[S]$) (at a constant enzyme concentration) vary in shape (Fig. 2.17) and may be hyperbolic or sigmoidal. Such graphs can be used to determine two useful constants: V_{max}, the maximum rate of reaction, and K_m (or better, $S_{0.5}$) the substrate concentration at which the reaction occurs at half-maximum velocity. K_m is the apparent Michaelis constant of the enzyme and is a measure of the affinity of the enzyme for its substrate ('affinity' $= 1/K_m$). For enzymes displaying hyperbolic saturation curves, the rate of reaction will be approximately proportional to substrate concentration when $[S]$ is less than the K_m. (The more complex sigmoidal curves are discussed later in the section on allosterism.)

The concentration of a substrate within the cell is in fact thought to be similar to the K_m of the enzyme which metabolizes it; the usual type of range for the substrate of enzyme A in Fig. 2.17 is indicated by the shaded area. A change in substrate concentration will usually lead to a change in the rate of reaction; this would not occur if the substrate

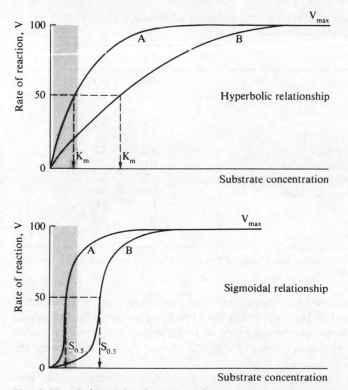

Fig. 2.17. Relationship between substrate concentration and rate of reaction for enzyme-catalysed reactions. K_m or $S_{0.5}$ is the concentration of substrate at which the rate of reaction is 0.5 of the maximum rate (V_{max}). The usual physiological range of substrate concentration for enzyme A (in both parts of the Fig.) is given by the shaded area.

concentration were saturating. Suboptimal substrate concentrations are one reason why the rate (flux) through a metabolic pathway is usually several-fold less than the activity of the least-active enzyme of the pathway. For example, in rat liver a rate of gluconeogenesis of 1.7μmol of pyruvate converted to glucose per min per g wet tissue was found, whereas the activities of the two least-active enzymes of the pathway (pyruvate carboxylase and phosphoenolpyruvate carboxy-kinase) were both 6.7 μmol/min per g tissue. The difference is even more extreme for glycolysis (Table 2.2), for which the least active enzyme (in the liver) is phosphofructokinase. However, the activity of this enzyme is subject to allosteric modification and its maximum activity *in vivo* (i.e. in the presence of saturating concentrations of substrates) would be less than that measured *in vitro*. During rapid bursts of metabolic activity, as occur in skeletal muscle during exercise, enzymes may become saturated with substrate and the rate of a

Table 2.2   Rate of glycolysis and activities of several glycolytic enzymes in rat liver and muscle

	Liver	Skeletal muscle
Rate of glycolysis	0.2†	0.17 (resting)
		17 (tetanized)
Hexokinase	0.7	1.8
Glucokinase	4.3	—
Phosphofructokinase	3.3	80
Fructosediphosphate aldolase	10	77
Glyceraldehyde-3-phosphate dehydrogenase	170	590
3-Phosphoglycerate kinase	150	340
Enotase	17	210
Pyruvate kinase	50	780
Lactate dehydrogenase	230	490

† All rates and activities are μmol/min per g tissue at 37° C and are taken from Scrutton and Utter (1968).

metabolic pathway may be the same as the activity of the least active enzyme. This has been observed for glycolysis in insect flight muscle. Glycogen, rather than blood glucose, is the major glycolytic precursor in tetanized muscle in the rat (Table 2.2), hence the rate can exceed the activity of hexokinase.

A further point is, that, at non-saturating concentrations of substrate, the rate at which the substrate would be metabolized by each of two enzymes with different K_m values would be determined by those K_m values (Fig. 2.17).

Metabolite concentrations in the cell are usually in the range of 1 μmol to 10 mmol/l. The cell contains many dissolved substances and their mean concentration cannot exceed the total solvent capacity of water. A low concentration of chemically reactive substances is advantageous as it reduces the probability of non-enzymic reactions occurring.

Cofactors
Some enzyme reactions require cofactors. These may be metal ions, for example:

muscle phosphorylase kinase	(calcium);
pyruvate kinase	(potassium);
tyrosinase	(copper);
all ATP-dependent enzymes	(magnesium).

Alternatively, cofactors may be organic molecules known as coenzymes; these are involved in group translocation and/or activation steps. Some examples are:

biotin	(carboxylation reactions);
pyridoxal phosphate	(amino group transfer);
NAD, NADP	(hydrogen atom transfer);
ATP	(phosphate transfer and activation steps);
CoA	(acyl group transfer and activation).

The total pool size of these coenzymes (e.g. free CoA plus acylated CoA) does not usually change but the proportion of coenzyme in different possible forms alters and may influence the rate of a reaction in which a particular form participates. The special rôle of ATP is considered later.

Product concentration

The release of product from the enzyme-product complex is not normally thought to be rate-limiting. However, the product of some reactions can inhibit the reaction. For example, glucose-6-phosphate can inhibit hexokinase.

Enzyme concentration

The average enzyme concentration in cells is approximately $1 \mu mol/l$ (range approximately 10 nmol to $100 \mu mol/l$). The concentration of some enzymes appears to change but slightly under various physiological conditions whereas that of others shows marked fluctation.

The quantity of an exzyme is determined by its rates of synthesis and degradation. Under steady-state conditions, the amount of an enzyme (*E*) is given by:

$$E = K_s/K_d$$

where K_s is a (zero-order) rate of synthesis and K_d is a (first-order) rate of degradation. All enzymes are 'turned-over' and both K_s and K_d can vary with physiological state leading to changes in the concentration of the enzyme (Table 2.3).

The principal means of varying the amount of an enzyme is by altering its rate of synthesis (Table 2.3). Enzyme (protein) synthesis is a complex process and may be regulated at various stages. The most important is undoubtedly the synthesis of mRNA (transcription). Not only is the rate of synthesis of each mRNA regulated but also, in any given eukaryotic cell, only a fraction of the possible mRNA are synthesized. Thus regulation at the level of transcription determines the metabolic capabilities of a cell. For example, only liver and kidney cells are able to synthesize glucose; and only mammary-gland cells can synthesize lactose, medium-chain fatty acids and casein. Changes at the

Table 2.3   Concentration and rate constants of synthesis and degradation of rat liver acetyl-CoA carboxylase in different physiological states

State	Enzyme concentration (E)	Rate constant of synthesis (K_s)	Rate constant of degradation (K_d)	K_s/K_d
Fed, balanced diet	1.00	1.00	1.00	1.00
Fasted	0.28	0.54	1.90	0.28
Fasted, re-fed a fat-free diet	3.76	4.05	1.07	3.78
Alloxan diabetic	0.53	0.59	1.00	0.59

Results are from Numa (1974) and are expressed as a fraction of the value obtained with rats fed a balanced diet.

level of transcription are responsible for the acquisition of new metabolic capabilities which form part of the overall process of differentiation. For example, phosphoenolpyruvate carboxykinase appears after birth in the hepatocyte permitting the initiation of gluconeogenesis; glucokinase appears at the onset of weaning in the rat hepatocyte enabling it to deal more efficiently with the increased flux of dietary glucose; and a variety of enzymes first appear just before or at the onset of lactation in the mammary epithelial cells to permit synthesis of milk constituents.

Transcription thus determines the complement and relative amounts of enzymes in cells. The factors which regulate transcription in eukaryotic cells are poorly understood compared with our knowledge of the systems operating in prokaryotic cells. However, it is clear that hormones exert some of their effects on metabolism at the level of transcription and it seems likely that some nutrients and/or their metabolites do also.

Regulation may occur during the translocation of mRNA from the nucleus to the cytosol, its association with ribosomes (initiation) and the subsequent synthesis of the peptide chain (translation); initiation may be an important stage for regulation by some hormones.

Regulation of enzyme amount (or perhaps 'effective' amount, i.e. conversion of an inactive peptide to an active enzyme) may also occur at the post-translational level. Apart from covalent modification (see below), the formation of an enzyme may require the association of several peptide chains (monomer units) to form a polymer (e.g. acetyl-CoA carboxylase); other enzymes operate as an enzyme complex, the formation of which involves the association of several dissimilar peptides (e.g. pyruvate dehydrogenase); some enzymes require the association of a prosthetic group (e.g. fatty acid synthetase); many enzymes probably have to be integrated into a membrane (e.g. adenylate cyclase).

Though the rate of enzyme degradation can vary, it appears to be a much less important means of altering enzyme amount than the rate of synthesis. However, it has recently been shown that during rapid accumulation of enzymes, such as at the onset of lactation in the mammary gland, there is not only an increase in the rate of synthesis but also a transient decrease in the rate of degradation (Fig. 2.18). The mechanisms responsible for the selective degradation of specific enzymes and their regulation are not known.

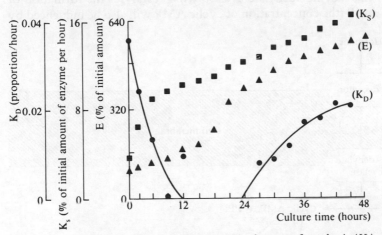

Fig. 2.18.   Changes in the concentration (E), the rate of synthesis (K_s) and the rate of degradation (K_D) of the enzyme fatty acid synthetase in mammary explants (pieces) maintained in organ culture. (From Mayer, 1978.)

Changing the amount of an enzyme is a relatively slow process (requiring several hours to effect) compared with other methods of altering the activity of an enzyme. It is regarded as 'coarse' control and is of importance in the long-term adaptation of metabolism to new physiological conditions such as prolonged fasting, changes of diet, birth, weaning, pregnancy and lactation.

Isozymes
Some enzymes exist in multiple forms or isozymes (e.g. hexokinase and lactate dehydrogenase). These isozymes usually have different properties (the four hexokinase isozymes, I, II, III and IV, have K_m for glucose of about 0.02, 0.2, 0.005 and 10 mmol/l). The proportions of the various isozymes vary from cell type to cell type and may change with age. Thus, varying the proportions of the various isozymes of a tissue provides another means of regulating metabolism within the cell; it is really another form of regulation at the level of transcription.

Covalent modification

A variety of enzymes are known to exist in active and inactive forms. Interconversion involves covalent modification, usually phosphorylation/dephosphorylation, but in some cases proteolytic cleavage.

Enzyme phosphorylation is catalysed by specific protein kinases, many of which are activated by cyclic AMP. The general features of the reaction are shown in Fig. 2.19. A hormone binds to a receptor and activates the enzyme adenylate cyclase which catalyses the formation of cyclic AMP (the concentration of cyclic AMP will also be influenced by

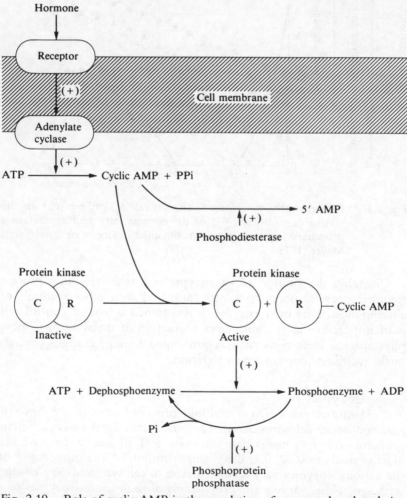

Fig. 2.19.   Role of cyclic AMP in the regulation of enzyme phosphorylation ($\xrightarrow{(+)}$: stimulation; PPi: pyrophosphate).

the activity of phosphodiesterase which degrades it; this enzyme is also thought to be under hormonal control). In the presence of cyclic AMP, the inactive protein kinase (which is thought to comprise a catalytic subunit (C) and a regulatory subunit (R)) dissociates. The catalytic subunit can now catalyse the ATP-dependent phosphorylation of its enzyme substrate. Dephosphorylation of the enzyme is catalysed by phosphoprotein phosphatase.

Phosphorylation can lead either to activation or to inactivation of an enzyme (Table 2.4), but it is important to note that enzymes catalysing

Table 2.4 Effect of cyclic AMP–dependent phosphorylation on the activity of various enzymes

Enzyme	Phosphorylated form
Glycogen phosphorylase	Active
Hormone-sensitive lipase	Active
Glycogen synthetase	Inactive
Glycerol phosphate acyltransferase	Inactive
Phosphofructokinase	Inactive
Pyruvate kinase	Inactive
Acetyl-CoA carboxylase	Inactive

the breakdown of energy stores (glycogen and triacylglycerols) are activated by phosphorylation whilst those involved in the deposition of the stores are inactivated. Thus changes in the concentration of cyclic AMP lead to a coordinated change in the pattern of metabolism – to synthesis or to degradation of energy reserves. This is depicted in Fig. 2.20, although the scheme has been much simplified, at least in the case of glycogen metabolism, which has been studied in most detail. The cyclic AMP-dependent kinase, for example, does not act directly

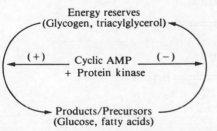

Fig. 2.20. Coordinating effects of cyclic AMP on the accumulation and mobilization of energy reserves ($\xrightarrow{(+)}$: stimulation; $\xrightarrow{(-)}$ inhibition).

on glycogen phosphorylase but instead activates glycogen phosphory kinase which in turn catalyses the phosphorylation of glycogen phosphorylase. Further levels of complexity have also been demonstrated.

Not all phosphorylation reactions involve a cyclic AMP-dependent protein kinase. Pyruvate dehydrogenase, which catalyses the synthesis of acetyl–CoA from pyruvate and has a critical rôle in the regulation of glucose utilization, also exists in an inactive phosphorylated form and an active dephosphorylated form. Interconversion of the two forms involves a specific phosphatase and kinase, but the latter is not affected by cyclic AMP. This may be due to pyruvate dehydrogenase being a mitochondrial enzyme and, therefore, not exposed to changes in the cyclic AMP concentration of the cytosol since the mitochondrial membrane appears to be impermeable to cyclic AMP. The factors which regulate the activation and inactivation of pyruvate dehydrogenase are not fully understood but it seems likely that Ca^{2+} has a key rôle in the activation process.

The importance of covalent modification of enzymes by phosphorylation lies in its rapidity (it requires only minutes) and its reversibility. A major change in enzyme activity can be effected without any change in the total amount of the enzyme. This is illustrated for pyruvate dehydrogenase in Fig. 2.21: in this study total activity rather than the total amount of enzyme was measured but the two would probably be indentical.

Enzyme activation can also be achieved by proteolytic cleavage. This mechanism, which differs from phosphorylation in that it is effectively irreversible, appears to be confined to digestive proteases. These enzymes are synthesized as inactive precursors (zymogens) which on secretion are cleaved to their active form. Three examples are given here.

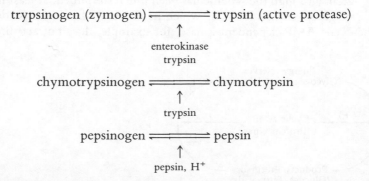

The cleavage reactions are catalysed by other proteases or, in the case of trypsinogen and pepsinogen, by the product, trypsin and pepsin, respectively.

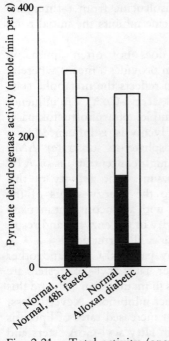

Fig. 2.21. Total activity (open bars) and the activity of the enzyme in the active state (solid bars) of pyruvate dehydrogenase of rat adipose tissue in different physiological and pathological states. (From Denton, Randle, Bridges, Cooper, Keibey, Pask, Stevenson, Stansbie and Whitehouse, 1975.)

Activation by proteolytic cleavage is not confined to enzymes. The hormone insulin is synthesized as a pro-hormone, pro-insulin, which is subjected to proteolytic cleavage in the Golgi apparatus of the pancreatic β-cells to yield the active hormone, and the apparently inactive residual C-peptide.

Allosteric modification

Some enzymes have sites (distinct from the active site) for the specific, reversible, non-covalent binding of substances which lead to changes in the activity of the enzyme. The effector substances are known as allosteric effectors and the enzymes as allosteric enzymes. Allosteric enzymes are usually large and often comprise several subunits. Allosterism provides an especially valuable mechanism for metabolic regulation since it provides a way by which the build-up of end-product of a sequence of reactions can influence the rate of the initial reaction in the series. Specific end-product inhibition has been demonstrated for the synthesis of a variety of amino acids in microorganisms (e.g. the synthesis of L-isoleucine from L-threonine involves five sequential reactions; L-isoleucine inhibits the initial reaction catalysed by threonine dehydrolase).

Such simple end-product inhibition does not often appear in mammalian metabolism; rather, allosterism provides a means whereby key substances, whose concentration often reflects the metabolic state of the cell (e.g. ATP, ADP, AMP, NADH, acetyl-CoA), can influence the rate of metabolic pathways. For example, phosphofructokinase, which has a key rôle in the regulation of glycolysis, is influenced by a series of allosteric effectors: fructose-6-phosphate (its substrate), AMP and ADP activate the enzyme; citrate and high concentrations of ATP (which is also a cofactor) inhibit the enzyme. The activity of this cytosolic enzyme is therefore sensitive to the energy status of the cytosol. A reduction in ATP concentration with a concomitant increase in ADP and AMP would increase the activity of the enzyme and result in an increased rate of glycolysis and hence ATP formation.

Acetyl-CoA carboxylase is inhibited by palmityl-CoA (and other long-chain fatty acyl-CoA esters). However, fatty acyl-CoA esters are not the final products of fatty acid synthesis in mammalian cells and this case cannot be regarded as true end-product inhibition. Nevertheless, impaired rates of fatty acid esterification or increased rates of lipolysis both lead to an accumulation of long-chain fatty acyl-CoA esters and hence to inhibition of acetyl-CoA carboxylase and fatty acid synthesis.

Apart from feed-back inhibition, feed-forward control can also occur and a reactant at an early stage of a sequence can alter the activity of a later step. For example, fructose-1,6-diphosphate, a glycolytic intermediate, activates pyruvate kinase.

Substrates can also act as allosteric effectors; as a result plots of reaction rate against substrate concentration are often sigmoidal in shape (Fig. 2.17). As the substrate concentration is increased the substrate binds to the allosteric site and alters the K_m of the enzyme for the substrate. With this type of mechanism, a small change in substrate concentration can lead to a much larger change in the rate of reaction than that observed for enzymes exhibiting classical Michaelis-Menten kinetics. In other words, the 'signal' of changing concentration is amplified. Fructose-6-phosphate has such an effect on phosphofructokinase (Fig. 2.22).

Allosteric effectors exert their effect by causing changes in the conformation of the enzyme. This usually results in a change in the K_m of the enzyme for its substrate (Fig. 2.22) but occasionally V_{max} is altered. For example, acetyl-CoA carboxylase is comprised of inactive subunits which aggregate in the presence of citrate to form the active polymer. Dissociation of the active polymer is induced by palmityl-CoA (see above) or by malonyl-CoA (the product of the reaction); all three substances are therefore allosteric effectors for this enzyme.

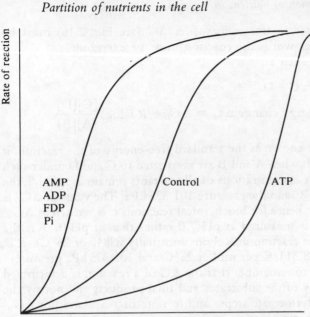

Fig. 2.22. Effects of allosteric effectors on the rate of phosphofructokinase reaction as a function of fructose-6-phosphate concentration (FDP: fructose-1,6-diphosphate).

Allosteric effects occur rapidly (usually within seconds) so they provide an almost instantaneous means of controlling the rate or direction of a metabolic pathway.

Free-energy, equilibria and the direction of metabolic flux

It has been shown in the preceding sections that the rates of reactions in cells are determined by the activities of enzymes (which may be regulated in various ways) and by the concentration of the reactants. Enzymes, however, do not alter the equilibrium constant of a reaction and hence the direction of the net flux remains unchanged. An appreciation of the manner in which the direction of flux through metabolic pathways is regulated requires consideration of some aspects of the thermodynamics of metabolism.

Free-energy
All reactions are reversible; enzymes accelerate the forward and backward reactions to the same extent and hence increase the speed at which equilibrium is attained. The direction of net flux is determined by the free-energy of the reactants, and for a reaction to occur there

must be a decrease in free-energy (i.e. ΔG (see Fig. 2.16) must be negative). In other words the reaction must be exergonic.

For a reaction such as:

$$A + B \rightleftharpoons C + D$$

the free-energy change $\Delta G = \Delta G_0 + RT \log_e \dfrac{[C][D]}{[A][B]}$.

ΔG_0 is a constant known as the standard free-energy of the reaction: it is the ΔG per mol, when A and B are converted to C and D under such conditions that the concentrations of all reactants remain at 1 mol/l; the temperature is 25 °C and the pressure 101.325 kPa. The value of ΔG_0 is dependent on pH; hence for biochemical reactions it is written as $\Delta G_0'$ to signify that it is measured at pH 7.0 rather than at pH 0. T is the temperature of the reaction in Kelvins (normally 298 K or 25° C); R is the gas constant (8.31 J/K per mol at 25° C and 101.325 kPa pressure).

It is important to remember that the ΔG of a reaction is determined by the free-energy of the substrates and final products and not by the free-energy of intermediate steps, and to note that ΔG and not $\Delta G_0'$ determines whether a reaction will proceed in a given direction. In general, reactions with a large negative $\Delta G_0'$ will occur under physiological conditions while those with a large positive $\Delta G_0'$ will not. There are, however, exceptions to these generalizations. For example, the reaction:

$$\text{fructose-1,6-diphosphate} \underset{\text{aldolase}}{\rightleftharpoons}$$
$$\text{glyceraldehyde-3-phosphate} + \text{dihydroxyacetone phosphate}$$

occurs despite a relatively high $\Delta G_0'$ (24 kJ/mol), because the concentrations of the reactants are very low (approximately 30, 20 and 150 μmol/l respectively) and so ΔG is negative.

In contrast, the following reaction does not occur under physiological conditions, despite having a lower $\Delta G_0'$ (14 kJ/mol), because at the intracellular concentrations of the components (approximately 1.5 and 0.1 mmol/l respectively) ΔG is positive.

$$\text{glucose} + \text{phosphate} \underset{\text{glucose-6-phosphatase}}{\rightleftharpoons}$$
$$\text{glucose-6-phosphate} + H_2O^{\dagger}$$

To maintain a glucose-6-phosphate concentration of 0.1 mmol/l by the above reaction, impossibly high glucose and phosphate concentrations would be required within the cell.

[†] Whenever water is a reactant or a product in a biochemical reaction, its concentration is arbitrarily set at 1.0 (actual concentration is approximately 56 mol/l).

The cell solves the dilemma of synthesizing glucose-6-phosphate from glucose by coupling the reaction to the hydrolysis of ATP, because, as stated above, it is the overall free-energy change that is the determinant. Hence:

$$\text{glucose} + \text{phosphate} \rightleftharpoons \text{glucose-6-phosphate} + H_2O$$
$$\Delta G_0' = 14 \, \text{kJ/mol}$$

$$\text{ATP} + H_2O \rightleftharpoons \text{ADP} + \text{phosphate}$$
$$\Delta G_0' = -31 \, \text{kJ/mol}$$

$$\text{glucose} + \text{ATP} \rightleftharpoons \text{glucose-6-phosphate} + \text{ADP}$$
$$\Delta G_0' = -17 \, \text{kJ/mol}$$

This third reaction is that catalysed by the enzyme hexokinase and the physiological concentrations of the components of the reaction are such that the reverse reaction will not occur in the cell.

ATP has a crucial rôle in metabolism since its free-energy of hydrolysis is sufficiently large to drive many important reactions which could not otherwise occur under physiological conditions. In some cases, as in the hexokinase reaction shown above, the phosphate (P_i) from ATP is transferred to a substrate. In others there is a coupling to a simple hydrolysis of ATP. For example:

$$\text{citrate} + \text{CoA} + \text{ATP} \xrightleftharpoons{\text{ATP-citrate lyase}} \text{oxaloacetate} + \text{acetyl-CoA} + \text{ADP} + P_i$$

and

$$HCO_3^- + \text{biotin}^\star + \text{ATP} \rightleftharpoons CO_2 \sim \text{biotin}^\star + \text{ADP} + P_i$$

Where biotin* is bound to carboxylating enzymes such as pyruvate carboxylase, propionyl-CoA carboxylase or acetyl-CoA carboxylase.

Some reactions require a greater energy input and so are coupled to the hydrolysis of ATP to AMP and pyrophosphate, for which $\Delta G_0'$ is $-42 \, \text{KJ/mol}$. For example:

$$\text{acetic acid} + \text{CoA} + \text{ATP} \xrightleftharpoons{\text{acetyl-CoA synthetase}} \text{acetyl-CoA} + \text{AMP} + \text{PPi}$$

$$\text{palmitic acid} + \text{CoA} + \text{ATP} \xrightleftharpoons{\text{palmityl-CoA synthetase}} \text{palmityl-CoA} + \text{AMP} + \text{PPi}$$

The reason for this is that the formation of these CoA compounds has a $\Delta G_0'$ of approximately $29 \, \text{kJ/mol}$. By coupling the reaction to hydrolysis of ATP to AMP an overall $\Delta G_0'$ of -13 kJ/mol is obtained, and the reaction is effectively irreversible under physiological conditions.

Apart from ATP, some reactions use other nucleotide triphosphates (GTP, UTP and CTP). For example:

$$\text{oxaloacetate} + \text{GTP} \xrightleftharpoons{\text{phosphoenolpyruvate carboxykinase}}$$

$$\text{phosphoenol pyruvate} + CO_2 + \text{GDP}$$

There are also a number of reactions in which a substrate is linked to the nucleotide phosphate itself:

$$\text{UTP} + \text{glucose-1-phosphate} \rightleftharpoons$$

$$\text{UDP-glucose} + \text{PPi}$$

(UDP-glucose is subsequently used for the synthesis of glycosidic bonds as in glycogen).

Thus, the energy derived from the hydrolysis of ATP and other nucleotide phosphates provides the energy required for the biosynthesis of a number of covalent bonds. These processes permit reactions to occur under physiological conditions which would otherwise be thermodynamically impossible, and avoid the problems which would arise with extremely high or low concentrations of reactants within the cell.

Equilibrium

Reactions move towards equilibrium; enzymes accelerate this process.

At equilibrium there is no net flux, and $\Delta G = 0$. Thus:

$$\Delta G_0' = -RT\log_e \cdot K_{eq} \quad (K_{eq} \text{ is the equilibrium constant}).$$

The quantitative relationship between $\Delta G_0'$ and K_{eq} is shown in Table 2.5

Most biochemical reactions in the cell are apparently at (or very near) equilibrium although in every metabolic pathway there is at least one step which is not at equilibrium, and thus the pathway as a whole is not at equilibrium.

As with $\Delta G_0'$, the magnitude of K_{eq} does not give a completely reliable indication as to whether the reaction is at equilibrium. For example, for the aldolase reaction, $\Delta G_0' = 24$ kJ/mol and $K_{eq} \approx 10^{-4}$, while for the lactate dehydrogenase reaction $\Delta G_0' = -25$ kJ/mol and $K_{eq} \approx 10^4$; but both reactions are thought to be at equilibrium. In general, enzymes which catalyse reactions at equilibrium have relatively-high activities (Table 2.2): all glycolytic reactions are thought to be at

Table 2.5   Quantitative relationship between the standard free-energy ($\Delta G_0'$)
and the equilibrium (K_{eq})

$\Delta G_0'$ (KJ/mol)	K_{eq}
17.1	0.001
5.69	0.1
0	0
− 5.69	1
−17.1	1000

equilibrium except those catalysed by hexokinase, phosphofructokinase
and pyruvate kinase.

Biochemical systems are 'open' and thus differ from 'closed' systems
normally encountered in thermodynamics. There can be no net reaction
at equilibrium in a 'closed' system but in a biochemical reaction as part
of a metabolic pathway there is net flux because of the constant addition
of increments of substrate and the removal of equivalent amounts of
product.

Enzymes catalysing the reactions which are at equilibrium cannot
directly influence either the rate of the pathway or the direction of flux.
They can, however, have an indirect effect. For example, the concentration of pyruvate in the cytosol is related to the concentration of
lactate, NAD and NADH:

$$\text{pyruvate} + \text{NADH} \xrightleftharpoons{\text{lactate dehydrogenase}} \text{lactate} + \text{NAD}.$$

Since this reaction is at equilibrium

$$K_{eq} = \frac{[\text{lactate}]}{[\text{pyruvate}]} \times \frac{[\text{NAD}]}{[\text{NADH}]}$$

the pyruvate concentration will depend on the total lactate + pyruvate
concentration and the [NAD]:[NADH] ratio of the cytosol. In the
liver, the pyruvate concentration is between 40 and 500 μmol/l while
the K_m of pyruvate carboxylase and pyruvate dehydrogenase for
pyruvate are approximately 400 and 40 μmol/l respectively. Therefore,
changes in the concentration of pyruvate caused by changes in the
equilibrium ratio of the lactate dehydrogenase reaction influence the
rate at which pyruvate is metabolized by these two enzymes.

Unidirectional reactions: regulation of the direction of metabolic flux

As stated previously, enzymes catalysing reactions which are at equilibrium cannot determine the direction of metabolic flux. However, some reactions are irreversible under physiological conditions because of restraints imposed by the concentrations of the participants. Such reactions are thus unidirectional because they keep moving towards a (physiologically) unattainable equilibrium. The enzymes which catalyse these reactions usually have relatively low activities (see examples in Table 2.2), are subject to covalent and/or allosteric modification and show the greatest changes in concentration in response to altering physiological conditions. They are therefore often referred to as *regulatory enzymes*. There are many examples since they are essential components of all metabolic pathways: hexokinase, phosphofructokinase, pyruvate kinase, glycogen synthetase, glycogen phosphorylase, acetyl-CoA synthetase, and pyruvate dehydrogenase.

Unidirectional reactions thus provide a means of determining the direction of metabolic flux through a pathway. They also allow (in fact, they are essential for) separate pathways for synthesis and degradation of cellular constituents. An example is:

$$\text{acetyl-CoA} \xrightleftharpoons[\substack{\text{fatty acid oxidation complex + palmityl-CoA} \\ \text{synthetase}}]{\text{acetyl-CoA carboxylase + fatty acid synthetase}} \text{palmitic acid}$$

For some pathways there may be common steps with different unidirectional enzymes at key positions, as in glycolysis and gluconeogenesis (Fig. 2.23). Unidirectional enzymes are usually found at strategic points in a pathway, often at the first step (e.g. hexokinase) and at branch points (e.g. pyruvate carboxylase and pyruvate dehydrogenase, Fig. 2.24).

Having separate (or partly separate) pathways for synthesis and degradation means that the rates of these processes can be under separate kinetic control (i.e. control by enzyme activity). Similarly, the proportions of a substance being metabolized by competing pathways can be under kinetic control. If there were only a single reversible pathway for synthesis and degradation, the net flux would be determined by the law of mass action. This would probably result in a greater variation in the concentrations of substances within the cell, and the variety of sophisticated controls which have evolved for regulating enzyme activity would be of no avail.

Futile cycles

One consequence of unidirectional reactions and pathways is the potential for futile cycles (sometimes called substrate cycles). For

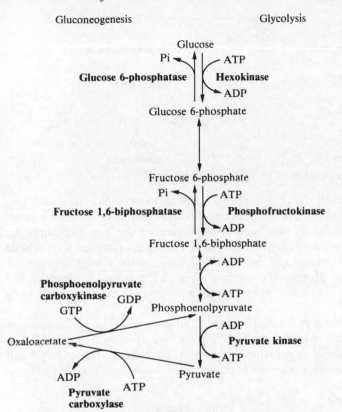

Gluconeogenesis   Glycolysis

Fig. 2.23. Pathways of glycolysis and gluconeogenesis showing key, unidirectional steps.

example:

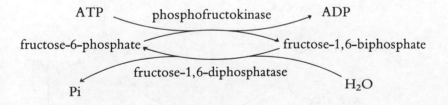

The net effect of the two reactions is:

$$H_2O + ATP \longrightarrow ADP + Pi$$

Operation of this cycle would therefore result in an apparent wastage
of ATP. Whether such cycles operate *in vivo* to any significant extent
is not certain. The enzymes involved are often subject to reciprocal

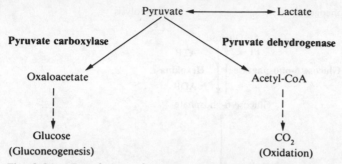

Fig. 2.24.   Regulation of pyruvate metabolism.

allosteric control (e.g. phosphofructokinase and fructose-1,6-diphosphatase) and operation in one direction can be favoured while the reverse direction is inhibited. Alternatively, the enzymes may be separated by compartmentation; for example, fatty acid synthesis occurs in the cytosol and fatty acid oxidation in the mitochondria. The two pools of glucose-6-phosphate (Fig. 2.15), should minimize the possibility of a futile cycle involving hexokinase and glucose-6-phosphate.

An apparently futile cycle occurs in adipose tissue in which some of the fatty acids released during lipolysis are re-esterified (Fig. 2.25). Also, as pointed out earlier, there is a continuous turnover of cell proteins. The exact purpose of these cycles is not clear but they may be

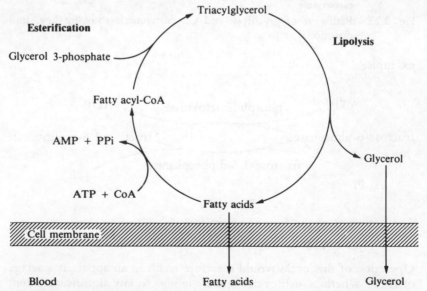

Fig. 2.25.   Triacylglycerol turnover: apparent futile-cycling in adipocytes.

of importance in metabolic regulation. For example, the cycling of fructose-6-phosphate and fructose-1,6-diphosphate increases the sensitivity of the rate of net fructose-6-phosphate phosphorylation to changes in AMP concentration (an allosteric activator of phosphofructokinase) and also results in a threshold effect (i.e. the AMP concentration has to rise above a certain threshold concentration before it affects the rate of net phosphorylation). Such a mechanism could be useful in tissues in which large changes in the rate of glycolysis may occur (e.g. skeletal muscle and liver) and these tissues have both enzymes. Smooth muscle, on the other hand, in which large changes in the rate of glycolysis are not a feature, lacks fructose-1,6-diphosphatase activity, and thus there is no cycling.

The Cori cycle has a well defined physiological function (Fig. 2.26) and, although wasteful in terms of ATP usage, provides a means of producing ATP in muscle when oxygen availability is reduced during excessive muscular activity.

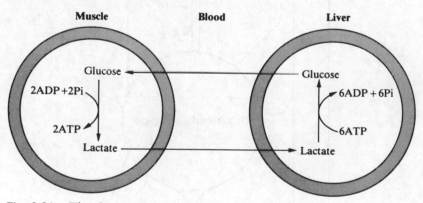

Fig. 2.26.   The Cori cycle (net: $4\,\text{ATP} \longrightarrow 4\,\text{ADP} + 4\,\text{Pi}$).

General features of metabolic pathways and the coordination of their regulation

Within the cell the activities of the various metabolic pathways have to be coordinated for the cell to maintain the concentration of its metabolites within certain limits and to preferentially carry out essential functions, for example, the maintenance of ionic gradients. Such aspects of coordinative control are considered in the present section.

Metabolic pathways: general features

Space does not permit a description of all the pathways of intermediary metabolism of cells but the basic features of anabolic and catabolic pathways are summarised in Fig. 2.27. Metabolism may be

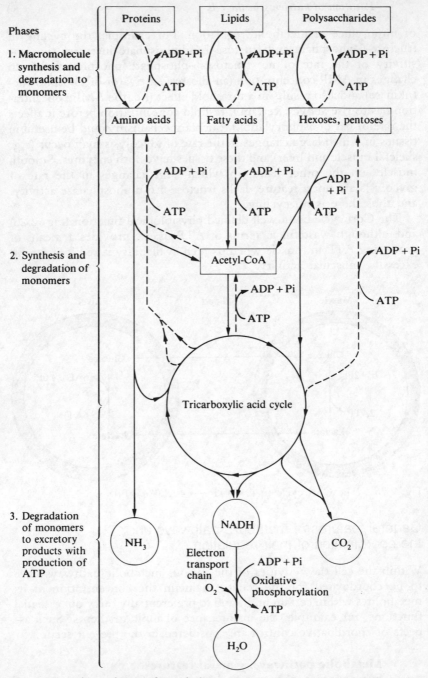

Fig. 2.27. Three phases of metabolism. (From Lehninger, 1975, with modification.) $\longrightarrow$ Catabolic pathways (leading to ATP production). $----\rightarrow$ Anabolic pathways (leading to ATP utilization).

viewed as comprising:

1. the synthesis and degradation of macromolecules (often polymers) (proteins, lipids, polysaccharides and nucleic acids) from, or to, simpler substances (amino acids, fatty acids, simple sugars, etc.);
2. the synthesis and degradation of simple substances to and from a few key intermediates (primarily acetyl-CoA and organic acids of the tricarboxylic-acid cycle);
3. the oxidation of acetyl-CoA to carbon dioxide via the tricarboxylic-acid cycle and the concomitant oxidation of hydrogen from this and other metabolic processes by the electron-transport chain leading to the production of ATP (oxidative phosphorylation).

Pathways of catabolism are convergent, with clearly defined starting materials but with a variety of end-products, whereas anabolic pathways are divergent and have distinct end-products but a variety of starting materials (Fig. 2.28). Figure 2.27 indicates the central rôle of the tricarboxylic-acid cycle in intermediary metabolism; since the reactions of the cycle are common to both catabolic and anabolic pathways, the tricarboxylic-acid cycle is sometimes called an amphibolic pathway.

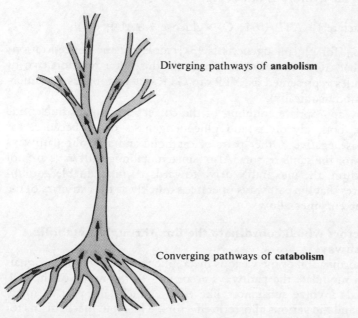

Diverging pathways of **anabolism**

Converging pathways of **catabolism**

Fig. 2.28. Characteristic patterns of catabolic and anabolic pathways. (From Lehninger, 1975, with modification.)

The flux through metabolic pathways is regulated by the key, unidirectional reactions located at the beginning of a pathway or at branch points; the activities of these enzymes are usually subject to a variety of controls as described earlier. The first reaction of some catabolic pathways involves an initial activation coupled to the hydrolysis of ATP, while anabolic pathways include one or more steps linked to hydrolysis of ATP or another trinucleotide phosphate. This is inevitable since for a given sequence, just as for an individual reaction, the free-energy change ΔG = (free-energy of products) $-$ (free-energy of substrates), and for the reaction to proceed ΔG must be negative. For example, glycolysis may be thought of as:

$$\text{glucose} \longrightarrow 2 \text{ lactate.}$$

For this reaction, ΔG is so greatly negative that the pathway can be used to produce some ATP, and in its final form may be summarized as:

$$\text{glucose} + 2\,\text{ADP} + 2\text{Pi} \longrightarrow 2\,\text{lactate} + 2\,\text{ATP} + 2\,H_2O$$
$$(\Delta G_0' = -136\,\text{kJ/mol})$$

For gluconeogenesis (the reverse) to occur the reaction has to be coupled to the hydrolysis of 6 ATP:

$$2 \text{ lactate} + 6\,\text{ATP} + 6\,H_2O \rightarrow \text{glucose} + 6\,\text{ADP} + 6\,\text{Pi}$$

In fact $\Delta G_0'$ for gluconeogenesis is 13kJ/mol, but the concentrations are such that ΔG is negative and large (in this latter reaction two of the molecules represented as ATP are GTP but this makes no difference thermodynamically).

Thus by appropriate coupling of the correct amount of nucleotide phosphate, both glycolysis and gluconeogenesis occur because, for each, ΔG is negative. Other pairs of catabolic and anabolic pathways take place for the same reason. Also, since metabolic pathways are not at equilibrium, the inexorable drive towards an unattainable equilibrium ensures that the pathways operate as quickly as the activities of the constituent enzymes allow.

Factors which coordinate the flux through metabolic pathways

Coordination of the various metabolic pathways requires signals which can modulate the pathways according to the needs of the cell. Such signals involve substances like ATP, which take part in many reactions, and the various allosteric effectors. The rapid mechanisms for modulating and coordinating metabolism operate against a background of slower changes in enzyme activity brought about by alterations in enzyme concentration in response, for example, to new physiological conditions.

Adenine nucleotides

ATP has a central rôle in the coordination of cellular metabolism and with other similar nucleoside triphosphates (Table 2.6) is essential to provide the energy needed for biosynthesis. Also, the initial steps in

Table 2.6   Nucleoside triphosphate requirements for the synthesis of macromolecules

Proteins	ATP, GTP
Polysaccharides	ATP, UTP
Lipids	ATP, CTP
Nucleic acids	ATP, GTP, UTP, CTP

the pathways of catabolism of sugars and fatty acids, pathways which are the main sources of ATP, involve an initial ATP-coupled activation step. ATP is required by all cells to provide the energy for the ion pumps of the plasma membrane that maintain the distinct ionic composition of cells and cell volume (Fig. 2.8), and in contractile cells ATP provides the energy for muscular contraction and hence mechanical work. Thus, to survive, a cell (and hence an organism) must have mechanisms for maintaining an adequate concentration of ATP.

ATP is produced in mammalian cells primarily by oxidative phosphorylation in the mitochondria. In this process hydrogen atoms provided by NADH or reduced flavin adenine dinucleotide are oxidized to water with the concomitant synthesis of ATP. For NADH, the overall reaction is:

$$NADH + H^+ + 3\,ADP + P_i + 0.5\,O_2 \longrightarrow$$
$$NAD^+ + 4\,H_2O + 3\,ATP \quad (\Delta G_0' = -129\,kJ/mol)$$

The reaction proceeds via a series of steps – the electron transfer chain.

ATP derived from oxidative phosphorylation can be exchanged for ADP from the cytosol by an ADP-ATP translocase in the mitochondrial inner membrane. ATP is also generated directly in the cytosol during glycolysis; however, the amount produced by this process is only approximately 5% of that produced by the complete oxidation of glucose.

$$glucose + 2\,ADP + 2\,Pi \longrightarrow 2\,lactate + 2\,ATP + 2\,H_2O \text{ (glycolysis)}$$

$$glucose + 6\,O_2 + 36\,ADP + 36\,Pi \longrightarrow 6\,CO_2 + 42\,H_2O + 36\,ATP$$
$$\text{(glycolysis + oxidative phosphorylation)}$$

The advantage of glycolysis is that it is independent of oxygen and thus provides a source of ATP under anaerobic conditions or when oxygen is in short supply, as during violent exercise.

ATP can be synthesized from ADP by the adenylate kinase reaction which is thought to be at equilibrium in the cell.

$$2\,ADP \rightleftharpoons ATP + AMP$$

The synthesis of other nucleoside triphosphates is dependent on ATP and is catalysed by the enzyme nucleoside diphosphate kinase:

$$ATP + XDP \rightleftharpoons ADP + XTP \text{ (where XDP is UDP, CDP or GDP).}$$

The production of ATP must be rapid and finely coordinated with its utilization since there is little storage of ATP; the molecule is essentially an energy carrier and its terminal phosphate group has a very high rate of turnover. Some cells have reservoirs of so-called 'high-energy' phosphate such as phosphocreatine.

$$ATP + creatine \xrightleftharpoons[]{creatine\ kinase} ADP + phosphocreatine$$

The enzyme, creatine kinase, is found primarily in muscle cells where its activity can provide sufficient energy for maintaining muscular contraction for several minutes.

ATP, ADP and AMP are all allosteric modulators of various reactions. AMP stimulates glycogenolysis, and both AMP and ADP stimulate glycolysis and the tricarboxylic-acid cycle, thereby promoting carbohydrate catabolism and ATP production. In contrast, ATP accumulation inhibits these processes (Fig. 2.29). The rate of ATP synthesis is therefore thought to be mediated by the relative concentrations of the adenine nucleotides rather than by the concentration of ATP alone. In other words, the energy state of the cell is reflected by the proportion of the adenine nucleotides present in the form of ATP. The precise relationships are not certain: two possibilities – 'energy charge' and 'phosphorylation potential' – have been proposed.

Atkinson (1977) proposed that the energy state of the cell be expressed by the ratio:

$$\frac{1}{2} \cdot \frac{[ADP] + 2[ATP]}{[AMP] + [ADP] + [ATP]}$$

He termed this the 'energy charge' of the cell, and it is a measure of the proportion of the total adenine nucleotide pool which is 'filled with high-energy phosphate'. If all were present as ATP, the energy charge would be 1.0. Atkinson (1977) suggested that the energy charge is the primary factor in the regulation of ATP production and, to a lesser extent, utilization. As shown in Fig. 2.30, the rates of ATP-generating reactions decrease and the rates of ATP-utilizing reactions increase as the energy charge increases. The intersection, where the rates of production and utilization of ATP are equal, corresponds to an energy charge

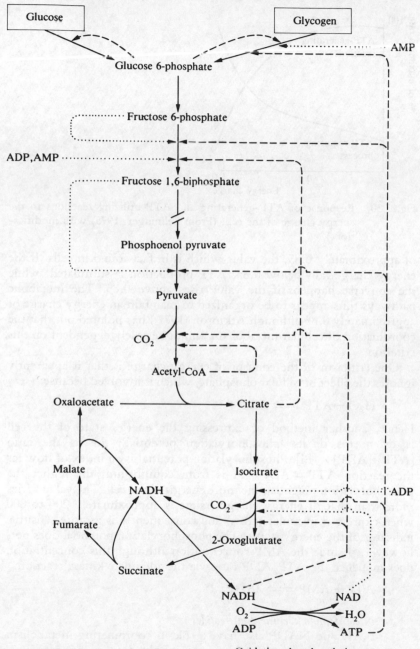

Fig. 2.29. Regulation of glycolysis, glycogenolysis and the tricarboxylic-acid cycle by adenine nucleotides and other intracellular signals (·······▶, stimulation; –––▶, inhibition).

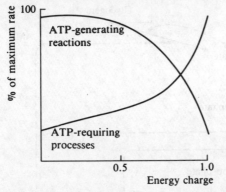

Fig. 2.30.   Response of ATP-generating and ATP-utilizing reactions to the
energy charge of the cell. (From Lehninger, 1975, with modification.)

of approximately 0.85, the value which is in fact found in cells. If the
energy charge falls below 0.85, ATP production is stimulated, while
the converse happens if the value rises above 0.85. The metabolic
pathways thus appear to be organized to maintain an energy charge of
approximately 0.85 although Atkinson (1977) has pointed out that the
coordination of cellular metabolism cannot be solely dependent on this
criterion.

One criticism of the concept of energy charge is that it apparently
ignores the effect of cellular phosphate, which is involved because:

$$H_2O + ATP \rightleftharpoons ADP + Pi$$

Hence, another method of expressing the energy state of the cell
is by means of its 'phosphorylation potential'; this is the ratio
$[ATP]:[ADP] \times [Pi]$. Phosphorylation potential is an index of how far
the reaction $ATP \rightleftharpoons ADP + Pi$ is from equilibrium; the higher the
phosphorylation potential, the more energized the cell. The value varies
more than that of energy charge (range is approximately 200 to 800
when expressed in molar terms) and consequently is a more sensitive
indicator of the energy status. The phosphorylation potential does not,
however, include the AMP concentration although this concentration
does influence the $ATP:ADP$ ratio via the adenylate kinase reaction:

$$ATP + AMP \rightleftharpoons 2ADP.$$

Nicotinamide adenine dinucleotides
NAD and NADP also have a rôle in coordinating metabolism
since, as hydrogen carriers, they are involved in many reactions.
Although apparently similar, they have distinct rôles. NADP, or at
least its reduced form, NADPH, is the principal source of hydrogen for
biosynthesis, in particular for fatty acid synthesis, whereas NAD, along

with flavin adenine dinucleotide, is the carrier of hydrogen produced during catabolism for subsequent oxidation by the electron transport chain. Thus the production of hydrogen for biosynthesis and that for oxidation are separated and can be regulated independently. Furthermore, most of the NADP is found in the cytosol while over 60% of the NAD is in the mitochondria.

The reaction is essentially:

$$Y\text{-reduced} + NAD(P)^+ \underset{}{\overset{Y\text{-dehydrogenase}}{\rightleftharpoons}} Y\text{-oxidized} + NAD(P)H + H^+$$

The quantities of nicotinamide adenine nucleotides within the cell are low. There is, therefore, a rapid turnover of their hydrogen, and the rates of production and utilization must be coordinated. In the cytosol, the various reactions involving NAD are thought to be at equilibrium, and changes in the NAD:NADH ratio would have effects in several different pathways. NADH is also an allosteric inhibitor of both phosphofructokinase and pyruvate dehydrogenase and a high NADH: NAD ratio in either the cytosol or the mitochondria would reduce the rate of acetyl–CoA synthesis from glucose and hence the rate of ATP production.

Metabolities

A number of metabolites can influence the activities of enzymes and therefore have a rôle as signals in coordinating metabolism (see also section on allosterism). Four examples will serve to illustrate the point.

1. Citrate: activates acetyl–CoA carboxylase and hence fatty acid synthesis; inhibits phosphofructokinase and hence glycolysis; and activates fructose-1,6–diphosphatase and hence gluco-neogenesis.
2. Glucose-6-phosphate: inhibits hexokinase and activates glycogen synthetase – hence the accumulation of glucose-6-phosphate will both retard its rate of formation from glucose and accelerate its conversion to glycogen.
3. Acetyl–CoA: inhibits pyruvate dehydrogenase; and activates pyruvate carboxylase – hence an accumulation of acetyl–CoA in the mitochondria will switch the point of entry into the tricarboxylic-acid cycle from acetyl–CoA to oxaloacetate (Fig. 2.24).
4. Palmityl–CoA: inhibits acetyl–CoA carboxylase and hence the rate of fatty acid synthesis, and inhibits citrate translocase and hence citrate efflux from the mitochondria.

Thus these four metabolites have an important rôle in coordinating changes in glucose and fatty acid metabolism.

It should be noted that early studies suggested that fatty acids and their acyl–CoA esters inhibited many enzymes but these effects were later shown to be due to a detergent effect of these substances when used at high concentrations.

Cyclic nucleotides and calcium

The cyclic nucleotides (cyclic AMP and cyclic GMP) and Ca^{2+} differ from the other substances described above in that they are thought to provide signals which are regulated by external factors (hormones and nerves). Cyclic AMP and cyclic GMP are synthesized from ATP and GTP respectively by the action of adenylate and guanylate cyclases. As shown in Fig. 2.20, cyclic AMP has an important rôle in the coordination of metabolism, especially in the regulation of the synthesis and utilization of energy stores (glycogen and tri-acylglycerol). The rôle of cyclic GMP is less well defined.

Ca^{2+} influences a variety of complex physiological processes (e.g. cell motility, muscle contraction, axonal flow, and secretion) and modifies the activities of various enzymes of intermediary metabolism. Ca^{2+} activates pyruvate, isocitrate and 2-oxoglutarate dehydrogenases of the mitochondria and so stimulates acetyl-CoA synthesis and oxidation; Ca^{2+} stimulates the activity of phosphorylase kinase, leading to increased glycogen phosphorylase activity (thus augmenting the effects of cyclic AMP); and Ca^{2+} stimulates cyclic AMP phosphodies-terase and thus can modulate the cyclic AMP concentration.

Cellular Ca^{2+} is compartmentalized, with separate pools in the cytosol and mitochondria, and with some Ca^{2+} bound to membranes. Hormones and nervous transmitters are thought to either increase Ca^{2+} uptake by the cell or alter the distribution within the cellular pools (a release of membrane-bound Ca^{2+} seems likely). A Ca^{2+} binding-protein, troponin C, was demonstrated in muscle cells, and its binding of Ca^{2+} is a key step in muscle contraction. More recently, a Ca^{2+}-binding protein called calmodulin has been found in the cytosol of a variety of cells. It is thought that an increase in cytosolic Ca^{2+} results in Ca^{2+} binding to calmodulin and that this complex activates such enzymes as phosphodiesterase and phosphorylase kinase. However, Ca^{2+} itself may directly activate the mitochondrial dehydrogenases listed above.

As has already been indicated, there is an interaction between Ca^{2+} and cyclic AMP in some systems (e.g. glycogen metabolism): details have not been fully resolved but a probable relationship is shown in Fig. 2.31.

Maintenance and productive processes at the intracellular level

In the introduction the distinction was made between the utilization of dietary constituents for 'maintenance' and 'production'. When dealing

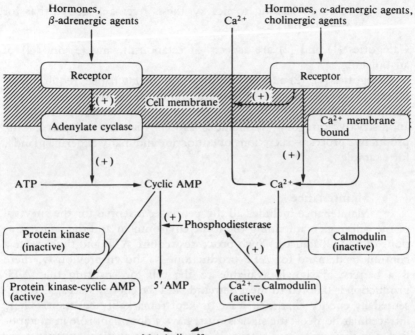

Fig. 2.31. Interrelationships between cyclic AMP and Ca^{2+} as second messengers of hormones and neurohumoral (cholinergic and adrenergic) transmitters ($\xrightarrow{(+)}$, stimulates).

with the coordination of metabolism within the cell in these terms, four basic processes must be considered:

1. breakdown of nutrients to provide ATP;
2. breakdown of nutrients to provide precursors (including NADPH) for biosynthesis (the supply and requirements of nutrients for the cell are most unlikely to correspond and the cell has to modify the nutrients to meet its requirements for biosynthesis);
3. biosynthesis of essential cellular constituents to replace those lost in turnover (i.e. replacement without net biosynthesis), or to alter the capabilities of the cell (e.g. increase in enzyme concentration, formation of additional membranes – although the latter may involve net synthesis, the processes are included as being essential for function);
4. biosynthesis of storage materials (e.g. lipid, glycogen), secretory materials (e.g. milk, egg constituents) and materials for increasing the number and/or the size of cells (growth and reproduction); in other words, biosynthetic

reactions leading to net synthesis over and above that for essential purposes.

Categories (1) and (2) are aspects of catabolism, and (3) and (4) of anabolism.

Categories (1), (2) and (3) comprise the 'maintenance' requirement, whereas (4) is the 'productive' process. These divisions are understandably not absolute: for (4) to occur there must be in increase in (1) and (2) and, strictly, category (4) includes aspects that are not part of the productive process – secretions of endocrine and many exocrine glands, for example.

Maintenance

Maintenance includes all the processes essential for the survival of the cell (e.g. maintaining the ionic environment and the concentrations of key substances.) Such processes require ATP and thus create a continuous demand for ATP production. As shown previously, there is a battery of signals available to the cell for ensuring that ATP production is tailored to meet demand, and the energy status, as represented by energy charge at least, is kept remarkably constant. These intracellular homeostatic signals must have a dominant rôle in metabolism and they provide a means of ensuring that available nutrients are preferentially directed towards ATP-producing processes when required.

Production

The direction of nutrients into anabolic pathways cannot be explained solely in terms of the energy status of the cell for, although a reduction in the energy status would curtail anabolic activity in favour of ATP production (see Fig. 2.30), anabolic processes occur without an apparent decrease in the energy charge. For net anabolic activity, therefore, nutrient availability must be in excess of that required for ATP production (which will be increased to meet the demands of the anabolic processes themselves) and there must be signals to indicate this excess availability in order that nutrients may be diverted into anabolic pathways. Although there is by no means a complete picture of all the signals involved, there are some examples of the types of mechanism which operate.

The flux through glycolysis is influenced by the energy status of the cell; hence, increased availability of glucose could lead to an increase in the glucose-6-phosphate concentration (assuming that the flux through glycolysis does not increase) and in turn to an activation of glycogen synthetase and an increased rate of glycogen deposition. Another example is that, if the availability of acetyl-CoA in the mitochondria begins to exceed the need for its oxidation, the accumulation of acetyl-CoA will inhibit pyruvate dehydrogenase and therefore the production of acetyl-CoA from pyruvate. At the same time, the acetyl-CoA will activate pyruvate carboxylase and result in greater oxaloacetate production, thereby increasing the pool of tricarboxylic-cycle acids available for anabolic pathways.

The cell, therefore, has signals, in addition to those concerned with the maintenance of the energy status, which direct metabolites into anabolic pathways when nutrient supply attains an appropriate level. Intracellular signals are not only dependent on nutrient availability within the cell, however. The cell is also sensitive to external signals provided by hormones and nervous transmitters, which modulate and coordinate metabolism in the body as a whole.

COORDINATION OF METABOLISM WITHIN THE WHOLE ANIMAL

Metabolism within the animal as a whole is coordinated by the endocrine (hormone) and nervous systems, which are closely interconnected: hormones can influence nervous activity and the nervous system is involved in the regulation of hormone secretion. In addition, hormones and neurohumoral transmitters (substances released from nerve-endings and having a localized activity) may have similar effects on the metabolism of tissues and the effects of both may be mediated by either cyclic nucleotides or calcium (Fig. 2.31). Some substances are, in fact, both hormones and neurohumoral transmitters.

Both the endocrine and the nervous system are sensitive to the metabolic status of the animal: they respond to the act of eating and to the quantity and nature (i.e. composition) of the diet; various nutrients in the blood can influence hormone secretion and also nervous activity.

Physiological states such as pregnancy and lactation modify the activity of the endocrine and nervous systems, resulting in alteration of the metabolism within the animal to meet the new requirement. In addition, the nervous system is sensitive to changes in the animal's environment and so provides a mechanism whereby bodily function can be modulated to meet the demands of such factors as cold or fear (these various relationships are summarized in Fig. 2.32).

The endocrine system

Hormones are a chemically diverse group of substances which are produced in trace amounts by the various endocrine glands of the body

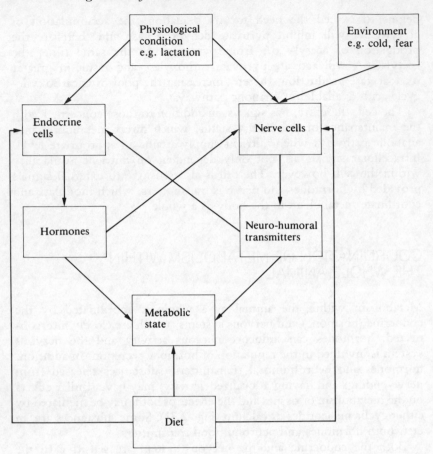

Fig. 2.32.   Interrelationships between the endocrine and nervous systems in the coordination of metabolism.

and secreted into the blood. They are *intercellular chemical messengers* of the body and as such are able to influence the metabolism of the various tissues and organs. Hormones thus have a crucial rôle in the integrated regulation of metabolism within the body and hence the partition of nutrients.

As shown in Table 2.7, hormones may be polypeptides, steroids or amino acid derivatives: classification of a substance as a hormone is on the basis of physiological rôle and origin rather than its chemical composition.

Most hormone producing (endocrine) cells are gathered together as discrete endocrine glands which are located in various parts of the body. Endocrine glands differ from other glands such as the mammary glands, salivary glands or sweat glands in that they are ductless and secrete their products directly into the blood. Endocrine glands often

Table 2.7   Chemical nature and origin of various hormones

Hormone	Chemical nature	Endocrine gland
Prolactin	Polypeptide	Anterior pituitary
Growth hormone (GH)	Polypeptide	Anterior pituitary
Thyrotropin (TSH)	Glyco-polypeptide	Anterior pituitary
Luteinizing hormone (LH)	Glyco-polypeptide	Anterior pituitary
Adrenocorticotropin (ACTH)	Polypeptide	Anterior pituitary
Oxytocin	Polypeptide	Posterior pituitary
Vasopressin	Polypeptide	Posterior pituitary
Insulin	Polypeptide	Pancreas
Glucagon	Polypeptide	Pancreas
Somatostatin	Polypeptide	Pancreas
Calcitonin	Polypeptide	Thyroid gland
Thyroxine	Amino acid derivative	Thyroid gland
Tri-iodothyronine	Amino acid derivative	Thyroid gland
Adrenalin (epinephrine)	Amino acid derivative	Adrenal medulla
Cortisol	Steroid	Adrenal cortex
Aldosterone	Steroid	Adrenal cortex
Testosterone	Steroid	Testis
Progesterone	Steroid	Ovary
Oestradiol	Steroid	Ovary

contain several different cell-types, each producing a specific hormone. In the islets of Langerhans in the pancreas for example, α-cells produce glucagon, β-cells produce insulin and D-cells produce somatostatin.

However, not all endocrine cells congregate to form glands. The gut produces a variety of hormones, e.g. gastrin, secretin, cholecystokinin (or pancreozymin), motilin, enteroglucagon, and gastric inhibitory peptide (or glucose-dependent insulin-releasing peptide), but the cells which produce these hormones are scattered over regions of the gut (e.g. Fig. 2.33). Although they are regarded as hormones and are released into the circulation, a number of gut hormones (e.g. neurotensin, vasoactive intestinal peptide, and substance P) are also found in nerve-endings and are released as neurohumoral transmitters on stimulation of the nerves. They are thought to comprise a *peptidergic system* analogous to the *cholinergic* and *adrenergic nervous systems* (see below). Also, the hormones of the posterior pituitary gland (oxytocin and vasopressin) are synthesized and secreted by nerve cells

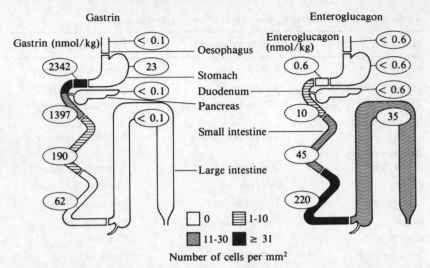

Gastrin   Enteroglucagon

Fig. 2.33.   The concentration of gastrin and enterglucagon and the numbers of
cells which secrete them in the different parts of the human
alimentary canal. The numbers in circles refer to the concentration
per kg tissue in that region of gut. The shading represents the
number of secreting cells per mm² of mucosal surface. (From
Bloom and Polak, 1978.)

originating in the hypothalamus, and are stored in the cells of the
posterior pituitary before release into the circulation.

In addition to the above, there are other substances such as prostaglandins and polyamines (e.g. spermidine) that are released into the
circulation and may influence events elsewhere in the body: however,
as they are not secreted by distinct endocrine cells, they are not
regarded as hormones.

The definition of a hormone is thus rather arbitrary; the important
point is that there are a variety of substances released into the circulation
which influence and coordinate the metabolism and function of remote
tissues.

Regulation of hormone secretion

The secretion of hormones is regulated by a variety of factors
including:

1. the nervous system;
2. other hormones;
3. nutrients in the blood or digestive tract;
4. metal ions.

Examples of these are shown in Table 2.8. Some stimuli affect the
secretion of a variety of hormones and the secretion of some hormones

Table 2.8 Examples of factors which regulate the secretion of hormones

	Substance/system	Effect	Hormone
1. Nervous system	Sympathetic nervous system	Stimulates	Adrenalin, glucagon
	Sympathetic nervous system	Inhibits	Insulin
	Parasympathetic nervous system	Stimulates	Insulin, pancreatic polypeptide, gastrin, somatostatin, glucagon
2. Hormones	Glucagon	Stimulates	Insulin, growth hormone
	Somatostatin	Inhibits	Insulin, glucagon, growth hormone
	Glucose-dependent insulin-releasing peptide (GIP)	Stimulates	Insulin, glucagon
3. Nutrients	Glucose	Stimulates	Insulin, GIP
	Glucose	Inhibits	Glucagon, growth hormone
	Propionic acid	Stimulates	Insulin
	Amino acids	Stimulate	Insulin, glucagon, growth hormone, cholecystokinin
4. Metal ions	Calcium	Stimulates	Calcitonin, cholecystokinin
	Calcium	Inhibits	Parathyroid hormone

is influenced by a variety of factors; thus regulation of hormone secretion is complex. As shown later, an individual hormone usually affects events in a number of tissues and often has more than one effect in a single cell. In addition, in the cell and in the body as a whole, the effects of one hormone are modulated by those of others and adaptation to a new environment or physiological state is likely to involve changes in the concentration of a variety of hormones in the blood. For example: insulin is a major anabolic hormone stimulating the synthesis of protein, glycogen and triacylglycerol, and its secretion is promoted by increased concentrations of precursors such as amino acids and glucose in the blood. Intake of food results in an increased availability of such nutrients but the body can pre-empt the increase in their concentration in the blood by stimulating insulin secretion via the parasympathetic nervous system and by the action of some gut hormones (secretion of the latter is stimulated by the presence of nutrients in the digestive tract). These effects are presumably to increase the efficiency of nutrient utilization during a meal. Food intake also stimulates a rise in the glucagon concentration in the blood, again due to the action of the parasympathetic nervous system and some gut hormones. The reason for this is not completely clear but, as glucagon promotes glucose production by the liver, it may be a mechanism to ensure that a pre-emptive release of insulin at the onset of a meal does not result in an undesirable fall in the blood glucose concentration. Eating, then, triggers a series of changes in the endocrine system which are designed to ensure an efficient utilization of ingested nutrients.

The anterior pituitary gland has a special rôle in the regulation of metabolism, for its hormones not only have direct effects on metabolism in their own right but control the secretion of hormones in several other endocrine glands (Table 2.9); also, somatomedin production by the liver is controlled by growth hormone.

The secretion of anterior pituitary hormones is controlled by specific releasing factors (e.g. thyrotropin releasing factor, TRH), which are small peptides released from nerve endings in the hypothalamus. The releasing factors are carried by a minute portal system to the anterior

Table 2.9   Rôle of anterior pituitary gland in regulation of hormone secretion

Anterior pituitary gland hormone	Target endocrine gland	Secondary hormone
Adrenocorticotropin (ACTH)	Adrenal cortex	Glucocorticosteroids
Thyrotropin (TSH)	Thyroid gland	Thyroxine, Tri-iodothyronine
Luteinizing hormone (LH)	Ovary (female) Testis (male)	Oestradiol Testosterone

pituitary gland where they stimulate the secretion of the appropriate hormone (except for prolactin which has a release-inhibiting factor). The secretion of anterior pituitary hormones is thus under neural control.

The secondary hormones such as cortisol or thyroxine, which are controlled by pituitary hormones, inhibit the secretion of their equivalent releasing factors, hence the concentration of the secondary hormones is subject to feed-back inhibition (Fig. 2.34). In addition, as shown in Table 2.8, other substances and hormones can modulate the secretion of the anterior pituitary gland hormones.

Mechanisms of hormone action

Receptors
All hormones, regardless of their chemical constitution, appear to have specific receptors in their target tissues. These receptors are

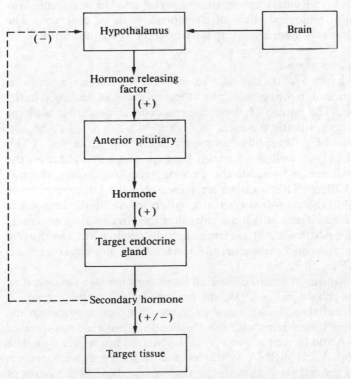

Fig. 2.34.   Rôle of anterior pituitary gland and hypothalamus in the regulation of hormone secretion ($\xrightarrow{(+)}$, stimulation; $\dashrightarrow$ $(-)$, inhibition).

located either on the outside of the plasma membrane (polypeptide hormones and catecholamine receptors) or within the cell (steroid and thyroid hormone receptors). Polypeptide and catecholamine hormones can thus interact with their receptors without entering the cell.

Hormone receptors are proteins and have a high affinity for their hormones (dissociation constants are approximately 10^{-10} to 10^{-9} mol/l). Receptors are very specific and probably interact with only a single hormone *in vivo*, although they bind other hormones at higher concentration *in vitro*. For example, the insulin receptor of adipocytes will also bind somatomedins but with a much lower affinity.

Some receptor-hormone interactions appear to exhibit negative co-operativity: that is, the mean affinity of the receptors for the hormone decreases as the amount of hormone bound increases. The physiological significance of negative cooperativity is uncertain but it may provide a buffer against very rapid changes in hormone concentration which are known to occur.

Not all the receptors for a hormone need to be occupied for the hormone to exert its maximum effect on a tissue. For example, only about 2% of the insulin receptors of adipocytes need to be occupied for the maximum biological effect of the hormone to be observed. The reason for the very large spare capacity of receptors is not known.

Subsequent events

The binding of a hormone to its receptor triggers a series of events which lead to the types of physiological changes described in the next section. The nature of these intermediate steps varies, and for some hormones it is still obscure.

A number of polypeptide hormones (including glucagon, TSH, ACTH and LH) as well as adrenalin bind to receptors located in the plasma membrane and activate the enzyme adenylate cyclase which is also located there. This leads to an increase in the concentration of cyclic AMP in the cytosol and so to a variety of metabolic changes as described earlier. These hormones thus alter the intracellular concentration of cyclic AMP without entering the cell; cyclic AMP can thus be regarded as a second messenger or intracellular messenger of such hormones (Fig. 2.19).

The mechanism of action of steroid hormones has also been studied in detail. As shown in Fig. 2.35, the hormone binds to its receptor in the cytosol and then the hormone-receptor complex migrates to the nucleus where it associates with the chromatin. This leads to increased rates of RNA and hence protein synthesis. Steroid hormones stimulate both ribosomal and mRNA synthesis: the former promotes protein synthesis in general (as occurs in the mammary gland at the onset of lactogenesis) while the latter results in increased rates of synthesis of specific proteins (Table 2.10).

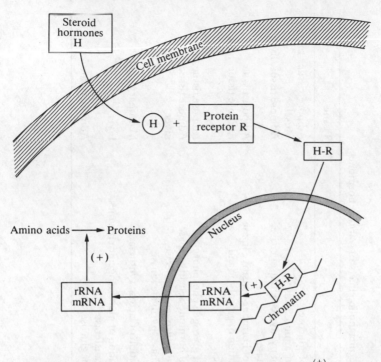

Fig. 2.35.   Mechanism of action of steroid hormones ($\xrightarrow{(+)}$ stimulation).

Although many metabolic effects of insulin have been demonstrated, the mechanisms responsible are still surprisingly obscure. Insulin receptors are found on the plasma membrane of target cells and studies with insulin bound covalently to agarose beads (which are too large to enter cells) suggested that the effects of insulin on membrane permeability and enzyme activity did not require the entry of insulin into the cell. This implied that there should be a second messenger for insulin by analogy with cyclic AMP. Insulin stimulates the uptake of Ca^{2+} and K^+ by cells and also causes the release of membrane-bound Ca^{2+} (insulin causes hyperpolarization of the plasma membrane and this is probably responsible for the changes in ion fluxes). Calcium ions probably mediate some of the effects of insulin but not all. Insulin can, under some circumstances, lower cyclic AMP concentration and raise cyclic GMP concentration but, again, not all the effects of insulin are paralleled by changes in cyclic nucleotide concentration. Also, one mechanism whereby insulin lowers the concentration of cyclic AMP involves the activation of a phosphodiesterase and this effect may well be due to Ca^{2+} (see Fig. 2.31). The effects of insulin may thus be mediated by changes in both Ca^{2+} and cyclic nucleotide concentrations, and possibly by other substances also. In addition, there is some

Table 2.10 Examples of the metabolic effects of various hormones

Hormone	Effect	Tissue
Insulin	Increased uptake of glucose	Adipose tissue, muscle
	Increased uptake of amino acids	Muscle
	Increased activity of pyruvate dehydrogenase, glycogen synthetase	Adipose tissue, liver
	Decreased activity of hormone-sensitive lipase	Adipose tissue
	Increased concentration of glycolytic and lipogenic enzymes	Adipose tissue, liver
Glucagon	Increased activity of glycogen phosphorylase	Adipose tissue, liver
	Increased activity of hormone-sensitive lipase	Adipose tissue
	Decreased activity of glycogen synthetase, phosphofructokinase, pyruvate kinase	Liver
Prolactin	Increased concentration of lactose synthetase	Mammary gland
Glucocorticoids	Increased concentration of gluconeogenic enzymes, tyrosine aminotransferase	Liver
	Decreased uptake of glucose	Adipose tissue

tentative evidence that insulin or the insulin-receptor complex may enter the cell.

Receptors for growth hormone and prolactin have been demonstrated on several cell types but further events are obscure and no 'second' messenger has been clearly demonstrated for these hormones. There is some evidence that prolactin may enter the mammary epithelial cell (this is the most likely source of the hormone in milk), and it has been shown to stimulate RNA synthesis in isolated nuclei from mammary epithelial cells, but the physiological significance of this observation is uncertain.

Metabolic effects of hormones

Direct effects
Hormones can influence the fate of nutrients in five main ways, by changing:
1. blood flow;
2. membrane permeability;
3. enzyme activity;
4. enzyme concentration;
5. secretion;

that is, by all the various mechanisms described in the earlier sections.

Blood flow is primarily regulated by the nervous system via neuro-humoral transmitters, but some effects are mediated by the hormone adrenalin. (The distinction between nervous and endocrine control is often very arbitrary.) Release of adrenalin leads to a reduced blood flow to the mammary gland, for example. Blood flow to the gut is increased by food intake and this may well be mediated by gut hormones as well as by the nervous system.

Examples of effects of hormones on membrane transport are shown in Table 2.10. One of the major effects of insulin is to increase the uptake of precursors for macromolecule synthesis by some tissues (e.g. adipose and muscle). However, the uptake of glucose by tissues which have an obligatory requirement for glucose (such as brain and red blood cells) is not regulated by insulin. Thus, when glucose availability is limited, blood insulin concentration falls, and the uptake of glucose by muscle and adipose tissue is reduced, whereas that by brain and red blood cells is unaffected, providing a powerful mechanism for regulating the partition of nutrients to meet the body's requirements.

Examples of effects of hormones on enzyme activity and concentration are also given in Table 2.10. As discussed elsewhere, effects on enzyme activity are mediated by changes in either the intracellular cyclic AMP concentration (e.g. glucagon), Ca^{2+} concentration, or both (e.g. probably insulin). The examples also show that a hormone can influence metabolism in more than one way. In addition, the effects of some hormones are the reverse of the effects of others (e.g. glucagon and insulin).

Hormones stimulate the release of substances from cells (e.g. glucose from liver, by glucagon; fatty acids and glycerol from adipose tissue, by adrenalin or glucagon), regulate secretions (e.g. the secretion of digestive enzymes and gastric juices is regulated by gut hormones) and control the release of other hormones.

Indirect or permissive effects of hormones

Apart from their direct effects, hormones may modify metabolism indirectly by altering the responsiveness of a tissue to other hormones. Removal of either the adrenal, thyroid or pituitary gland greatly reduces the ability of adrenalin or noradrenalin to stimulate lipolysis in adipose tissue. Cortisol, thyroxine, tri-iodothyronine and growth hormone are all required to maintain the maximum lipolytic response to catecholamines and are said to have a 'permissive' effect in this instance. Similarly, glucocorticoid hormones are required for the initiation of lactogenesis by prolactin in a variety of species, and oestradiol makes tissues (e.g. uterus) more sensitive to progesterone.

Conversely, hormones may prevent the effect of another hormone. For example, the high concentration of progesterone during pregnancy prevents the premature initiation of lactogenesis by prolactin.

These permissive effects are probably due to the numbers of hormone receptors and the amounts of intermediates such as adenylate cyclase being under hormonal control.

The number of receptors for a hormone in a tissue is not constant and varies with age (e.g. Fig. 2.36), or physiological state (e.g. Fig. 2.37). The decrease in the number of insulin receptors of adipocytes with age is probably at least partly responsible for the decrease in responsiveness of the tissue to insulin which occurs with ageing. Likewise, the increase in the number of insulin receptors during pregnancy should facilitate fat deposition which occurs at this time. There is evidence for a loss of progesterone receptors from the mammary epithelial cells during early lactation, providing a possible explanation for the inability of progesterone to inhibit established lactation.

Some hormones modulate the numbers of their own receptors. Both growth hormone and insulin reduce the numbers of their respective receptors; the fall in the number of insulin receptors of adipocytes during ageing is accompanied by increased serum insulin concentration. There are also examples of hormones affecting the number of receptors for a different hormone. Oestradiol, for example, stimulates the number of progesterone receptors in a variety of tissues (e.g. uterus, mammary gland and adipose tissue). Apart from this, interactions

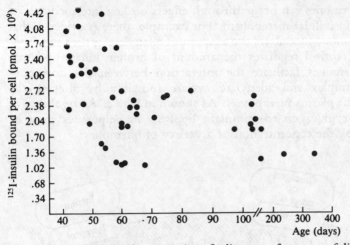

Fig. 2.36.   Insulin-binding capacity of adipocytes from rats of different ages. (From Olefsky and Reaven, 1975.)

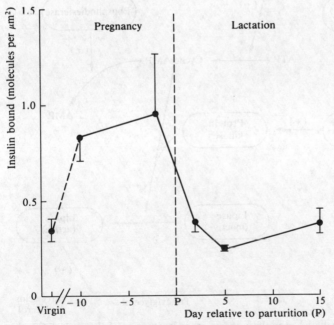

Fig. 2.37.   Number of high-affinity insulin receptors per μm^2 of cell surface of rat adipocytes during pregnancy and lactation. (From Flint, Sinnett-Smith, Clegg and Vernon, 1979.)

between hormones can occur through effects on key intermediates or key points in cellular metabolism. For example, there is evidence that growth hormone modulates the amount of adenylate cyclase in adipocytes, that cortisol regulates the amount of protein kinase and that thyroid hormones facilitate the interaction between the hormone-receptor complex and adenylate cyclase (possibly by altering the fluidity of the plasma membrane). As shown in Fig. 2.38, the ability of adrenalin or glucagon to stimulate lipolysis in adipocytes may be influenced by the concentration of a variety of hormones.

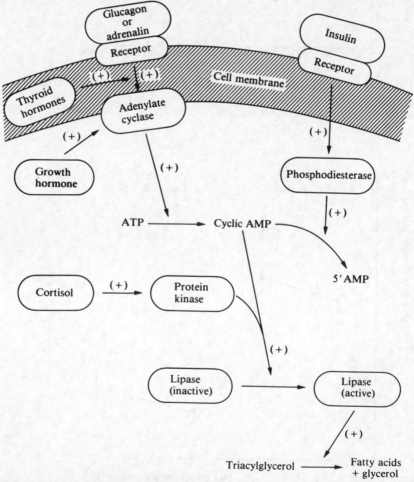

Fig. 2.38.   Postulated modulations by other hormones of the stimulation by glucagon and adrenalin of the rate of lipolysis in adipose tissue ($\xrightarrow{(+)}$, stimulation).

Hormones and the coordination of metabolism

Hormones can influence metabolism, and hence the partition of nutrients, in a variety of different ways but the various effects of different hormones are related so that there is a coordinated response within the body to a given change in physiological condition.

As an example, the rôle of insulin and glucagon in the regulation of glucose metabolism may be considered. Insulin stimulates the utilization of glucose by peripheral tissues (e.g. muscle and adipose tissue) as a source of energy and promotes the accumulation of reserves of glycogen and lipid. Glucagon, on the other hand, stimulates the mobilization of the reserves of glycogen and lipid, it increases the rate of gluconeogenesis and it promotes a switch from the use of glucose to a use of fatty acids as a source of energy. Diets rich in carbohydrate increase the concentration of insulin and decrease the concentration of glucagon in the blood, whereas fasting, or feeding low-carbohydrate diets, has the reverse effect. As shown in Fig. 2.39, changes in the amount and the composition of the diet lead to changes in the molar ratio of insulin to glucagon in the blood, and hence in the rates of glucose utilization and production. Ruminants, which as a result of rumen fermentation have in effect a low-carbohydrate diet, have molar insulin:

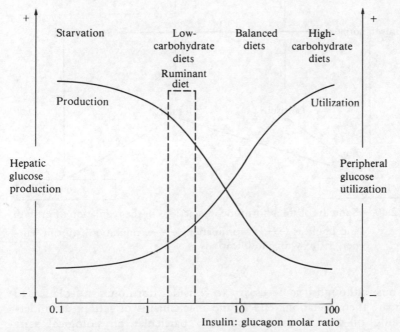

Fig. 2.39. Relationship between glucose metabolism and the plasma insulin: glucagon molar ratio.

glucagon ratios of approximately 2. Ruminants have a relatively high rate of glucose production by the liver and a low rate of glucose utilization by peripheral tissues. However, although the regulation of glucose metabolism can be explained in terms of the insulin:glucagon ratio of blood, fasting and various dietary regimes will alter the blood concentrations of other hormones, which will also influence glucose metabolism (e.g. glucocorticoids).

Similarly, in ruminants during pregnancy and lactation, the energy balance of the animal is reflected by the insulin:growth hormone ratio (the ratio decreases if the animal is in negative energy balance). As growth hormone antagonizes the effects of insulin on adipose tissue, such a change in the ratio of these two hormones should facilitate the mobilization of lipid reserves. In contrast, insulin and growth hormone are both thought to be required for growth in the immature animal. A scheme of probable hormone interrelationships modifying growth and lipolysis is shown in Fig. 2.40; this scheme, which certainly is a simplification of the actual interrelationship *in vivo*, emphasizes the complexity of the interactions.

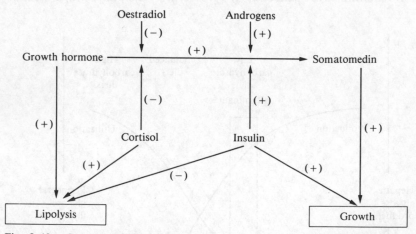

Fig. 2.40.   Some (probable) hormone interactions in the regulation of growth and lipolysis ($\xrightarrow{(+)}$, stimulation; $\xrightarrow{(-)}$, inhibition). (From Turner, 1978, with modifications.)

Thus, although it is necessary to consider hormones in isolation to elucidate their metabolic effects and mechanisms of action, an understanding of what is happening in a particular physiological state requires knowledge of the effects of all the hormones involved and their various interactions.

The nervous system

The autonomic nervous system provides an important means of regulating metabolism. Sensory nerves monitor the concentration of metabolites in extracellular fluid either centrally or at selected sites in the body (e.g. the hepatic portal blood in ruminants). The CNS integrates this information together with that from other sources (e.g. the external environment, other body-regulation systems – thermoregulatory, water balance, etc.) and 'decides' the overall metabolic strategy (e.g. reproduction) as well as providing minute-to-minute control of many metabolic processes. Information from the CNS (i.e. motor pathways) can be directed to influence metabolism by three major routes.

1. Nervous impulses can stimulate or inhibit specific neurosecretory neurons to alter the secretion of hypothalamic hormone-releasing factors, which in turn control the synthesis and release of hormones from the anterior pituitary. Some neurosecretory products may themselves act as hormones in the general circulation, for example, oxytocin and vasopressin from the posterior pituitary, and adrenalin from the adrenal medulla.
2. Vasomotor nerves can alter blood flow through a tissue or organ and thereby influence metabolism.
3. Neurotransmitters may influence the cells of a tissue or organ directly. While control by such means is well established for some organs, little work has been done on organs of central importance in metabolic regulation, although many such organs (e.g. liver and pancreas) are innervated and it is possible that under normal physiological conditions metabolism and hormone release are directly controlled by autonomic nerves.

Neural influences may, of course, also affect metabolism indirectly. Changes in gut motility affect absorption of nutrients, for example.

The motor nerves of the autonomic nervous system can be divided into three categories. The first is the parasympathetic system in which the transmitter released at the final site of action is acetylcholine (these final (post-ganglionic) neurons are referred to as being cholinergic, and acetylcholine is referred to as a cholinergic agent). The second is the sympathetic system in which the transmitter is usually noradrenalin (an adrenergic agent). The third is the recently-discovered peptidergic system in which peptides act as the transmitter; it may be of particular importance in the control of the alimentary canal and associated organs.

Pharmacological studies have shown that the adrenergic system can be classified according to the type of receptor (α or β) present on the target tissues (e.g. the smooth muscles of blood vessels and of the alimentary canal). The major circulating adrenergic agent adrenalin and the major local transmitter noradrenalin have different potencies at different sites depending on the type of receptor present. Some tissues appear to have only α-receptors (e.g. cerebral and skin blood vessels), some have only β-receptors (e.g. heart), while others have both α and β (e.g. blood vessels of the intestinal viscera and intestinal smooth muscle). Activation of one type of receptor usually has a different effect from activation of the other. Thus, in the blood vessels of the abdominal viscera, stimulation of the α-receptors leads to contraction of the smooth muscle and hence to vasoconstriction, whereas stimulation of the β-receptors leads to relaxation and vasodilation. This classification cannot be applied with any degree of certainty to the metabolic effects of adrenergic agents.

In general, the parasympathetic system provides local nervous control to discrete organs or tissues. By contrast, the sympathetic system not only varies its output from minute to minute to control function in response to changes in the external and internal environments but, acting as a whole, it can discharge massively as part of the animal's 'fight or flight' response to an external stimulus. In fright (and rage) all sympathetically-innervated structures are stimulated simultaneously and adrenalin is released into the circulation from the adrenal medulla. The overall effects are well-known: heart rate increases; blood flow is directed from the skin and abdominal viscera to the skeletal muscles; the spleen (in many species) contracts and more red blood cells enter the circulation; and the bronchioles dilate and the blood glucose concentration rises.

FURTHER READING

Atkinson, D. E., 1977. *Cellular Energy Metabolism and its Regulation*. Academic Press, New York.

Davson, H., 1970. *A Textbook of General Physiology*, 4th edn., Vol. 1, Ch. VIII, IX and XII Churchill, London.

Davson, H., 1970. *A Textbook of General Physiology*, 4th edn., Vol. 1, Chs VIII, IX and XII. Churchill, London.

Hochochka, P. W. and Somero, G. N., 1973. *Strategies of Biochemical Adaptation*. W. B. Saunders, Philadelphia.

Lehninger, A. L., 1975. *Biochemistry: the Molecular Basis of Cell Structure and Function*. 2nd edn. Worth, New York.

Newsholme, E. A. and Start, C. 1973. *Regulation in Metabolism*. Wiley, Chichester.

REFERENCES

Alkinson, D.E., 1977. *Cellular Energy Metabolism and its Regulation*. Academic Press, New York.

Bloom, S. R. and Polak, J. M., 1978. Gut hormone overview. In *Gut Hormones* (ed. S. R. Bloom), pp. 3–17. Churchill Livingstone, Edinburgh.

Denton, R. M., Randle, P. J., Bridges, B. J., Cooper, R. H., Keibey, A. L., Pask, H. T., Stevenson, D. L., Stansbie, D. and Whitehouse, S., 1975. Regulation of mammalian pyruvate dehydrogenase *Mol. & Cell. Biochem.* **9**: 27–53.

Flint, D. J., Sinnett-Smith, P. A., Clegg, R. A. and Vernon, R. G., 1979. Role of insulin receptors in the changing metabolism of adipose tissue during pregnancy and lactation in the rat, *Biochem. J.* **182**: 421–7.

Krstić, R. V., 1979. *Ultrastructure of the Mammalian Cell: an Atlas*. Springer-Verlag, Berlin.

Kuhn, N. J., Carrick, D. T. and Wilde, C. J., 1980. Lactose synthesis: the possibilities of regulation, *J. Dairy Sci.* **63**: 328–36.

Lehninger, A. L., 1975. *Biochemistry: the Molecular Basis of Cell Structure and Function*. 2nd edn. Worth, New York.

Linzell, J. L., 1971. Techniques for measuring nutrient uptake by the mammary gland. In *Lactation* (ed. I. R. Falconer), pp. 261–79. Butterworth, London.

Mayer, R. J., 1978. Hormonal factors in lipogenesis in mammary gland. In *Vitamins and Hormones: Advances in Research and Applications* (ed. R. S. Harris), Vol. 36, pp. 143–63. Academic Press, New York.

Numa, S., 1974. Regulation of lipogenesis in animal tissues. In *Current Topics in Enzyme Regulation* (ed. B. L. Horecker), Vol. 8, pp. 197–246.

Olefsky, J. M. and Reaven, G. M., 1975. Effects of age and obesity on insulin binding to isolated adipocytes, *Endocrinology* **96**: 1486–98.

Scrutton, M. C. and Utter, M. F., 1968. The regulation of glycolysis and gluconeogenesis in animal tissues, *A. Rev. Biochem.* **37**: 249–302.

Singer, S. J. and Nicholson, G. L., 1972. The fluid mosaic model of the structure of cell membranes, *Science, Wash., D.C.* **175**: 720–31.

Turner, M. R., 1978. Effect of diet and age on hormone function, *Proc. Nutr. Soc.* **37**: 295–9.

3 THE REGULATION OF NUTRIENT SUPPLY WITHIN THE BODY

R. G. Vernon and M. Peaker

All higher animals ingest food in discrete meals and associated with this there are short-term variations in the rate of entry of nutrients into the body. Additionally, the composition of the mixture of nutrients absorbed from the gut varies with the diet, and does not coincide exactly with the body's requirements for the maintenance of essential functions and activities, or for the productive processes such as growth, reproduction and lactation. Consequently the body has to adjust continuously to variations in the amount and composition of the nutrient supply, and it does this in several ways.

When nutrient supply is in excess of the immediate requirements, some nutrients may be stored within the body for mobilization and use at a later time. Considerable stores of energy-providing nutrients in the form of fat can be accumulated. Some glucose is stored as glycogen and a short-fall in amino acid supply can be met by proteolysis, primarily in liver and skeletal muscle. Certain tissues, for example liver and muscle, can oxidize a wide variety of substrates and their oxidative metabolism readily adjusts to accommodate variations in nutrient availability. Other tissues are more exacting in their needs: for example, red blood cells and, in some species, brain cells, have a specific requirement for glucose for oxidation. Nutrient supply to an individual tissue is controlled by the blood supply, by factors that affect nutrient uptake and especially by the composition of the circulating blood. The last is modulated through the metabolism of individual tissues, the liver in particular, in response to the demands of the body as a whole. The precision of regulation varies with the individual nutrient and for certain substances, glucose for example, there is a considerable degree of homeostatic control, and blood glucose concentration is maintained within narrow limits. In contrast, the blood concentration of some substances, acetate for example, can fluctuate markedly, the blood concentration generally reflecting the rate of uptake from the gut.

This chapter deals with the transport of nutrients in the body and with the mechanisms that permit adjustment to short-term variations in nutrient supply. Other mechanisms that modulate metabolism in the longer term, and dictate the overall strategy of nutrient use for growth, fattening, reproduction and lactation, are considered in later chapters.

TRANSPORT OF NUTRIENTS

The main vehicle for the transport of nutrients within the body is the blood; all tissues have an arterial supply and venous drainage, and the volume of blood supply is usually closely related to the metabolic activity of the particular tissue. In addition, there is a second and more restricted means of transport which is provided by the lymphatic system.

Blood

In birds and mammals blood returning from all parts of the body is mixed during passage through the heart and lungs, and arterial blood from whatever source, with the exception of the pulmonary artery, is identical in composition. The composition of venous blood, however, varies with the site of sampling since it is affected by the activity of the organs and tissues being drained, through the removal of substances or their addition to the blood. For blood that truly represents the nutrient supply to the tissues, therefore, sampling must be from an arterial site, although for some substances the concentration in mixed venous blood from the right atrium or pulmonary artery is sufficiently close to that of arterial blood for all practical purposes.

The difference between the composition of arterial blood and that draining an organ provides a powerful experimental technique for studying nutrient uptake (or output) by an organ *in vivo*. If C_a is the concentration of a substance in arterial blood (weight per unit volume), C_v that in venous blood, and Q the rate of blood flow (volume per unit time), then, according to the Fick principle:

$Q(C_a - C_v)$ = uptake (weight per unit time) or, if negative, output.

A special case is the hepatic portal system. Blood from the intestines does not enter the general circulation directly but enters the liver via the hepatic portal vein and its capillaries. Blood from the liver (not derived entirely from the portal vein since the hepatic artery also supplies blood to the liver) then enters the general circulation via the hepatic vein. In birds there is an additional complication – the presence of a renal portal system which has connexions with the hepatic portal system.

By combining isotopic-tracer techniques with measurements of blood flow and of arterial, hepatic portal and hepatic venous concentrations, it is possible to obtain comprehensive data on the fate of absorbed nutrients in animals in different physiological states. An example of the results of applying such techniques is shown in Fig. 3.1.

Lymph

Lymph may be regarded as an overspill of interstitial fluid from a tissue. For most tissues the rate of lymph flow is very low in relation to the rate of blood flow and for quantitative purposes transport via the lymph may be ignored. Intestinal lymph, however, is of great importance since the triacylglycerols formed by the intestinal cells from absorbed lipids do not enter the hepatic portal vein to any great extent but instead enter the intestinal lymphatic vessels; these vessels eventually connect with the general blood supply in the region of the heart.

Form of nutrients in blood and lymph

In blood plasma, some nutrients occur in free solution (e.g. glucose and amino acids) while some are bound to plasma proteins (e.g. many fatty acids and calcium) and are in equilibrium with the free form. Strong binding is particularly important when the free form is toxic, for example iron is transported bound to transferrin.

Esterified fatty acids have a very low solubility in water and are transported as lipoproteins. These lipid–protein complexes are spherical particles with a core of neutral lipid (triacylglycerols and cholesteryl esters), and with phospholipids and unesterified cholesterol in association with proteins forming a monolayer on the outside. The lipoproteins vary in size and density since the ratio of lipid to protein increases as size increases. The largest, which are 80 to 500 nm in diameter and arise in the intestine and are transported in intestinal lymph, are known as chylomicrons. Various fractions of lipoproteins can be obtained from blood plasma by centrifugation and these fractions are named according

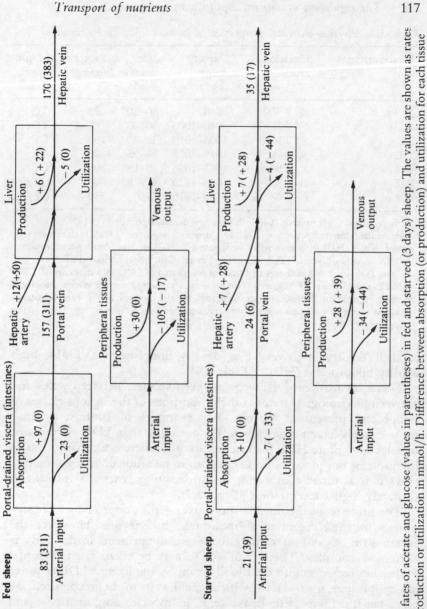

Fig. 3.1. Metabolic fates of acetate and glucose (values in parentheses) in fed and starved (3 days) sheep. The values are shown as rates of flow, production or utilization in mmol/h. Difference between absorption (or production) and utilization for each tissue is equal to net production or appearance in blood. (After Bergman, 1975.)

Table 3.1   Physico-chemical properties of human lipoprotein classes

Ultracentrifugal class[†]	Flotation rate[‡]	Density range (kg/m^3)	Size range (nm)	Protein (g/kg)	Major lipid class[†]
Chylo.	$S_f^0 > 400$	940	80–500	20	TG
VLDL	S_f^0 20–400	940–1006	30–80	80	TG
IDL	S_f^0 12–20	1006–1019	25–30	150	CE
LDL	S_f^0 0–12	1019–1063	16–25	220	CE
HDL$_1$	$F_{1.20}$ 9–20	1063–1090	10–13	300	CE
HDL$_2$	$F_{1.20}$ 3.5–9	1090–1120	8.5–10	400	CE/PL
HDL$_3$	$F_{1.20}$ 0–3.5	1120–1210	7–9	550	CE/PL

[†] Abbreviations: Chylomicron (Chylo.); very low density lipoprotein (VLDL); intermediate density lipoprotein (IDL); low density lipoprotein (LDL); high density lipoprotein 1 (HDL$_1$); high density lipoprotein 2 (HDL$_2$); high density lipoprotien 3 (HDL$_3$); triacylglycerol (TG); cholesteryl ester (CE); phospholipid (PL).

[‡] S_f^0 rate is defined as Svedbergs of flotation, measured at 26°C in a medium of 1.745 molal NaCl (density 1063 kg/m³). Flotation rates corrected for the effects associated with concentration dependence are indicated by the symbol S_f^0. F rate denotes a flotation rate measured at any other density, signified by a subscript, e.g. $F_{1.20}$. (After Puppione, 1978.)

to their density, e.g. very low density lipoproteins (VLDL), high density lipoproteins (HDL) (Table 3.1).

There are marked differences between species, between sexes and between physiological states in the proportions of the various classes of lipoprotein present in plasma. For example, in contrast to man most animals have proportionately more HDL than LDL; in humans, females have more HDL than males. In cattle there is a density class of lipoproteins not present in other species so far studied; in non-lactating cows it is a minor component but in lactating cows it is present in relatively high concentration (Table 3.2).

The proteins of the outside monolayer – the apoproteins – are important for the recognition of lipoproteins by enzymes. However, the metabolism of, and interactions between, lipoproteins in the body is extremely complex. The fate of VLDL may be taken as an example. Following secretion into the bloodstream by the liver, VLDL acquires an apoprotein from HDL which enables it to be recognized by extra-hepatic lipoprotein lipase (e.g. in muscle, adipose tissue and mammary gland). This enzyme cleaves the fatty acids from the triacylglycerols leaving a remnant particle which may either be removed by the liver or may acquire more cholesteryl esters plus another, different apoprotein from HDL. This scheme with further ramifications is illustrated in Fig. 3.2.

The red blood cell contains substances of nutritional importance but the concentrations vary markedly with species, individual and develop-

Table 3.2 Serum lipoprotein concentrations (mg/100 ml)

	Flotation rate intervals (see Table 3.1)						
	S_f^0 100–400	S_f^0 20–100	S_f^0 12–20	S_f^0 0–12	$F_{1.20}$ 9–20	$F_{1.20}$ 3.5–9	$F_{1.20}$ 0–3.5
Cow							
Lactating	0	0	0	118	334	509	87
Dry†	—	—	—	—	4	217	70
Coypu	120	0	1	87	0	20	45
Hamster							
male	66	47	8	69	7	197	36
Rabbit							
female	0	16	10	66	0	26	83
Human							
Male	28	87	38	368	0	54	222
Female	6	42	19	302	0	172	264

† No analysis on the LDL. (After Puppione, 1978)

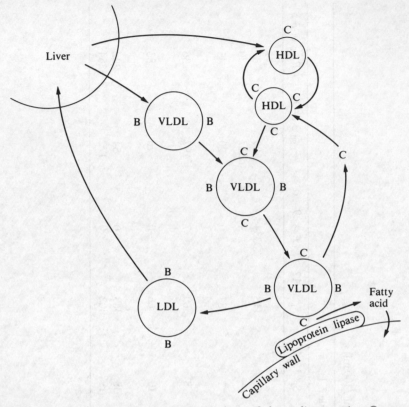

Fig. 3.2.   Simplified scheme for metabolism of plasma lipoproteins: O, central lipid core; B, apoprotein B; C, apoprotein C. For other abbreviations see Table 3.1.

mental state. Thus most adult sheep have virtually no glucose in their erythrocytes but glucose is found in some individuals and is a normal component in the red blood cells of foetal sheep. Some substances may be at similar concentrations in red blood cells and blood plasma, e.g. acetate in ruminants, but their presence in the cells is only of major metabolic importance if the permeability of the cell membrane is sufficiently high for significant transport of the substance into or out of the red blood cell to occur during the passage of blood through a capillary. Transport of amino acids in the red blood cell has usually been considered to be of negligible metabolic importance since, when measured *in vitro*, the permeability of the red blood cell membrane to amino acids is low. However, there have been suggestions that in some organs amino acids may pass directly from red blood cells to interstitial fluid during passage of the cells through the capillaries.

Blood composition

Since the concentrations of a substance in blood cells and blood plasma are not usually the same, blood composition is influenced by the ratio of the volume of cells to the volume of plasma; the concentrations of nutrients in plasma are usually more informative about metabolism than the concentrations in whole blood.

For some important nutrients homeostatic mechanisms operate to maintain concentrations in plasma constant over a wide range of dietary or metabolic inputs, although concentrations may change significantly during the daily feeding-cycle, e.g. glucose concentration is maintained relatively constant but rises after a meal in simple-stomached animals. For these substances, the concentrations of which are controlled within close limits, concentrations below a given lower limit are seen only during gross dietary insufficiency or in diseased states. The steady-state concentration (and the lower limit of concentration) may, however, differ widely between species: plasma glucose concentrations are typically 5 mmol/l in man, 3.6 mmol/l in cattle and sheep, 5.3 mmol/l in pigs and 15 mmol/l in chickens.

Physiological state is an important determinant of blood plasma composition. Stress leads to a rapid, temporary rise in the concentrations of glucose, lactate and free fatty acids. Starvation and dietary change lead to more permanent alterations, as may factors such as pregnancy, lactation, environmental temperature, stage of oestrous cycle and stage of development. Typical values for the concentrations of blood constituents of major metabolic importance in several species are given in Table 3.3.

METABOLISM OF SPECIFIC ORGANS

Liver

In mammals, nutrients absorbed from the diet, with the exception of lipids which enter the circulation via the lymphatic system, must pass through the liver before they enter the general circulation. The liver thus has a key rôle in modulating the proportions of absorbed nutrients reaching the peripheral circulation; all the metabolic pathways outlined in Fig. 2.27 are important in the liver. In particular, it has the vital rôle of maintaining the blood glucose concentration within narrow limits since it can not only take up and store excess glucose as glycogen but it can also produce glucose, both from its reserves and by gluconeogenesis. The liver is the site of ketone body and urea production

Table 3.3   Concentrations (mg/l) of some blood constituents in the goat, cow and pig. (After Linzell, 1974)

	Goat	Cow	Pig
Blood			
Glucose	460	500	560
Acetate	90	90	20
Lactate	70	80	130
Plasma			
3-Hydroxybutyrate	60	50	10
Acetoacetate	3	6	6
Triacylglycerols	220	90	320
Free fatty acids	90	80	4
Phospholipids	1600	800	550
Cholesterol	370	230	170
Cholesterol esters	1000	1830	240
Free glycerol	3.4	n.d.[†]	n.d.
Methionine	3	3	8
Phenylalanine	7	7	21
Leucine	21	22	43
Threonine	10	10	27
Lysine	21	12	42
Arginine	25	13	41
Isoleucine	18	17	30
Histidine	10	10	24
Valine	28	31	49
Glutamate	19	9	62
Tyrosine	10	7	26
Asparagine	9	4	6
Proline	26	8	45
Ornithine	11	9	19
Aspartate	3	2	4
Alanine	17	16	37
Glutamine	37	26	64
Glycine	69	18	51
Citrulline	19	12	n.d.
Serine	14	9	17
Total amino acids[‡]	380	250	630

[†] n.d. = not determined.

[‡] Individual values totalled; some (e.g. tryptophan) were not determined.

and has a critical rôle in lipoprotein and chloesterol metabolism. The liver secretes a number of substances including blood proteins, bile salts and the somatomedin hormones. It also degrades blood proteins, including peptide hormones, and has an important rôle in the elimination of toxic substances from the body.

Protein metabolism

Some dietary amino acids are taken up by the liver during the absorptive period and stored as protein for later use. Apart from the synthesis of liver proteins, amino acids are used for the synthesis of secretory proteins such as albumin and low molecular weight substances such as choline and bile salts. Amino acids are also degraded in the liver, the carbon being used primarily for gluconeogenesis or for oxidation while the amino group is eliminated as urea. The various pathways are summarized in Fig. 3.3.

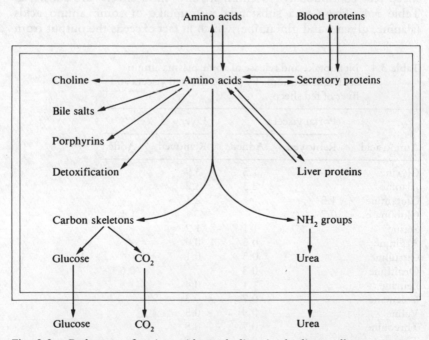

Fig. 3.3. Pathways of amino acid metabolism in the liver cell.

Amino acid uptake

For amino acid uptake by the liver both passive and sodium-dependent active transport systems have been described. These are often referred to as the L-type and the A-type systems from their preference for leucine and alanine respectively, but both systems have a broad, overlapping specificity for amino acids. The active transport systems are unidirectional and are of critical importance for uptake since it normally occurs against a concentration gradient. The passive (facilitated diffusion) systems have a high capacity for amino acid exchange and are important for transport out of the cell. The transport systems are not saturated at physiological concentrations of amino acids; hence the rate of uptake is directly related to the blood plasma concentration and will vary with the protein content of the diet and the time after a meal.

Amino acid uptake by the active transport systems is increased by insulin, glucagon, growth hormone, glucocorticoids and catecholamines. Cyclic AMP mimics the effects of glucagon and catecholamines but it is not thought to be an obligatory intermediate. During fasting the capacity of the active transport systems increases; these systems are especially important for the uptake of glucogenic amino acids.

The rates of net uptake of a number of amino acids by the liver of sheep fed 'continuously' to eliminate any 'meal effects' are shown in Table 3.4. There is a substantial net uptake of some amino acids (alanine, glycine and glutamine) which in fact exceeds the output from

Table 3.4   Net uptake and release of some plasma amino acids and ammonia by portal-drained viscera and liver of fed sheep.

Amino acid	Portal viscera Removed	Portal viscera Added	Liver Removed	Liver Added
Glycine		1.5	3.9	
Alanine		2.3	3.2	
Glutamine	1.5		2.1	
Glutamate	0.2			1.1
Serine		1.1	1.2	
Arginine		0.3	0.9	
Citrulline		0.5	0.1	
Ornithine		0.3		0.6
Leucine		1.1	0.4	
Isoleucine		0.7	0.3	
Valine		0.9	0.5	
Threonine		0.7	0.8	
Tyrosine		0.6	0.9	
Phenylalanine		0.8	1.1	
Ammonia		29.0	30.3	

Values in mmol/h. All rates, except citrulline and valine removal by liver, were significantly different from zero. Mean body weight of sheep was 50 kg and all were fed 800 g of alfalfa pellets per day at 1-h intervals. Mean portal and hepatic plasma flows were 1.3 and 1.6 l/min. (From Bergman and Heitmann, 1978.)

the gut; this reflects the transfer of these amino acids from peripheral tissues to the liver. In contrast, there is little uptake of the branched-chain amino acids (leucine, isoleucine and valine) and a net output of glutamate and the urea-cycle intermediate, ornithine. The relative rates of net uptake of the individual amino acids do not reflect their concentration in portal blood. Other factors are involved such as the affinity of the translocases for the different amino acids, the relative rates of metabolism of the amino acids and their rates of efflux. The sheep liver differs from that of non-ruminants in its high rates of uptake of glutamine and glycine, but in other respects there appears to be little difference between species.

There is a much greater absorption of ammonia from the gut and uptake by the liver in ruminants than in non-ruminants; this is due to the metabolism of rumen microorganisms which degrade ingested protein.

Protein synthesis and degradation

Protein synthesis takes place in the cytosol and requires ribosomes (which contain ribosomal RNA (rRNA)), messenger RNA (mRNA), transfer RNA (tRNA), amino acids, ATP, GTP and various enzymes. Synthesis of all types of RNA occurs in the nucleus and some modifications occur prior to their release into the cytosol. Formation of ribosomes involves association of rRNA with approximately 70 different proteins. Ribosomes comprise a small (40S) and a large (60S) subunit (40S and 60S refer to their behaviour on density-gradient centrifugation). rRNA comprises approximately 87% of the total RNA of the cell, tRNA approximately 7% and mRNA 1%. Changes in the total RNA content of the cell are thus thought to reflect changes in rRNA concentration.

The various stages of protein synthesis in the cytosol are shown in Fig. 3.4. After release from the nucleus the mRNA binds the 40S and then the 60S subunits of the ribosome (initiation). The transit of the ribosome along the mRNA chain as the nascent polypeptide chain is extended is called 'elongation' whilst the release of the fully formed peptide chain and the ribosome from the mRNA is known as termination. Several ribosomes are usually attached to the mRNA chain giving rise to a polysome. Ribosomes on release have to dissociate into the two subunits before re-attachment to another mRNA chain. Hormones can alter the amount of rRNA and hence the total rate of protein synthesis in the tissue; they can also regulate the synthesis of specific mRNA species. Initiation and elongation are also thought to be subject to hormonal control.

In contrast to the relatively detailed knowledge of protein synthesis, understanding of mechanisms of protein degradation is crude. All proteins are degraded but at widely differing rates (Tables 3.5 and 3.6).

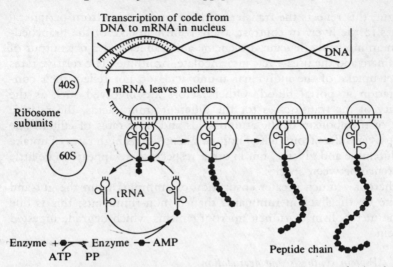

Fig. 3.4. A general outline of the mechanism of protein synthesis. Amino
acids (●) undergo activation by ATP and amino acid-activating
enzymes to form aminoacyl-tRNA. These molecules are then used
by the ribosomes to provide the appropriate amino acids for addition
into the growing polypeptide chain which is being built up according to the sequence of bases contained in the RNA. (From Manchester, 1976.)

Table 3.5   Average half-lives ($t_{1/2}$) of cytosol and
mitochondrial proteins of rat liver and
muscle

	$t_{1/2}$ (days)	
	Liver	Muscle
Cytosol proteins	0.9	10.7
Mitochondrial proteins	1.8	9.0
Myofibrils	—	22.6

(Results from Waterlow, Garlick and Millward, 1978.)

Table 3.6   Half lives ($t_{1/2}$) of some cytosol proteins of
rat liver

Protein	$t_{1/2}$ (days)
Tyrosine amino transferase	0.06
Phosphoenolpyruvate carboxykinase	0.30
Glucokinase	1.0
Aldolase	5.0
Lactate dehydrogenase	3.5–6.0

(Results from Waterlow et al., 1978.)

Table 3.7 Diurnal changes in liver protein turnover in meal-fed rats

Time (h)	Food intake	Total liver protein† (g)	Synthesis rate (% per day)	Breakdown rate (% per day)
0	↑	8.57	} 44	} 0
2				
4	↓			
6				
8		10.16	} 42	
10				
12				} 45
14				
16		10.20	} 48	
18				
20				} 120
22			} 64	
24		8.34		

† Expressed as g/kg initial body weight. (From Waterlow *et al.*, 1978.)

Both the rate of degradation of a tissue fraction and the rates of degradation of individual enzymes can change in response to novel physiological situations, and are subject to hormonal control.

All cells contain proteolytic enzymes. These are sequestered in membrane-bound vesicles (lysosomes) along with other degradative enzymes. Proteolysis is thought to occur in vesicles sometimes called autophagosomes; these may be formed by lysosomes fusing with preformed vacuoles or by lysosomes producing pseudopodia-like protrusions which engulf a portion of cellular material. Autophagosomes can be big enough to contain mitochondria. Conditions such as fasting that result in increased rates of proteolysis are associated with increased numbers of autophagosomes. Their numbers are also modulated by hormones: glucagon increases and insulin decreases their numbers in liver.

The autophagosome mechanisms can account for gross changes in the rate of proteolysis but do not appear to have the specificity necessary to account for the different rates of degradation of individual enzymes. The explanation for these effects is still lacking but one possibility is that lysosomes bind proteins with different affinities, resulting in different rates of uptake and hence degradation within the vesicle.

The protein concentration of the liver is not constant; it increases during the absorptive period and decreases during the post-absorptive phase (Table 3.7). Starvation and the feeding of diets containing inadequate amounts of protein lead to a loss of liver protein. In starvation, the liver can lose up to 40% of its protein, mostly during the first few days, after which liver protein is maintained while net proteolysis occurs in peripheral tissues.

Although the liver contains less than 6% of the total body protein, it is a major site of protein synthesis. Current estimates suggest that in the rat approximately 25% of whole-body protein synthesis occurs in the liver (Table 3.8) and this is similar to the contribution made by skeletal muscle. Lower values for liver protein synthesis have been obtained in the cow but these are underestimates since they do not include the 30 to 40% of the protein synthesized in the liver that is secreted as plasma protein.

The high rate of protein synthesis is balanced by a high rate of degradation giving the liver proteins much higher rate of turnover than, say, the muscle proteins (Table 3.5); turnover rates are especially high for certain of the liver enzymes involved in metabolic regulation (Table 3.6). In addition to the liver proteins, the liver is responsible for the degradation of plasma proteins including peptide hormones; insulin is secreted by the pancreas into the portal vein and approximately half of the insulin is removed by the liver and fails to reach the general circulation.

Table 3.8   Liver and muscle protein and rate of protein synthesis in rats and cows, as a percentage of whole-body protein and protein synthesis.

	Rat		Cow	
	Liver	Muscle	Liver	Muscle
Protein content	5	40	1.5–2.0	50–60
Protein synthesis	24	26	>6[†]	16

[†] Does not include secretory proteins. (Results from Waterlow *et al.*, 1978 (cf. Table 3.7); Lobley, Milne, Lovie, Reeds and Pennie, 1980; McNurlan, Pain and Garlick, 1980.)

The rate of synthesis of liver (i.e. non-secreted) proteins does not appear to be stimulated by amino acid influx or by insulin, and does not change following a meal (Table 3.7). The amino acid activating enzymes which catalyze the formation of amino acyl-tRNA have a high affinity for amino acids (K_m in the μmol/l range) and are probably normally saturated with substrate. However, insulin decreases and glucagon increases the rate of protein degradation and it should be noted that the variation in protein content of the liver after a meal is due more to changes in the rate of proteolysis than to changes in the rate of protein synthesis (Table 3.7).

Fasting for 2 days or feeding protein-deficient diets does, nonetheless, reduce the rate of protein synthesis in rat liver. Changes are usually small and are almost always less than half of the previous rate, reflecting the fact that the rate of total protein synthesis is the mean of many individual rates, some of which increase and some of which decrease in response to a change in physiological state. The fall in the rate of total protein synthesis on fasting for 2 days is paralleled by a fall in the RNA content of the liver suggesting that it is due to a diminished number of ribosomes.

Synthesis of secretory proteins appears to be maintained over a 2-day fast in the rat but this too is decreased during a prolonged fast or during protein deprivation. Albumin is the major component of the secretory protein and its synthesis accounts for approximately 10% of total liver protein synthesis.

Changes in the concentration and rates of synthesis and degradation in response to changing physiological states have been described for a number of hepatic enzymes in the rat and other non-ruminants. Acetyl-CoA carboxylase (Table 2.3) is representative of the key enzymes of glucose utilization and fatty acid synthesis, the amount of which increases in response to feeding high-carbohydrate diets and falls in response to fasting or feeding low-carbohydrate diets. In contrast, the amounts of the key enzymes of gluconeogenesis and amino acid catabolism decrease in response to high-carbohydrate diets and increase on fasting and on feeding low-carbohydrate diets. Changes in amounts of enzyme are usually matched by changes in the rate of enzyme synthesis (in contrast to total protein synthesis) but changes in the rate of degradation can also be important (Table 2.3). Gluconeogenic enzymes and the enzymes of amino acid catabolism in general have higher rates of turnover than the key enzymes of glucose utilization whilst for the enzymes of the glycolytic pathway that are common to both glucose utilization and synthesis rates of turnover are low (Table 3.6).

Hormones, especially glucocorticoids, insulin and glucagon, have important rôles in regulating the amounts of specific liver enzymes (Table 3.9). Glucocorticoids stimulate the synthesis of gluconeogenic enzymes and enzymes of amino acid metabolism, thus ensuring that their concentrations are maintained in the post-absorptive state when there is a general loss of liver protein. Insulin stimulates the synthesis of glucokinase; this effect and those of glucocorticoids are dependent on RNA synthesis. In contrast, the effects of insulin and glucagon on tyrosine aminotransferase synthesis, and glucagon on phosphoenolpyruvate carboxykinase synthesis, are thought to be at the level of initiation.

Table 3.9   Effects of hormones on the concentration of some liver enzymes

Enzyme	Hormone		
	Glucocorticoid	Insulin	Glucagon
Tyrosine aminotransferase	↑ †	↑	↑
Phosphoenolpyruvate carboxykinase	↑	↓	↑
Glucokinase	↑ ‡	↑	↓ §

† ↑ Increased concentration; ↓ Decreased concentration.
‡ In presence of insulin and glucose.
§ Antagonizes effect of insulin.

Amino acid catabolism

The liver is the major site of amino acid catabolism within the body and is virtually the only tissue which synthesizes urea, the major excretory form of nitrogen in mammals. Other tissues which catabolize amino acids (e.g. muscle and intestinal mucosal cells) release the amino group into the blood as another amino acid, usually glutamine and alanine, or as ammonia. The toxicity of NH_3 restricts this latter mechanism, although NH_3 is released into hepatic portal blood by the intestinal mucosal cells as well as being absorbed from the gut.

The initial reaction in the catabolism of most amino acids involves transamination with 2-oxoglutarate.

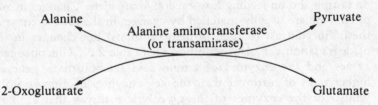

The reaction is reversible under physiological conditions and is used for the synthesis of non-essential amino acids. The liver has high levels of amino acid transferases for all the relevant amino acids except the branched-chain acids (leucine, isoleucine and valine). For these acids, transamination is thought to occur primarily in peripheral tissues, especially muscle. Some of the branched-chain keto acids produced are released into blood and taken up by the liver, which has greater amounts of branched-chain keto acid dehydrogenase (required for de-gradation of the carbon skeleton) than peripheral tissues. Thus the cata-bolism of these amino acids takes place partly in one tissue and partly in another.

The carbon skeletons of the amino acids are broken down in the liver to three major products: pyruvate, tricarboxylic acid-cycle intermedi-ates or acetyl-CoA (Fig. 3.5). Amino acids yielding acetyl-CoA are described as ketogenic and the others as glucogenic since their metabo-

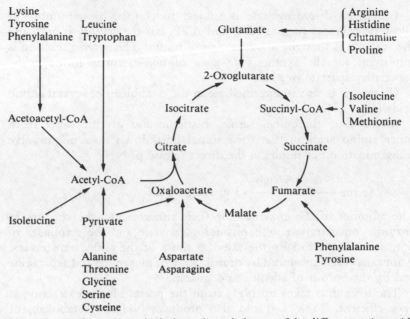

Fig. 3.5. Pathways by which the carbon skeletons of the different amino acids enter the tricarboxylic acid cycle.

lites can be used for gluconeogenesis. Acetyl–CoA is probably oxidized but may also be used for biosynthesis.

Concentrations of amino acid aminotransferases increase during the post-absorptive period and are high during starvation and in pathological conditions such as diabetes; high-protein diets also increase their concentration. The enzymes have high turnover rates (Table 3.6) and their synthesis is stimulated by glucocorticoids, glucagon and insulin (Table 3.9). The affinity for amino acids of aminotransferases is much lower than of the amino acid–activating enzymes of protein synthesis. Hence amino acid catabolism will increase as the intracellular concentration of the amino acids increases.

Amino acid transamination requires a supply of 2-oxoglutarate. This is regenerated from glutamate by the action of glutamate dehydrogenase, which catalyzes the reaction:

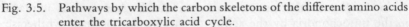

NAD (or NADP) + glutamate $\longleftrightarrow$
    2-oxoglutarate + NADH (or NADPH) + NH$_4^+$

The enzyme is located in the mitochondria whereas the aminotransferases are primarily cytosolic so translocation of glutamate and 2-oxoglutarate across the mitochondrial membrane is required (see Fig. 2.11).

Glutamate dehydrogenase is subject to control by a number of allosteric effectors such as ADP and ATP, but the activity is high and the reaction is thought to be near equilibrium. The reverse reaction is important for the synthesis *de novo* of non-essential amino acids, especially aspartate (see below).

Glutamate is also an intermediate in the catabolism of several amino acids (Fig. 3.5).

Methionine, threonine, serine, histidine and glycine differ from other amino acids in that their initial breakdown does not involve transamination but results in the direct release of NH_3:

$$\text{Serine} \xrightarrow{\text{Serine dehydrolase}} \text{Pyruvate} + NH_3.$$

The affinities of the enzymes for their amino acids, the changes in enzyme concentration with physiological state and the responses to hormones are essentially the same as those of the aminotransferases. Ammonia is also produced by deamination of glutamine and asparagine and by catabolism of adenine and guanine.

The liver thus takes up NH_3 from the portal blood (extraction is very efficient, Table 3.4) and also produces NH_3 by catabolism of amino acids and other nitrogenous compounds. Ammonia is activated in the mitochondria by the action of carbamyl phosphate synthetase:

$$2ATP + CO_2 + NH_3 + H_2O \longrightarrow \text{Carbamylphosphate} + 2ADP + P_i.$$

Carbamylphosphate is metabolized in the urea cycle with the release of urea as shown in Fig. 3.6. Carbamylphosphate supplies one amino group of urea, the second coming from aspartate (Fig. 3.6). The cycle releases fumarate which is converted to oxaloacetate and thence to aspartate by the action of aspartate ,aminotransferase (this provides a second mechanism for regenerating 2-oxoglutarate from glutamate). The urea cycle thus requires equal amounts of NH_3 and glutamate. In the non-ruminant, glutamate production normally exceeds that of NH_3 and there must be an appropriate proportioning of glutamate metabolism. By contrast, in the fed ruminant, due to the high rate of absorption from the gut, NH_3 production is greater than that of glutamate, and glutamate has to be produced by the reversal of the glutamate dehydrogenase reaction. An additional complication in both ruminants and non-ruminants is that some glutamate is released from the liver (as glutamine, it acts as carrier of amino groups from peripheral tissues). Aspartate aminotransferase, like glutamate dehydrogenase, is an active enzyme and the reaction is thought to be at equilibrium; therefore, the concentrations of aspartate, glutamate and NH_3 are linked by equilibrium reactions.

The main regulatory reaction of urea production is thought to be the synthesis of carbamylphosphate. Carbamylphosphate synthetase is

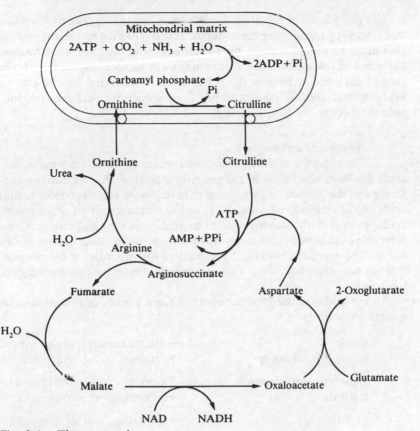

Fig. 3.6. The urea cycle.

activated by physiological concentrations of acetyl glutamate which is produced by the following reaction.

$$\text{Glutamate} + \text{acetyl-CoA} \underset{\text{Acylase}}{\overset{\text{Synthase}}{\rightleftharpoons}} \text{Acetylglutamate}$$

The synthase is activated by arginine and inhibited by propionyl-CoA; the K_i of propionyl-CoA is approximately $0.7\,\text{mmol/l}$, hence its physiological significance is uncertain.

Apart from these 'fine' controls of urea synthesis, the amounts of the enzymes of the urea cycle change in response to alterations in the protein content of the diet. The capacity of the cycle for urea production is high, however, and is unlikely to become inadequate for the removal of NH_3 under normal physiological conditions with diets containing moderate levels of natural proteins. Urea is released from the liver and excreted via the kidneys.

The net release of ornithine by the liver and the uptake of citrulline and release of arginine by the kidneys in sheep has led to the suggestion that in ruminants part of the urea cycle occurs in the kidney. However, the rates of release of these constituents are small compared with the rate of urea production in the sheep liver as indicated by the rate of NH_3 uptake, and the contribution of the kidney to total urea production is likely to be less than 10%.

Amino acid metabolism

The capacity of the liver for the synthesis of non-essential amino acids has been alluded to in the preceding section. As the aminotransferase and the glutamate dehydrogenase reactions are reversible, amino acids can be synthesized using NH_3 or the amino group of other amino acids, provided the appropriate keto acids can be synthesized. Considerable exchange of amino groups between amino acids is thought to occur. The reactions provide a mechanism for modulating the proportions of non-essential amino acids absorbed to meet the requirements of tissues.

Amino acids are used for the synthesis of a variety of low molecular weight substances:

serine   → ethanolamine⎤ phospholipid
serine + methionine   → choline   ⎦ synthesis

aspartate + glutamine + glycine → purines   ⎤ nucleic acid
asparate   → pyrimidines ⎦ synthesis

glycine   → glycocholic acid⎤ bile acid
                                                          ⎦ synthesis.

Glycine is also used in detoxification reactions. For example, ruminants absorb benzoic acid, a product of microbial metabolism in the rumen. This is detoxified by conversion to hippuric acid:

Glycine + benzoic acid ⟶ Hippuric acid.

Production of hippuric acid is possibly the reason for the relatively high rates of glycine uptake by the ruminant liver.

Carbohydrate metabolism
Glucose uptake and activation

Glucose crosses the plasma membrane of the liver cell by facilitated diffusion. Since the translocase has a low affinity for glucose, the rate of translocation is proportional to glucose concentration over the physiological range but is sufficient to ensure near equilibration of glucose across the membrane. The direction of net flux depends on the glucose concentration in portal blood. In the perfused dog liver a switch from uptake to output occurs when the portal concentration falls below 6 mmol/l. The liver glucose translocase does not appear to be under direct endocrine control.

Within the hepatocyte, glucose is activated by phosphorylation to glucose-6-phosphate. The reaction is catalysed by hexokinase which has a high affinity for glucose, but the reaction is inhibited by glucose-6-phosphate. In some mammals, which normally receive substantial amounts of glucose from the diet, there is an additional isoenzyme of hexokinase known as glucokinase. This isoenzyme has a low affinity for glucose (K_m 10 to 15 mmol/l) and in species possessing the enzyme the rate of phosphorylation is proportional to glucose concentration over the physiological range. The isoenzyme is not inhibited by glucose-6-phosphate and its synthesis is induced by insulin. Glucokinase is absent from ruminant and avian liver.

Glucose-6-phosphate can be metabolized by various pathways (Fig. 3.7).

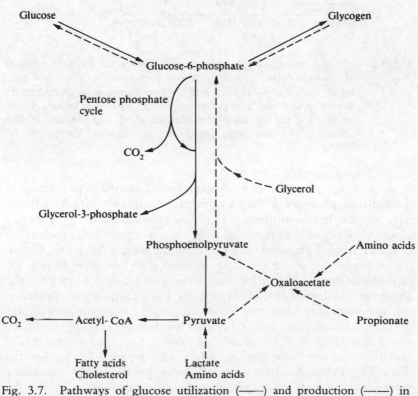

Fig. 3.7. Pathways of glucose utilization (———) and production (- - -) in liver.

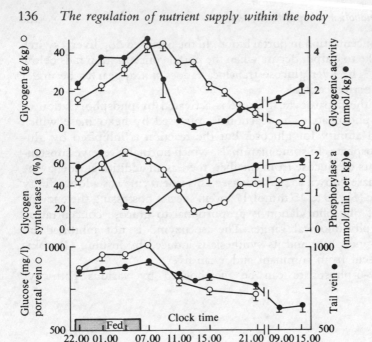

Fig. 3.8.   Periodic changes in glycogen content, glycogenic activity, activities of phosphorylase *a* and glycogen synthetase *a* (as % of total synthesis, *a* plus *b*) in liver, and the concentration of glucose in the hepatic portal vein and peripheral blood (tail vein) of rats during feeding and fasting. Rats were allowed access to food until 06.00 h on day 2 and then were fasted. (From Shikama, Yajima and Vi 1980.)

Glycogen metabolism

Glycogen is a readily accessible store of glucose-6-phosphate. In the fed state glycogen stores comprise approximately 50 g/kg of total liver weight. In non-ruminants receiving adequate amounts of dietary glucose, glycogen is deposited during the absorptive period when the concentration of glucose in the portal blood is high (Fig. 3.8). Glycogen is broken down and glucose released from the liver during the post-absorptive period when the portal glucose concentration falls. Synthesis and degradation of glycogen is thus an important mechanism for maintaining a relatively constant glucose concentration in the peripheral blood (Fig. 3.8). Glycogen breakdown also occurs during stress, providing 'fuel' for muscle. However, the glycogen reserves of the liver are not large and are effectively depleted by a 24-h fast (Fig. 3.8). Prolonged starvation or consumption of diets containing inadequate amounts of glucose require the production of glucose by gluconeogenesis (see below). The importance of liver glycogen is that it provides a buffer against sudden changes in blood glucose concentration, and at the beginning of a fast it provides a source of glucose while the gluconeogenic capacity of the liver is increased.

The pathways of glycogen synthesis and degradation (glycogenolysis) are shown in Fig. 3.9. The regulation of these processes is complex and their study has contributed greatly to the understanding of metabolic control in general.

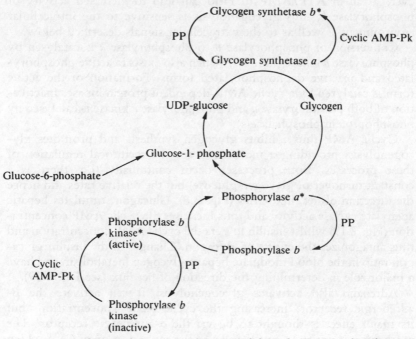

Fig. 3.9. Regulation of glycogen synthesis and degradation (PP, phosphoprotein phosphatase; cyclic AMP-Pk, cyclic AMP–dependent protein kinase;*, phosphorylated form).

Glycogen synthesis is catalysed by glycogen synthetase, an enzyme which exists in an active dephosphorylated form (synthetase *a*) and an effectively inactive phosphorylated form (synthetase *b*). Inactivation (conversion of *a* to *b*) is catalysed by a cyclic AMP–dependent protein kinase whilst activation is catalysed by phosphoprotein phosphatase. The apparent inactivity of glycogen synthetase *b* is due to its regulation by allosteric effectors, glucose-6-phosphate and the adenine nucleotides, which activate and inhibit it respectively. The concentrations of the effectors *in vivo* are such that the *b* form is effectively inactive. Conversion of *b* to *a* results in a loss of sensitivity to these allosteric effectors.

Glycogenolysis is catalysed by phosphorylase. This enzyme also exists in two forms, but in this case it is the phosphorylated form which is active (phosphorylase *a*) while the dephosphorylated form (phosphorylase *b*) is normally inactive. Again the inactivity of phosphorylase *b* arises from control by allosteric inhibitors (glucose-6-phosphate and ATP) and activators (AMP and phosphate). The concentrations of these substances *in vivo* normally render the enzyme inactive, while phosphorylation results in a loss of sensitivity to allosteric control. However, a fall in ATP/AMP to ratio can lead to increased activity of phosphorylase *b*; thus glycogenolysis is sensitive to the intracellular environment as well as to the extracellular signals described below.

Conversion of phosphorylase *b* to phosphorylase *a* is catalysed by phosphorylase *b* kinase (Fig. 3.9) which also exists in active phosphorylated and inactive dephosphorylated forms. Formation of the active form is catalyzed by a cyclic AMP-dependent protein kinase. Inactivation of both phosphorylase *a* and phosphorylase *b* kinase is catalysed by phosphoprotein phosphatase(s).

Cyclic AMP thus inhibits glycogen synthesis and promotes glycogenolysis, providing a mechanism for the reciprocal regulation of these processes. Both processes occur continually (i.e. there is a constant turnover of glycogen glucose) but the relative rates and hence the direction of net flux varies (Fig. 3.8). Glucagon stimulates hepatic adenylate cyclase activity and thus increases the cyclic AMP concentration (Fig. 2.19) whilst insulin lowers the cyclic AMP concentration and thus antagonizes the effects of glucagon. Changes in the insulin:glucagon ratio in the blood modulate hepatic glycogen metabolism and have a major rôle in determining the direction of net flux (see Fig. 2.39).

Adrenalin also activates glycogenolysis. It can activate the β-adrenergic receptor, increasing the cyclic AMP concentration, but its major effect is thought to be via the α-adrenergic receptor. The mechanism is not clear, but changes in the concentration of Ca^{2+} which activates phosphorylase kinase (see Fig. 2.31), are involved. Other hormones such as vasopressin, oxytocin and angiotensin also stimulate glycogenolysis but the physiological significance is not known. Glucose *per se* reduces the rate of glycogenolysis; the mechanism appears to involve the binding of glucose to phosphorylase *a*, thereby rendering the enzyme more susceptible to inactivation by phosphoprotein phosphatase.

Further metabolism of glucose-6-phosphate

Glucose-6-phosphate may be metabolized via the pentose phosphate cycle to produce NADPH for biosynthetic reactions and ribose for nucleic acid synthesis. NADPH production is the major function of the cycle and the flux is probably determined by the demand for NADPH. This demand will be high if the liver is synthesizing fatty acids, an activity important only in the livers of animals receiving adequate amounts of carbohydrate in the diet. Fasting or feeding of low-carbohydrate diets results in a reduction in the amounts of glucose-6-phosphate dehydrogenase and 6-phosphogluconate dehydrogenase, the key enzymes of the pathway. The major fate of glucose-6-phosphate, however, is metabolism via the glycolytic pathway (Figs. 3.7, 2.23, and 2.29). Some triose phosphate is channelled off for glycerolipid synthesis but the bulk is converted to pyruvate. Pyruvate is translocated into the mitochondria where it is converted to acetyl-CoA by pyruvate dehydrogenase. Acetyl-CoA is either oxidized to carbon dioxide in the tricarboxylic acid cycle or used for synthesis, primarily of fatty acids, and cholesterol.

The rate of glycolysis is subject to a variety of allosteric controls (Fig. 2.29): it is sensitive to the energy state of the cell and to the oxidation of other substances, especially fatty acids (the other major source of energy in the liver). Oxidation of fatty acids, by increasing the energy state (i.e. the energy charge or phosphorylation potential, see Ch. 2) of the cell and also by increasing the NADH:NAD and acetyl-CoA:CoA ratios, inhibits the rate of glycolysis and the conversion of pyruvate to acetyl-CoA. Control of the latter reaction is of crucial importance because it leads to an irreversible loss of carbon from the pool of glucose and glucogenic precursors. Acetyl-CoA can be transported to other organs as ketones or stored as fatty acids, but it cannot be converted back to glucose and ultimately it is oxidized to carbon dioxide (Fig. 3.10). The pyruvate dehydrogenase reaction is thus a metabolic Rubicon and its restriction is of great importance in glucose conservation in species such as ruminants, which obtain little glucose from the diet, and in all species during starvation.

The key glycolytic enzymes, and phosphofructokinase, pyruvate kinase and pyruvate dehydrogenase, can be inactivated by phosphorylation. For the first two, cyclic AMP-dependent protein kinases are involved and the proportion of the enzymes in the active state appears to depend on the insulin: glucagon ratio in the blood. Calcium and not cyclic AMP is thought to be the major factor influencing the proportion of pyruvate dehydrogenase that is in the active state.

In general, hepatic glycolysis occurs in animals receiving adequate amounts of dietary carbohydrate in the absorptive period and probably during the early post-absorptive period, when glucose is available from glycogen. During the late post-absorptive period, in starvation and in animals receiving low-carbohydrate diets, hepatic glycolysis is suppressed and gluconeogenesis is the dominant pathway. Ruminants fall into the latter category because, although they receive a high-carbohydrate diet, microbial fermentation in the rumen results in little glucose being absorbed, and in these species there is no net glucose utilization in the liver (Fig. 3.1).

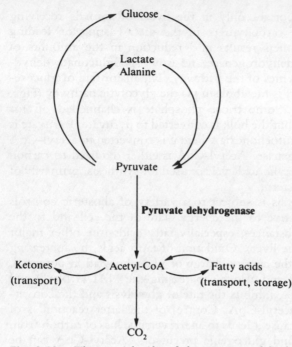

Fig. 3.10.   The crucial rôle of the pyruvate dehydrogenase reaction in the regulation of glucose utilization.

Gluconeogenesis

During fasting or in animals fed low-carbohydrate diets, gluconeogenesis is the source of glucose since glycogen reserves are soon depleted. In ruminants over 90% of glucose may be produced by gluconeogenesis, and in ruminants fed high-roughage diets the proportion is probably near to 100%. The liver synthesizes approximately 80% of the glucose, the remainder arising from the kidney; this reflects the fact that these organs alone possess the enzyme glucose-6-phosphatase, which hydrolyzes glucose-6-phosphate to glucose.

Glucose is required by the brain where it is the main fuel for ATP production; glucose is oxidized by the pentose phosphate pathway for NADPH production; during pregnancy and lactation glucose is transferred to the foetus or used for lactose production (in the lactating ruminant lactose synthesis accounts for more than 50% of the glucose produced). All of these processes involve an irreversible loss of glucose from the body and hence increase the demand for gluconeogenesis. The need for gluconeogenesis is reduced in the ruminant, however, by the utilization of acetate rather than glucose for lipid synthesis and for oxidation. Similarly, in non-ruminants, which normally receive adequate amounts of dietary glucose, fasting results in both an increase in the rate of gluconeogenesis and a reduction in the rate of glucose utilization by peripheral tissues.

Glucose can be synthesized from a number of precursors, their relative importance depending on their availability. Lactate, glycerol and some amino acids (especially alanine) are important precursors in all species. In the ruminant, large amounts of propionate are absorbed from the rumen, and it is the major precursor (Table 3.10). Propionate

Table 3.10 Fraction of glucose synthesized from various metabolites in fed mature sheep (± s.e. where available). In (a) estimation was by infusion of ^{14}C-labelled substrate and comparison of specific radioactivities of glucose and substrate. In (b) estimation was by comparison of the ratio of hepatic output of glucose (or glucose turnover as estimated by isotope dilution) to hepatic uptake of substrate. Values in parenthesis indicate the numbers of studies. (From Lindsay, 1978.)

	(a) Isotope dilution	(b) Hepatic uptake
Propionate	0.42 ± 0.056(4)	0.41(2)
Isobutyrate + valerate	–	0.05(1)
Lactate	0.19 ± 0.064(3)	0.22 ± 0.068(3)
Glycerol	0.047(1)	0.04(2)
Alanine	0.05(2)	0.07 ± 0.020(3)
Glutamine	0.05(2)	0.05(2)
Serine	0.008(1)	0.02(2)
Glycine	0.01(1)	0.05(2)
Aspartate	0.005(1)	0.01(2)
Threonine	0.006(2)	0.015(2)

is extracted from portal blood with a high efficiency and little passes into the general circulation. Amino acids and glycerol for gluconeogenesis may be derived from dietary protein and lipid respectively, and in the ruminant some lactate is formed from propionate metabolism in the rumen epithelium. In all species, during fasting there is an increase in the supply of glycerol from the mobilization of adipose tissue, and amino acids are released by proteolysis initially in the liver and then in muscle. Some glucose synthesis can be accounted for by substrate recycling (Fig. 3.10). Lactate is formed from glucose in peripheral tissues (the Cori cycle, Fig. 2.26) and there is an analogous alanine cycle (Fig. 3.19); alanine is used to transport amino groups from muscle to the liver whilst its carbon, like that of lactate, is derived from glycolysis. In the ruminant, recycling accounts for approximately 10% of glucose production whilst in the rat in the post-absorptive state it is approximately 20%.

The contribution of amino acids to gluconeogenesis in the fed ruminant is still uncertain, with estimates ranging from 10 to 30% of total glucose production. Most amino acids are classified as glucogenic since their carbon can theoretically be used for gluconeogenesis (Fig. 3.5) but few appear to make a significant contribution in the fed ruminant. Alanine and glutamine (which is also released from muscle and other tissues, Fig. 3.17) are the most important amino acids in this respect. However, during food deprivation when propionate is not available, amino acids must be the major precursors for net glucose production.

The main pathway of gluconeogenesis is essentially the reverse of glycolysis (Fig. 3.7 and Fig. 2.23) with independent enzymes to overcome certain effectively irreversible steps; these enzymes are referred to as the key gluconeogenic enzymes. The various precursors feed into the pathway at different points. Glycerol is converted to glycerol-3-phosphate by glycerol kinase, an enzyme found mainly in liver, and also in the kidney and intestinal mucosal cells. Lactate and some amino acids (Fig. 3.5) are first converted to pyruvate, which is translocated into the mitochondria where it is converted to oxaloacetate by pyruvate carboxylase. Oxaloacetate is also produced from propionate and glucogenic amino acids, which are degraded to tricarboxylic acid cycle intermediates (Fig. 3.5). Oxaloacetate cannot cross the mitochondrial membrane and is therefore converted to malate or aspartate, which can be translocated. In the cytosol oxaloacetate is regenerated from these precursors and converted to phosphoenolpyruvate by phosphoenolpyruvate carboxykinase, and thence to glucose-6-phosphate (Fig. 3.7 and Fig. 2.23). As discussed in Ch. 2 (Fig. 2.15) there is evidence that glucose-6-phosphate is first incorporated into glycogen before release as glucose.

A switch from a high-carbohydrate to a low-carbohydrate diet, or to fasting, results in an increased capacity for gluconeogenesis in non-ruminants; this is associated with increased amounts of the key gluconeogenic enzymes. Fasting does not change the capacity for gluconeogenesis in ruminant liver since virtually all glucose is produced by gluconeogenesis under normal feeding conditions. Glucose output in fact falls on fasting in the ruminant, owing to the reduced availability of propionate, which indicates the importance of substrate supply. This is further emphasized by the 2 to 3 fold increase in hepatic glucose output near parturition in ruminants, which appears to be due to an increased food intake and an increased rate of portal blood flow (and hence substrate supply), without any important change in the gluconeogenic capacity of the liver.

Glucagon, glucocorticoids and insulin modulate gluconeogenesis; the last inhibits while the others increase the rate. The effects of these hormones on the synthesis of gluconeogenic enzymes, amino acid uptake and proteolysis have been described above. In addition, glucocorticoids stimulate and insulin inhibits proteolysis in muscle, thereby modulating the supply of amino acids to the liver. The insulin:glucagon ratio also largely determines the proportion of the key glycolytic enzymes in the active state, which again will influence the rate of gluconeogenesis. Thus the three hormones regulate the rate of gluconeogenesis by a number of mechanisms. In addition, the energy for gluconeogenesis is provided by fatty acid oxidation, which will inhibit glycolysis by various allosteric mechanisms described earlier, and which, by increasing the acetyl-CoA to CoA ratio in the mitochondria, will increase the flux of pyruvate to oxaloacetate and inhibit its conversion to acetyl-CoA.

Lipid metabolism
Fatty acid uptake
The rate of fatty acid uptake by the liver is proportional to the concentration of fatty acids in the blood. In ruminants, the extraction ratio is approximately 0.15; it is higher in non-ruminants, possibly due to the relatively slower rates of blood flow. Hormones have no direct effect on the rate of fatty acid uptake and no translocase has been identified.

The liver does not secrete a lipoprotein lipase and thus does not have direct access to the fatty acids of chylomicron lipids. The liver does, however, take up and recycle the remnants of lipoproteins (Fig. 3.2), probably by pinocytosis.

Fatty acid synthesis
The liver is an important site of fatty acid synthesis in some species, and glucose is the major precursor (Table 3.11). This process is of negligible importance in ruminant liver and in the livers of all species when fasting. In rats it appears that glycogen glucose rather than blood glucose is used.

Table 3.11 Major sites of fatty acid synthesis and its major precursors in different species

Species	Sites of synthesis	Precursor
Rat	Liver, adipose tissue	Glucose
Rabbit	Liver, adipose tissue	Glucose, acetate
Guinea-pig	Adipose tissue	Acetate
Pig	Adipose tissue	Glucose
Ruminant	Adipose tissue	Acetate
Man, birds	Liver	Glucose

The synthesis of acetyl–CoA from glucose has been described above whilst its translocation into the cytosol as citrate and regeneration by the ATP–citrate lyase reaction are shown in Fig. 2.12. Acetyl–CoA is converted to malonyl–CoA and thence to palmitic acid by the reactions catalyzed by acetyl–CoA carboxylase and fatty acid synthetase respectively (Fig. 3.11); the latter reaction requires a supply of NADPH. NADPH is produced mainly by the pentose phosphate pathway in the rat with some being produced by the oxidation of malate by NADP–malate dehydrogenase (malic enzyme); the latter reaction is more important in birds since they have a low pentose phosphate cycle activity.

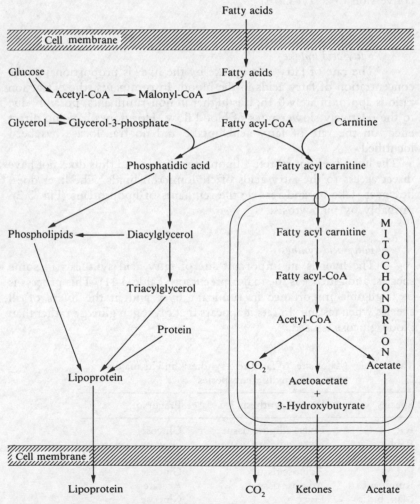

Fig. 3.11.   Pathways of fatty acid metabolism in liver cells.

Hepatic fatty acid synthesis from glucose is dependent on the rate of glycolysis and occurs only in animals receiving adequate amounts of glucose during the absorptive period. Fasting or feeding low-carbohydrate diets results in a loss of the key enzymes of fatty acid synthesis including ATP-citrate lyase (Table 2.3). Apart from these 'coarse' controls fatty acid synthesis is subject to allosteric controls since acetyl-CoA carboxylase is inhibited by long-chain fatty acyl-CoA esters, and is activated by citrate and CoA (the rôle of citrate as a physiological activator is uncertain).

Acetyl-CoA can also be synthesized from acetate:

$$\text{Acetate} + \text{CoA} + \text{ATP} \xrightarrow{\text{Acetyl-CoA synthetase}} \text{Acetyl-CoA} + \text{AMP} + \text{PPi.}$$

Acetyl-CoA synthetase is found in the liver of a number of species including ruminants. Despite this, fatty acid synthesis from acetate is negligible in ruminant liver and there is little or no net hepatic uptake of acetate, which is surprising in view of the relatively high concentrations of acetate in portal blood (Fig. 3.1).

Fatty acid metabolism

Fatty acids synthesized *de novo* or taken up from the blood are first activated by formation of their CoA esters; the reaction is essentially the same as that for synthesis of acetyl-CoA from acetate. The activating enzymes have a low affinity for fatty acids, hence the rate of activation is proportional to fatty acid concentration over the physiological range.

The fatty acyl-CoA esters may be used for lipid synthesis (esterification), or they may be taken up by the mitochondria and either oxidized to carbon dioxide or converted to ketones (Fig. 3.11). The proportions metabolized by these pathways depend on the physiological state (Table 3.12); in addition the total rate of fatty acid metabolism during fasting is increased due to the increased fatty acid concentration in the blood.

Table 3.12 Proportion of oleic acid esterified or converted to ketones and CO_2 in hepatocytes from fed and fasted rats. (From Whitelaw and Williamson, 1977.)

	Proportion of total fatty acid taken up	
Product	Fed	Fasted
Esterified	0.72	0.38
Ketones	0.17	0.57
CO_2	0.11	0.05

Esterification

The glycerol-3-phosphate required for fatty acid esterification (Fig. 3.11) may be obtained from glucose or from glycerol and other gluconeogenic precursors, depending on the physiological state. In adipose tissue, the initial enzyme of esterification, glycerol phosphate acyltransferase, is converted to an inactive form by a cyclic AMP-dependent protein kinase, but it is not yet clear if such a mechanism operates in liver also. Phosphatidic acid may be converted to phospholipids or triacylglycerols but the mechanisms regulating the proportions of these products are unclear. Phospholipids and triacylglycerols are the major products in ruminant and rat liver respectively.

Little lipid is stored in the liver except in some pathological conditions including ketosis ('fatty liver'). Most of the lipids synthesized are associated with specific proteins and are secreted as lipoproteins (Fig. 3.2).

In non-ruminants, fasting decreases the concentration of glycerol-3-phosphate, and the activities of glycerol phosphate acyltransferase and phosphatidate phosphohydrolase (which converts phosphatidic acid to diacylglycerol) (Fig. 3.11), all of which should contribute to a reduced rate of esterification.

Oxidation and ketogenesis

Entry of fatty acids into the mitochondria requires their conversion to acyl carnitine esters catalysed by carnitine acyltransferase; once in the mitochondria the fatty acyl-CoA is regenerated (see Fig. 2.13). This translocation is dependent on an adequate supply of carnitine. Carnitine concentration increases in ruminant liver on fasting and is thought to have a key rôle in increasing ketogenesis during fasting in these species, but this is no longer thought to be an important mechanism in the rat. In the latter it has been shown that malonyl-CoA, an intermediate of fatty acid biosynthesis (Fig. 3.11), inhibits carnitine acyltransferase, providing a mechanism for limiting fatty acid oxidation and ketogenesis when the rate of fatty acid synthesis is high. Glucagon and fasting both reduce the malonyl-CoA concentration. The role of malonyl-CoA has not been investigated in ruminant liver but it seems unlikely to be important in view of the low rate of fatty acid synthesis. There is some evidence that glucagon may stimulate the uptake of acylcarnitine by mitochondria, and during fasting carnitine acyltransferase activity increases. Thus there are a number of mechanisms by which the flux of fatty acids into mitochondria and to esterification can be modulated, and their relative contribution probably varies between species.

Within the mitochondria fatty acyl-CoA are oxidized to acetyl-CoA by β-oxidation. This also yields NADH and $FADH_2$, which are used by the electron transport chain for oxidative phosphorylation. The effects of increased acetyl-CoA and NADH concentration on glucose metabolism have already been discussed. Acetyl-CoA is oxidized to carbon dioxide by the tricarboxylic acid cycle, but if its rate of production exceeds the rate of oxidation excess acetyl-CoA is converted to the ketones, acetoacetate and 3-hydroxybutyrate. In ruminants some acetyl-CoA is hydrolysed to acetate or stored as acetylcarnitine, but the capacity for the latter is very limited. The increased rates of ketogenesis during fasting are promoted both by the redirection of a greater proportion of fatty acids into the mitochondria, coupled with an increased rate of fatty acid uptake by the liver, both of which increase dramatically the rate of acetyl-CoA production. It has also been suggested that the rate of acetyl-CoA oxidation may decrease due to a loss of oxaloacetate for increased gluconeogenesis. Whether there is a decrease in acetyl-CoA oxidation is not certain and clearly a decrease is not essential in view of the massive increase in acetyl-CoA production. Increased fatty acid uptake by the mitochondria promotes ketogenesis *per se*, since it reduces the concentration of free CoA, which inhibits the first reaction of ketogenesis (Fig. 3.12). The product of this reaction, acetoacetyl-CoA, inhibits both its synthesis and its conversion to

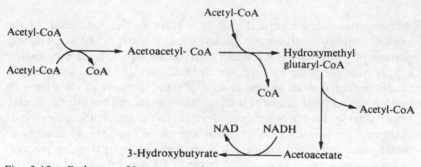

Fig. 3.12. Pathway of ketogenesis from acetyl-CoA.

hydroxymethyl glutaryl-CoA. The final product, acetoacetate, is in equilibrium with 3-hydroxybutyrate and these substances are released into the blood since the liver lacks the enzymes required to utilize them. In ruminants 3-hydroxybutyrate is also produced from butyrate by the rumen epithelium, accounting for the relatively high concentrations of ketones in the blood of fed ruminants.

Although ketogenesis can be viewed as a means of removing excess acetyl-CoA, ketones have an important rôle in the metabolism of the animal. They are oxidized by a number of tissues including muscle and the mammary gland, and in man they are utilized by the brain during fasting, thereby reducing the requirements for glucose. Ketones also act as metabolic signals since at high physiological concentrations they inhibit fatty acid release from adipose tissue and thereby limit their own rate of production. In ruminants, ketone production can become excessive, resulting in disorders such as ketosis in cattle and pregnancy toxaemia in sheep.

Cholesterol metabolism

The liver is the major site of cholesterol synthesis in most mammals; ruminants are an exception in that the intestinal mucosa and possibly adipose tissue are the major sites. The precursor is cytosolic acetyl-CoA. The rate-limiting step in the complex pathway of cholesterol synthesis involves hydroxymethyl glutaryl-CoA reductase (mitochondrial hydroxymethyl glutaryl-CoA produced during ketogenesis is not available for cholesterol synthesis). The reductase is subject to end-product inhibition by cholesterol and so the pathway is modulated by dietary cholesterol (this is very low in ruminants). Cholesterol is a key constituent of all membranes. It is also needed for lipoprotein production, the synthesis of cholesterol esters, bile acids and elsewhere in the body, steroid hormones.

Adipose tissue

Adipose tissue has a central rôle as a store in the regulation of the animal's energy metabolism. Excess 'energy' is deposited as fat during periods of plenty and is released as fatty acids when the dietary energy supply is inadequate to meet the animal's needs. Such a capacity is clearly essential if an animal is to withstand periods of starvation or periods when food intake is inadequate to meet requirements, as may occur during late pregnancy and early lactation. Futhermore, it is necessary for animals which eat discrete meals since the availability of dietary nutrients for oxidation will vary throughout the day whereas energy requirements may not. A cycle of fat deposition and mobilization may therefore occur, supplementing the cycle of glycogen build-up and breakdown in the liver. In rats fed once-daily, for example, there is a progressive change from glucose to fatty acid oxidation during the course of the day (Table 3.13).

Table 3.13   Metabolic fuel and respiratory quotient during the absorptive and post-absorptive periods in meal-fed rats. (From Leveille, 1970.)

Period	Time after the start of the daily meal (h)	Metabolic fuel	Respiratory quotient
Absorptive	0–8	Ingested glucose	>1.0
Post-absorptive	8–14	Glycogen + lipid	0.85
Post-absorptive	14–24	Lipid	0.73

Fat is a better energy store than glycogen or protein since its energy value is greater (approximately 38 MJ/kg compared with approximately 18 MJ/kg for carbohydrate and protein) and it is also hydrophobic, thus stored fat contains little free water whereas glycogen and protein are heavily hydrated. Hence the energy stored per kilogram fresh weight is approximately 33 MJ for fat compared with approximately 4 MJ for glycogen and protein. In a large animal the reserves of glycogen and of fat are usually adequate to meet the resting requirements for less than 24 h and for several months, respectively.

Adipose tissue is situated at a number of sites in the body – under the skin, and around the kidneys and other abdominal organs. The metabolic capabilities of the various depots are similar (with the exception of brown adipose tissue which has a special rôle in heat production) and it is not clear if the various depots have specific rôles. Periods of undernutrition seem to result in a greater utilization of subcutaneous than abdominal fat although there may be quantitative differences between species and breeds (see Chs. 7 and 12).

Lipid synthesis

The pathways of triacylglycerol and fatty acid synthesis in adipose tissue are the same as in liver (Fig. 3.11); these pathways and their regulation are described in greater detail in Ch. 7.

The adipocyte plasma membrane is freely permeable to fatty acids. Unlike the liver, adipose tissue secretes a lipoprotein lipase, and chylomicron and VLDL triacylglycerols are thought to be the major source of preformed fatty acids. Adipose tissue can also synthesize fatty acids, and the tissue is the major site of fatty acid synthesis in some species, including ruminants and pigs (Table 3.11). Glucose and acetate are the major precursors of acetyl-CoA for fatty acid synthesis (Table 3.11). Glucose oxidation via the pentose phosphate pathway supplies over half of the NADPH needed for fatty acid synthesis; the rest is obtained by oxidation of malate and isocitrate. The relative importance of these two substrates depends on species and diet.

Glycerol-3-phosphate is also synthesized from glucose since glycerol kinase activity is very low in adipose tissue. Thus glycerol released during lipolysis cannot be further metabolized by the tissue.

The relative contributions of lipoprotein triacylglycerols, acetate and glucose to the fatty acids used for fat synthesis depend on their availability from the diet and the endocrine status of the animal and, in particular, on the plasma insulin concentration. Glucose uptake by adipose tissue is stimulated by insulin. This effect is of greatest importance in young non-ruminant animals, which have a high capacity for glucose utilization for fatty acid synthesis. In ruminants, the rate of glucose utilization by adipose tissue is low and probably satisfied by the basal rate of glucose uptake (i.e. the rate in the absence of insulin). The conversion of glucose to acetyl–CoA (in the cytosol) is regulated by insulin, glucagon and adrenalin as described for the liver (except that adipocytes lack a glucokinase), and fatty acid oxidation again inhibits glycolysis. Acetyl–CoA carboxylase is inhibited by fatty acyl–CoA esters and activated by insulin, partly through a lowering of the concentration of the CoA esters. Insulin and adrenaline both stimulate phosphorylation of acetyl–CoA carboxylase, but at different sites on the molecule, leading to increased and decreased activity of the enzyme respectively.

The uptake of acetate by adipocytes does not appear to involve a carrier. The rate of fatty acid synthesis from acetate in ruminants is also proportional to concentration over the physiological range. The reason for the very low rate of fatty acid synthesis from glucose in ruminant adipose tissue is not fully understood. It has been attributed to the low ATP–citrate lyase activity of the tissue but recent evidence indicates that pyruvate dehydrogenase activity is low also. In addition, the rate of glycolysis is low and most pyruvate produced is released as lactate thus conserving glucose and glucogenic carbon for essential purposes (Fig. 3.10).

Insulin stimulates the synthesis of adipose tissue lipoprotein lipase, and the effect is increased by glucocorticoids and antagonized by catecholamines.

Fatty acids for triglyceride synthesis are activated by conversion to their CoA esters. The rate of fatty acid esterification is proportional to the fatty acid concentration over the physiological range. Glycerol phosphate acyl-transferase is subject to inactivation by cyclic AMP-dependent phosphorylation. This is promoted by adrenalin and antagonized by insulin. There is evidence that other enzymes of glycerolipid synthesis may be regulated in a similar manner. Triacylglycerols are the major products and they are stored in membrane-bound fat-droplets.

Lipolysis

Lipolysis is regulated by hormone-sensitive lipase. The products are glycerol, virtually all of which is released into the blood, and fatty acids, some of which are released and some of which are re-esterified (see Fig. 2.25). Release of fatty acids is dependent on the availability of their carrier, albumin, in the blood and is reduced at plasma fatty acid concentrations above 1 mmol/l due to the progessive filling of the carrier binding sites. This leads to an accumulation of fatty acids in the adipocyte and an inhibition of lipolysis. High physiological concentrations of 3-hydroxybutyrate also inhibit the rate of lipolysis.

The major factors which modulate the rate of lipolysis, however, are hormones and the sympathetic nervous system acting via its major neurotransmitter, noradrenalin. Glucagon and catecholamines (acting via their β-receptors) activate adenylate cyclase and hence hormone-sensitive lipase via a cyclic AMP-dependent protein kinase (see Figs. 2.19 and 2.38). These effects are modulated by other hormones such as tri-iodothyronine, glucocorticoids and growth hormone. Insulin is the principal antilipolytic hormone; its mechanism of action is not fully understood but it operates in part through antagonism of the rise in cyclic AMP, caused by other hormones through activation of phospho-diesterse (Fig. 2.38). There is marked variation between species in response to lipolytic hormones; glucagon appears to be weakly lipolytic in mammals, especially in ruminants, while the catecholamines are strongly lipolytic: the reverse is true in birds.

Coordination of metabolism

Both esterification and lipolysis occur at the same time so there is a continuous turnover of lipid (Fig. 2.25), and the relative rates of the two processes determine whether there is net deposition or mobilization. The fall in the insulin to glucagon ratio during the post-absorptive period leads to a progressive increase in the rate of lipolysis, and hence fatty acid availability within the tissue. This results in a decreased rate of glycolysis, and reduced pyruvate dehydrogenase and acetyl-CoA carboxylase activities. These and other mechanisms described above result in a rapid fall in the rate of fatty acid synthesis. In addition, there is a reduction in activity of the enzymes of esterification, and more fatty acids are released into the blood. If the concentrations of fatty acids or of their metabolite, 3-hydroxybutyrates in the plasma becomes very high, they will begin to inhibit lipolysis. In addition to these mechanisms which modulate the metabolism in response to nutrient availability, in emergencies the sympathetic nervous system can activate lipolysis very rapidly, regardless of the insulin concentration, to provide fatty acid for use by other tissues, particularly muscle.

Muscle

Muscle accounts for 40 to 50% of body weight and 40 to 60% of body protein (Table 3.8). During muscle growth there is a substantial net uptake of amino acids for protein synthesis, while fasting leads to proteolysis and a net efflux of amino acids for gluconeogenesis. Muscle, however, is not a reserve of protein analogous to adipose tissue since continued proteolysis leads to a deterioration in the structure of muscle and in its capacity for physical work.

Skeletal muscle also presents a problem in the overall regulation of nutrient utilization by the body; although its rate of nutrient oxidation (per gram of tissue) is relatively low during periods of rest, the rate increases dramatically during periods of rapid movement. In man, for example, during heavy work total oxygen consumption increases approximately eight-fold, mostly due to increased oxidation in skeletal muscle (Table 3.14). Muscle metabolism can therefore impose a considerable drain on the nutrient supply; the ability to meet this demand can be vital, particularly in the wild where it can mean the difference between survival and death!

Table 3.14 Relative amounts of oxygen consumed by the whole body, skeletal muscle and cardiac muscle in man at rest and during heavy work. (From Lehninger, 1975.)

	At rest	Heavy work
Skeletal muscle	0.30	6.95
Cardiac muscle	0.11	0.40
Rest of body	0.59	0.65
Total	1.00	8.00

There are several types of muscle:
1. skeletal muscle comprises the majority: it is responsible for external physical work and its metabolic rate varies with workload;
2. cardiac muscle is continuously active and its metabolic rate increases during physical work; and
3. smooth muscle (e.g. in the wall of the gastrointestinal tract) is mainly responsible for peristaltic movements within the body.

Skeletal muscle is further classified into 'white' and 'red' muscle. White muscle has a poor blood supply and relatively few mitochondria. During physical exertion it depends on glycogenolysis and anaerobic glycolysis for ATP production; it can therefore function at maximum capacity for only short periods (pheasant wing muscles and the leg muscle of the cheetah are examples of this type). Red muscle (and cardiac muscle), on the other hand, has a rich blood supply and many mitochondria; it is capable of aerobic oxidation and can oxidize acetate, fatty acids and ketones as well as carbohydrates; it is capable of sustained activity (e.g. in long–distance running).

Energy metabolism
Muscle cells have small reserves of ATP in the form of phosphocreatine which are used during the initiation of muscular con-

traction. These are rapidly exhausted, however, necessitating the production of ATP by oxidative phosphorylation or glycolysis.

The pathways for the conversion of glucose and fatty acids to acetyl-CoA have been described above for the liver. Red muscle and cardiac muscle also have the enzymes required for the conversion of ketone bodies to acetyl-CoA (Fig. 3.13) and an acetyl-CoA synthetase for conversion of acetate to acetyl-CoA. In addition, muscle secretes a

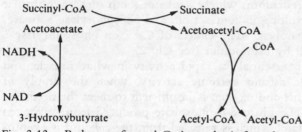
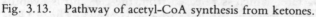

Fig. 3.13.   Pathway of acetyl-CoA synthesis from ketones.

lipoprotein lipase and hence has access to chylomicron and VLDL triacylglycerol fatty acids. Acetyl-CoA is oxidized to carbon dioxide via the tricarboxylic-acid cycle.

The choice of substrate for oxidation depends on availability: the rate of uptake and metabolism of acetate, fatty acids and ketones is dependent on their plasma concentration, while glucose uptake is insulin-dependent; ketones, if available, are thought to be the preferred substrate. Oxidation of acetate, ketones or fatty acids inhibits glycolysis, the inhibition arising from changes in the concentrations of allosteric effectors of glycolysis, especially citrate, acetyl-CoA and glucose-6-phosphate (see Fig. 2.29). These mechanisms are important, for they ensure that glucose oxidation in muscle is minimized, thus conserving the body's supply. As activity of red muscle increases its nutrient requirements for oxidation are met by increased rates of lipolysis in adipose tissue and by glycogenolysis in the liver. These processes are stimulated by the sympathetic nervous system via noradrenlin and adrenalin respectively. In addition, adrenalin increases cardiac output and blood flow to muscle. Thus the muscle receives a coordinated increase in nutrient flux.

Some glucose is stored in muscle as glycogen; the concentration is less than in liver and is higher in white than in red muscle. Glycogen synthesis is stimulated by insulin and inhibited by adrenalin. The enzymes of glycogen metabolism and their properties are essentially the same as in liver (Fig. 3.9) and, as in liver, adrenalin exerts its effect via β-adrenergic receptors and cyclic AMP. Insulin stimulates the conversion of glycogen synthetase *b* to synthetase *a* but the mechanism is not clear; insulin does not alter the cyclic AMP concentration or antagonize the effects of adrenalin. Glycogen phosphorylase activity is very high in muscle, especially white muscle, and the conversion of phosphorylase *b* to *a* during glycogenolysis is stimulated by adrenalin (though not by glucagon as in liver). Cyclic AMP acts as the intracellular signal for this effect, which is not antagonized by insulin.

Glycogenolysis is also stimulated by Ca^{2+}. Muscular contraction is initiated by the cholinergic system. This causes a release of Ca^{2+} from the sarcoplasmic reticulum which activates both the myofibrillar ATPase system, resulting in contraction, and phosphorylase *b* kinase, stimulating glycogenolysis. The effects of Ca^{2+} on phosphorylase *b* kinase are mediated by calmodulin (see Ch. 2).

Glycogenolysis is essential for rapid activity in white muscle, and also in red muscle during extreme activity, when the supply of blood-borne nutrients and oxygen is insufficient to meet the needs for ATP production. The glucose-6-phosphate produced from glycogen is converted to lactate, which is released from the cell and is eventually reconverted to glucose in the liver (the Cori cycle). The ATP is produced anaerobically, while there is no net loss of carbon from the 'glucose plus glucogenic precursor' pool. Glycogenolysis can support rapid activity for short periods, however, hence the short flight-time of the pheasant and the sprint of the cheetah.

The potential threat to the plasma nutrient pool by the massive oxidative capacity of muscle is thus averted by the use of endogenous glycogen reserves during short periods of intense muscular activity, and by concomitant lipolysis in adipose tissue and hepatic glycogen-olysis during long-term exercise.

Protein metabolism

The basic pathways of amino acid and protein metabolism in muscle are summarized in Fig. 3.14. Some aspects, especially protein synthesis and degradation, are considered in Ch. 7, and are described only briefly here.

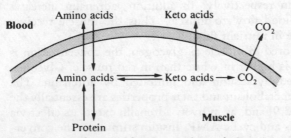

Fig. 3.14.   Pathways of amino acid metabolism in muscle.

Amino acid uptake

Amino acid uptake by muscle occurs by active (A-type) and passive (L-type) facilitated diffusion as described for the liver. The properties and probable roles of the A and L systems of muscle and liver appear similar and are not considered further.

A number of hormones stimulate amino acid uptake by muscle (Table 3.15). All, with the exception of tri-iodothyronine, which is thought to stimulate the L-type translocase, stimulate the A-type translocase, as in liver. The effects of growth hormone are seen only in young animals; they are thought to represent a direct action of the hormone, i.e. they are not mediated by somatomedins.

Table 3.15 Effects of hormones on amino acid uptake, protein synthesis and degradation in skeletal muscle. (Data mostly from Goldberg, Tischler, De Martino and Griffin (1980), with additional data for amino acid uptake from Guidotti, Borghetti and Gazzola (1978))

Hormone	Amino acid uptake	Protein synthesis	Protein degradation	Net effect
Insulin	↑ †	↑	↓	Anabolic
Growth Hormone	↑	↑	No effect	Anabolic
Tri-iodothyronine				
(Euthyroid levels)	↑	↑	↑	Anabolic
(Hyperthyroid levels)	?	↑	↑ ↑	Catabolic
Glucagon	?	↓	?	Catabolic
Glucocorticoids	↓	↓	↑	Catabolic
Catecholamines	↓	No effect	↑	Catabolic

† ↑, stimulation; ↓, depression.

Protein synthesis and degradation

Muscle makes a substantial contribution to total protein synthesis (Table 3.8) primarily because of its large mass of protein. Mean turnover rates of muscle proteins are markedly lower than those of liver (Tables 3.5 and 3.8). In the fed animals changes in the rate of net protein deposition in response to feeding are thought to be due to changes in the rate of protein synthesis rather than to proteolysis as in the liver. As shown in Fig. 3.15, fasting reduces the rate of synthesis but there is little net loss of protein for about 2 days, after which proteolysis increases with a concomitant loss of protein.

The rates of protein synthesis and degradation are regulated by hormones (Table 3.15); hormones which stimulate amino acid uptake also stimulate protein synthesis. Net protein synthesis is also promoted by physical work and by the amino acid leucine, although the physiological significance of the latter effect is uncertain. Glucocorticoids inhibit amino acids uptake and increase the rate of proteolysis, and thus

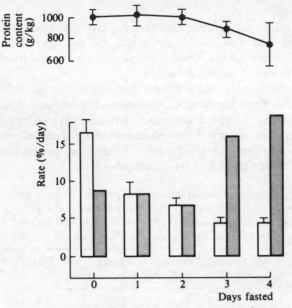

Fig. 3.15.   Changes in the protein content and rates of protein synthesis (□) and degradation (▨) in skeletal muscle of young rats during a 4-day fast (bars indicate s.e.). (From Waterlow *et al.*, 1978, p. 633.)

the availability of amino acids for gluconeogenesis. The effects of tri-iodothyronine are complex and depend on the initial concentration of the hormone in the plasma (Table 3.15). In man the rate of proteolysis in muscle decreases during prolonged starvation and this is thought to be due to a reduction in plasma tri-iodothyronine concentration; there could also be similar hormone-linked reductions in the rate of lipolysis in adipose tissue (Fig. 2.38) and in basal metabolic rate. During starvation, hypothyroid animals survive longer and lose less weight than normal animals (Fig. 3.16), presumably because the low plasma levels of tri-iodothyronine reduce the rate of use of body reserves.

Amino acid metabolism

Apart from their utilization for protein synthesis, there is extensive metabolism of some amino acids in muscle. The tissue is a major site of glutamine and alanine synthesis and has an important rôle in the catabolism of the branched-chain amino acids (leucine, isoleucine and valine).

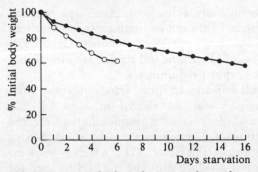

Fig. 3.16. Weight loss during prolonged starvation in normal (●) and thyroidectomized (○) rats. (After Goldberg, De Martino and Chang,
1978.)

For animals in the fed state there is a small net uptake of a number of
amino acids by muscle but there is also a net output of alanine and
glutamine (Fig. 3.17). Fasting results in a net output of most amino
acids (Fig. 3.17) but the outputs of alanine and glutamine are greater
than could be anticipated from the amino acid composition of muscle
protein; only 25 to 30% of alanine released is thought to come from

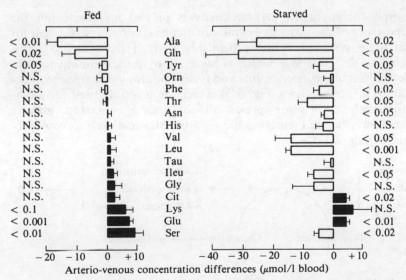

Fig. 3.17. Arterio–venous concentration differences across the hind limbs of
fed and starved sheep. Bar graphs represent the means ± s.e. of the
mean in μmol/l blood for determinations on 10 fed sheep and five
starved sheep. The figures alongside each bar graph give the
probability that the mean value differs from zero. A probability of
>0.1 is indicated by NS. (From Ballard, Filsell and Jarrett, 1976.)

proteolysis. There is proportionately a low output of aspartate and asparagine, and in non-ruminants (but not in ruminants) of branched-chain amino acids. There is also a net uptake of glutamate (Fig. 3.17). For skeletal muscle the outputs of glutamine and alanine are similar, but in cardiac muscle glutamine output predominates.

Metabolism of amino acids requires an initial transamination, catalysed by specific aminotransferases. As shown in Fig. 3.18, 2-oxoglutarate is the acceptor and glutamate the product. In the liver, the primary means of regeneration of 2-oxoglutarate is by the action of glutamate dehydrogenase with the release of NH_3, which is used for urea synthesis. Muscle does not produce urea and the NH_3 is used for glutamine synthesis while some amino groups are transferred to pyruvate by alanine transaminases (Fig. 3.18). Glutamine and alanine are therefore considered to be carriers of amino groups to the liver and kidneys.

The sources of alanine and glutamate carbon are not known with certainty. Pyruvate for alanine synthesis is probably derived from glucose and glycogen. Pyruvate may also be synthesized from other amino acids which can be metabolized to oxaloacetate (Fig. 3.5) by the sequence:

$$\text{oxaloacetate} \longrightarrow \text{phosphoenolpyruvate} \longrightarrow \text{pyruvate}.$$

Phosphoenolypyruvate carboxykinase is present in muscle but the importance of the pathway is still a matter of controversy. Carbon for glutamine synthesis is most probably derived from amino acids, including the glutamate which is taken up by muscle during fasting. Metabolism of aspartate, valine and isoleucine also yields tricarboxylic-acid cycle intermediates (Fig. 3.5) which are probably used for glutamine synthesis. In some species, although not in ruminants, glucose carbon may be used, entering the tricarboxylic-acid cycle as oxaloacetate (cf. Fig. 2.23).

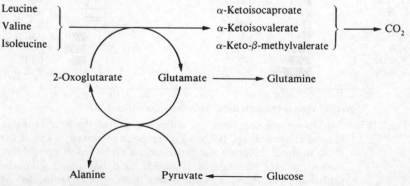

Fig. 3.18.   Metabolism of branched-chain amino acids in muscle.

Table 3.16   Net uptake and release of alanine and
glutamine (mmol/h per animal) by
tissues of fed, non-pregnant sheep.
(From Bergman and Heitmann, 1978.)

Tissue	Alanine	Glutamine
Liver	3.2	2.1
Kidney	0.7	−1.5
Portal-drained viscera	−2.3[†]	1.5

[†] Denotes release.

Alanine released from muscle is mainly taken up by the liver (Table 3.16) where it is used for gluconeogensis (see above). In fed sheep, glutamine is taken up by the liver and intestinal mucosa, whilst in non-ruminants little glutamine is taken up by the liver, and intestinal mucosa is the major site of removal. In the mucosa, glutamine is mainly oxidized with the release into the portal blood of NH_3 which is taken up by the liver; there is also some production of alanine from glutamine. There is a net output of glutamine by the kidney in fed sheep, but this changes to a net uptake during fasting when the NH_3 released from glutamine is used to maintain acid-base balance. The relationships between the organs in the metabolism of these amino acids in sheep is illustrated in Fig. 3.19.

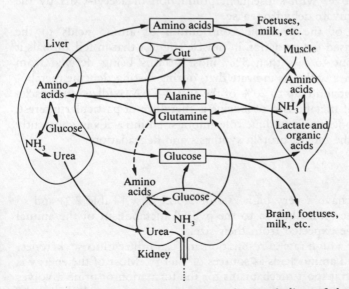

Fig. 3.19.   Inter-organ relationships in the metabolism of alanine and gluta-mine in the sheep. (From Bergman and Heitmann, 1978.)

Muscle, and other peripheral tissues, such as adipose tissue, kidney and mammary gland, are thought to be the main sites of metabolism of the branched-chain amino acids; liver has little capacity for branched-chain amino acid metabolism possibly because hepatic activities of appropriate transferases are low.

Initial transamination takes place in the cytosol (Fig. 3.18) and the amino group is removed as alanine or glutamine. The fate of the carbon skeleton is less certain. Subsequent metabolism involves decarboxylation within the mitochondria, catalyzed by a branched-chain keto acid dehydrogenase (the reaction is analogous to that of pyruvate dehydrogenase). The activity of this enzyme is low in muscle, although it increases several-fold on fasting, seemingly due to activation: some of the branched-chain keto acids are released from muscle and are taken up by liver, which has an active dehydrogenase. The eventual products of their metabolism are acetyl-CoA (leucine), succinyl-CoA (valine) and both (isoleucine) (Fig. 3.5). In muscle succinyl-CoA is probably used for glutamine synthesis while acetyl-CoA is oxidized. It should be remembered that net oxidation of succinyl-CoA to carbon dioxide by the tricarboxylic-acid cycle, like that of other tricarboxylic-acid cycle acids, requires initial conversion to acetyl-CoA. This could occur via the sequence:

Succinyl-CoA $\longrightarrow$ oxaloacetate $\longrightarrow$

phosphoenolpyruvate $\longrightarrow$ pyruvate

described above, with subsequent production of acetyl-CoA by the action of pyruvate dehydrogenase.

Estimates of the probable contribution of amino acids to the acetyl-CoA used for oxidation in muscle suggest that in fed animals it would amount to less than 5%, most of this being derived from leucine. Studies with rats indicate that, during fasting, leucine metabolism may contribute up to 20% of the acetyl-CoA oxidized in muscle. Regulation of metabolism of leucine is therefore of particular interest, especially in view of its unique rôle amongst amino acids in apparently modulating the rate of protein synthesis and degradation.

Kidney

The kidneys have a very high rate of blood flow (Table 2.1) and so make a greater contribution to the overall metabolism of the animal than might be expected from their size.

They have a high rate of respiration and can utilize glucose, ketones, fatty acids and amino acids as sources of energy. Most of the energy is required for transport mechanisms for the formation of urine involves active transport. Urine formation occurs in two stages. Initially, the blood plasma is filtered through the glomeruli of the kidney cortex. All solutes (except macromolecules such as proteins) pass into the renal tubules from which some substances such as glucose, amino acids, Na^+, Cl^- and hence water are reabsorbed into the blood, so the glomerular filtrate is concentrated 50 to 100-fold by the time it passes from the kidneys to the bladder. Uptake of Na^+ involves active transport. Reabsorption of glucose and amino acids occurs against a concentration gradient and so involves Na^+-dependent active transport. In contrast, NH_3 and H^+ are secreted from the blood into the glomerular filtrate against a concentration gradient. Other substances, such as urea, are neither secreted nor absorbed against a gradient, and their relatively high concentration in urine is due to the concentration of the glomerular filtrate. The kidney, then, has a key rôle in regulating the composition of the blood; waste products such as urea are removed from the blood while desired substances are retained. The removal of H^+ by the kidney is important in maintaining the acid–base balance of the blood.

Apart from its rôle in urine production, the kidney is also a site of gluconeogenesis and contributes approximately 20% of glucose production in fasting animals. The gluconeogenic precursors and the pathways are the same as in the liver except that in the ruminant propionate is not available as a precursor because of its prior removal by the liver.

The kidney has a rôle in amino acid metabolism (Fig. 3.19 and Table 3.16). Some of the alanine taken up is used for gluconeogenesis and some is released as serine. Some glutamine is taken up in most species and deaminated, although in the fed sheep a net output of glutamine was observed (Table 3.16).

Brain and other tissues

Other tissues of the body differ from those described above in that they do not contribute to the overall nutrient economy of the body. Their effects arise from their demands on the nutrient pool. All tissues require a source of energy, amino acids for protein synthesis and fatty acids for membrane synthesis. Some tissues have a special requirement for minor nutrients (e.g. the thyroid gland needs iodine).

The brain and the nervous system in general have an important requirement for glucose, which is effectively the sole source of energy in the fed state. Glucose uptake is continuous since reserves of glycogen in nervous tissue are trivial, and glucose is oxidized to carbon dioxide via the glycolytic pathway and the tricarboxylic-acid cycle. Glucose uptake is insulin-independent and so it can occur even when plasma insulin concentration falls to very low levels, as in starvation. The rate of ATP production by the nervous system is high (approximately 20% of total oxygen utilization occurs in the brain in man) and is primarily required to fuel ion pumps which maintain the gradients for the membrane potential. During fasting, the brain of some species (e.g. man, rat) but not others (e.g. sheep) develops the capacity to oxidize ketones; this capacity provides an important mechanism for glucose conservation. The brain also has a considerable requirement for fatty acids, particularly the essential fatty acids, for phospholipid synthesis, especially in young animals.

INTEGRATION OF METABOLISM IN THE WHOLE ANIMAL

Metabolism in normally fed animals depends on the nature of the diet and the pattern of feeding. Animals that consume their food as a single meal once daily will show marked diurnal variations in metabolism and for the latter part of the day will be effectively fasting. This necessitates the build-up of reserves of glycogen, protein and lipid during the absorptive period for use during the post-absorptive period (Fig. 3.8; Tables 3.7 and 3.13). In contrast, animals which graze or nibble continually show much less diurnal variation in their metabolism and have less need to accumulate 'short-term' reserves, although reserves are still needed in case of starvation or under-nutrition.

Metabolic coordination

Insulin and glucagon have a major rôle in the coordination of metabolism. Feeding increases the secretion of both hormones, but insulin especially, and hence there is a rise in the insulin:glucagon ratio (Fig. 3.20). The extent of the increase in plasma insulin concentration and insulin:glucagon ratio depends on the nature of the diet and is greatest in non-ruminants receiving carbohydrate-rich food (Fig. 2.39). Animals that eat discrete meals show much larger changes in the insulin:glucagon ratio than animals that nibble or graze throughout the day. This is of importance since a high insulin:glucagon ratio promotes the accumulation of tissue reserves.

   Although the insulin:glucagon ratio has a key rôle in the regulation of liver and adipose tissue metabolism, it is not important for metabolic regulation in all tissues. Muscle responds to insulin but not to glucagon, and for this tissue it is the insulin concentration in blood which is important; other tissues, such as the brain, do not respond to either hormone. A further complication is that the various component/pathways of metabolism differ in their sensitivity to a given

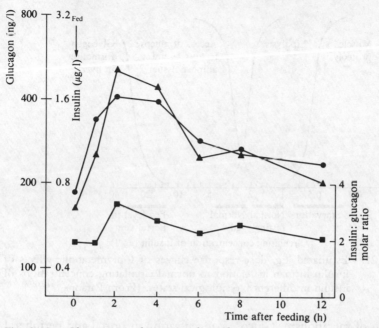

Fig. 3.20.   Changes in plasma insulin, glucagon and the insulin : glucagon molar ratio in sheep following a meal of lucerne chaff (400 g) and oat grain (400 g) (fed once daily) (▲, insulin; ●, glucagon, ■, insulin: glucagon ratio). (From Bassett, 1975.)

hormone (Fig. 3.21). The fall in the insulin concentration during the post-absorptive period permits lipolysis but still prevents proteolysis in muscle; the concentration has to be very low, as in starvation, for muscle proteolysis to occur.

Fasting results in an increase in blood glucocorticoid concentration which modifies muscle and liver metabolism, promoting gluconeogenesis, while a fall in blood tri-iodothyronine during prolonged starvation reduces the breakdown of body tissues and slows the basal metabolic rate, increasing the animal's ability to survive. Other hormones also modify metabolism to suit the demands of a particular physiological state, e.g. prolactin during lactation, and placental lactogen and progesterone during pregnancy; catecholamines have a special rôle in providing an override mechanism in times of emergency.

Metabolism in the absorptive period

Simple-stomached animals: high-carbohydrate diets

Consumption of high-carbohydrate diets leads to high insulin: glucagon ratios in the absorptive period, and insulin dominates the

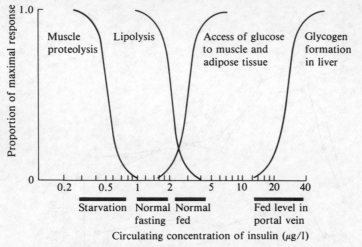

Fig. 3.21.   Estimated $\log_e$ dose–response curves of four metabolic effects of insulin in man in relation to normal circulating concentrations of insulin in different physiological states. (From Parsons, 1976.)

pattern of metabolism. Glucose concentration in portal and peripheral blood is high, and free fatty acid concentration in the blood falls rapidly, due to an inhibition of lipolysis and a high rate of re-esterification in adipose tissue.

Glucose uptake and concentration in the liver rises while the rate of free fatty acid uptake falls; there is a reduction in the concentration of cyclic AMP and an increased net synthesis of glycogen (Fig. 3.8). The rate of glycolysis and the activity of pyruvate dehydrogenase, and thus the rate of glucose oxidation, increase, and glucose becomes the major source of energy. Glucose carbon is used for fatty acid synthesis and fatty acids are diverted towards esterification rather than oxidation; the lipids so formed are released as lipoproteins. Gluconeogenesis and proteolysis are reduced, the latter change leading to a net deposition of protein (Table 3.7). Some oxidation of amino acids also occurs and there is an associated synthesis of urea. Overall there is an increase in the net synthesis of macromolecules, with glucose oxidation as the major source of energy and glucose carbon a major precursor for biosynthesis (Fig. 3.22).

Glucose uptake by the insulin–sensitive peripheral tissues such as muscle and adipose tissue is also increased. Glucose oxidation becomes the main source of energy in resting muscle while in adipose tissue glucose is used for fatty acid synthesis. Fatty acids are also obtained from VLDL triacylglycerols by adipose tissue and are deposited as fat. Amino acid uptake and protein synthesis increase in muscle.

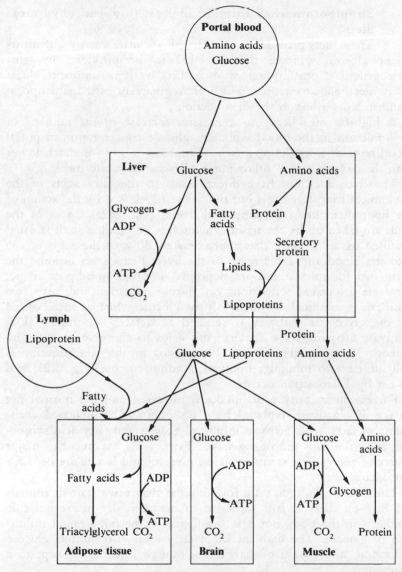

Fig. 3.22. Some major metabolic pathways of liver, muscle, adipose tissue and brain in animals given a high-carbohydrate diet.

As the animal moves into the post–absorptive state, glucose utilization is maintained for a period by hepatic glycogenolysis but the gradual fall in the insulin:glucagon ratio results in an increased release of fatty acid from adipose tissue and a switch to fatty acid utilization (see below).

Simple-stomached animals: high fat (low-carbohydrate) diets

These diets provide an animal with adequate energy but insufficient glucose; glucose therefore has to be provided by gluconeogenesis. Consumption of such diets by non-ruminants elicits many metabolic adaptations which are reminiscent of the situation in ruminants described in the next section.

A high-fat meal leads to a massive increase in the number of chylomicrons in the blood while the glucose concentration in portal blood remains low; the plasma insulin:glucagon ratio is much lower than that which occurs following a high-carbohydrate meal.

The liver does not have direct access to the fatty acids of the chylomicra triacylglycerols but the acids are released by the action of the lipoprotein lipase in peripheral tissues (Fig. 3.23). Most of the acids are taken up by the tissues themselves but studies with isolated perfused tissues suggest that approximately 30% of the acids escape into the blood and are carried to the liver. Fatty acids become the main fuel for muscle and are deposited as lipids in adipose tissue; there are associated restrictions on glucose oxidation and fatty acid synthesis is inhibited. Virtually all the glucose which is metabolized by the glycolytic pathway is released as lactate, indicating a low pyruvate dehydrogenase activity; this helps to conserve glucose and glucogenic carbon (Fig. 3.10). The plasma insulin concentration is still sufficient to minimize lipolysis in adipose tissue (Fig. 3.21) and so net lipid deposition occurs.

For the liver, fatty acid uptake is increased and the normal net uptake of glucose is replaced by a net ouput. The increased availability of fatty acids helps to inhibit glycolysis and fatty acid synthesis, and stimulate gluconeogenesis. Fatty acids become the major source of energy whilst amino acids, glycerol and lactate are used for gluconeogenesis.

The insulin:glucagon ratio found in the absorptive state in animals fed high-fat diets is still sufficient to maintain net macromolecule synthesis in the body but it is insufficient to permit general utilization of glucose. The high intake of fatty acids also inhibits glucose utilization, and so gluconeogenesis, although essential, is kept to a minimum.

Ruminant animals: high-carbohydrate (low-fat) diets

These diets are typical of those given to adult ruminants but as a consequence of rumen fermentation the animal receives energy in the form of short-chain fatty acids with little glucose. The proportions of acetate and propionate produced during rumen fermentation depend on the diet: high-forage diets tend to give a high

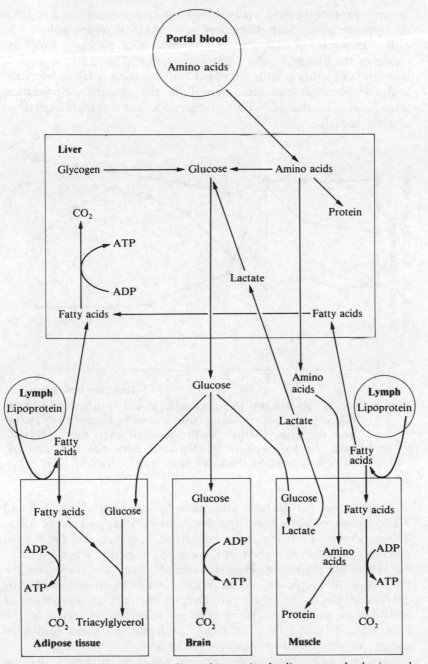

Fig. 3.23.   Some major metabolic pathways in the liver, muscle, brain and adipose tissue of animals fed a high-fat low-carbohydrate diet.

acetate : propionate ratio whereas high-concentrate diets tend to have the opposite effect. Such differences have metabolic repercussions.

In ruminants consumption of a discrete meal evokes a small increase in the plasma insulin : glucagon ration (Fig. 3.20); there is a large rise in plasma volatile fatty acid concentration, a fall in free fatty acid concentration and little change in the glucose concentration (Fig. 3.24). The changes tend to be smaller, but more prolonged, in grazing animals.

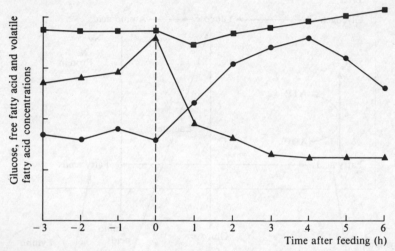

Fig 3.24.   Plasma glucose (■), free fatty acid (▲) and volatile fatty acid (●) concentration after feeding sheep a meal of lucerne chaff (400 g) and oat grain (400 g). Sheep were fed once daily. Ordinate scale: 0–0.6 g/l, glucose; 0–400 μmol/l, fatty acids; 0–2.0 mmol/l, volatile fatty acids. (Redrawn from data of Bassett, 1974).

There is no net glucose utilization by the liver (Figs. 3.1 and 3.25), gluconeogenesis being the dominant pathway of glucose metabolism. Propionate is the major precursor, however, and the rate of glucose production is highest in the absorptive period when propionate availability is greatest. High-concentrate diets, which increase the proportion of propionate in the rumen, result in an enhanced production of glucose by the liver. Despite the high concentration of acetate in the portal blood there is no net utilization of acetate by the liver (Fig. 3.1) and fatty acids are probably the main source of energy, as described in the preceding section.

Liver glycogen has a less important rôle in ruminant than in non-ruminant animals since feeding and the absorption of substrates from the gut tend to be more continuous. In meal-fed animals

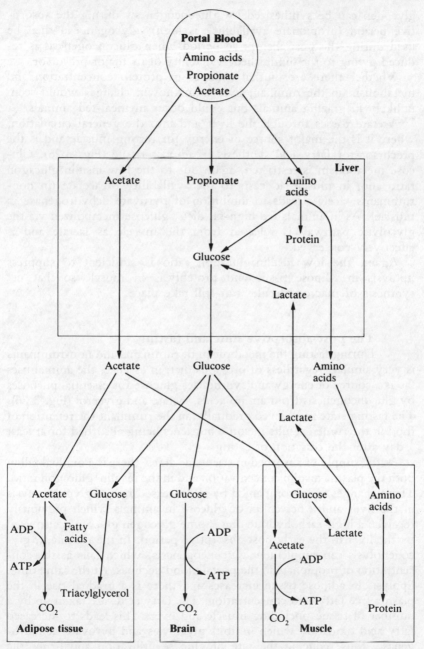

Fig. 3.25.   Some major metabolic pathways of liver, muscle, brain and adipose tissue of fed ruminants.

glycogen can be synthesized by gluconeogenesis during the absorptive period (propionate availability is high); glycogen can then be used during the post-absorptive period when gluconeogenesis is reduced owing to the diminished availability of its major precursor.

Whether there are diurnal changes in protein concentration and metabolism in the ruminant liver is unknown; changes would seem unlikely in grazing animals but could occur in meal-fed animals.

Acetate passes through the liver and into the general circulation, where it is the major source of energy for resting muscle and is the precursor for fatty acid synthesis in adipose tissue (Fig. 3.25). Glucose metabolism is restricted, again due to the low insulin:glucagon ratio and, in muscle at least, to the availability of acetate (in non-ruminants, acetate leads to inhibition of pyruvate dehydrogenase in muscle). As in animals fed high-fat diets, glucose metabolized via the glycolytic pathway is released from the muscle as lactate and is effectively conserved.

Again, the low insulin:glucagon ratio is sufficient to suppress lipolysis in adipose tissue and proteolysis in muscle so that net synthesis of macromolecules can still take place.

The post-absorptive state and fasting

During fasting the metabolism of ruminants and non-ruminants is very similar, regardless of previous diet; in essence, the animal uses fat as a source of energy and synthesizes glucose for essential purposes by gluconeogenesis from amino acids, lactate and glycerol (Fig. 3.26). The fasting state is achieved gradually; in the ruminant the retention of food in the rumen results in some nutrients being absorbed for at least 1 day after the cessation of eating.

As the supply of absorbed nutrients declines, there is a gradual fall in both the plasma insulin concentration and in the insulin:glucagon ratio. These changes are accompanied by an increased rate of glycogenolysis in the liver and a net efflux of glucose in animals which previously received a high-carbohydrate diet. Some glycogen glucose is also used by the liver in the early post-absorptive period. In the ruminant, glycogenolysis can supplement gluconeogenesis, which falls as the concentration of propionate in the portal blood declines. At the same time, lipolysis in adipose tissue increases and there is a gradual rise in the plasma free fatty acid concentration. The fatty acids are taken up by a number of tissues including muscle and liver. This leads to increased fatty acid oxidation which inhibits glycolysis and pyruvate dehydrogenase, thus reducing the rate of glucose utilization and hence the need for a high rate of gluconeogenesis. The fall in insulin and/or the insulin:glucagon ratio also contributes to a sharp decrease in the rate of glucose utilization in tissues such as the liver, muscle and adipose tissue.

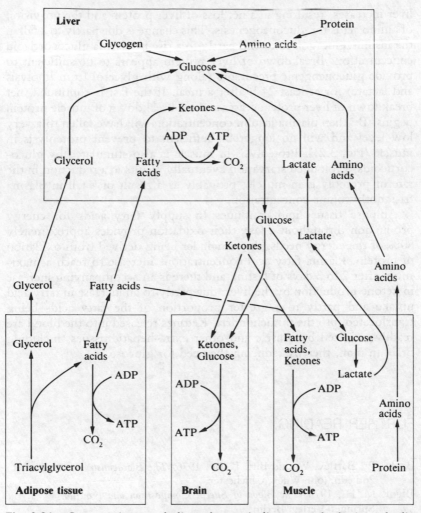

Fig. 3.26.   Some major metabolic pathways in liver, muscle, brain and adipose tissue during fasting.

In the ruminant, the plasma acetate concentration falls during the post-absorptive period, thereby diminishing the rate of acetate oxidation in muscle, which again switches to fatty acid oxidation. Fatty acid synthesis in adipose tissue also declines sharply.

Glycogen reserves in the liver last for less than 1 day, and in animals previously given a high-carbohydrate diet the capacity for gluconeogenesis increases; the key gluconeogenic enzymes and also the enzymes of amino acid catabolism have turnover times of a few hours and their concentrations can be increased very rapidly. Proteolysis in liver increases, resulting in a net loss of liver protein and the provision of amino acids for gluconeogenesis. This change is due partly to a fall in the insulin:glucagon ratio and partly to a rise in plasma glucocorticoid concentration. Breakdown of liver protein appears to be sufficient to provide gluconeogenic precursors (along with glycerol from lipolysis and lactate) for at least 24 h after a meal. If the fast is continued, net breakdown of liver protein ceases and net breakdown of muscle protein begins. By then plasma insulin concentration will have fallen to a very low level and will no longer be sufficient to prevent proteolysis in muscle (Fig. 3.21). Proteolysis in muscle is also stimulated by glucocorticoids. Prolonged starvation eventually results in a reduction in the rate of proteolysis in muscle, probably as a result of a fall in plasma tri-iodothyronine concentration.

Adipose tissue lipid continues to supply fatty acids for energy production throughout a fast; their oxidation provides approximately 80% of the energy needs, the remainder being derived from oxidation of protein. Plasma fatty acid concentrations increase to reach a maximum after 2 to 3 days of fasting and there is an accompanying increase in ketone production by the liver, due partly to an increase in fatty acid uptake and partly to a greater proportion of the fatty acids being translocated into the mitochondria. Ketones released into the blood are readily oxidized by muscle and other extra-hepatic tissues, including brain in man, thereby reducing the need for glucose.

FURTHER READING

Banks, P., Bartley, W. and Birt, L. M., 1976. *The Biochemistry of the Tissues*. 2nd edn. John Wiley, Chichester.

Blunt, M. H., 1975. *The Blood of Sheep: Composition and Function*. Springer-Verlag, Berlin.

Christie, W. W., 1981. *Lipid Metabolism in Ruminant Animals*. Pergamon Press, Oxford.

Evered, D. F., 1981. Advances in amino acid metabolism in mammals, *Biochem. Soc. Trans.* **9**: 159–69.

Garland, P. B. and Hales, C. N., 1978. *Substrate Mobilization and Energy Provision in Man, Biochem. Soc. Symp., No. 43*. Biochemical Society, London.

Goldberg, A. L. and Chang. T. W., 1978. Regulation and significance of amino acid metabolism in skeletal muscle, *Fedn Proc. Fedn Am. Socs exp. Biol.* **37**: 2301–6.

Krebs, H. A., Hems, R and Lund, P., 1973. Some regulatory mechanisms in the synthesis of urea in the mammalian liver, *Adv. Enzyme Regul.* **11**: 361–77.

Further reading 173

Lindsay, D. B., 1979. Metabolism in the whole animal, *Proc. Nutr. Soc.* **38**: 295–301.

Lindsay, D. B., 1980. Amino acids as energy sources, *Proc. Nutr. Soc.* **39**: 53–9.

McDonald, I. W. and Warner, A. C. I., 1975. *Digestion and Metabolism in the Ruminant*. New England Publishing Unit, Armidale.

Munro, H. N., 1970. *Mammalian Protein Metabolism,* Vol. IV. Academic Press London.

Newsholme, E. A. and Start, C., 1973. *Regulation in Metabolism*. John Wiley, Chichester.

Robinson, A. M. and Williamson, D. H., 1980. Physiological roles of ketone bodies as substrates and signals in mammalian tissues, *Physiol. Rev.* **60**: 143–87.

Ruckebusch, Y and Thivends, P., 1980. *Digestive Physiology and Metabolism in Ruminants*. MTP Press, Lancaster.

Trenkle, A., 1978. Relation of hormonal variations to nutritional studies and metabolism of ruminants, *J. Dairy Sci.* **61**: 281–93.

Vernon, R. G., 1980. Comparative aspects of lipid metabolism in monogastric, pre-ruminent and ruminating animals, *Biochem. Soc. Trans.* **8**: 291–2.

Waterlow, J. C., Garlick, P. J. and Millward, D. J., 1978. *Protein Turnover in Mammalian Tissues and in the Whole Body*. North Holland, Amsterdam.

REFERENCES

Ballard, F. J., Filsell, O. H. and Jarrett, I. G., 1976. Amino acid uptake and output by the sheep hind limb, *Metabolism* **25**: 415–18.

Bassett, J. M., 1974. Diurnal patterns of plasma insulin, growth hormone, corticosteroid and metabolite concentrations in fed and fasted sheep, *Aust. J. biol. Sci.* **27**: 167–81.

Bassett, J. M., 1975. Dietary and gastro-intestinal control of hormones regulating carbohydrate metabolism in ruminants. In *Digestion and Metabolism in the Ruminant* (ed. I. W. McDonald and A. C. I. Warner), pp. 383–98. University of New England Publishing Unit, Armidale.

Bergman, E. N., 1975. Production and utilization of metabolites by the alimentary tract as measured in portal and hepatic blood. In *Digestion and Metabolism in the Ruminant* (ed. I. W. McDonald and A. C. I. Warner), pp. 292–305. University of New England Publishing Unit, Armidale.

Bergman, E. N. and Heitmann, R. N., 1978. Metabolism of amino acids by the gut, liver, kidneys and peripheral tissues, *Fedn Proc. Fedn Am. Socs exp. Biol.* **37**: 1228–32.

Goldberg, A. L., De Martino, G. and Chang, T. W., 1978. Release of glucogenic precursors from skeletal muscle. In *Regulatory Mechanisms of Carbohydrate Metabolism* (ed. V. Esmann), pp. 347–58. Pergamon Press, Oxford.

Goldberg, A. L., Tischler, M., De Martino, G. and Griffin, G., 1980. Hormonal regulation of protein degradation and synthesis in skeletal muscle, *Fedn. Proc. Fedn Am. Socs exp. Biol.* **39**: 31–6.

Guidotti, G. G., Borghetti, A. F. and Gazzola, G. C., 1978. The regulation of amino acid transport in animal cells, *Biochim. biophys. Acta* **515**: 329–66.

Lehninger, A. L. 1975. *Biochemistry: the Molecular Basis of Cell Structure and Function*. 2nd edn. Ch. 30. Worth, New York.

Leveille, G. A., 1970. Adipose tissue metabolism: influence of periodicity of eating and diet composition, *Fedn Proc. Fedn Am. Socs exp. Biol.* **29**: 1294–1301.

Lindsay, D. B., 1978. Gluconeogenesis in ruminants, *Biochem. Soc. Trans.* **6**: 1152–6.

Linzell, J. L., 1974. Mammary blood flow and methods of identifying and measuring precursors of milk. In *Lactation: a Comprehensive Treatise*, Vol. I (ed. B. L. Larson and V. R. Smith), pp. 143–225. Academic Press, New York.

Lobley, G. E., Milne, V., Lovie, J. M., Reeds, P. J. and Pennie, K., 1980. Whole body and tissue protein synthesis in cattle, *Br. J. Nutr.* **43**: 491–502.

McNurlan, Margaret A., Pain, Virginia M. and Garlick, P. J., 1980. Conditions that alter rates of tissue protein synthesis *in vivo*, *Biochem. Soc. Trans.* **8**; 283-5.

Manchester, K. L., 1976. Hormonal control of protein metabolism. In *Protein Metabolism and Nutrition* (ed. D. J. A. Cole, K. N. Boorman, P. J. Buttery, D. Lewis, R. J. Neale and H. Swan), pp. 35–47. Butterworth, London.

Parsons, J. A., 1976. Endocrine pharmacology. In *Peptide Hormones* (ed. J. A. Parsons), pp. 67–82. Macmillan Press, London.

Puppione, D. L., 1978. Implications of unique features of blood lipid transport in the lactating cow, *J. Dairy Sci.* **61**: 651–9.

Shikama, H., Yajima, M. and Ui, M., 1980. Glycogen metabolism in rat liver during transition from the fed to fasted states, *Biochim. biophys. Acta* **631**: 278–88.

Whitelaw, Emma and Williamson, D. H., 1977. Effects of lactation on ketogenesis from oleate or butyrate in rat hepatocytes, *Biochem. J.* **164**: 521–8.

Section 2

THE ROLE OF NUTRIENT SUPPLY IN THE REGULATION OF METABOLISM

4 PHYSIOLOGY OF REGULATION OF FOOD INTAKE

J. M. Forbes

It is a characteristic of living things to take in substances from outside the organism to maintain their organized state. Most plants and some animals must accept more or less passively those nutrients that become available to them, but in higher vertebrates food must be actively sought, ingested and digested before it can be of use to the animal. Such animals have had to develop a drive to seek and eat food, which competes with other drives, such as those for water and reproduction. For the animal to indulge in more than one such activity at any one time is physically impossible, so that the individual has to eat sufficient food at each meal to satisfy nutrient requirements during the subsequent period when other drives may predominate, or until the source of the next meal is identified. The evolution of the drive to eat has, therefore, been accompanied by a subsequent drive not to eat; the hungry animal searches for food, but the satiated animal ignores it.

These short-term factors must in some way be linked to the longer-term regulation of energy balance because it is a matter of common observation that most adult individuals of most species match their energy intake quite closely with their energy output. Under some circumstances energy output can be varied: for example, caged rats given access to an exercise wheel, which they normally turn approximately 1000 times a day, greatly reduce the amount of energy spent in exercise when a lesion is made in the ventromedial hypothalamus, so that they gain weight rapidly even when restricted to their pre-operative level of food intake (Kennedy and Mitra, 1963). Farm animals do not normally indulge in such voluntary exercise and their capacity to regulate energy balance by controlling energy output is small and not usually considered to be of significance. It must, therefore, be by alterations of meal size and frequency that farm animals regulate their energy balance, and there must be a feedback mechanism whereby feeding behaviour comes under the influence of body weight or composition. The fat depots have long been known to be important in this feedback and several theories have been proposed to account for the relative constancy of fat content in the mature rat and human. In particular, a neural set-point has been proposed (Hervey, 1969) with which the current body fat content is compared, and the error used to stimulate or inhibit food intake. The existence of such a set-point is in doubt, however, and no satisfactory feedback mechanism from adipose tissue has yet been demonstrated. The alternative to a set-point theory is one which postulates that the relative constancy of body weight and composition is due to a balance between hunger and satiety factors (Wirtshafter and Davis, 1977). This latter idea is particularly attractive in relation to those species of farm animals which have been selected for rapid growth and fat deposition, and which continue to fatten if fed *ad libitum* on high quality foods.

CENTRAL NERVOUS INVOLVEMENT

Animals use one or more of the special senses to detect food; the decision whether to eat or not is made by the brain, dependent on the current state of energy supply from the gut, the competition from other drives and the previous experience of the food in question. Conversely, feeding stops when a satiating quantity of food has been eaten, this presumably being detected by the brain. The idea that there are two brain centres, one involved in the initiation, the other in the cessation of feeding, developed when Hetherington and Ranson (1940) demonstrated that damage to the ventromedial nucleus of the hypothalamus of the cat caused over-eating and obesity, while lesions in the adjacent lateral area of the hypothalamus of the rat caused under-eating, followed in some cases by death. More recently, attention has been turned to studies in farm animals. Chickens and pigs eat more and become excessively fat following electrical lesions of the ventromedial nuclei; this might be of practical significance in geese where fatty liver (*foie gras*) is a delicacy. Goats eat excessively following similar lesions and fill their rumens to the extent that breathing becomes difficult. Two attempts at causing such 'hypothalamic hyperphagia' in sheep have failed (see Baile and Forbes, 1974), but whether this was because of the small size of the lesions in relation to the size of the brain is not known.

Figure 4.1 is an annotated photograph of a cross-section through the brain of a sheep, showing the areas mentioned in the text. Administration of barbiturate anaesthetics into the ventromedial area or ventricles stimulates feeding in pigs, chickens, sheep and goats, probably by reducing the activity of the 'satiety centre' (Baile and Forbes, 1974). Lateral hypothalamic lesions cause sustained hypophagia in goats, while electrical stimulation of this area in goats induces an immediate feeding response. Stimulation of the ventromedial nucleus in this species, as in small mammals, prevents feeding even in hungry animals. This evidence has led to the two-centre hypothesis in which the balance between a satiety centre (the ventromedial nucleus) and a hunger centre (the lateral hypothalamus) is postulated to control feeding. The discovery of direct neural links between the two centres (Arees and Mayer, 1967) strengthened the hypothesis, but could not compensate for the fact that it was based mainly on evidence derived from experiments with animals in which significant areas of the brain had been destroyed.

Attention was then turned to the involvement of chemical transmitters in the brain following the demonstration of Grossman (1968) in rats that crystals of noradrenalin, a major neural transmitter, placed in the hypothalamus caused hyperphagia; whereas carbachol, an analogue of the natural transmitter acetylcholine, caused anorexia but stimulated drinking. More refined techniques enabled very small volumes of solutions of transmitters to be injected into the hypothalamus and adjacent areas of the brain, and confirmed the stimulatory effects of noradrenalin on feeding (Grossman, 1968). The picture is by no means clear, however, as areas as far from the classical feeding and satiety centres as the amygdala respond to noradrenalin, and the hyperphagia induced in the rat in the day-time by lateral hypothalamic injections of noradrenalin becomes hypophagia when the injections are made at night.

In farm animals, most work of this type has been performed with sheep. Baile and his colleagues developed techniques for injecting into the basal fore-brain and confirmed the stimulatory effect on feeding of noradrenalin injections at many sites (Baile, 1974). At other sites isoproterenol was effective; this is a synthetic catecholamine which affects different receptors from those stimulated by noradrenalin. These effects could be eliminated by prior injection of a specific blocking agent, and modified by injections of prostaglandins, which are also present naturally in the brain. Parallel experiments in which carbachol, another stimulator, was injected into the hypothalamus showed a dose-related stimulation of feeding during 1 h after injection, which was blocked by the specific antagonist, atropine, but not by the adrenergic blockers phenoxybenzamine and LB 46 (*dl*-4-(2-hydroxy-3-isopropyl-amino-proxy)-indol) (Fig. 4.2; see Baile, 1974). Drinking was stimulated in only isolated cases; these results are quite different from those obtained in the rat, but similar to those observed in the rabbit given intrahypothalamic carbachol.

In pigs, isoproterenol injected into the ventromedial hypothalamus temporarily depressed food intake (Jackson and Robinson, 1971).

The placement of guides to enable injections to be made into specific areas of the brain is technically difficult and, in large animals, it is

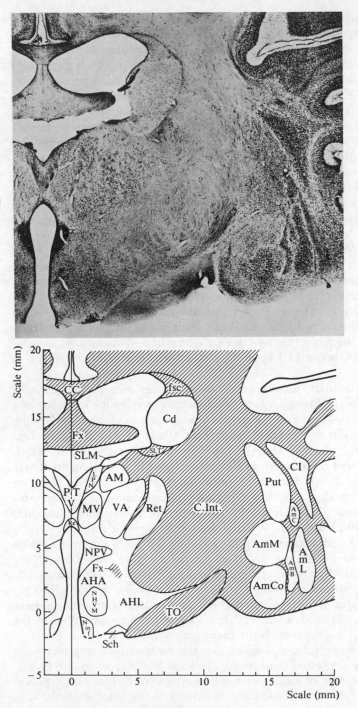

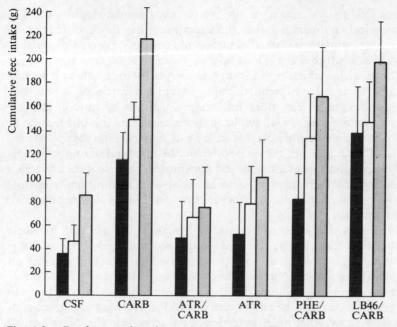

Fig. 4.2. Food eaten by sheep during 30 min ■, 1 h □ and 2 h ▨ after
hypothalamic injections of 1 μl synthetic cerebrospinal fluid (CSF)
or 1 μl synthetic cerebrospinal fluid containing 28 nmol carbachol
(CARB), 28 nmol atropine (ATR), 120 nmol phenoxybenzamine
(PHE), and 120 nmol LB46 (see Baile, 1974.)

Fig. 4.1. Photograph and diagram of a vertical section through the fore-brain
of a sheep (Richard, 1967). NHVM, ventromedial nucleus of
hypothalamus; AHL, lateral hypothalamic area; TO, optic tract;
dashes indicate position of attachment of pituitary gland. (Other
abbreviations are: CC, corpus callosus; Fx, fornix; FSC, fasciculus
sub-callosus; Cd, nucleus condatus; StT, stria terminalis; SEM, stria
medullaris thalami; AM, nucleus anterior mediatis; LPN, nucleus
lateratis posterior; PVT, nucleus paraventriculus thalami; MV,
nucleus medialis; Re, nucleus renniers; VA, nucleus ventralis anterior; Ret, nucleus reticularis; NPV, nucleus paraventricularis
hypothalami; AHA, area hypothalamica anterior; N. inf., nucleus
infundibuli; SCL, nucleus suprachiasmaticus; C. int., capsula in-
terna; Put, putamen; Cl, claustrum; AmC, nucleus amygdala centra-
lis; AmM, nucleus amygdala medialis; AmL, nucleus amygdala
lateralis; AmB, nucleus amygdala basalis; AmCo, nucleus amygdala
corticalis.)

impossible to be certain of the site being stimulated until there is histological confirmation after the experiment has finished. It is much easier to cannulate the lateral ventricle and to allow injected material to be carried with the continuous flow of cerebrospinal fluid through the third ventricle, which runs through the hypothalamus where it is contiguous with the extracellular fluid. Sheep and cattle prepared with ventricular guides eat more following injections of noradrenalin or isoproterenol (Baile, 1974), whilst in sheep, carbachol inhibits feeding in contrast to the hyperphagia that follows its injection into hypothalamic tissue. Whether any of these responses to the injection of unphysiologically large amounts of likely neural transmitters represent the activation of pathways which are involved in the control of feeding under normal physiological conditions, or whether they are purely pharmacological, is unknown.

Neurones are exposed to other substances in addition to their endogenous transmitters and it has long been considered that satiety is induced by a direct action of the absorbed products of a meal on sensitive areas of the brain. Thus, Mayer (1955) used the selective uptake of gold thioglucose by the ventromedial nucleus in mice to support the idea that the satiety centre could actively take up glucose. It was later shown that micro-injections of glucose into the ventromedial nucleus were only effective in stopping feeding when insulin was available, presumably to stimulate the uptake of glucose into the sensitive cells. Conversely, the inhibitor of glycolysis, 2-deoxy-D-glucose, when injected ventricularly in doses too small to have any effect when given systemically, stimulated feeding in rats. It seems, therefore, that some neurones involved in the feeding circuit of the brain are directly sensitive to the uptake or utilization of glucose.

Some steroid hormones can also cross the blood-brain barrier and are actively taken up by the brain. Oestradiol, the major oestrogen produced by the ovarian follicle at oestrus, is taken up by the hypothalamus, where it is responsible for depressing food intake and for inducing oestrous behaviour (Wade, 1972). In castrated male sheep, injections of oestradiol into a lateral ventricle significantly depress the weight of food eaten in the subsequent hour, and continuous intravenous infusion also causes hypophagia, except when the dose is very low, and intake is slightly increased.

It is not easy to see how all these experimental results, which depend so much on species, dose and time of day, can be integrated into a general hypothesis of the rôle of the brain in the control of food intake. The hypothalamus is not, however, isolated from the rest of the brain or the rest of the body. Indeed, the lateral area of the hypothalamus is part of a major route, the medial fore-brain bundle, which carries information in both directions between the higher conscious centres of the brain and the lower autonomic centres. The 'hunger centre' is thus ideally situated to play a major rôle in controlling feeding behaviour, which is an intersection between conscious and autonomic activity. The ventromedial hypothalamic nucleus, although not part of such a major neural pathway as the lateral area, is intimately involved with the neuroendocrine control of secretion of anterior pituitary hormones, especially growth hormone. Lesions of the 'satiety centre' reduce the secretion of growth hormone thereby increasing the insulin to growth hormone ratio which will enhance lipogenesis, and the resulting increased energy requirements will stimulate food intake; insulin treatment of intact rats also causes increases in lipogenesis and food intake. Hyperphagia might, therefore, be a secondary rather than the primary result of lesions of the ventromedial nucleus.

PERIPHERAL RECEPTORS

The brain is well buffered and protected from changes in the availability of substrates. It is not, therefore, in a good position to detect the relatively small changes in, say, blood glucose concentration which would be necessary if it were the only organ involved in the control of food intake. It is far more likely that the brain integrates signals from peripheral receptors in order to make the decision as to whether or not the animal needs to eat.

Oropharyngeal receptors

Jaw fatigue or salivary secretion are not thought to limit the size of a meal, because removal of food from the stomach before it has time to exert any chemical effect there results in very long periods of voluntary feeding both in rats and cattle (see Balch and Campling, 1962). The taste and texture of food are used to identify a food: these may be innate responses, or the animal may have learned to associate a particular food with a pleasant or unpleasant sequel. Palatability is an important determinant of food intake in some circumstances, as was elegantly demonstrated in the sheep by Greenhalgh and Reid (1967) who offered half of the daily ration by mouth and introduced the remainder via rumen cannulae. When straw was offered and dried grass introduced through the cannula daily intake was only 23.5 g DM per $kg^{0.73}$, whereas when dried grass was offered and straw introduced, total intake was 48.8 g/$kg^{0.73}$ per day. In both experimental treatments the total food entering the rumen via the two routes consisted of 500 g dried grass and

500 g straw per kg, and the digestibility of the total diet was unaffected by the method of feeding.

Stomach receptors

The stomach is a reservoir for ingested food; the more the animal eats at any meal, the fuller the stomach becomes. Stretch receptors are progressively stimulated and stomach distension in the absence of chemical factors may inhibit feeding, as when a balloon is inflated in the stomach of the dog (see Balch and Campling, 1962). Because of the very slow passage of food from the fore-stomachs, ruminants given forages are particularly susceptible to rumen distension (see Ch. 11), and stretch receptors have been identified electrophysiologically in the rumen wall (Leek and Harding, 1975).

There is little evidence that chemoreceptors in the wall of the gastric stomach are directly involved in the cessation of feeding, but the rumen wall is undoubtedly sensitive to the production of volatile fatty acids in the rumen. For example, injection of 30 mmol sodium acetate or propionate into a rumen pouch depressed food intake, while concurrent injection of local anaesthetics blocked these effects (Fig. 4.3; Martin and Baile, 1972). Although behavioural studies such as this argue for a specific effect of acetate on rumen wall chemoreceptors, electrophysi-

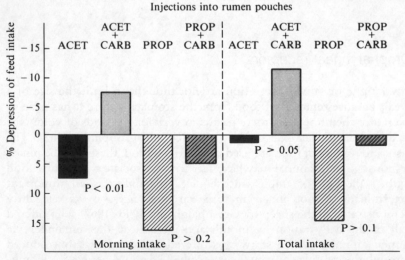

Fig. 4.3.   The effect on food intake of injections into rumen pouches, in sheep and goats of 30 ml of 1.0 M sodium acetate (ACET) or propionate (PROP), with or without 12 mg carbocaine (CARB) (Martin and Baile, 1972).

ological studies show that the rumen mechanoreceptors, which are also chemosensitive, respond to the pH of the acid solutions irrespective of the nature of the acid used.

Intestinal receptors

Distension of the intestines may become a factor limiting food intake when food passes more rapidly than usual from the stomachs of the ruminant, as with ground foods, but chemical rather than physical stimulation of the duodenal wall is more likely to play a rôle in satiation with normal diets. This has been well described for the rabbit, where infusion of 10 ml of isotonic glucose solution reduced food intake by 6 J per J of glucose infused (Novin, 1976). In the sheep, lactic acid is particularly effective in inhibiting food intake when infused into the duodenum, while glucose does not appear to be involved in the control of intake in ruminants. Injection of glucose solution into the duodenum of chickens had an inhibitory effect on feeding for some 10 min while the same amount of sorbitol, which is not absorbed, prevented feeding for approximately 1 h; this suggests that in chickens duodenal distension or osmotic stimulation is more important than the chemical effect of absorbed glucose. Glucose infusion into the duodenum of the pig 3 min after the start of a meal depresses food intake, but this effect is blocked by vagotomy (Table 4.1).

Table 4.1 Effect of infusion of 250 ml of glucose solution (150 g/l) in intact or vagotomized pigs (Stephens and Heron, 1979)

| | | | Food intake (g) | | | |
| | | | Day before infusion | | Day of infusion | |
No. of pigs	Vagus	Time of infusion	Mean	s.e.	Mean	s.e.
11	Intact	10 min before start of meal	1060	170	1019	162
4	Sectioned	3 min after start of meal	940	50	912	106
14	Intact	3 min after start of meal	782	41	445	27

Hepatic receptors

All material absorbed from the digestive tract passes to the liver via the hepatic portal vein, with the exception of the fat transported by the lymphatic system. The liver is also a major regulator of energy metabolism in the short term, maintaining a supply of glucose when energy requirements exceed energy supply from the gut, and replenishing its reserves of glycogen when the supply of absorbed metabolites exceeds the current demands of the rest of the body. Thus the liver is well situated to act as a major source of information on the current metabolic status of the animal and recent evidence suggests that it does fulfil such a rôle, transmitting information to the brain via the vagus nerve. Russek has championed the cause of the liver in the control of feeding for many years (Russek and Grinstein, 1974), since his observations that various experimental manipulations of liver uptake or release of glucose, or liver glycogen content, were correlated with changes in food intake in rats and dogs. Glucose receptors have been identified electrophysiologically in guinea-pig liver, and electron microscopy shows nerve endings close to some hepatocytes, which could detect passage of metabolites into or out of these cells by monitoring changes in membrane potential. In the overnight fasted rabbit, glucose infusion into the portal vein depresses the amount eaten when food is offered to intact animals, but has no effect in vagotomized animals (Novin, 1976). In the chicken, there is a dose-related depression in food intake during 3-h portal infusions of solutions of glucose (5 to 60 g/l) at 1.2ml/min (Fig. 4.4); chickens do not survive total vagotomy and it will be

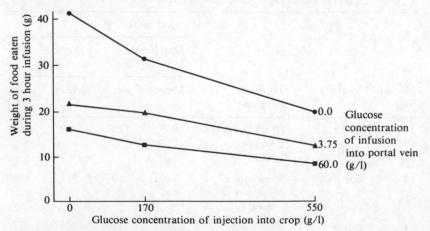

Fig. 4.4.   The effect of a 3-h infusion of glucose solutions into crop and hepatic portal vein on the concurrent food intake of growing cockerels (Shurlock and Forbes, 1981).

necessary to devise a method of more local denervation of the liver in order to demonstrate whether the feeding response to portal glucose infusions is mediated via the nervous system.

There is no consistent effect of glucose on feeding in ruminants, irrespective of site of infusion. However, propionate, which is almost entirely taken up by the liver and converted to glucose, does depress intake, particularly when infused into the ruminal vein (see Baile and Forbes, 1974). Three-h infusions of sodium propionate into the portal vein of sheep caused a dose-related depression of food intake, with complete cessation of feeding when the dose was 1.2 mmol/min. This is somewhat greater than the rate of absorption of propionate from the rumen after a large meal of a concentrate food, so that the liver's exposure to propionate does not by itself account for physiological satiety. The route of the signal from liver to brain in the sheep was investigated by section of the hepatic plexus of nerves, which runs in the wall of the hepatic artery and is a tributary of the vagus nerve. Of seven sheep recovering fully from the operation, three were later shown to be at least 95% liver-denervated and these three animals did not stop eating during 3-h infusions into the portal vein of sodium propionate at 1.2 mmol/min (Fig. 4.5). The rôle of propionate and the liver in the control of feeding in the sheep seems, therefore, to be parallel to that of glucose and the liver in the simple-stomached laboratory mammal.

INITIATION AND TERMINATION OF MEALS

Meal initiation

The glucostatic theory of the control of feeding envisaged that a meal was initiated when blood glucose concentration, or glucose utilization rate by a sensitive tissue, fell below a critical level; that is, the animal was stimulated to eat when its supply of energy-yielding substrates from the previous meal was falling below energy demand. It has been established that plasma insulin concentrations have fallen to a low level before the onset of spontaneous meals, both in rats and sheep, which supports the concept of feeding in response to low nutrient availability. Another sign of impending or actual energy deficit, at least in sheep, is a rise in growth hormone secretion. In sheep accustomed to free access to a complete pelleted food, withdrawal of food for 8 h results in an increase in the size and frequency of growth hormone secretory episodes, within approximately 3 h; plasma growth hormone levels fall immediately food is made available again. In these and other animals growth hormone peaks, presumably due to mild energy deficit, have been observed to precede spontaneous meals in a large proportion of

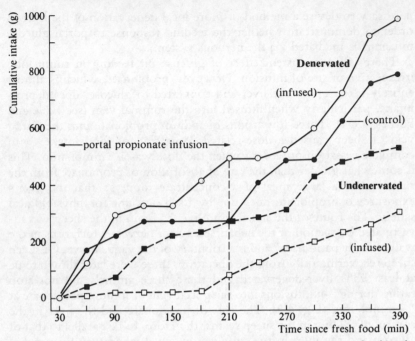

Fig. 4.5.   The effect of denervation of the liver on the depression in food intake
induced by infusion of 1.2 mmol/min sodium propionate into the
portal vein from 30 to 210 min after offering fresh food (Anil and
Forbes, 1980) (□——□, undenervated, infused with propionate;
■——■, undenervated, control infusion; ○——○, denervated, infused with propionate, ●——●, denervated, control infusion).

cases (Forbes, 1980), supporting the contention that feeding starts in
response to impending energy deficit.

There are other, external, factors that can induce feeding. Offering
fresh food, or food more palatable than that previously available, will
often induce feeding, and animals accustomed to being fed at a particular time of day will undergo a voluntary fast for several hours
rather than eat the remainder of the previous day's offering. Social
feeding is also common; sheep in adjacent individual pens often take
'spontaneous' meals in unison, as do those in a flock outside.

Once started, feeding continues at a relatively constant rate which
depends on the size of the animal, the ease of prehension and the
palatability of the food.

Meal termination

There is compelling evidence that feeding terminates in response to the
signals from the stomach, intestines, liver and (possibly) brain, which

were dealt with earlier. The ingestion of food results in progressive distension and, after a delay (the length of which will be characteristic of the food) the appearance of soluble products of digestion that will affect the receptors in gut wall, liver and brain. The sum total of these negative feed-back signals, when collated with the positive influences of palatability and social feeding, will determine whether the animal continues to eat, or stops eating. There will be some cases where one of these signals is of overriding importance: with a bulky food stomach distension will account for meal termination, and with a high-carbohydrate food glucose absorption can explain satiation. In most instances, however, the sum of two or more signals is likely to be the satiating factor (Fig. 4.6).

This theory of meal termination is superficially less attractive than one in which a single satiety factor is postulated. Thus, the glucostatic (Mayer, 1955) and thermostatic (Brobeck, 1948) theories have received much attention in the past and, more recently, a single gut hormone, cholecystokinin, has been invoked as the satiety factor (Smith, Gibbs and Young, 1974); infusions of cholecystokinin into the cerebroventricles of sheep at rates as low as 0.01 pmol/min depressed food intake by

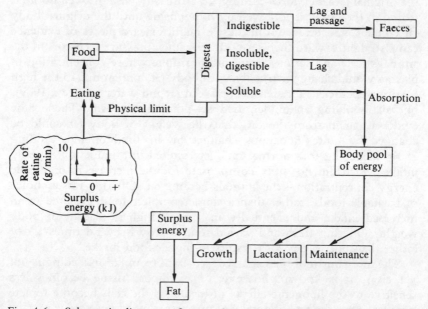

Fig. 4.6. Schematic diagram of a simulation model of the control of food intake in sheep. Rate of eating is switched from 0 to 10 g/min when the 'surplus' in energy supply has fallen to less than a lower threshold. Eating continues until the 'surplus' in energy supply exceeds another, higher, threshold, at which point it is switched from 10 to 0 g/min.

35%. In the absence of a single satiety factor that can be shown to be involved in the termination of feeding under all circumstances, there must, for the time being at least, be reliance on the facts so far established and acceptance of a multi-factor theory of satiety. Such a theory cannot easily be stated verbally, but can be expressed by means of simulation models, such as those described later in this chapter.

MAINTENANCE OF ENERGY BALANCE

In the introductory remarks it was observed that many adult animals maintain a relatively constant body weight and composition over long periods of time. This implies that there is a long-term control of food intake (or energy output) which must be intimately linked with the short-term control of feeding. It has been clear for many years that body fat is a key component in this respect. Under-feeding or surgical removal of fat in rats results in compensatory hyperphagia to restore the original fat level; force-feeding, to artificially raise the weight of fat stored in the body, is followed by hypophagia until the original body fat content is restored. From these straightforward pieces of evidence came straightforward theories both frivolous (pressure receptors in the animal's feet) and serious (a steroid hormone whose concentration in plasma would change markedly with body fat content due to the high partition coefficient for steroids between fat and water: Hervey, 1969), but all involving an unidentified set-point mechanism. Then came evidence, again from the rat, that the weight of body fat could be changed by quite innocuous changes in the food offered. Adding 250 g fat per kg to a normal rat diet resulted in a reduction in daily intake which did not fully compensate for the increase in digestible energy concentration – the animals became fat. Offering rats a choice of palatable foods, rather than a single complete food, resulted in an increased intake and eventually in a new, higher, plateau of body weight. Offering fresh and varied food to cows several times a day rather than once a day also results in higher food intake.

The mechanism of the negative feed-back from fat on feeding is not yet clear. It is known, however, that adipose tissue becomes less sensitive to the lipogenic effects of insulin as the cells become replete with fat. Thus the rate of uptake of precursors by adipose tissue may be reduced as the animal fattens, leaving higher concentrations in the blood to induce earlier satiety. Growth hormone and adrenalin might also be involved, as lipolytic agents.

Whatever the feed-back from fat, it appears to interact with the other satiety signals, and the resultant food intake and body weight is determined by the balance between these factors, rather than being fixed; 'settling point' is a more appropriate concept than 'set point' (Wirtshafter and Davis, 1977).

Most of the research into body fat and food intake has been carried out with the rat because of its ease of management and carcass analysis (the whole animal can be subject to ether extraction in a giant Soxhlet thimble). Little relevant work has been done with farm animals but, in those species which have been selected for fast rate of weight gain without particular regard to the composition of that gain, the negative feed-back from fat to feeding seems to have been attenuated. Although there is a definite negative relationship between body fat and food intake in sheep when fed *ad libitum* on a concentrated ration for long periods, they continue to deposit fat, albeit at a declining rate, even when 600 g/kg of their body weight is accounted for by adipose tissue. Pigs, similarly, achieve massive bulk when fed *ad libitum*, and cattle deposit considerable amounts of fat if offered a high quality food when they have low demands for energy for growth and lactation. The absence in ruminants of an obvious plateau to body weight has been used to support the notion that cattle and sheep have lost the ability to use a function of body fat as one of the signals controlling food intake. The observation that fat cattle and sheep eat less than thin ones was explained by the competition for abdominal space between abdominal fat and rumen capacity. This cannot, however, be the whole truth because, even with concentrated diets where gut distension is unlikely to have an important effect on feeding, there is an effect of fatness on food intake which is proportional to the concentration of digestible energy in the food. Direct evidence on the manner in which fat affects feeding in the ruminant is sparse. Surgical removal of the tails of growing fat-tailed sheep, which contained 1.9 kg fat, resulted in no difference in the quantity of fat in other depots when the sheep were slaughtered and compared with control animals 1.5 years later. Prior underfeeding of cows results in hyperphagia when the animals are allowed free access to food (Bines, Suzuki and Balch, 1969). Unfortunately, direct measurements of body fat have not been made in this type of experiment and one can only speculate that the effect of fat on feeding may be similar in farm animals to that in the rat, but modified by the effects of artificial selection for rapid rates of fattening.

Physiological changes such as growth, pregnancy and lactation are normally accompanied by the appropriate changes in food intake, so that body weight is maintained. Sometimes, however, physical limits intervene, as in the pregnant ruminant where gut capacity is reduced (Forbes, 1970), or in the high yielding cow where, despite the large abdominal capacity, energy requirements are so high that they cannot be met fully by current food intake, even when a high-quality food is offered. A further complication at oestrus and late pregnancy is the intake-depressing effect of oestrogens (Forbes, 1970), probably acting on hypothalamic receptors.

INTEGRATION INTO WORKING HYPOTHESES

The conclusion that the control of food intake is multifactorial has led to the construction of various types of models, some of which, because of the number of factors involved, are computationally complex and most-conveniently written as computer programs. The full range of such models has been covered in detail elsewhere (Booth, 1978) and only the most physiological approach will be dealt with in this chapter.

From the results of a wide range of experiments, Booth (1978) concluded that rats start to eat when the supply of energy-yielding substrates from the gut and the adipose tissues falls below a threshold which is related to the energy requirements of the animal, and that they stop eating when energy supply exceeds another threshold. Based on this concept he constructed a model in which energy flow from the gut was calculated at frequent intervals using absorption curves derived from direct measurements, and the contribution of energy from adipose tissues was made to correspond to that normally observed in laboratory rats (negative during the night and positive during the day). The energy requirements for heat production were subtracted from the total energy flow and the remaining energy was compared with the hunger and satiety thresholds: if below the hunger threshold, feeding was switched on; if above the satiety threshold, feeding was switched off. By successive iterations, predictions of feeding behaviour were made which were close to observed feeding patterns of rats (Table 4.2).

Table 4.2   Feeding pattern parameters observed in rats and those derived from a model of the feeding behaviour of the rat (Toates and Booth, 1974)

	Real rat	Modelled rat	
		Mean	s.e.
Dark phase			
Total intake (g in 12 h)	13.0	13.3	1.6
Size of meal (g)	2.6	2.1	0.4
Meal-to-meal interval (min)	137	100	15
Light phase			
Total intake (g in 12 h)	8.5	6.4	0.9
Size of meal (g)	2.0	2.2	0.9
Meal-to-meal interval (min)	154	282	73

A comparable model for the ruminant has subsequently been developed in which more emphasis is placed on physical limitation of food intake (Forbes, 1980; Fig. 4.6). Feeding was switched on when absorbed energy fell below energy requirements by more than a threshold value, which could be varied in different simulation experiments, and feeding stopped when energy supply exceeded requirements by another threshold value. These thresholds were incorporated in the acknowledgement that whilst energy flow *per se* was probably not monitored by the animal, the levels and flows of several substances, each related to the provision of energy, were monitored. Variation of the thresholds over quite a wide range (from 0 to 0.5 kJ/min) had little effect on the predictions of feeding behaviour, indicating that an animal does not need to monitor energy flow with great accuracy in order to control its food intake.

With a medium-quality forage of digestibility 0.65, offered to a mature sheep of moderate fatness, the model predicted a daily intake of 1 550 g dry matter, eaten in 10 meals in seven periods of feeding. A comparable sheep in reality ate 1 415 g in 13 meals grouped into seven periods of feeding (Fig. 4.7). Increasing fatness, programmed to reduce gut capacity, depressed daily intake and predicted smaller, more

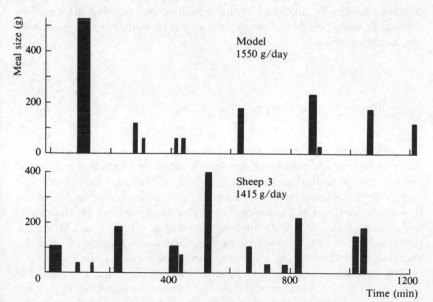

Fig. 4.7. Predictions of meal size and frequency by the model outlined in Fig. 4.6, with parameters set for a mature, moderately fat sheep and a diet of 0.65 DM digestibility; and observed meal pattern of a mature, moderately fat sheep (sheep 3) offered dried grass/barley pellets.

frequent, meals. Increasing the energy requirements was predicted to give increased intake, again with more frequent small meals, because physical limitation became more dominant as the energy requirements became less easy to meet. With this moderate-quality food, live-weight loss was predicted for sheep with metabolizable energy requirements greater than 12 MJ/day, equivalent to the energy requirement for maintenance and a milk yield of approximately 2 l/day. Appropriate changes in energy requirements, gut capacity and rate of eating were used to simulate growth and pregnancy and, in each case, predicted changes in daily intake were similar to those observed in experiments with animals. Changing the parameters used to describe the food, to simulate poor quality forage, concentrates, grinding of the food and restricted food availability, all gave predicted changes in food intake which were similar to those observed experimentally. The meal patterns generated during each of these simulations were compared with observed patterns, where available, and showed qualitative agreement.

It is likely, therefore, that the principles on which the rat and ruminant models are based are reasonable: that feeding starts in response to a relative deficit of energy to supply requirements, and stops when an excess occurs (or is seen as likely to occur) unless physical limitations intervene. The computer model thus provides a complex quantitative hypothesis, which is capable of experimental testing, and can be modified in the light of more detailed information derived from experimental work; it is an aid to, rather than a substitute for, understanding.

DEFICIENCIES AND TOXICITIES

The discussion so far has centred on the control of energy intake because there is little evidence for specific appetites for other macronutrients, except water and sodium. It is well known, however, that dietary deficiencies of protein, minerals or vitamins cause, as one of the first signs, reduced food intake. Clearly, this would not be the case if the intake of any of these constituents were controlled; in that case a protein-deficient diet would be eaten in increased quantities, and the excess energy thereby consumed would be deposited as fat.

The protein content of the food below which voluntary intake is depressed varies according to the animal's protein requirements, but for mature pigs and chickens it is approximately 100 g/kg, and for ruminants, which can recycle nitrogenous compounds, approximately 70 g/kg. Often it is one essential amino acid which is limiting and addition of this to the diet in small quantities results in increased food intake. Thus, in the ruminant, where methionine is often the first limiting amino acid, infusion into the duodenum, or inclusion in the food in a form which will protect it against rumen degradation, prevents the depression of intake caused by feeding a marginally protein-deficient diet. A more general protein deficiency can be alleviated in all species by feeding a high-protein supplement or, in the ruminant, by feeding urea or other soluble nitrogenous compounds. In this latter case the extra nitrogen available to the rumen microorganisms restores their ability to digest cellulose and increases the rate of passage through the rumen, thereby possibly alleviating a physical limitation on intake. The difference between nitrogen deficiency in the rumen and protein deficiency in the animal was clearly demonstrated by Egan and Moir (1965), who offered sheep straw with a crude protein content of only $40\,g/kg$. They then injected either $70\,g$ casein, $21.5\,g$ urea or $22\,g$ propionic acid into the duodenum, the latter quantities to be isonitrogenous and isocaloric, respectively, with the casein. The results are given in Table 4.3, and it can be seen that there was an

Table 4.3   Effects of treatments upon voluntary DM intake, measured as excess over mean intake on days 1 to 5 (before infusion) observed on days 6 to 8 (after infusion); see text for quantities infused (Egan and Moir, 1965)

Treatment	Mean DM intake for days 1–5 (g/day)	Mean increments in intake (g) over mean for days 1–5		
		Day 6	Day 7	Day 8
Control (phosphate)	565	−16	−1	+39
Casein	576	+135[†]	+74	−18
Urea	585	+49	+142[‡]	+60
Propionate	570	−6	+27	−11

[†] Significantly different from control on the same day ($P < 0.01$).
[‡] Significantly different from control on the same day ($P < 0.05$).

elevation of intake caused by ruminal urea which was accompanied by increased rates of digestion and passage, while that caused by duodenal casein occurred despite decreases in both cellulose digestion and passage of undigested particles. The implication is that urea primarily relieved a physical limitation while casein, infused at a site where its amino acids could be absorbed without degradation, relieved a metabolic limitation. To support this latter suggestion, Egan (1965) later showed that there was a more rapid rate of removal of acetate from blood in the duodenal casein-infused sheep compared with controls. It is possible, therefore, that lower food intake in protein-deficient animals is due to a reduction in energy requirements caused by a deceleration of one or more metabolic pathways. This idea is supported by the observation that exposure of rats offered a protein-deficient diet to cold environments caused sufficient increase in intake to alleviate the signs of protein deficiency.

Diets which are excessively high in protein content are also eaten by rats in smaller quantities than normal diets and this may be associated with a reduced rate of stomach emptying because parenteral infusion of amino acids inhibits gastric motility.

Most of the work on effects of protein and amino acids on food intake has been performed with animals offered a single food. An alternative and probably more useful approach is the technique of self-selection (Anderson, 1977). Rats offered the choice of high-carbohydrate and high-protein diets selectively increased their energy intake when exposed to colder environments, without changing their protein intake.

Another aspect of the involvement of amino acids in the control of feeding is their rôle in the central nervous system, particularly as precursors of neurotransmitters. In rats given a diet in which threonine was the limiting amino acid, infusions of threonine into the carotid artery stimulated food intake more than similar infusions into the jugular vein (Rogers and Leung, 1973). Similarly, with histidine-deficient chickens infusion of histidine was more effective into the carotid artery than into the jugular vein (Boorman, 1979). The uptake of tyrosine, a precursor of the catecholamines (an important group of neural transmitters), is related to plasma levels of several amino acids which affect food intake, and it is reasonable to suggest that changes in plasma amino acid concentrations or ratios, as affected by absorption, might be directly involved in meal initiation and termination. Again, self-selection from a range of foods may be a particularly relevant experimental approach to the further study of the rôle of neurotransmitters and their precursors in the control of food intake since it might help to avoid the complication of competition between the appetite for energy and that for protein, encountered when a single mixed food is given (Anderson, 1977).

A specific appetite for calcium has been demonstrated in the laying hen, which controls its calcium and energy intakes independently when given a choice of foods (Hughes, 1979). Appetites for zinc, phosphorus, thiamine and methionine, as well as for protein, have also been demonstrated in the fowl.

Animals suffering from a specific deficiency show more exploratory behaviour and chew at a variety of novel materials, but it has not been proved unequivocally that sheep, cattle or pigs have specific appetites for any mineral other than sodium (Pamp, Goodrich and Meiske, 1976). They may learn that ingestion of a particular material alleviates the discomfort caused by the deficiency, but then continue to eat greater quantities of that material than are necessary for the deficiency to be remedied.

PRACTICAL CONSIDERATIONS

Poultry

Birds compensate for the dilution of the energy concentration of the diet, and undergo voluntary hypophagia following fattening induced by forced feeding or insulin injections (Lepkovsky, 1973). They may, therefore, be said to control their energy intake in a manner analogous to that in mammals, although less is known of the mechanisms in the bird. Egg-laying strains of chicken do not eat during the hours of darkness although broiler chickens do eat at night. Increased energy expenditure, as in egg-laying birds or in those exposed to cooler environments, causes a compensatory increase in food intake and adult body weight is normally maintained at a relatively constant level. Efficiency of egg production from food declines at environmental temperatures below a critical temperature of approximately 20 °C because food intake is increased, and also above approximately 25 °C because both food intake and egg production are reduced under mild heat-stress.

In the hope that they can select a protein to energy ratio suited to their nutritional requirements, hens have been offered a choice of protein-rich and energy-rich foods, but have not been able to make an appropriate selection (Summers and Leeson, 1979). Offering a calcium-rich material separately from an otherwise balanced ration, however, resulted in the selection of a calcium intake that was suited to the birds' needs.

Pigs

The high rate of fattening of domestic pigs is well-known and it can be deduced that any feed-back mechanisms from fat to the controlling centres of feeding are not as sensitive as those in rats or humans. This insensitivity presumably arose during selection for rapid weight gain at a time when fat was readily accepted as a human food. Now that fat is disliked by many people, the pig's propensity to fatten is normally counteracted in farming practice by restricted feeding, which is expensive in terms of the pigman's time. The possibilities of limiting digestible energy intake by dilution of the diet have been investigated by Owen and Ridgman (1967), who found that weight gains from 27 to 50 kg live weight were depressed by the inclusion of 200 g sawdust or 300 g oat food per kg in an otherwise standard diet but, from 50 to 118 kg, the pigs compensated for the dilution, and weight gains and fat deposition were unaffected. Introduction of a diluted food at a later age gave a temporary reduction in food intake, but this was not considered to be of commercial importance.

A chemical approach to preventing excessive fattening in pigs has also been investigated by Wyllie and Owen (1978), who extracted an intake-depressing substance from the urine of satiated (but not hungry) pigs, but this has not yet been tried on a large scale. In the long term, the problem of over-fatness in pigs could be alleviated by selection of successive generations against fat synthesis, whilst trying to maintain the capacity for rapid muscle deposition.

Ruminants

Over-eating is rarely a problem with ruminants; the difficulty is more often that their production of meat or milk is limited by physical restraints on the intake of forages. The interactions between the metabolic and physical controls of feeding discussed earlier are such that the relationship between voluntary food intake and food quality is biphasic, with a positive slope for poor- and moderate-quality foods and a negative slope for good-quality foods. Figure 4.8 is a summary of

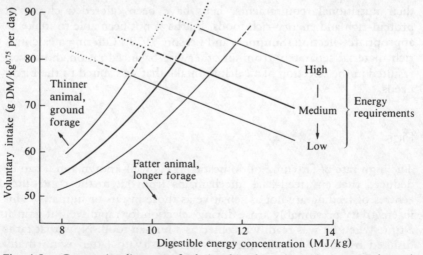

Fig. 4.8.   Composite diagram of relationships between voluntary intake and animal and food factors in ruminants (see text for explanation).

these relationships, which are derived from the work of Conrad, Pratt and Hibbs (1964) and Baumgardt (1970), amongst others. At any given digestibility on the 'physical' part of the curve, intake will be lower for fat animals and higher for ground foods; on the 'metabolic' section, intake will be related to the nutrient requirements of the animal. Thus the intersection of the two lines, which was at a DM digestibility of 0.67 for cows yielding moderate amounts of milk (Conrad *et al.*, 1964), may vary quite widely, being considerably lower than this figure for animals with relatively low energy requirements offered a ground, pelleted food. Prediction of voluntary intake for a given type of animal offered a specified food will not be accurate because many of the factors underlying the control of food intake are not quantitatively documented. This is demonstrated by attempts to predict the food intake of dairy cows throughout lactation from their metabolizable energy requirements and the physical limitations on intake (Forbes, 1977); qualitative agreement with observed patterns of intake was achieved, but the quantitative agreement was not good. For the present, for predictive purposes, multiple correlations of food intake against food quality, milk yield, live weight and live-weight change must be relied on and these are considered more fully in Ch. 11.

CONCLUSIONS

Farm animals, like other species of mammals and birds, control their food intake primarily by monitoring the yield of energy from each meal, which gives an approximate balance between energy requirements and energy intake in the short term. In the long term, there are feed-backs from body fat reserves which modulate the short-term controls to provide long-term stability of body weight and composition. Cattle, sheep, pigs and possibly broiler chickens have been selected for rapid body weight gain which may have resulted in relative insensitivity to fatness by those mechanisms which control food intake. Changes in food intake and meal patterns associated with growth, pregnancy, lactation, fattening and brain lesions are consistent with the hypothesis that energy supply is monitored as a means of controlling food intake.

Deficiencies of specific nutrients cause depression of food intake, possibly by limiting the rate of energy utilization; specific, inborn appetites for water and sodium have been demonstrated but other deficiencies may be corrected by the animal learning that ingestion of a particular material alleviates the discomfort caused by the deficiency.

The sensory qualities of a food will provide inputs to the brain which will be integrated with inputs from gut, liver and other sensitive areas to determine whether, and at what rate, an animal eats. The control of food intake is thus multifactorial but should be capable of rational explanation once the level of stimulation of all the relevant receptors can be defined for any given situation. It is not surprising that prediction of food intake has proved to be difficult.

FURTHER READING

Baldwin, B. A., 1976. Quantitative studies on taste preference in pigs, *Proc. Nutr. Soc.* **35**: 69–73.
Bell, F. R., 1976. Regulation of food intake, *Proc. Nutr. Soc.* **35**: 63–7.
Boorman, K. W. and Freeman, B. M., 1979. *Food Intake Regulation in Poultry*. Longman, Edinburgh.
Goatcher, W. D. and Church, D. C., 1970. Review of some nutritional aspects of the sense of taste, *J. Anim. Sci.* **31**: 973–81.
Jones, G. M., 1972. Chemical factors and their relation to feed intake regulation in ruminants: a review, *Can. J. Anim. Sci.* **52**: 207–39.

REFERENCES

Anderson, G. L., 1977. Regulation of protein intake by plasma amino acids. In *Advances in Nutritional Research* (ed. H. H. Draper), pp. 145–66. Plenum Press, New York.
Anil, M. H. and Forbes, J. M., 1980. Feeding in sheep during intraportal infusions of short-chain fatty acids and the effect of liver denervation, *J. Physiol., Lond.* **298**: 407–14.
Arees, E. A. and Mayer, Jean, 1967. Anatomical connections between medial and lateral regions of the hypothalamus concerned with food intake, *Science, Wash.*, D.C. **157**: 1574–5.
Baile, C. A., 1974. Putative neurotransmitters in the hypothalamus and feeding, *Fedn Proc. Fedn Am. Socs exp. Biol.* **33**: 1166–75.
Baile, C. A. and Forbes, J. M., 1974. Control of feed intake and regulation of energy balance in ruminants, *Physiol. Rev.* **54**: 160–214.
Balch, C. C. and Campling, R. C., 1962. Regulation of voluntary food intake in ruminants, *Nutr. Abstr. Rev.* **32**: 669–86.
Baumgardt, B. R., 1970. Control of feed intake in the regulation of energy balance. In *Physiology of Digestion and Metabolism in the Ruminant* (ed. A. T. Phillipson), pp. 235–53. Oriel Press, Newcastle upon Tyne.

Bines, J. A., Suzuki, S. and Balch, C. C., 1969. The quantitative significance of long-term regulation of food intake in the cow, *Br. J. Nutr.* 23: 695–704.

Boorman, K. N., 1979. Regulation of protein and amino acid intake. In *Food Intake Regulation in Poultry* (ed. K. N. Boorman and B. M. Freeman), pp. 87–126. Longman, Edinburgh.

Booth, D. A., 1978. Prediction of feeding behaviour from energy flows in the rat. In *Hunger Models : Computable Theory of Feeding Control* (ed. D. A. Booth), pp. 227–78. Academic Press, London.

Brobeck, J. R., 1948. Food intake as a mechanism of temperature regulation, *Yale J. Biol. Med.* 20: 545–52.

Conrad, H. R., Pratt, A. D. and Hibbs, J. W., 1964. Regulation of feed intake in dairy cows. I. Change in importance of physical and physiological factors with increasing digestibility, *J. Dairy Sci.* 47: 54–62.

Egan, A. R., 1965. Nutritional status and intake regulation in sheep. IV. The influence of protein supplements upon acetate and propionate tolerance of sheep fed on low quality chaffed oaten hay, *Aust. J. agric. Res.* 16: 473–83.

Egan, A. R. and Moir, R. J., 1965. Nutritional status and intake regulation in sheep. I. Effects of duodenally infused single doses of casein, urea and propionate upon voluntary intake of a low-protein roughage by sheep, *Aust. J. agric. Res.* 16: 437–49.

Forbes, J. M., 1970. The voluntary food intake of pregnant and lactating ruminants: a review, *Br. vet. J.* 126: 1–11.

Forbes, J. M., 1977. Development of a model of voluntary food intake and energy balance in lactating cows, *Anim. Prod.* 24: 203–14.

Forbes, J. M., 1980. Hormones and metabolites in the control of food intake. In *Digestive Physiology and Metabolism in Ruminants* (ed. Y. Ruckebusch and P. Thivend), pp. 145–60. MTP Press, Lancaster.

Greenhalgh, J. F. D. and Reid, G. W., 1967. Separating the effects of digestibility and palatability on food intake in ruminant animals, *Nature, Lond.* 214: 744.

Grossman, S. P., 1968. Hypothalamic and limbic influences on food intake, *Fedn Proc. Fedn Am. Socs exp. Biol.* 27: 1349–60.

Hervey, G. R., 1969. Regulation of energy balance, *Nature, Lond.* 222: 629–31.

Hetherington, A. W. and Ranson, S. W., 1940. Hypothalamic lesions and adiposity in the rat, *Anat. Rec.* 78: 149.

Hughes, B. O., 1979. Appetite for specific nutrients. In *Food Intake Regulation in Poultry* (ed. K. N. Boorman and B. M. Freeman), pp. 141–69. Longman, Edinburgh.

Jackson, H. M. and Robinson, D. W., 1971. Evidence for hypothalamic α and β andrenergic receptors involved in the control of food intake in the pig, *Br. vet. J.* 127: li–liii.

Kennedy, G. C. and Mitra, J., 1963. Body weight and food intake as initiating factors for puberty in the rat, *J. Physiol., Lond.* 166: 408–18.

Leek, B. F. and Harding, R. H., 1975. Sensory nervous receptors in the ruminant stomach and the reflex control of reticulo-ruminal motility In *Digestion and Metabolism in the Ruminant* (ed. I. W. McDonald and

A. C. I. Warner), pp. 60–76. University of New England Publishing Unit, Armidale.

Lepkovsky, S., 1973. Hypothalamic-adipose tissue interrelationships, *Fedn Proc. Fedn Am. Socs exp. Biol.* **32**: 1705–8.

Martin, F. H. and Baile, C. A., 1972. Feed intake of goats and sheep following acetate or propionate injections into rumen, ruminal pouches, and abomasum as affected by local anesthetics, *J. Dairy Sci.* **55**: 606–13.

Mayer, Jean, 1955. Regulation of energy intake and the body weight: the glucostatic theory and the lipostatic theory, *Ann. N.Y. Acad. Sci.* **63**: 15–43.

Novin, D., 1976. Visceral mechanisms in the control of food intake. In *Hunger: Basic Mechanisms and Clinical Implications* (ed. D. Novin, Wanda Wyrwicka and G. A. Bray), pp. 357–67. Raven Press, New York.

Owen, J. B. and Ridgman, W. J., 1967. The effect of dietary energy content on the voluntary intake of pigs, *Anim. Prod.* **9**: 107–13.

Pamp, D. E., Goodrich, R. D. and Meiske, J. C., 1976. A review of the practice of feeding minerals free choice, *Wld Rev. Anim. Prod.* **12** (4): 13–8.

Richard, P., 1967. *Atlas Stereotaxique du Cerveau de Brebis.* Institut National de la Rechoche Agronomique, Paris.

Rogers, Q. R. and Leung, P. M. B., 1973. The influence of amino acids on the neuroregulation of food intake, *Fedn Proc. Fedn Am. Socs exp. Biol.* **32**: 1709–19.

Russek, M. and Grinstein, S., 1974. Coding of metabolic information by hepatic glucoreceptors. In *Neurohumoral Coding of Brain Function* (ed. R. D. Myers and R. R. Drucker-Colin), pp. 81–97. Plenum Press, New York.

Shurlock, T. G. H. and Forbes, J. M., 1981. Evidence for hepatic glucostatic regulation of food intake in the domestic chicken and its interaction with gastrointestinal control, *Br. Poult. Sci.* **22**: 333–46.

Smith, G. P., Gibbs, J. and Young, R. C., 1974. Cholecystokinin and intestinal satiety in the rat, *Fedn Proc. Fedn Am. Socs exp. Biol.* **33**: 1146–9.

Stephens, D. B. and Heron, F., 1979. The attenuation of the suppression of appetite resulting from intraduodenal infusions of glucose by vagotomy in young pigs, *Proc. Nutr. Soc.* **38**: 46A (Abstr.).

Summers, J. D. and Leeson, S., 1979. Diet presentation and feeding. In *Food Intake Regulation in Poultry* (ed. K. N. Boorman and B. M. Freeman), pp. 445–69. Longman, Edinburgh.

Toates, F. M. and Booth, D. A., 1974. Control of food intake by energy supply, *Nature, Lond.* **251**: 710–1.

Wade, G. N., 1972. Gonadal hormones and behavioural regulation of body weight, *Physiol. Behav.* **8**: 523–34.

Wirtshafter, D. and Davis, J. D., 1977. Set points, settling points and the control of body weight, *Physiol. Behav.* **19**: 75–8.

Wyllie, D. and Owen, J. B., 1978. Anorexigenic substances and voluntary food intake in the pig, *Anim. Prod.* **26**: 19–29.

5   FOETAL AND NEONATAL METABOLISM

Anne Faulkner

Satisfactory growth of the foetus and newborn animal is dependent on adequate nutrition to supply fuels for energy production and building materials for new tissue. Undernutrition during development can result in growth retardation and deformities, some of which cannot be compensated for by increased food intake during later development. In the mammal, the supply of food to both the foetus and newborn animal is derived from the mother; the foetus receives its nutrients directly from the maternal circulation via the placenta and the newborn animal receives its nutrients in milk via the mammary gland. Adequate nutrition is, therefore, dependent on both maternal nutrition and the efficiency with which nutrients are transferred from the mother to the offspring.

FOETAL NUTRITION

Immediately after fertilization the zygote is free in the uterus and absorbs its foodstuffs directly from the surrounding fluids. The developing animal gains little weight during this time. When implantation occurs, the formation of embryonic membranes enables the embryo to obtain nutrients from the maternal circulation via the placenta.

The placenta

The placenta is a union of foetal and maternal tissues for the purpose of nutrient transport and it is able to transfer gases and metabolites to and from the foetus as well as eliminating waste products and synthesizing hormones (Wynn, 1975). The transfer of nutrients across the placenta is dependent on several factors, such as the blood flow across the uterine and umbilical circulations, the permeability of the placenta to different substrates and the concentration of substrates in the maternal and foetal blood (Girard, Pintado and Ferre, 1979).

Placental blood flow

Placental blood flow increases towards the end of pregnancy as a result of increased maternal and foetal cardiac output and decreased vascular resistance. Uterine and umbilical blood flows keep pace with the growth of the uterus and foetus throughout gestation despite the reduced placental growth that occurs in some species before birth. This increased flow is needed to meet the increased nutrient requirements of the foetus in late gestation. The importance of an adequate uterine blood flow has been demonstrated experimentally. Artificially induced reduction of the placental vascular supply in sheep and rats produced growth retardation and reduced birth weights (Wigglesworth, 1966; Creasy, de Swiet, Kahanpää, Young and Rudolph, 1973). Hormones may also regulate placental blood flow: an increase in plasma progesterone is known to reduce uterine blood flow in early pregnancy (Caton, Abrams, Lackore, James and Barron, 1973).

In the placenta the two blood supplies are separated by membranes. The number of membranes varies with species, being least in primates and rodents and greatest in ruminants and pigs (Amoroso, 1961). The number of membranes separating the two circulations does not appear to influence the efficiency of nutrient transport. The efficiency of nutrient transfer across the placenta is influenced by the relationship of the maternal and foetal circulations. In the sheep placenta, the directions of blood flow in maternal and foetal capillaries are parallel (i.e. concurrent flow). This arrangement appears to be less efficient than the countercurrent flow seen in the rabbit placenta.

Placental permeability and substrate concentrations

Several mechanisms have been described for the transport of substrates across the placenta (Widdas, 1961; Dancis and Schneider, 1975; Miller, Koszalka and Brent, 1976).

Simple diffusion is the transfer of substrates down a chemical concentration gradient at rates which are compatible with Fick's laws of diffusion and the physiochemical properties of the substrate. No energy expenditure is required. Substrates transferred across the placenta in this way include lactate, urea and acetate. Gases (oxygen and carbon dioxide) cross the placenta by diffusion, but the transfer of oxygen to the foetal circulation is facilitated by the greater affinity of foetal haemoglobin for oxygen (Wood, Pearce, Clegg, Weatherall, Robinson,

Thorburn and Dawes, 1976). Transfer of carbon dioxide from the foetal maternal circulation is facilitated by the simultaneous uptake of oxygen.

Facilitated diffusion is the transfer of a substrate down a chemical concentration gradient at rates in excess of those predicted by the laws of simple diffusion, but requiring no expenditure of energy. Glucose, the major metabolic fuel of the foetus, is transferred by facilitated diffusion, which probably involves a carrier molecule crossing the placental membranes (Dancis and Schneider, 1975). The placental transfer is specific for glucose, other hexoses being transferred across the placenta at much slower rates. Transport of glucose across the placenta is a function of the concentration difference of glucose between maternal and foetal blood. Insulin may also have a direct effect on placental glucose transport as specific receptors for insulin have been detected in placental membranes (Girard *et al.*, 1979).

Active transport is the transfer of substrates against a chemical concentration gradient and requiring the expenditure of energy. Amino acids are transported in this way. Their concentration is generally greater in foetal blood than in maternal blood. Glutamate appears to be the only amino acid which is transferred from the foetus to the maternal circulation, and there is little net transport of the other acidic amino acids (Battaglia and Meschia, 1978) (Fig. 5.1).

Electrolytes and water-soluble vitamins are also transported actively across the placenta. Data from work on the pig indicate an active

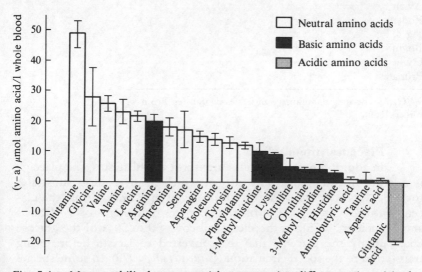

Fig. 5.1. Mean umbilical veno-arterial concentration differences ($v - a$) in the ovine foetus (bars indicate s.e.). (From Lemons, Adcock, Jones, Naughton, Meschia and Battaglia, 1976.)

transport of sodium ion from the foetal to the maternal circulation (Barnes, 1976).

Transport of large molecules. Large molecules, such as triglycerides, phospholipids and cholesteryl esters, do not cross the placenta. Free fatty acids can cross the placenta by diffusion from the maternal to foetal circulation in some species (e.g. rabbit and guinea pig, and, to a lesser extent, rat and sheep) but the magnitude of this transfer is small (Girard *et al.*, 1979). However, a lipoprotein lipase capable of hydrolysing free fatty acids from triglyceride has been detected in the placentae of some species, and may indicate an extraction and transfer of free fatty acids from triglycerides by the placenta (Elphick and Hull, 1977). Maternal proteins and polypeptides cross the placenta slowly or not at all. The gamma globulins are the exception, and they are transferred rapidly to the foetus in some species (e.g. primates) by a mechanism involving pinocytosis. There appears to be minimal transfer of gamma globulins in ruminants; the resulting deficit of the immunoglobulins is compensated for by absorption of proteins from colostrum postnatally (Dancis and Schneider, 1975) (Table 5.1).

Table 5.1   Routes of passive transfer of immunoglobulins from mother to foetus

Species	Route of transfer		
	Yolk	Placenta	Colostrum or milk
Avian	+		
Rodent	+	−	+
Pig	−	±	+
Bovine	−	±	+
Ovine	−	−	+
Primates	−	+	−

+, Transfer occurs; ±, minimal transfer; −, no transfer. From Miller (1966).

Placental metabolism

In addition to its rôle in the transport of substrates, the placenta is a large, metabolically active organ which itself requires substrates for energy production and growth. It has been estimated that the placenta utilizes up to 30% of the oxygen delivered to it (Dancis and Schneider, 1975). In the sheep and cow, 30 to 50% of the glucose taken up by the placenta may be converted to lactate before being transferred to the foetal circulation (Girard *et al.*, 1979). In some species (sheep, goat, cow, pig and horse) a part of the glucose taken up by the placenta is converted to fructose which is transferred to, and accumulates in, the foetal blood. No transfer of fructose back to the maternal circulation appears to occur. In rodents the placenta can store glucose as glycogen for use by the foetus in late pregnancy and during periods of maternal undernutrition (Dawes and Shelley, 1968).

The placenta of the sheep grows rapidly in early and mid-pregnancy but reaches maximum weight at approximately two-thirds of the way through the gestation period, after which it remains constant or declines slightly (Barcroft, 1946). The foetus grows steadily until the end of gestation (Fig. 5.2). There is a positive correlation between foetal weight and placental weight at birth, and surgical reduction of the size of the placenta during pregnancy results in reduced birth weights in sheep (Alexander, 1964). Reduced placental weight may be caused by maternal undernutrition in early pregnancy, but partial compensation for this can occur if extra food is given in late pregnancy. This implies either an improvement in placental function, or an increase in placental

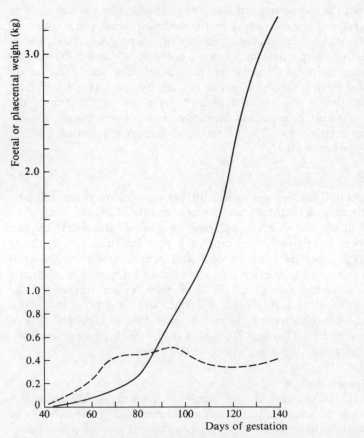

Fig. 5.2. Growth of the sheep foetus and placenta during gestation (——, foetal weight; — — —, placental weight). (From Barcroft, 1946.)

weight beyond the stage of gestation at which maximum placental weight is normally seen in the sheep (Robinson, 1977).

The placenta also has a rôle as an endocrine organ and has the capacity to synthesize a number of hormones. The hormones produced by the placenta vary with different species but include steroid hormones (oestrogens and progesterone) and polypeptide hormones (chorionic gonadotrophin and placental lactogen) (Thau and Lanman, 1975).

Carbohydrate metabolism in the foetus

Glucose

Glucose, derived from the maternal circulation, is the major substrate for the foetus and can also be metabolized by the uterus. The very high rates of glucose uptake by the pregnant uterus can account for up to 70% of the total glucose turnover of the pregnant ewe (Silver, 1976). In the sheep, cow and horse, between 40 and 50% of this glucose may be used directly by the foetus, the remainder being metabolized by the uterus. Glucose is used by the foetus for energy production (being the essential energy precursor in the brain), the synthesis of energy reserves and the biosynthesis of new tissue. Glucose carbon can account for 23% of the total carbon requirement of the foetus (Girard *et al.*, 1979).

Glucose oxidation

Although the foetus requires little energy for movement, digestion, respiration and temperature control, its rate of oxidative metabolism is high. In the sheep, goat, cow and horse, the foetal oxygen consumption is relatively constant at 7 to 8 ml/min per kg body weight. This contrasts with the postnatal period, when oxygen consumption is related to surface area rather than body weight. Glucose oxidation accounts for 50 to 70% of the oxygen uptake in the foetus of the fed ruminant (Table 5.2) but, when the pregnant ewe is starved, the contribution of glucose to oxidative metabolism falls to approximately 30% (Table 5.2) (Girard *et al.*, 1979). Amino acids are oxidized increasingly during maternal starvation.

Glycogen storage

In all species studied, the mammalian foetus accumulates glycogen during the latter half of gestation (Dawes and Shelley, 1968). In the lung and cardiac muscle the glycogen content reaches a maximum at approximately half-way through the gestation period, falling during the latter part of gestation (Fig. 5.3). It has been suggested that these

Table 5.2   Metabolic balance in foetuses of different
species

Substrates	Foetal O_2 uptake used in oxidizing substrates			
	Sheep		Calf	Horse
	Fed	Fasted	Fed	Fed
Glucose	50	30	60	70
Lactate	25	15	40	–
Amino acids	20	60	10	–
Acetate	5	–	10	–
Glycerol	–	1	–	–

Values were obtained in unstressed, chronically catheterized foetuses (from Girard *et al.*, 1979) and in some cases
represent slight overestimates.

tissues act as a temporary glycogen store for the foetus during the latter
part of gestation, and mobilization of cardiac glycogen is also observed
during hypoxia (Shelley, 1961). In the liver and skeletal muscle, the
glycogen content increases throughout gestation (Fig. 5.4) and acts as
an energy reserve for the newborn animal. This energy store may be
particularly important in the young pig, which has very little body fat
at birth (Mersmann, 1974).

The storage of glycogen in the foetus is dependent upon hormonal
control. In the rabbit, foetal decapitation prevents glycogen storage in
the foetal liver, and injection of corticosteroids and growth hormone or
prolactin restore glycogen deposition. Hypophysectomy or adrenalectomy of the sheep foetus also reduces the glycogen content of the
foetal liver but deposition can be restored to normal in these animals by
infusing cortisol alone (Girard *et al.*, 1979). The onset of glycogen
deposition in the liver cannot be attributed to the increase in activity of
the biosynthetic enzymes at this time. In the guinea-pig, all enzymes
required for glycogen synthesis are present before glycogen deposition
occurs (Walker, 1968).

Fat storage

Glucose can also be metabolized by the foetus for the synthesis
of triglycerides. In the adult ruminant, glucose carbon is not used for
the synthesis of fatty acids: acetate fulfils this rôle. However, the foetal
ruminant resembles the non-ruminant in that it has the capacity to
synthesize lipids from glucose in the liver (Ballard, Hanson and
Kronfeld, 1969), and the rate of lipid synthesis from glucose in foetal
adipocytes is twice that of the adult (Vernon, 1980).

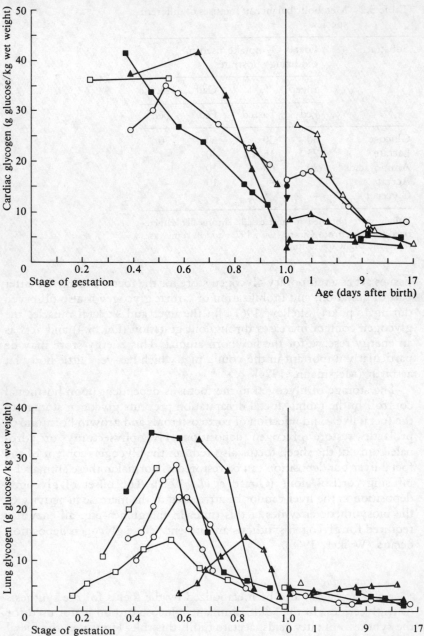

Fig. 5.3.   Glycogen content of the foetal heart and the foetal lungs of various species (□, main; ■, monkey; ▲, guinea-pig; ○, sheep; △, rat; ●, pig; ▼, cat; ▲, rabbit). (From Shelley, 1961.)

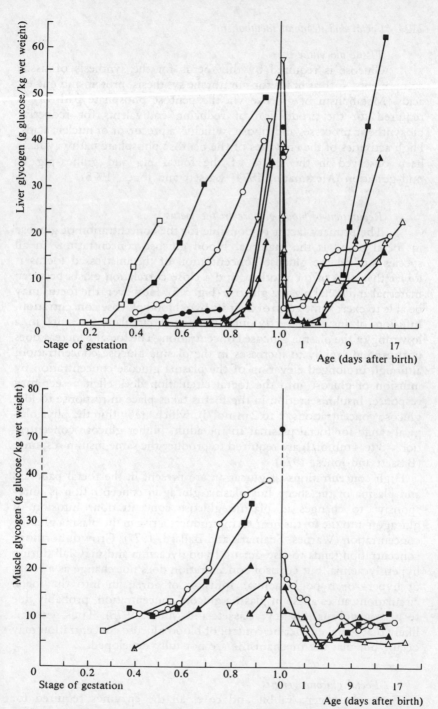

Fig. 5.4. Glycogen content of the foetal liver and the foetal muscle of various species (▽, dog; other symbols as for Fig. 5.3). (From Shelley, 1961.)

Tissue biosynthesis

Glucose is required by the foetus for the synthesis of tissue components, such as lipids for membrane synthesis, protein and nucleic acids. Metabolism of glucose via the pentose phosphate pathway is required for the production of reducing equivalents for reductive biosynthetic processes and ribose, which is a precursor of nucleic acids. High activities of the enzymes of the pentose phosphate pathway have been observed in the livers of the foetal pig and guinea-pig in mid-gestation (Mersmann, 1974; Bassett and Jones, 1975).

Regulation of blood glucose in the foetus

The primary factor responsible for the concentration of glucose in foetal blood is the maternal blood glucose concentration. In all species studied the glucose concentration of the unstressed foetus is lower than that of the mother, and a close correlation exists between maternal and foetal plasma glucose (Fig. 5.5). However, the foetus may be able to exert some control over its own blood glucose concentration. Infusion of insulin directly into the foetal circulation results in a lowering of the plasma glucose concentration. The foetal pancreas does not respond rapidly to increases in the plasma glucose concentration, although prolonged elevation of the plasma glucose concentration by infusion of glucose into the foetal circulation does elicit a secretory response. Insulin secretion in the foetus takes place in response to low glucose concentrations (1 to 2 mmol/l), which are within the physiological range for foetal plasma. In the adult, higher glucose concentrations (3 to 4 mmol/l) are required to produce the same insulin response (Bassett and Jones, 1975).

High concentrations of glucagon are present in the foetal pancreas and plasma of the sheep but plasma glucagon concentration is unresponsive to changes in plasma glucose concentration. Infusion of glucagon into the foetus near term produces a rise in the plasma glucose concentration (Warnes, Seamark and Ballard, 1977). Growth hormone concentration tends to rise during hypoglycaemia and may fall during hyperglycaemia, but cortisol concentration does not change as a result of hyper- or hypoglycaemia. Infusion of adrenalin into the foetal circulation causes a rise in plasma glucose concentration, probably due to glycogenolysis (Shelley, Bassett and Miller, 1975). Thus it seems likely that foetal endocrine control of blood glucose concentration may occur, but that the mechanisms are not fully developed.

Foetal gluconeogenesis

In the sheep, rabbit and cow, all the enzymes required for glucose synthesis are present in the foetal liver near term. Reports differ as to whether this capacity for glucose synthesis is actually utilized by

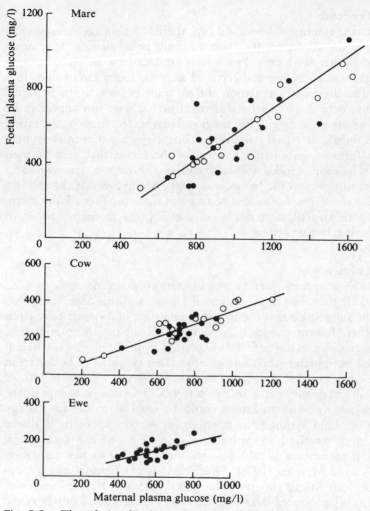

Fig. 5.5. The relationship between maternal and foetal plasma glucose levels in the mare, cow and sheep (○, values from conscious animals; ●, values from anaesthetized preparations). (From Silver, Steven and Comline, 1973.)

the foetus before birth but, if glucose synthesis by the foetus does occur, the rates reported would account for only 5% of the total glucose required by the foetus. There does seem to be a discrepancy between the reported values for the glucose requirement of the sheep foetus and the umbilical uptake of glucose, and glucose synthesis by the foetal liver may be required to provide the extra glucose needed in addition to that obtained from the maternal circulation (Girard *et al.*, 1979).

Fructose

In the ruminant, horse and pig, there is a high concentration of fructose in foetal plasma, the concentrations being three to four times higher than that of glucose. Fructose is produced by the placenta from maternal plasma glucose and secreted into the foetal circulation. It is confined to the foetal circulation and no transfer back to the maternal circulation occurs. In the foetal lamb, fructose does not appear to be utilized to any great extent, but the foetal plasma fructose concentration may fall during maternal starvation. Thus it appears that fructose may act as a form of carbohydrate store for the foetus that may be used during starvation. Under normal conditions, however, fructose has a very low turnover in the foetus and a very limited rate of metabolism (Girard *et al.*, 1979). Some loss of fructose from the foetal kidney into the amniotic and allantoic fluids surrounding the foetus is known to occur during late gestation.

Lactate

In most species, foetal plasma lactate concentrations are two- to three-fold higher than in the maternal plasma and this observation has led to the suggestion that the foetus is in a state of hypoxia relative to the mother. Recent studies have shown that, in the sheep and cow, lactate is transferred to the foetal circulation from the placenta, where it is formed from maternal plasma glucose. This synthesis of lactate from glucose occurs under aerobic conditions and is not a result of lack of oxygen in either the foetus or the placenta. The fate of lactate in the foetus is not yet known but it could be used as a fuel for energy production, lipid synthesis or possibly for gluconeogenesis. If all the lactate were oxidized to carbon dioxide, 25% of the total foetal oxygen consumption would be accounted for by lactate oxidation (Battaglia and Meschia, 1978). Short periods of maternal oxygen deprivation can result in rises in foetal plasma lactate, and this endogenously produced lactate appears to be metabolized slowly as the original plasma lactate concentrations are not restored for some time (Silver, 1976).

Glycerol

Glycerol has been shown to cross the placenta to the foetal circulation in the rat and rabbit but not in the sheep. It seems unlikely that glycerol could contribute significantly to the metabolic needs of the foetal ruminant (Girard *et al.*, 1979). Glycerol can be released into the foetal plasma of the lamb following lipolysis of triglycerides from foetal adipose tissue, and infusion of catecholamines into foetal sheep and rabbits causes a consistent rise in plasma glycerol concentrations (Hull, 1975a).

Fatty acid metabolism in the foetus

Short-chain fatty acids

The adult ruminant relies on the production of VFA (i.e. acetate, propionate and butyrate) by the rumen microorganisms for much of its carbon and energy requirements. There is no evidence that propionate or butyrate cross the placenta to the foetal circulation, but acetate does cross the placenta and may be an important fuel for the foetal ruminant. In the foetal cow, plasma acetate concentrations correlate with those of the mother, and acetate uptake by both the foetus and the uterus has been detected (Table 5.2). Thus acetate metabolism may make a small but significant contribution to the energy requirement of the foetus. In the ruminant, ketone bodies, acetoacetate and 3-hydroxybutyrate do not appear to cross the placenta or to be metabolized by foetal tissues even though their concentrations increase rapidly in maternal blood during starvation (Silver, 1976).

Long-chain fatty acids
The origin of fatty acids

The origin of the foetal lipids can be either the maternal circulation or synthesis *de novo* within the foetus. All mammalian foetuses studied have the capacity to synthesize lipid from glucose in the liver and adipose tissue, although this capacity is small in the foetal pig (Mersmann, 1974). There is an obligatory requirement for placental transfer of the essential fatty acids for such processes as growth of the brain and nervous tissue. In some species (rabbit, rat and primates) the essential fatty acids form a higher fraction of the total fatty acids in the foetus than they do in the mother (Hull, 1975b), but in the ovine foetus the concentrations of essential fatty acids are low. In the rabbit and guinea-pig, significant quantities of fatty acids cross the placenta and may provide a substantial source of energy as well as a major portion of the lipid in the foetal body. In ruminants placental transfer could account for only a small proportion of the foetal lipid, and the greater part must originate from synthesis of fatty acids from glucose and acetate in the foetus.

Lipid stores

The amount of fat in the foetus varies considerably depending on the species studied (Table 5.3). The fatty acids are stored as triglyceride in the tissues of the foetus (liver, skeletal muscle, and white and brown adipose tissue). The accumulation of lipid in the ovine foetus takes place early in gestation and reaches a maximum several weeks before birth (Fig. 5.6). The rate of lipid accumulation declines near term. Perirenal and abdominal adipose tissue consists mainly of

Table 5.3   Lipid stores in the full-term
              foetuses of several species

Species	Body fat (g/kg body weight)
Man	160
Guinea-pig	100
Rabbit	60
Sheep	30
Calf	30
Foal	20
Pig	10
Rat	10

From Girard *et al.* (1979).

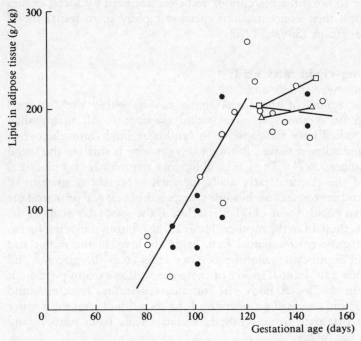

Fig. 5.6   The accumulation of lipid in the ovine foetus (o, single foetus; •,
            twin foetus; △, foetus of ewe, subjected to under-nutrition; □, foetus
            of ewe given a high-energy diet *ad libition*). (From Alexander, 1978.)

brown adipose tissue (i.e. adipose tissue with a large vascular supply
and high mitochondrial content), and subcutaneous deposits are predominantly white adipose tissue in foetal sheep. The subcutaneous fat
regresses during the latter part of gestation and can disappear by full
term. The rate of regression of the foetal subcutaneous adipose tissue is
hastened by maternal starvation, indicating that the foetal lamb can

utilize this energy store during periods of undernutrition. Liver and skeletal muscle have a low lipid content in the ovine foetus and this also decreases near term (approximately 50 g/kg of tissue falling to 15 g/kg) (Alexander, 1978).

This pattern of lipid accumulation in mid-gestation in the ovine foetus *in vivo* is similar to the pattern of development of the lipogenic enzymes observed in smaller animals (Jones and Ashton, 1976). Fatty acid synthetase, acetyl-CoA carboxylase and ATP-citrate lyase in the foetal guinea-pig all reach maximum activity in mid-gestation, falling in activity near term. In the pig, lipogenic activity appears to be low in the foetus in late gestation (Mersmann, 1974).

The deposition of fat in the foetal tissues appears to be hormonally controlled. Hypophysectomized ovine foetuses are born with thick layers of subcutaneous fat (Alexander, 1978). Decapitation or thyroidectomy of foetal rabbits also results in lipid accumulation and this can be prevented by injecting thyroxine into the foetal circulation. Therefore the deposition of fat appears to be regulated by thyroid hormones under pituitary control (Girard *et al.*, 1979). Lipolysis of foetal adipose tissue is also influenced by circulating hormones. Catecholamines injected into foetal sheep cause an increase in the circulating levels of glycerol and free fatty acids (Jones, 1976). However, the activity of the sytems for fatty acid oxidation is low in foetal tissues, but rises rapidly after birth (Hull, 1975b).

Steroids

Cholesterol and cholesterol derivatives cross the placenta of most species by diffusion and are utilized by the foetus. The foetus also exhibits a high rate of cholesterol biosynthesis *de novo*. In the rat approximately 110 g/kg of the cholesterol in the foetal body is derived from the maternal circulation (Noble, 1979). The cholesterol is utilized for tissue biosynthesis and also for the synthesis of steroid hormones. Some steroid hormones (e.g. cortisol) cross the placenta but it is unlikely that the transfer rate is sufficient to satisfy the foetal requirements, and foetal synthesis of cortisol from glucose and acetate does occur.

Nitrogen metabolism in the foetus

Amino acids

The amino acids that cross the placenta to the foetal circulation are used to build new tissue and as fuel for energy production. In the foetus of the ruminant especially, the total quantity of amino acids transferred is greatly in excess of that required to satisfy the estimated growth rate, and oxidation of amino acids could account for 20 to 60% of the total oxygen consumption of the foetus (Table 5.2). An estimated 0.65 g nitrogen per kg per day is required for ovine foetal growth but amino acid uptake by the foetal lamb was estimated at 1.5 g nitrogen per kg per day. The amino acids transferred to the foetus include all the essential amino acids plus those which the foetus is incapable of synthesizing in amounts adequate for protein synthesis. Some amino acids may be formed by transamination within the foetal tissues as there is no net transport of the acidic amino acids (aspartate and taurine) and glutamate is transferred from the foetal to the maternal circulation (Battaglia and Meschia, 1978) (Fig. 5.1).

Nitrogen excretion

The transfer of glutamate from the foetal to the maternal circulation may represent a form of nitrogen excretion for the foetus. High oxidation rates of amino acids result in the production of waste nitrogen which has to be excreted by the foetus. Excretory nitrogen crosses the placenta mainly as urea and ammonia. The concentration of urea in foetal plasma is greater than that in the maternal plasma and urea crosses the placenta by diffusion. In the foetal sheep the rate of excretion of urea is approximately four times that of the adult (corrected for body weight differences) and it has been calculated that 20% of the foetal oxygen consumption in late gestation could be required to sustain the observed rate of urea production (Battaglia and Meschia, 1978). There appear to be considerable species differences in the rate of foetal urea formation. The foetal rat and rabbit have low rates of transaminase activity and urea production, whereas in foetal ruminants and pigs transaminase activity and urea formation are substantial (Jones, 1976).

Proteins

Maternal proteins are transferred across the placenta despite their large molecular size, but there is considerable selectivity in the process. Gamma globulins are extensively transferred in some species (primates) but others, including ruminants, appear to receive the immunity by absorption of protein from colostrum postnatally (Table 5.1).

The vast proportion of protein present in the foetus at birth is synthesized within the foetus. The total protein content of the foetus increases during gestation from 50 g/kg in the small embryo to 270 g/kg in the newborn animal (Fig. 5.7) (Blaxter, 1964). Very high rates of protein synthesis are seen in all foetal tissues but different growth rates occur in the various organs at different stages of development. Thus, at 72 days gestation the foetal sheep liver is twice the

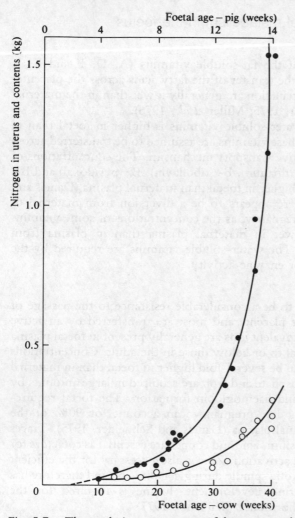

Fig. 5.7. The total nitrogen content of the uterus and its contents in pregnant pigs (o) and cows (●). (From Blaxter, 1964.)

weight of the gut but, at term, the gut is heavier than the liver. The requirement for different amino acids probably changes as a result of these different growth rates of various organs. The amino acid composition of the foetal calf at 20 weeks is different from that at 40 weeks (Synderman, 1978). In addition to protein synthesis for cell growth, the foetus also synthesizes secretory proteins. The production of plasma proteins is one of the first functions to develop in the foetal liver (Young, 1975) and the foetus can supply all its requirements for polypeptide hormones.

Vitamin and mineral metabolism in the foetus

Vitamins

The transfer of the fat-soluble vitamins (A, D, E and K) is assumed to resemble the transfer of the fatty acids across the placenta. The levels in foetal circulation are generally lower than in the maternal (Dancis and Schneider, 1975; Miller *et al.*, 1976).

The level of the water-soluble vitamins is higher in foetal than in maternal plasma and these vitamins are assumed to be transferred across the placenta by an active transport mechansim. The concentrations of folic acid, vitamin B_1 (thiamin), B_2 (riboflavin), B_6 (pyridoxal) and B_{12} are two- to four-fold higher in foetal than maternal plasma (Dancis and Schneider, 1975). There appears to be a diversion from maternal to foetal needs during pregnancy, as the concentrations of some vitamins (B_6 and B_{12}) are lower in maternal plasma than in plasma from non-pregnant adults. The water-soluble vitamins are required by the foetus as cofactors for enzyme activity.

Minerals

There appears to be a considerable resistance to the passage of electrolytes across the placenta and most are transferred by an active mechanism. The monovalent ions are generally present in foetal plasma at concentrations equal to or below those in the adult. Concentrations of the divalent ions can be several-fold higher in foetal than in maternal plasma. Calcium, phosphate and iron are required in large amounts by the foetus for bone and haemoglobin formation. The foetal requirement for iron during late pregnancy can account for 90% of the turnover in the maternal plasma (Dancis and Schneider, 1975). Traces of manganese, magnesium, zinc and copper are essential as cofactors for enzyme synthesis and activation. Zinc is also necessary for the efficient functioning of the mitotic spindle during cell division and therefore has an essential rôle during development. Iodine is required for the synthesis of thyroid hormones (Williams, 1977).

Maternal nutrition and foetal growth

Maternal metabolism changes during pregnancy. Lipid stores in maternal adipose tissue increase over the first two-thirds of the gestation period, but towards the end of pregnancy lipolysis in adipose tissue increases and there is a rise in plasma concentrations of free fatty acids (Hull, 1975b). In general, malnutrition in the mother results in the production of foetuses of low body weight at birth (Wallace, 1948). This effect is greater if the malnutrition occurs in late rather than early pregnancy. Because of the mobilization of maternal energy stores during late pregnancy, the foetuses of animals in poor body condition, or of young animals which had not reached their mature body size at mating, are more susceptible to maternal malnutrition than the foetuses of mature animals in good body condition (Robinson, 1977).

Undernutrition in early pregnancy

In view of the small size of the foetus in early gestation it is not surprising that maternal undernutrition has little effect on foetal size at this stage of development. Very little effect on foetal weight was observed in a number of studies in which ewes were subjected to restricted food intake during the first half of pregnancy (Robinson, 1977). However, placental weight may be reduced by maternal undernutrition in early pregnancy and some inhibition in placental function may result in a high rate of abortion.

Undernutrition in late pregnancy

The foetal lamb gains approximately 850, 500 and 250 g/kg of its birth weight in the last 8, 4 and 2 weeks of gestation respectively. Maternal undernutrition at this time can have a large effect on foetal birth weight (Fig. 5.8) (Wallace, 1948). Birth weight also decreases as

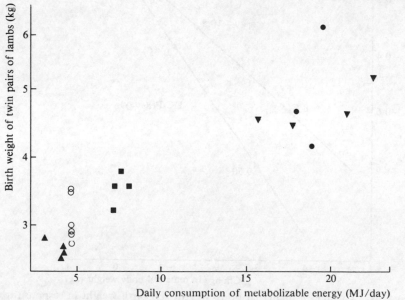

Fig. 5.8.   Effects of maternal nutrition on foetal birth weight in sheep (●, super-maintenance; ■, maintenance; ▲, sub-maintenance; ▼, high-plane; ○, low-plane). (From Wallace, 1948.)

the litter size increases suggesting that, with large litters, there is a restriction in nutrient supply to the foetus even in well nourished mothers (Blaxter, 1961). Even with small litters, mobilization of both maternal and foetal energy reserves (glycogen and lipid) generally occurs before birth, suggesting that the high energy requirements of the foetus at term cannot be met from maternal food intake alone. Decreased maternal protein intake also affects foetal growth even when energy intake is adequate. If the amino acid supply to the foetus is reduced, foetal protein synthesis is decreased and long-term growth retardation may occur. With either maternal protein or energy deficiency, mobilization of maternal body reserves occurs and there is a greater effect on the maternal than on the foetal body weight (Fig. 5.9). The mother can sustain the foetus at the expense of her own body tissues but this ability is less in the case of protein deficiency than it is for energy deficiency. Sustaining the foetus during periods of under-nutrition can result in lowering of the maternal plasma glucose concentrations and raising maternal plasma fatty acid and ketone body

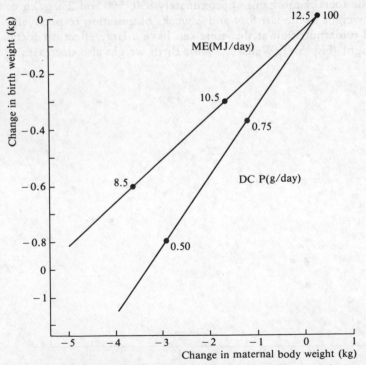

Fig. 5.9.   Changes in maternal body weight and birth weight in response to reduction in the dietary digestible crude protein or metabolizable energy (upper line, reduced ME; lower line, reduced dietary crude protein DCP). (From Robinson, 1977.)

concentrations, which can be fatal in extreme cases (i.e. pregnancy toxaemia).

Foetal compensation for maternal undernutrition

The foetus can alter its metabolism to a certain extent to compensate for changes in maternal nutrition. Starvation of the pregnant ewe results in a shift from glucose to amino acid oxidation in the foetal tissues (Girard *et al.*, 1979). Mobilization of foetal lipid and glycogen reserves, and possibly adaptation to fructose metabolism, can also occur during starvation. Blood supplies to various organs can be altered, following injury to the utero-placental circulation, in order to maintain the supply of glucose and oxygen to the brain and heart (Table 5.4) (Creasy *et al.*, 1973). When foetal growth retardation does occur there is a sparing of some organs such as the brain, heart and kidneys at the expense of other organs such as liver, thymus, spleen and skeletal muscle (Creasy *et al.*, 1973).

Table 5.4   Measurement of the distribution of foetal cardiac output. (From Creasy *et al.*, 1973)

Organ	Proportion of cardiac output	
	Control	Restricted utero-placental circulation
Brain	0.034	0.068
Gut	0.066	0.108
Liver	0.005	0.005
Kidney	0.031	0.050
Lung	0.054	0.017
Placenta	0.419	0.291

Trace element deficiency

Deficiencies of the trace elements in maternal diets can adversely affect foetal development. Maternal copper deficiency can cause abnormal foetal brain development (demyelination and cavitation of the cerebrum in the most severe cases and lack of coordination of movement in milder cases) and weakness of the bone resulting in skeletal defects (Williams, 1977). Severe manganese deficiency leads to a high abortion rate or short postnatal survival times. Shortening of the bones of the legs may occur due to manganese deficiency, together with abnormal pancreatic tissue growth, and loss of balance due to defective development of the inner ear (Williams,

1977). Severe zinc deficiency has widespread effects on foetal development including deformities of the tail and legs, defective lungs and urigenital system and gross brain malfunction. Iron deficiency results in anaemia, and mobilization of maternal iron reserves to accommodate foetal requirements makes maternal anaemia common in human pregnancy. Iodine deficiency causes abortions or stillbirths; in less severe cases the newborn animal may be weak and hairless. Calcium deficiency can affect skeletal size and development and the rate of calcium transfer across the placenta in late gestation may limit foetal size in ewes bearing large litters.

MATERNAL ADAPTATIONS TO PREGNANCY

Supporting foetal growth imposes an increased demand on the metabolism of the pregnant animal. As the growth of the foetus is greatest during the latter part of pregnancy, the demands on the mother are also greatest at this time; the energy cost to the mother in early and mid pregnancy is thought to be slight. The foetus requires sources of energy and precursors for tissue biosynthesis. In the ewe it has been estimated that the energy cost in late pregnancy is approximately 38 kJ/kg per day (Lindsay, 1973) and that the pregnant uterus removes approximately 40 g amino acids per day (Lindsay, 1971). To accommodate these demands, there is an increase in food intake during pregnancy, although food intake may be restricted in very late pregnancy.

The increase in food intake may, to some extent, account for the changes in weight of the non-reproductive organs of the pregnant animal. In both the rat and the ewe there is an increase in the weight of the liver and gastro-intestinal tract in late pregnancy. In well-nourished ewes the increases can be of the order of 30%; in ewes maintained on a low plane of nutrition a lower but consistent increase in the weight of the liver and gastro-intestinal tract is observed (Robinson, McDonald, McHattie and Pennie, 1978). The increase in liver weight appears to be associated both with cell enlargement and with increased cell numbers.

Carbohydrate metabolism in pregnancy

Glucose is the principal energy source of the pregnant uterus and it has been suggested that up to 70% of the glucose turnover in the ewe is removed by the foetus near term. Therefore, in late pregnancy, the utilization of glucose by the pregnant animal increases substantially. In the simple-stomached animal the glucose is absorbed from the diet and there is no apparent increase in the rate of gluconeogenesis. In the ruminant, which absorbs little dietary glucose, the increased requirement is met almost entirely from increased rates of gluconeogenesis in the liver and kidney (Bergman, 1973). When these requirements are high (as in ewes carrying more than one lamb) rates of gluconeogenesis may be inadequate and blood glucose levels fall.

In the ewe, rates of gluconeogenesis increase approximately twofold in late pregnancy. In non-pregnant animals gluconeogenesis can be related to the energy intake, and it appears that the increased rates of gluconeogenesis in pregnancy may be a consequence of the increased food intake rather than of pregnancy *per se* (Lindsay, 1973). Ewes on a fixed food intake show only slight increases in glucose entry rate as pregnancy proceeds. Therefore, substrate supply, together with the increase in liver size, appears to be the principal regulator of glucose synthesis in the liver of the pregnant ruminant. Of the known precursors of glucose, there appears to be no change in the proportion of glucose derived from amino acids but propionate may be relatively more important in the pregnant than in the non-pregnant animal (Lindsay, 1971).

There are indications that during pregnancy, to accommodate the increased demand for glucose by the foetus, glucose utilization by maternal tissues is decreased in ruminant and simple-stomached animals. The increase in the rate of gluconeogenesis in the pregnant ewe is insufficient to meet the demands of the pregnant uterus, and the normal requirements of the extra-uterine tissues and glucose contribution to carbon dioxide production in the extra-uterine tissues has been calculated to fall in late pregnancy from 10 to 20% or less. Mobilization of fat depots probably supplies the additional energy for metabolism in the extra-uterine tissue. It has been proposed that endocrine factors, especially insulin and progesterone secretion, regulate glucose utilization by the extra-uterine tissues in late pregnancy (Lindsay, 1971 and 1973).

Nitrogen metabolism in pregnancy

The high rate of protein synthesis in the foetus in late pregnancy requires a supply of amino acids from the maternal circulation. In the rat, supplies of amino acids are accumulated as maternal protein in early pregnancy for use during periods of rapid foetal growth (Naismith and Morgan, 1976). During early and mid pregnancy, when foetal requirements are low, the dam retains nitrogen in muscle to give an increase in lean tissue of 8.5%. In late pregnancy, the protein reserve is mobilized irrespective of the protein intake of the mother, indicating that muscle breakdown at this time is hormonally controlled. There is no net gain in protein in the maternal rat as a result of pregnancy (Naismith and Morgan, 1976). Although such detailed studies have not been performed in the pregnant ruminant, available data suggest a similar mechanism may operate. During the last 8 weeks of pregnancy in the ewe there is a redistribution of protein in the body. Non-carcass protein decreases in ewes maintained on high or low planes of nutrition; carcass protein tends to remain constant, but this is due to the inclusion of the udder with the carcass. Allowing for the substantial growth of the udder in the last weeks before parturition, there is substantial breakdown of muscle protein in ewes in late pregnancy (Robinson et al., 1978).

In addition to the mobilization of muscle protein to meet the nitrogen demands of the foetus, the ewe appears to become more efficient in utilizing digested nitrogen as pregnancy advances. This is reflected in a decrease of approximately 50% in the calculated intakes of apparently digested nitrogen required for zero nitrogen balance, from mid pregnancy to parturition (Robinson and Forbes, 1967). An explanation for this increased efficiency may be that the rate of recycling of urea to the digestive tract is higher in pregnant than in non-pregnant sheep (Nolan and Leng, 1970). An increase in efficiency of absorption of amino acids from the digestive tract may also occur. The rate of oxidation of amino acids in the tissues appears to be unchanged as the contribution of amino acids to carbon dioxide is unaffected by pregnancy.

Lipid metabolism in pregnancy

The deposition and mobilization of fat during pregnancy is also a biphasic process. During early and mid pregnancy lipid reserves accumulate, and during late pregnancy and early lactation these reserves are mobilized. The timing of the mobilization depends on the species, the number of foetuses carried and the plane of nutrition of the pregnant or lactating animal. The pregnant ewe carrying more than one lamb may have to mobilize fat depots several weeks before parturition, whereas the well fed dairy cow will not require this additional energy source until just prior to term. In both cases, substantial portions of the lipid deposited during pregnancy may be utilized after parturition to maintain milk production. The increase in lipid stores in pregnancy is due to an increase in the volume of the adipocytes rather than to an increase in adipocyte number. Changes in adipocyte volume during pregnancy have been observed in the cow, rat, goat, and sheep (Flint, Sinnett-Smith, Clegg and Vernon, 1979; Vernon, 1980) and are associated with increased rates of lipid synthesis within the cell. There are also changes in the activities of the enzymes involved in fatty acid synthesis and esterification. Decreases in the activities of acetyl-CoA carbo-xylase and glucose-6-phosphate and NADP-malate dehydrogenase were found in adipose tissue from goats during late pregnancy. The rate of fatty acid esterification in cattle reaches a peak just before term (Vernon, 1980).

The factors regulating lipid metabolism in pregnancy have still to be elucidated. Plasma insulin levels decrease in late pregnancy in the sheep, cow and rat, and this may contribute to the mobilization of lipid at this time. In non-ruminants the insulin to glucagon ratio appears to regulate lipid metabolism in adipose tissue, but in ruminants it has been suggested that the insulin to growth hormone ratio is an important regulator during pregnancy and lactation (Vernon, 1980). Progesterone may also have a rôle in regulating lipolysis in late pregnancy, as it has been shown to be ketogenic in the rat (Lindsay, 1973).

Ketone bodies are produced from free fatty acids taken up by the liver. In late pregnancy in the ewe, when energy demands may exceed food intake, excessive mobilization of fat depots can lead to the accumulation of pathological quantities of ketones in the blood (i.e. pregnancy toxaemia). Several factors appear to be responsible for this condition. An inadequate supply of carbohydrate in the form of glucose results in a fall in blood glucose and insulin concentrations. As blood glucose falls, increasing quantities of free fatty acids are mobilized and are taken up by the liver. Changes in the liver itself lead to an increased proportion of the fatty acids being converted to ketone bodies with the subsequent development of ketosis; loss of appetite exacerbates the condition. The key rôle of glucose in the development of ketosis is evident from the therapeutic effects of administering intravenous glucose to animals with pregnancy toxaemia. The pregnant ruminant, and the sheep in particular, is susceptible to ketosis (Ch. 9) because of its high requirements for glucose and its complete dependence on gluconeogensis to fulfil this need.

NEONATAL NUTRITION

At birth the food supply to the developing animal changes dramati-cally. From existing on a 'diet' composed of a continuous supply of amino acids and carbohydrate (mainly in the form of glucose), the newborn animal has to adapt to a milk diet with a high fat and protein content. Nutrients are no longer transferred directly to the circulation in a pre-digested form and the neonatal animal has to establish rapidly a system for the digestion and absorption of nutrients. In addition, food intake in postnatal life is intermittent, demanding more sophisticated regulation of the concentration of nutrients, such as glucose, in blood.

The utilization of nutrients must also change. Tissue growth still continues at a rapid rate but the newborn animal has the new problem of maintaining body temperature. This requires an increase in oxidative metabolism, especially in view of the high ratio of surface area to body weight of the young animal compared with the adult.

Development of the gastro-intestinal tract

Taste buds appear on the tongue of the foetal lamb during the first third of the gestation period and the taste system is functional over the last third of gestation. Swallowing begins at approximately 80 days of gestation in the sheep, and towards term the foetus may swallow as much as 700 ml of amniotic fluid each day (Bradley and Mistretta, 1973).

All sections of the gastro-intestinal tract can be detected in the embryo and are present at birth. However, the stage of development of the individual sections at birth differs, as does their rate of growth in the neonatal period (Fig. 5.10) (Wardrop and Coombe, 1960). The abomasum and small intestines of the ruminant are functional at birth and, during the 1st week after birth, the abomasum has the fastest growth rate of all the parts of the alimentary tract. The weight of the abomasum as a proportion of the total stomach weight begins to decrease as the rumen develops; the rumen has the fastest growth rate of the compartments stomach (Fig. 5.11) during the period from 2 to 8 weeks after birth. The changes in sizes of the compartments stomach reflect the diet during this period. In the neonatal ruminant an oesophageal groove ensures that milk bypasses the rumen and enters the abomasum directly but, later, solid food is eaten and enters the rumen.

Milk clots rapidly on entering the stomach and clot formation is necessary for milk retention in the stomach, allowing slow digestion to occur. Within 2 h of suckling, the clot has been digested to the extent of allowing half the stomach contents to pass into the small intestine. The remaining, predominantly fatty, material passes to the intestine 3 to 4 h after feeding.

In ruminants and non-ruminants alike the small intestine is well developed at birth and will actively absorb glucose and some amino acids (Wilson and Lin, 1960).

Carbohydrate metabolism in the neonatal animal

Mobilization of carbohydrate reserves at birth

Immediately after birth the concentration of glucose in the blood of the neonatal animal tends to fall. Rapid mobilization of the glycogen

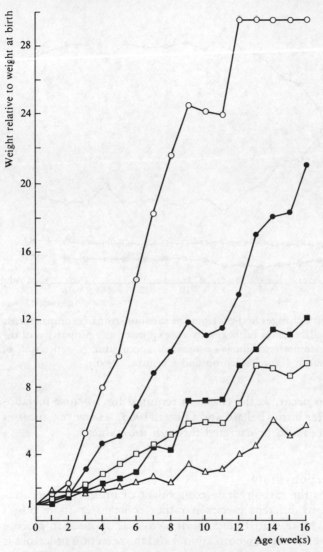

Fig. 5.10. Changes in weights of the stomachs of the lamb after birth: results are expressed relative to their weights at birth (○, rumen; ●, reticulum; ■, omasum, □, small intestine; △, abomasum). (From Wardrop and Coombe, 1960.)

reserves of the liver and skeletal muscle occurs to maintain the blood concentration (Fig. 5.4). Glycogenolysis appears to precede, rather than be a result of, the drop in the blood glucose concentration, and the glycogen content of the liver and muscle falls dramatically within 24 h of birth. Some utilization of fructose, which accumulates in foetal

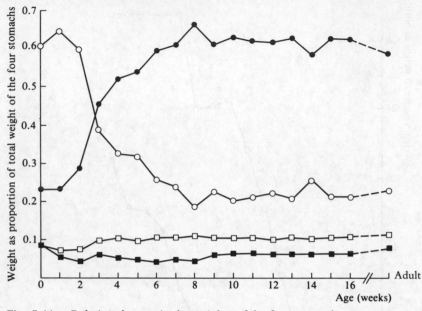

Fig. 5.11. Relative changes in the weights of the four stomach compartments of the lamb after birth: results are expressed as a proportion of the total stomach weight (●, rumen; ○, abomasum; □, reticulum; ■, omasum). (From Wardrop and Coombe, 1960.)

blood, may also occur, as the enzymes required for fructose metabolism develop after birth (Ballard and Oliver, 1965). However, most of the fructose appears to be excreted through the kidneys.

Milk carbohydrate

Lactose is the carbohydrate component of milk. Its concentration in milk from different species is rather constant at about 50 g/l (Blaxter, 1961). No essential function of lactose as opposed to glucose has been observed in the newborn animal and the secretion of lactose is probably to facilitate storage in the maternal mammary gland (Walker, 1968). The importance of milk lactose as an energy source for the neonatal animal depends on the fat content of the milk. The proportion of the total calories derived from lactose varies from 0.6 in the horse, to 0.3 in the goat and cow, and 0.2 in the sheep and pig (Blaxter, 1961).

Digestion of carbohydrates

The ability to digest lactose develops during gestation and is fully functional at birth. The enzyme, lactase, which hydrolyses lactose to glucose and galactose, is present in the intestines at high activity during early neonatal life (Dahlqvist, 1961). Active absorption of glucose and galactose by the intestinal mucosa is also present at birth (Wilson and Lin, 1960). When solid food is taken, the activity of lactase in the intestines decreases slowly while the activities of other carbohydrate-digesting enzymes increase (e.g. maltase, trehalase and amylase). These events appear to be hormonally regulated by thyroxine and glucocorticoids, as adrenalectomy and thyroidectomy delay the changes (Walker, 1968).

Control of blood glucose concentrations in the newborn animal

Although glucose is available in the diet as lactose, the neonatal animal can also synthesize glucose in the liver and kidney from glycerol, lactate, galactose and amino acids. The enzymes required for glucose synthesis are present in the liver of the foetal sheep, but active gluconeogenesis does not occur *in vivo* until immediately after birth and the gluconeogenic enzymes increase in activity postnatally (Warnes *et al.*, 1977). This synthesis of glucose, together with the ingestion of glucose as lactose, enables glycogen reserves to be replenished in the tissues of the neonatal animal in the first few weeks after birth (Ballard and Oliver, 1965). Glycogen stores and gluconeogenesis are required by the newborn animal in order to maintain a constant blood glucose concentration between meals.

The regulation of the blood glucose concentration in the neonatal animal develops quickly and is under endocrine control as in the mature animal. Immediately after birth there is a fall in plasma insulin and a rise in plasma glucagon concentration. Large increases in plasma insulin concentration are seen in young lambs during the period after feeding when plasma glucose concentration increases. There is also an immediate transitory increase in insulin concentration following sucking, which is probably reflex in origin (Shelley *et al.*, 1975).

Nitrogen metabolism in the neonatal animal

The newborn and sucking animal has a very rapid growth rate which requires a high rate of protein synthesis, although species differences can be seen and these generally relate to the maturity of the animal at birth (Mersmann, 1974). The amino acids required for protein synthesis are derived from the milk proteins. The supply of essential amino acids in milk is more than sufficient to meet the growth requirements of the young animal (Table 5.5). In the newborn pig and puppy, 900 g/kg of

Table 5.5 Amino acid intake and incorporation into protein in the piglet while it doubles its birth weight (7 days)

	Arg	His	Ile	Leu	Lys	Met	Phe	Thr	Try	Val	Tyr	Cys
Total intake of amino acid in sow's milk (g)	23.5	9.2	17.2	32.8	30.4	5.6	14.4	14.4	–	20.4	–	5.6
Incorporation of amino acid into body tissue of piglets (g)	10.1	4.0	5.8	10.9	12.0	2.9	6.1	6.1	1.3	9.3	4.2	1.9

From McCance and Widdowson (1964).

the protein nitrogen absorbed is found to be incorporated into tissue protein in the first few days after birth (McCance and Widdowson, 1964).

Digestion and absorption of protein

Gamma globulins can be transmitted to the newborn animal in the colostrum (i.e. the first milk produced after birth, which is rich in protein). The immunoglobulins are absorbed intact by passing through cells of the gut into the lymphatic system and reaching the circulation via the thoracic duct. The colostrum of the cow and pig contains a trypsin inhibitor which protects the immunoglobulins from proteolysis in the intestines. In the pig, the cells which absorb the intact protein molecules close within 24 h of birth and no further absorption takes place (McCance and Widdowson, 1964). Closure appears to be regulated by glucocorticoids.

Proteolysis of the milk proteins occurs under the action of rennin and trypsin, and the amino acids released are actively absorbed in the intestines. Over 800 g/kg of the milk protein is absorbed by the intestines. In the pig, active absorption of amino acids is present at birth and increases three-fold during the sucking period (Mersmann, 1974). Development of pepsin activity in the stomach of pigs and calves is dependent on the ingestion of solid food, while rennin activity decreases after birth. Tryptic activity is present in newborn pigs and changes little with age (Blaxter, 1961).

Nitrogen excretion

Catabolism of protein and amino acids in the neonatal animal requires a functional kidney, as excretory nitrogen can no longer be transferred to the maternal circulation via the placenta. The kidney develops during gestation and some urine may be excreted by the foetal lamb into the amniotic and allantoic fluids late in gestation. Renal function may not be completely developed at birth: young puppies cannot concentrate their urine as efficiently as adult dogs and amino acids may be lost in urine. In addition, urea accumulates in the blood of the neonatal animal in the 1st day after birth (McCance and Widdowson, 1964). Amino acid transaminases and urea-cycle enzymes develop immediately after birth in those species which lack the enzymes during foetal life (Jones, 1976).

Lipid metabolism in the newborn animal

Changes at birth

At birth the plasma of the ruminant has a very low concentration of unesterified fatty acids. Within 1 h of birth there is a large increase in their concentration, which continues over the next few hours. The origin of these unesterified fatty acids is the adipose tissue, which is mobilized rapidly in response to reduced environmental temperatures and catecholamine release during birth. Within 72 h of birth the concentrations of the unesterified fatty acids in plasma fall until they may account for less than 50 g/kg of the total fatty acids present (Noble, 1979). With the onset of sucking the concentration of plasma triglycerides, phospholipids, cholesterol and cholesteryl esters increases rapidly.

Digestion of milk fat

Milk clots rapidly as it enters the stomach and most of the milk fat is entrapped in the casein coagulate of the milk clot. Lipid hydrolysis occurs in the stomach under the action of the pregastric esterase, which is mixed with the milk on swallowing. Estimates of the extent of lipid hydrolysis in the stomach range from 200 g to 650 g/kg of the total lipid offered, probably depending on the retention time. On entering the small intestine the pregastric esterase activity falls, and bile and pancreatic lipase complete the process of lipid digestion. Immediately after birth the concentration of lipase in the pancreas and its rate of secretion into the intestine are low, but both increase considerably within the first few days after birth. The rate of absorption of fatty acids from the small intestine is at a maximum during early life (Noble, 1979).

Essential fatty acids in the newborn animal

Polyunsaturated fatty acids are essential for cellular membrane formation and function, and for the synthesis of prostaglandins. Deficiency results in reduced growth rates and skin disorders. Tissues and plasma from young non-ruminants (rabbits and pigs) have a high content of polyunsaturated fatty acids which have been supplied from the maternal circulation via the placenta. Neonatal ruminants have a very low body content of essential fatty acids and, in comparison with non-ruminants, might be classified as deficient in essential fatty acids. However, no signs of deficiency are observed under normal circumstances. In lambs reared on ewe's milk there is a gradual accumulation of essential fatty acids into tissues during the first weeks after birth, even though ewe's milk is not rich in essential fatty acids. The young ruminant appears to be more efficient than the non-ruminant in absorbing and retaining dietary essential fatty acids during the first weeks after birth. However, it has been suggested that practical advantages might be gained by artificially increasing the supply of essential fatty acids to newborn ruminants exposed to adverse conditions (multiple births, high infection risks and environmental stress) (Noble, 1979).

Brown adipose tissue

Brown adipose tissue is a characteristic tissue of the newborn animal and has an important rôle in thermoregulation immediately after birth. The newborn animal has a thinner coat and less subcutaneous fat than the adult and, therefore, there is a higher rate of heat loss. In addition, all animals are born wet and substantial heat loss occurs due to evaporation especially when birth occurs in the open. Non-ruminants accumulate large amounts of brown adipose tissue around and between the muscles of the neck and back. Ruminants have large deposits in the abdominal cavity and around large blood vessels.

The darker colour of the brown adipose tissue compared with white adipose tissue is due to its greater density of mitochondria and plentiful blood supply. Exposure of the newborn animal to cold leads to non-shivering heat production. This is achieved by sympathetic nervous stimulation of brown adipose tissue which results in lipolysis and oxidation of long-chain fatty acids within the tissue. The oxidation of the free fatty acids is not dependent on ATP formation as it is in other tissues, and appears to be regulated by a degree of uncoupling of respiration from phosphorylation. Ruminants, unlike non-ruminants, have very little white adipose tissue in early life, and brown adipose tissue appears to fulfil some of the functions of white adipose tissue in the newborn ruminant. Whereas only white adipose tissue is mobilized during fasting in the newborn rabbit, the lamb mobilizes fat from brown adipose tissue in response to fasting as well as to cold exposure. In lambs and calves brown adipose tissue tends to lose its characteristic features during the first 2 to 3 weeks after birth and brown adipose cells are converted to white adipose tissue (Hull, 1966; Noble, 1979).

Metabolism of lipid after birth

The oxidation of fatty acids, which is low in the foetal tissues, increases rapidly after birth when milk fat becomes available (Hull, 1975b). The proportion of total energy supplied by milk fat shows considerable species variation, being 0.7 to 0.8 in the pig, sheep and cow, but only 0.3 to 0.4 in the horse.

During the first 3 to 4 weeks of postnatal life there is a rapid increase in adipose tissue mass. In the lamb, lipid content of the body increases from 20 to 90 g/kg during the first weeks after birth. Dietary fatty acids are the major precursors of this growing lipid store and fatty acids synthesized *de novo* represent less than 30 g/kg of those esterified in the lamb during the first 17 days after birth (Vernon, 1980). The activities of the enzymes of fatty acid synthesis in the non-ruminant, which are high in foetal liver and adipose tissue, decrease during the sucking period and rise again on weaning (Mersmann, 1974; Jones and Ashton, 1976). The deposition of lipid in the newborn animal appears to be hormonally regulated by growth hormone. Hypophysectomized lambs have an increased rate of lipid deposition but treatment with growth hormone reduces the rate of lipid storage.

Mineral metabolism in the newborn animal

Milk provides most of the trace elements required by the newborn animal and the concentration of the trace elements in colostrum is often much higher than in milk. However, the quantities supplied may not be adequate for the high requirement of the growing animal, and mobilization of body reserves may be necessary to meet the deficit. In the newborn animal there is a fall in the concentration of iron in the fat-free body during the suckling period due to the depletion of the inorganic iron content of the liver and spleen. Iron deficiency is a special consideration in stall-fed pigs. The pig has a low iron content at birth with no appreciable liver reserves; on open pasture iron can be obtained from the soil, but in stall-fed pigs anaemia may develop unless an iron supplement is given. Although not as susceptible as pigs, lambs and calves can also develop iron deficiency when raised on milk-based diets. The copper content of the milk is also low and mobilization of the liver reserves of the neonatal animal may be required. Calcium, which is needed in large quantities for skeletal growth, is present in high concentrations in milk (Blaxter, 1961).

Malnutrition in newborn animals

Energy and protein undernutrition

The first weeks after birth are characterized by high growth rates, and undernutrition during this period can cause growth retardation and abnormalities. The newborn animal is dependent on the supply of milk from the mother and growth rates are related to milk intake (Fig. 5.12). Large litters can result in reduced availability of milk for individual animals, and restriction of maternal food reduces milk yield and the growth of the newborn animal. Animals with a high potential for lactation may mobilize body reserves to maintain milk yield.

The effects of undernutrition at different stages of development vary with species. The pig appears to be most susceptible during early postnatal life. Whereas in the dog and rat maternal protein deficiency during pregnancy results in a permanent retardation of brain development in the foetus, in the pig maternal protein deficiency has only a marginal effect on the development of the foetal brain. However, a protein-deficient diet given to pigs 3 to 12 weeks after birth produces

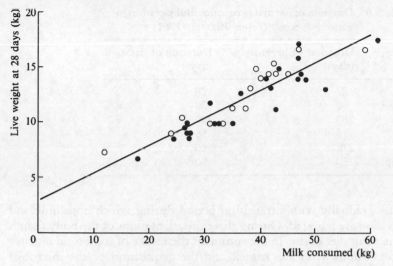

Fig. 5.12. The relationship between live weight of the lamb and total amount of milk consumed (o, Suffolk; ●, Border Leicester × Cheviot). (From Wallace, 1948.)

permanent changes in the neurons and neuroglial cells, and restricted food intake for the 1st year of life produces a permanent reduction in the cellular content of the brain (Cheek, 1975).

Trace element deficiency

Deficiency of trace elements during early development can cause growth abnormalities. Iron deficiency in pigs causes laboured and irregular breathing (thrumps) and loss of appetite, piglets lose weight and some die. Copper deficiency can result in anaemia as well as skeletal abnormalities, and changes in the pigmentation and growth of hair and wool. Manganese deficiency causes impaired growth and abnormalities of bone, often resulting in lameness and difficulty in standing. Zinc deficiency causes growth retardation and dwarfism with shortening of the bone length. Selenium is also required for growth, and deficiency can result in muscular dystrophy in lambs, calves and rabbits, and subcutaneous haemorrhages in chicks. High levels of some trace elements are toxic and also result in growth abnormalities (Schutte, 1964).

Weaning

The duration of the sucking period varies from species to species (Table 5.6). Unlike the changes at birth, the change to an adult diet

Table 5.6   Duration of normal pregnancy and lactation in
             various species. (From Blaxter, 1961)

	Duration of pregnancy (days)	Duration of lactation (days)
Rat	22	28
Rabbit	30	30
Man	280	180
Pig	115	56
Ox	278	60
Sheep	150	50

occurs gradually with a transition period during which both milk and solid food are ingested. During this time adaptations of the body tissues to the adult diet occur. In the ruminant the intake of solid food initiates the development of the rumen and the acquisition of the microbial population of the rumen. An all-milk diet during this time retards the development of the rumen but has no effect on the growth of the abomasum. The development of the rumen is accompanied by an increased ability to absorb and metabolize short-chain fatty acids, which are produced in the rumen as a result of microbial fermentation. The stimulus for development of the ruminant stomach appears to be the presence of VFA (particularly butyrate) in the developing rumen. Propionate becomes the major precursor of glucose synthesis in the liver, and peripheral tissues adapt to the utilization of acetate for energy production and lipid biosynthesis.

In the non-ruminant, weaning involves a change from a diet rich in fat to one in which carbohydrates are the major energy source. Intake of solid food is required for the development of the carbohydrate-digesting enzymes (e.g. sucrase and maltase), as well as for the elongation of microvilli in the epithelial cells of the small intestine (Walker, 1968). With the increasing intake of carbohydrate, gluconeogenesis is reduced (Bassett and Jones, 1975), and there is an increase in the biosynthesis of the fatty acids *de novo* in the liver and adipose tissue (Mersmann, 1974).

REFERENCES

Alexander, G., 1964. Studies on the placenta of the sheep, *J. Reprod. Fert.*
    7: 289–322.
Alexander, G., 1978. Quantitative development of adipose tissue in foetal
    sheep, *Aust. J. biol. Sci.* **31**: 489–503.

Amoroso, E. C., 1961. Histology of the placenta, *Br. med. Bull.* **17**: 81–90.

Ballard, F. J., Hanson, R. W. and Kronfeld, D. S., 1969. Gluconeogenesis and lipogenesis in tissue from ruminant and nonruminant animals, *Fedn Proc. Fedn Am. Socs exp. Biol.* **28**: 218–31.

Ballard, F. J. and Oliver, I. T., 1965. Carbohydrate metabolism in liver from foetal and neonatal sheep, *Biochem. J.* **95**: 191–200.

Barcroft, Sir Joseph, 1946. *Researches on Perinatal Life*, Vol. 1. Blackwell, Oxford.

Barnes, R. J., 1976. Water and mineral exchange between maternal and foetal fluids. In *Fetal Physiology and Medicine* (ed. R. W. Beard and P. W. Nathenielsz), pp. 194–214. Saunders, London.

Bassett, J. M. and Jones, C. T., 1975. Fetal glucose metabolism. In *Fetal Physiology and Medicine* (ed. R. W. Beard and P. W. Nathanielsz), pp. 158–72. Saunders, London.

Battaglia, F. C. and Meschia, G., 1978. Principal substrates of fetal metabolism, *Physiol. Rev.* **58**: 499–527.

Bergman, E. N., 1973. Glucose metabolism in ruminants as related to hypoglycemia and ketosis, *Cornell Vet.* **63**: 341–62.

Blaxter, K. L., 1961. Lactation and the growth of the young. In *Milk: the Mammary Gland and its Secretion* (ed. S. K. Kon and A. T. Cowie), Vol. II, pp. 305–61. Academic Press, New York.

Blaxter, K. L., 1964. Protein metabolism and requirements in pregnancy and lactation. In *Mammalian Protein Metabolism* (ed. H. N. Munro and J. B. Allison). Vol. II, pp. 173–223. Academic Press, New York.

Bradley, R. M. and Mistretta, Charlotte M., 1973. The sense of taste and swallowing activity in foetal sheep. In *Foetal and Neonatal Physiology*, *Proc. Sir Joseph Barcroft Centenary Symp.* (ed. R. S. Comline, K. W. Cross, G. S. Dawes and P. W. Nathanielsz), pp. 77–81. Cambridge University Press, Cambridge.

Caton, D., Abrams, R. M., Lackore, L. K., James, G. B. and Barron, D. H., 1973. Effects of progesterone administration on the rate of uterine blood flow of early pregnant sheep. In *Foetal and Neonatal Physiology, Proc. Sir Joseph Barcroft Centenary Symp.* (ed. R. S. Comline, K. W. Cross, G. S. Dawes and P. W. Nathanielsz), pp. 286–7. Cambridge University Press, Cambridge.

Cheek, D. B., 1975. Maternal nutritional restriction and fetal brain growth. In *Fetal and Postnatal Cellular Growth* (ed. D. B. Cheek), pp. 111–31. Wiley, New York.

Creasy, R. K. de Swiet, M., Kahanpää, K. V., Young, W. P., and Rudolph, A. M., 1973. Pathophysiological changes in the foetal lamb with growth retardation. In *Foetal and Neonatal Physiology, Proc. Sir Joseph Barcroft Centenary Symp.*(ed. R. S. Comline, K. W. Cross, G. S. Dawes and P. W. Nathanielsz), pp. 398–402. Cambridge University Press, Cambridge.

Dahlqvist, A., 1961. Intestinal carbohydrases of a new-born pig, *Nature, Lond.* **190**: 31–2.

Dancis, J. and Schneider, H., 1975. Physiology: transfer and barrier function. In *The Placenta* (ed. P. Gruenwald), pp. 98–124 MTP Press, Lancaster.

Dawes, G. S. and Shelley, Heather J., 1968. Physiological aspects of carbohydrate metabolism in the foetus and newborn. In *Carbohydrate*

Metabolism and its Disorders (ed. F. Dickens, P. J. Randle and W. J. Whelan), Vol. 2, pp. 87–121. Academic Press London.

Elphick, M. C. and Hull, D., 1977. Rabbit placental clearing-factor lipase and transfer to the foetus of fatty acids derived from triglycerides injected into the mother, *J. Physiol., Lond.* **273**: 475–87

Flint, D. J., Sinnett-Smith, P. A., Clegg, R. A. and Vernon, R. G., 1979. Role of insulin receptors in the changing metabolism of adipose tissue during pregnancy and lactation in the rat, *Biochem. J.* **182**: 421–7.

Girard, J., Pintado, E. and Ferre, P., 1979. Fuel metabolism in the mammalian fetus, *Annls. Biol. anim. Biochim. Biophys.* **19** (1B) : 181–97.

Hull, D., 1966. The structure and function of brown adipose tissue, *Br. med. Bull.* **22**: 92–6.

Hull, D., 1975a. Storage and supply of fatty acids before and after birth, *Br. med. Bull.* **31**: 32–6.

Hull, D., 1975b. Fetal fat metabolism. In *Fetal Physiology and Medicine* (ed. R. W. Beard and P. W. Nathanielsz), pp. 105–20. Saunders, London.

Jones, C. T., 1976. Fetal metabolism and fetal growth, *J. Reprod. Fert.* **47**: 189–201.

Jones, C. T. and Ashton, I. Karen, 1976. Lipid biosynthesis in liver slices of the foetal guinea pig, *Biochem. J.* **154**: 149–58.

Lemons, J. A., Adcock, E. W., Jones, M. D., Naughton, M. A., Meschia, G. and Battaglia, F. C., 1976. Umbilical uptake of amino acids in the unstressed foetal lamb, *J. clin. Invest.* **58**: 1428–34.

Lindsay, D. B., 1971. Changes in the pattern of glucose metabolism in growth, pregnancy and lactation in ruminants, *Proc. Nutr. Soc.* **30**: 272–7.

Lindsay, D. B., 1973. Metabolic changes induced by pregnancy in the ewe. In *Production Disease in Farm Animals* (ed. J. M. Payne, K. G. Hibbitt and B. F. Sansom), pp. 107–14. Baillière Tindall, London.

McCance, R. A. and Widdowson, Elsie., 1964. Protein metabolism and requirements in the newborn. In *Mammalian Protein Metabolism* (ed. H. N. Munro and J. B. Allison), Vol. II, pp. 225–45. Academic Press, New York.

Mersmann, H. J, 1974. Metabolic patterns in the neonatal swine, *J. Anim. Sci.* **38**: 1022–30.

Miller, J. F. A. P., 1966. Immunity in the foetus and the new-born, *Br. med. Bull.* **22**: 21–6.

Miller, R. K., Koszalka, T. R. and Brent, R. L., 1976. The transport of molecules across placental membranes. In *Cell Surface Review* (ed. G. Poste), Vol. 1, pp. 145–223. North Holland, New York.

Naismith, D. J. and Morgan, B. L. G., 1976. The biphasic nature of protein metabolism during pregnancy in the rat, *Br. J. Nutr.* **36**: 563–6.

Noble, R. C., 1979. Lipid metabolism in the neonatal ruminant, *Prog. Lipid Res.* **18**: 179–216.

Nolan, J. V. and Leng, R. A., 1970. Metabolism of urea in late pregnancy and the possible contribution of amino acid carbon to glucose synthesis in sheep, *Br. J. Nutr.* **24**: 905–15.

Robinson, J. J., 1977. The influence of maternal nutrition on ovine foetal growth, *Proc. Nutr. Soc.* **36**: 9–16.

Robinson, J. J. and Forbes, T. J., 1967. A study of the protein requirements of the mature breeding ewe. 2. Protein utilization in the pregnant ewe, *Br. J. Nutr.* **21**: 879–91.

Robinson, J. J., McDonald, I., McHattie, I. and Pennie, K., 1978. Studies on reproduction in prolific ewes. 4. Sequential changes in the maternal body during pregnancy, *J. agric. Sci., Camb.* **91**: 291–304.

Schutte, K., 1964. *The Biology of the Trace Elements*. Lippincott, Philadelphia.

Shelley, Heather J., 1961. Glycogen reserves and their changes at birth and in anoxia, *Br. med. Bull.* **17**: 137–43.

Shelley, Heather J., Bassett, J. M. and Miller, R. D. G., 1975. Control of carbohydrate metabolism in the foetus and newborn, *Br. med. Bull.* **31**: 37–43.

Silver, Marian, 1976. Fetal energy metabolism. In *Fetal Physiology and Medicine*. (ed. R. W. Beard and P. W. Nathanielsz) pp. 173–93. Saunders, London.

Silver, Marian, Steven, D. H. and Comline, R. S., 1973. Placental exchange and morphology in ruminants and the mare. In *Foetal and Neonatal Physiology, Proc. Sir Joseph Barcroft Centenary Symp.* (ed. R. S. Comline, K. W. Cross, G. S. Dawes and P. W. Nathanielsz), pp. 245–71. Cambridge University Press, Cambridge.

Synderman, S. E., 1978. Protein and amino acid metabolism. In *Perinatal Physiology* (ed. U. Stave), pp. 383–95. Plenum Medical, New York.

Thau, R. B. and Lanman, J. T., 1975. Endocrinological aspects of placental function. In *The Placenta* (ed. P. Gruenwald), pp. 125–44. MTP Press, Lancaster.

Vernon, R. G., 1980. Lipid metabolism in the adipose tissue of ruminant animals, *Prog. Lipid Res.* **19**: 23–106.

Walker, D. G., 1968. Developmental aspects of carbohydrate metabolism. In *Carbohydrate Metabolism and its Disorders* (ed. F. Dickens, P. J. Randle and W. J. Whelan), Vol. 1, pp. 465–96. Academic Press, London.

Wallace, L. R., 1948. The growth of lambs before and after birth in relation to the level of nutrition. Part I, *J. agric. Sci., Camb.* **38**: 93–153 (references 399–401).

Wardrop, I. D. and Coombe, J. B., 1960. The post-natal growth of the visceral organs of the lamb. I. The growth of the visceral organs of the grazing lamb from birth to sixteen weeks of age, *J. agric. Sci., Camb.* **54**: 140–3.

Warnes, Deidre M., Seamark, R. F. and Ballard, F. J., 1977. The appearance of gluconeogenesis at birth in sheep. Activation of the pathway associated with blood oxygenation, *Biochem. J.* **162**: 627–34.

Widdas, W. F., 1961. Transport mechanisms in the foetus, *Br. med. Bull.* **17**: 107–11.

Wigglesworth, J. S., 1966. Foetal growth retardation, *Br. med. Bull.* **22**: 13–5.

Williams, R. B., 1977. Trace elements and congenital abnormalities, *Proc. Nutr. Soc.* **36**: 25–32.

Wilson, T. H. and Lin, E. C. C., 1960. Active transport by intestines of fetal and newborn rabbits, *Am. J. Physiol.* **199**: 1030–2.

Wood, W. G., Pearce, K., Clegg, J. B., Weatherall, D. J., Robinson, J. S., Thorburn, G. D. and Dawes, G. S., 1976. Switch from foetal to adult haemoglobin synthesis in normal and hypophysectomised sheep, *Nature, Lond.* **264**: 799–801.

Wynn, R. W., 1975. Principles of placentation and early human placental development. In *The Placenta* (ed. P. Gruenwald), pp. 18–34. MTP Press, Lancaster.

Young, M., 1975. The accumulation of protein by the fetus. In *Fetal Physiology and Medicine* (ed. R. W. Beard and P. W. Nathanielsz), pp. 59–79. Saunders, London.

6   EGG FORMATION IN POULTRY

A. B. Gilbert and R. Anne Pearson

The complete shelled egg is the sole reproductive product in birds. Consequently, the avian embryo is enclosed in a discrete package which must contain all the nutrients for the production of a viable chick, unlike the mammal in which a continuous supply of nutrients is available from the mother.

Information about the general structure and composition of the egg is available for many avian species (Romanoff and Romanoff, 1949) but essentially only the chicken egg has been studied in any detail (Gilbert, 1971b and 1979). This account must therefore deal almost exclusively with the hen and, although other birds are likely to be similar, it cannot be unequivocally accepted that all aspects of the relationship between nutrition and egg production will be identical throughout the avian group.

The unincubated hen's egg weighs approximately 60 g and contains approximately 40 g water, 7 g protein, 7 g lipid, 0.4 g carbohydrate, 2.5 g minerals and 3 g of non-metallic elements. It consists of three basic parts: the colloquial yolk (the oocyte), forming just over 300 g/kg of the egg; the white (albumen), approximately 600 g/kg; and the calcified shell (approximately 80 g/kg). None of these components are homogeneous, either structurally or chemically (Romanoff and Romanoff, 1949; Gilbert, 1971b and 1979; Freeman and Vince, 1974). The yolk contains nearly all (990 g/kg) of the lipid material of the egg (the remainder occurring almost entirely in the cuticle of the shell), 470 g/kg of the protein (as lipoproteins) and approximately 250 g/kg of the water. The albumen contains the remainder of the water, 500 g/kg of the egg protein and some minerals. The shell appears to be almost anhydrous but has 960 g/kg of the mineral material of the egg, mainly as calcium carbonate.

ANATOMY AND PHYSIOLOGY OF EGG FORMATION

The following account is based on many reviews of the functional anatomy and endocrinology of reproduction in birds, but in particular on several chapters in Bell and Freeman (1971), and on Lofts and Murton (1973), Gilbert (1979), Follett and Robinson (1980), and Wingfield and Farner (1980).

In contrast to mammals, there is only one functional ovary and oviduct in most avian species; the organs on the right side usually remain vestigial in the adult. However, in common with mammals, the single ovary has the dual rôle of steroidogenesis and gametogenesis.

Steroidogenesis has many biochemical features in common with mammals, although the cells responsible for producing each class of steroid may not always be homologous. Moreover, the post-ovulatory follicle does not produce progesterone (it is not truly a corpus luteum) and, instead, progesterone is produced by the pre-ovulatory follicles. During a short period in the daily ovulatory cycle there is a surge in progesterone production by these follicles and plasma levels are considerably raised.

A characteristic feature of the avian ovary is the sequential development of the follicles such that each follicle is approximately 24 h less mature than the one immediately preceding it. This hierarchical arrangement of the follicles causes the typical 'bunch of grapes' appearance of the ovary. Ovulation of the largest follicle in the hierarchy occurs, with the interval between ovulations usually slightly greater than 24 h. Within approximately 15 min of ovulation the liberated secondary oocyte is actively engulfed by the infundibulum of the oviduct. Because albumen deposition occurs almost immediately the egg enters the oviduct, sperm penetration takes place outside the oviduct in the so-called 'ovarian pocket', a part of the abdominal cavity. This penetration by the spermatozoa then brings about the final maturation division of the female pro-nucleus.

Once in the oviduct, the remaining elements of the egg are produced, a process lasting approximately 24 h. The oviduct is formed of five distinct regions, each having a specific function. The infundibulum is the most cranial region of the oviduct; its main function is to engulf the shed oocyte, but it has some secretory activity and also contributes material to the egg white. However, the main mass of the proteinaceous material of the oviduct is produced by the magnum, the largest part of the oviduct, with well developed glandular elements. The albumen when first formed is very gelatinous and it only takes on its characteristic 'egg-white' appearance when a watery fluid is added in the shell gland. After approximately 3 h in the magnum the egg passes to the isthmus where, during the next approximately 1.5 h, the fibrous shell-membranes are formed. These give the egg its characteristic shape – a shape often erroneously thought to be conveyed by the calcified shell.

For the majority of the time that the egg is in the oviduct it is in the shell gland (18 to 20 h), a region with several complex functions. The gland produces the watery fluid which is added to the albumen, produces the organic material of the shell, secretes the calcified part of the shell and adds the final covering (the cuticle) to the egg. Few, if any, of these functions can be ascribed with certainty to a particular group of cells within the organ.

The vagina is involved in the 'bearing-down reflex' associated with oviposition and it also contains, in a specialized cranial region, the tubular 'sperm–host glands'. In these gland-like structures sperm can survive for long periods and, for this reason, a single insemination will lead to the production of fertile eggs for approximately 10 days in the chicken, and longer in some other species. Nevertheless, the spermatozoa must travel throughout the entire oviduct before ovulation to reach the oocyte soon after ovulation.

The endocrinology of reproduction in birds (Fig. 6.1) has many features similar to those in mammals; however there is no distinct oestrous cycle, pregnancy does not occur, and the action of many of the hormones may appear unfamiliar to a mammalian endocrinologist. Moreover, since birds do not have mammary glands, the hormones which are usually associated with lactation have other rôles, although their actions are mainly outside the scope of the present subject.

Little is known of the endocrinology before sexual maturation, although steroidogenesis occurs even in the embryo. The main factor that leads to the development of sexual maturity seems to be a steadily increasing daylength, i.e. period of daylight, which, through mechanisms not entirely understood, initiates changes in the output of gonadotropin releasing factors (GnRF). These bring about release of the pituitary gonadotropins which, in turn, cause a general rise in steroid production by the ovary. The steady rise in circulating oestrogen ultimately depresses the plasma levels of LH at a time which coincides with the first ovulation (Williams and Sharp, 1977). However, before this occurs the continuous production of the sex steroids brings about the multitude of changes required for reproduction to occur: among these are the development of the secondary sexual characters (mainly under regulation by oestrogens and androgens), changes in calcium uptake mechanisms in the gut (oestrogens), formation of the endosteal bone (androgens and oestrogens), growth and differentiation of the oviduct (androgens, oestrogens and progesterone), breakdown of the septum dividing the oviduct from the cloaca (oestrogens), spreading of the pubic bones (oestrogens) and changes in lipogenesis in the liver associated with the production of the yolk lipoproteins (oestrogens).

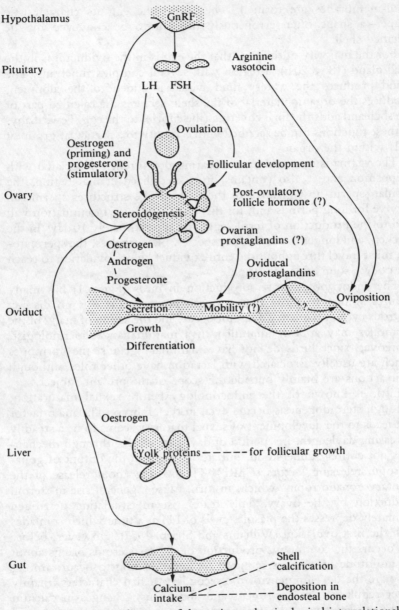

Fig. 6.1.   Schematic diagram of the major endocrinological interrelationships in the control of ovarian and oviducal function (GnRF: gonadotropin releasing factors).

During the daily ovulatory cycles which follow sexual maturation, follicular maturation depends mainly on FSH, although LH may also be important. However, the main function of LH is to bring about ovulation of the mature follicle. The initial stimulus for LH release appears to be the transition from daylight to darkness, although the actual release of LH may occur some hours later. Also, LH acts on the granulosa cells causing an increased output of progesterone. This hormone (not oestrogen as in mammals) has the positive feed-back effect, via the hypothalamus, of reinforcing the stimulus for LH release, and the interaction of the two hormones culminates in an ovulatory surge of LH of short duration. As yet there is no understanding of the way in which LH acts within the follicle to bring about ovulation.

Few of the mechanisms relating to the control of oviduct function are known (see also Gilbert, 1980), although generally protein synthesis and the secretion of albumen depend mainly on the oestrogens. However, formation of at least one specific protein (avidin) requires progesterone. Prostaglandins may play an important rôle in the transport of the egg through the oviduct and in oviposition. Although the evidence is not entirely unequivocal, the oxytocic hormone (arginine vasotocin in the bird) appears to be important in oviposition, and certain neural mechanisms appear also to be involved.

A summary of the endocrine changes at the end of the laying period is complicated by the differences between domestic and wild species: the overall decline in egg production of domestic birds with age during the first laying year appears to be physiologically different from the sudden cessation of egg production in wild birds when the optimum clutch size for the species is reached. The former may be more akin to the general state of photo-refractoriness which occurs in wild birds with the end of a laying season, and is usually accompanied by an at least partial moult. In contrast, the attainment of a complete clutch is followed by incubation behaviour. In both cases a reduction in circulatory steroids and LH occur, but with incubation there is a marked rise in prolactin. This may inhibit the stimulating effect of LH on ovarian steroidogenesis. The 'pause day' (when no egg is laid) between sequences of egg-laying in domestic species is different again from either of these cases. The pause is caused by a feature of the hierarchical development of follicles in the ovary: there is usually no mature follicle present on the preceding day and hence ovulation and the subsequent development of the egg does not occur.

The major components of yolk are produced by the liver in response to oestrogenic stimulation. The materials consists mainly of lipoproteins and phosphoproteins and these characteristically appear in the blood as the hen approaches reproductive age. Little is known of the mechanisms for their incorporation into the oocyte (Gilbert, 1980) except that they appear to enter mainly without change, a situation contrasting with the uptake of lipids into adipocytes (Hillyard, White and Pangburn, 1972; Gornall and Kuksis, 1973; Holdsworth, Mitchell and Finean, 1974). Recently, the anatomical features associated with the uptake of very low density lipoprotein (VLDL), phosvitin and globulins have been described (Roth, Cutting and Atlas, 1976; Yukso and Roth, 1976; Perry, Gilbert and Evans, 1978a and b; Evans, Perry and Gilbert, 1979), and the route by which these materials enter the oocyte is known. In the first, early stages of yolk accumulation, yolk of a different nature (so-called 'white' yolk) is deposited: its origin is obscure but possibly it is formed within the granulosa cells (see Gilbert, 1979).

Unlike yolk, the proteins of albumen are synthesized within the glandular cells of the oviduct. So far, approximately 40 proteins have been identified (Feeney and Allison, 1969) but only a few have been clearly linked with specific cells responsible for their production: this small group of proteins includes avidin, lysozyme, ovalbumin, ovotransferrin (conalbumin) and ovomucoid (see Gilbert, 1979 and 1980).

The shell consists of an organic matrix laid down upon the shell membranes (see Gilbert, 1979 and 1980) and within this meshwork are the calcite crystals. Since the shell-forming region of the oviduct is unable to store calcium, there is a continuous removal of this mineral from the blood (Hodges, 1969). On the other hand, like the protein of albumen, the organic material is produced by the oviducal cells (Gilbert, 1979 and 1980).

The production of a shelled egg imposes a considerable strain on the calcium metabolism of the hen since each shell contains approximately 2 g of calcium, a quantity equivalent to 10% of the total mass of the element in the body. For this reason the uptake mechanisms within the gut are extremely efficient and approximately 2 g of calcium can be removed each day from a diet containing levels of calcium in excess of 30 g/kg. These mechanisms are oestrogen-dependent and may involve a calcium-binding protein (Wasserman, Corradino, Fullmer and Taylor, 1974). The calcium removed from the diet is used directly for shell calcification or it may be deposited in the specialized endosteal bone to be mobilized later when required. Although the endosteal bone was once thought to be a major reserve store for calcium, recent evidence indicates that the bone may hold sufficient calcium for only two eggs; its function seems mainly to be for the short-term placement of calcium removed from the gut during periods when shelling is not taking place.

Because the loss of calcium in the shell is so extreme, there are regulatory mechanisms on egg formation which operate when dietary calcium intake is insufficient. These mechanisms do not so much bring about the production of eggs with deficient shells, for this would be a wasteful process in reproduction; instead, they influence ovarian function so that the output of oocytes is directly related to the number which can be properly shelled with the calcium that is available to the bird (Gilbert, Peddie, Mitchell and Teague, 1981).

THE EFFECTS OF NUTRITION ON EGG FORMATION

Given an adequate supply of nutrients, a disease-free hen in a thermo-neutral environment will produce eggs of a relatively constant composition and physical size. If these eggs are fertile and incubated correctly then most will hatch after 21 days to produce a viable chick. Any variations in the egg will lead to a reduction in the chances of a viable chick being produced. This chapter is largely concerned with the effect of nutrition on the ability of the hen to produce eggs that will give rise to viable offspring; however, the rôle of nutrition in egg production is a complex one and is related to the many components of the environment which interact to influence the physiological performance of the bird.

What is seldom realized is that the turnover of material during reproduction in domestic avian species is enormous. A reasonable production for a commercial laying strain of hen is approximately 280 eggs during the first laying season (lasting approximately 1 year): since each egg weighs approximately 60 g, the total material voided by the hen is of the order of 15 kg, a mass about 10-times her body weight. No other domestic species has such a reproductive capacity (Gilbert, 1971a). As a consequence of this, a greater proportion of the nutrient intake is directly related to reproductive effort in the bird than in any other domestic animal, and any variation in the dietary intake could be expected to have profound effects on egg production. When the nutritional environment is not suited to optimal egg production, the hen could respond in several ways: it could reduce the size and/or number of eggs produced while maintaining the ideal composition, or it could modify the composition while maintaining output; alternatively, it could adopt a compromise by changing the size, number and composition of the eggs. The responses that occur under specific nutritional circumstances, the manner in which they are related to the physiology of egg formation, and their effect on the production of a viable chick are considered below. The major nutritional influences on egg formation are represented schematically in Fig. 6.2.

Starvation

Not surprisingly the complete removal of all or of some specific items (e.g. calcium and sodium) from the diet rapidly leads to a complete

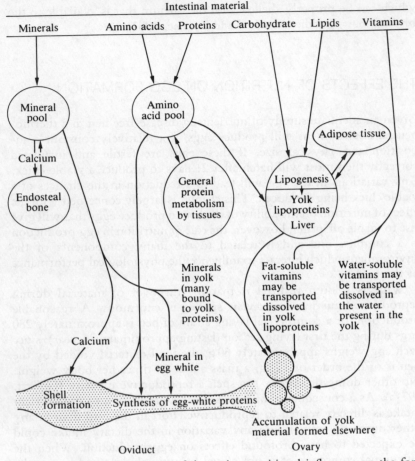

Fig. 6.2.   Schematic diagram of the major nutritional influences on the formation of an egg.

cessation of egg production (Morris and Nalbandov 1961; Gilbert, 1973; Whitehead and Shannon, 1974; Douglas, Harms and Nesbeth, 1978). With complete starvation the ovary rapidly becomes atretic and regresses; however, in the case of calcium deficiency this is not so, and both the ovary and oviduct remain almost normal (Gilbert and Blair, 1975). Whatever the immediate physiological effect of nutritional deprivation may be, the response of the ovary is undoubtedly mediated through the pituitary output of gonadotropins. Injection of gonadotropins to birds supplied only with water and oyster shell (Morris and Nalbandov, 1961), or to birds fed a normal diet but without calcium (Taylor, Morris and Hertelendy, 1962), maintains daily ovulation patterns.

'Energy' intake

It is not easy to relate the results of experiments in which the energy intake has been altered to specific physiological effects. Birds of commercial layer strains appear able to adjust their voluntary food intake to meet their daily energy requirements (Morris, 1968; Cherry, 1979). Consequently, when very high energy diets are fed, voluntary food intake could be so reduced as to lead to a deficiency in intake of a specific nutrient in the diet.

Ultimately, high-energy diets will lead to an unbalanced nutrient supply and the general over-production of lipid material that the liver utilizes to produce yolk lipoproteins. The increased yolk weight relative to the other components of the egg could be a reflexion of this (Gardner and Young, 1972), particularly since the composition of the yolk remains unaltered. Energy deficiencies lead to a reduced egg-size and ultimately a reduction in egg numbers but, again, this may simply be a reflexion of general dietary deficiencies rather than a specific effect of energy *per se*.

Unlike the laying strains, broiler breeders (the parents of meat-type chicks) do not appear to exert such a rigid regulation of their energy intake and excessive deposition of fat within the adipose tissue results if these birds are allowed food *ad libitum*. This is associated with depressed egg production and decreased fertility but the direct causes of these effects have not been established (Fuller, Potter and Kirkland, 1969; Chaney and Fuller, 1975). It may be that reduced egg output results from an increase in internal laying (i.e. the oviduct fails to accept the oocyte after ovulation) (A. J. Evans and A. B. Gilbert, unpublished results); since yolk material is rapidly removed from the body cavity (Sturkie, 1955) this situation can only lead to an exacerbation of the obesity. However, if internal laying is the cause, the effects are probably related to mechanical than physiological factors.

Protein

There is a considerable amount of protein in both yolk and albumen and the laying hen obtains the amino acids required for the synthesis of egg protein from the diet, although she would appear to be able to utilize tissue protein reserves in the short-term when dietary amino acids are in short supply (Harms, Moreno and Damron, 1971). However, protein reserves are limited and, in the long-term, overall dietary deficiencies of total proteins or their amino acids are associated with reductions in egg size and number. In cases of marginal deficiency egg size only is reduced, but in severe deficiency egg production may cease altogether. When protein intake is reduced or a particular amino acid is limiting, the amino acid composition of the egg protein remains unchanged but the total amount of protein synthesized is reduced, with an overall decrease in the amount of each amino acid lost in eggs.

The response to a change in the intake of protein or of a particular amino acid is often complicated by indirect effects of the alteration in diet on egg formation. Increasing additions of a limiting amino acid to a diet marginally deficient in that amino acid have progressively decreasing effects on egg output as amino acid requirements for egg production are met. However, dietary excesses of one or more of the essential amino acids can have detrimental effects on performance and excess dietary protein seems to increase the requirements for other essential nutrients. For example, the vitamin B_{12} requirement for hatchability appeared to increase when the protein content of a diet given to breeding birds was increased from 160 to 320 g/kg (Patel and McGinnis, 1977).

Free amino acids account for approximately 16 mg of the nitrogenous fraction of the egg and, unlike egg protein, the quantities of these individual amino acids seems to be a function of the amounts present in plasma and hence ultimately of their availability in the diet.

The lack of any effect of dietary protein on the composition of egg protein is not surprising since the embryo requires certain amino acids for development: leucine, methionine, lysine and phenylalanine are essential while arginine, trytophan, valine and tyrosine may also be (see Freeman and Vince, 1974). Hence an egg deficient or unbalanced in amino acids would be detrimental to embryonic development. Since all the egg proteins are synthesized specifically an unbalanced content is unlikely, although the total amount available may vary and may cause a reduction in egg size. This effect makes it difficult to assess the direct effects of protein and amino acid intake on hatchability although, surprisingly, in view of the amino acids that are apparently essential for embryo development, dietary deficiencies of trytophan, lysine (Ingram, Cravens, Elvehjem and Halpin, 1951a) or methionine (Ingram, Cravens, Elvehjem and Halpin, 1951b) did not appear to affect the hatchability of eggs produced.

Lipid

Nearly all of the lipid in the egg is present in the yolk. Synthesis of the yolk lipoproteins occurs in the liver and under normal circumstances the main precursors are the break-down products of dietary carbohydrates. Nevertheless, some dietary lipid may be used and in adverse dietary conditions there may be mobilization of lipid from the adipose tissue. Yolk lipid is the major source of energy for the developing embryo and it accounts for between 840 and 980 g/kg of the material oxidized (Romanoff and Romanoff, 1949); for this reason it could be argued that the relative proportions of the major components of yolk are unlikely to be affected by the composition of the diet. Also, since the uptake of these major components appears to take place by a specific mechanism (via the coated vesicles) (Roth *et al.*, 1976; Yukso and Roth, 1976; Perry and Gilbert, 1979), the composition of the lipid supply for yolk formation is assured: only the quantity of the major yolk components passing into the oocyte appears to be capable of regulation at the level of the ovary. The experimental evidence available suggests that the lipid content of the egg is not sensitive to the dietary lipid intake (for example, see Vogtmann and Clandinin, 1975): even high-fat diets do not affect total egg-yolk lipid, although the proportions of egg-yolk fatty acids can often be related to the fatty acid composition of the dietary triglycerides (Chen, Common, Nikolaiczuk and MacRae, 1965; Sell, Choo and Kondra, 1968). However, lipogenesis decreases as dietary fat levels increase in most animals (Masoro, 1962) and, if this is also true in the bird, as dietary fat content increases the liver may use proportionally more dietary fat for synthesis of yolk material. Under these circumstances dietary unsaturated fatty acids appear more suitable precursors than saturated fatty acids (Chen *et al.*, 1965; Weiss, Naber and Johnson, 1967).

Despite these general conclusions there is no doubt that certain fatty acids are essential in diets for laying hens if they are to produce viable offspring. These acids, e.g. linoleic and arachidonic acids, are derived predominantly from vegetable oils and are stored in the body for some time so that dietary deficiencies are not always immediately apparent. Nevertheless, the amount of linoleic (and arachidonic) acid found in the yolk is ultimately related to the intake in the diet, and dietary deficiencies of linoleic acid are associated with a marked reduction in egg production, egg size, and the proportion of dry matter and lipid content of the yolk. This is accompanied by a reduction in fertility and an increase in early embryo mortality (Menge, Calvert and Denton, 1965; Calvert, 1967; Menge, 1968; Guenter, Bragg and Kondra, 1971). In a severe deficiency of either linoleic or arachidonic acid the acids could not be detected in the yolk and hatchability was reduced to zero (Menge *et al.*, 1965).

In contrast to the major yolk lipoproteins, there are minor lipid components of yolk which do appear to be directly related to the quantities present in the diet. For example, high dietary levels of cholesterol bring about high levels of cholesterol in blood plasma and in the yolk (Chung, Rogler and Stadelman, 1965), but not all plasma cholesterol is derived from the diet and the type of dietary fat may influence cholesterol production in the bird. Thus a high dietary level of safflower oil results in a high output of cholesterol by the liver (Weiss *et al.*, 1967).

It seems likely that subtances such as cholesterol accumulate in the oocyte incidentally with other components because the specific mechanisms for the uptake of the major components are not selective. For example, the pinocytotic coated vesicles which are involved in the uptake of VLDL and phosvitin would probably include an aqueous fraction and consequently dissolved water-soluble substances. The concentration of the soluble substances within the coated vesicle will depend on their concentration in the tissue fluid in the space surrounding the oocyte, and this in turn will depend mainly on their concentration in blood plasma.

Vitamins

There are certain other constituents which also appear to enter the yolk incidentally along with the main yolk components, although the mechanisms for the transfer of all the constituents may not be identical. Jeroch (1971a, b and c, and 1972), in a series of experiments on vitamin B_2 requirements, was able to show a relationship between dietary intake of the vitamin and the production of a viable offspring by a breeding hen. Chick development during the 1st week of life was determined mainly by the vitamin B_2 obtained from the egg during development, and this depended on the parental vitamin B_2 intake. The concentrations of vitamins A, E and K, pantothenic acid, nicotinic acid, pyridoxine, folic acid and biotin in the egg have also been shown to be dependent upon their concentration in the diet (see Scott, Nesheim and Young, 1976). This suggests that the bird has no specific mechanism for ensuring that adequate quantities of vitamins are present in the egg, which is surprising in view of the essential nature of the vitamins in normal development of the embryo, hatching and survival of hatched chicks (Scott *et al.*, 1976).

The methods by which the vitamins enter the oocyte are not known, although the water-soluble ones, bound to their carrier proteins (Farrell, Buss and Clagett, 1970; Sonneborn and Hansen, 1970; White, Dennison, Della Fera, Whitney, McGuire, Meslar and Sammelwitz, 1976), are likely to enter with water, possibly through the pinocytotic vesicles; and the lipid-soluble ones (A, D, E and K) are almost certain to enter dissolved in the lipid fraction of yolk, for which there are specific transport mechanisms.

Inorganic ions

The effect of variations in the dietary intake of inorganic ions on egg production is complicated by the fact that most of the ions have widespread effects on physiological processes in the body and particularly on those associated with the heart, muscle and nerve. Consequently, there are extremely efficient mechanisms of regulation to maintain the ionic balance in blood plasma constant to within very narrow limits. Moreover, some ions, such as magnesium, may interfere with the uptake of other ions from the gut. In addition to this, some of the yolk proteins possess efficient binding properties, particularly for the divalent ions. Hence variations in the levels of the bound ions in the blood plasma may reflect their relative availability from the diet or the relative concentration of the yolk proteins, and the latter may, in turn, be affected by dietary ionic concentration. Also, although both yolk and albumen contain appreciable quantities of inorganic material, by far the greatest requirement for inorganic constituents is for shell formation. For these reasons it is extremely difficult to determine whether a particular response within the reproductive system to a specific ion deficiency is a secondary consequence of an effect elsewhere or whether it represents a primary effect.

Notwithstanding these considerations, the concentrations of ions within the yolk or albumen tend to reflect their concentrations in the diet. Consequently, the first effects of changes in the mineral composition of the diet appear in the composition of the egg and only if a deficiency is severe enough will it eventually cause a fall in egg numbers. The exceptions are calcium and sodium; both these ions appear to have a primary effect on egg output rather than on egg composition (Gilbert, 1973; Whitehead and Shannon, 1974), although composition may be affected also.

In a similar way to the vitamins, it appears that most of the ions in the egg (except for those in the shell) are present in concentrations proportional to dietary intake. This is not unexpected since most ions (e.g. sodium and potassium) enter passively into the egg in the large quantities of water present. Furthermore, most of the divalent ions (calcium, magnesium, zinc, etc.) of the yolk are transported bound to the lipoproteins (see Gilbert, 1971b). Under normal dietary conditions these mechanisms must be relatively efficient because the ionic composition of the egg is important for the development of the embryo. For example, a maternal iron deficiency has a marked impact on egg yolk iron, iron status of the embryo and embryonic survival (Morck, 1978). Similarly, a maternal selenium deficiency will depress hatchability and the viability of the offspring (Latshaw, Ort and Diesem, 1977). A direct relationship has been established between the iodine content of the maternal diet and true iodine content of the thyroids of the embryos: when breeding hens are given iodine-deficient diets, hatchability is depressed, hatching time prolonged and absorption of the yolk sac is retarded (Rogler, Parker, Andrews and Carrick, 1961).

If the normal passive methods for transport into the egg were not adequate, evolutionary pressure on such a vital aspect of reproduction would surely have been sufficient to lead to the development of more-specific uptake mechanisms.

CONCLUSIONS

Variations in the diet can be expected to have profound effects, both direct and indirect, on the production of shelled eggs because a large proportion of the nutrient intake of domestic birds is directly related to reproduction. However, it is not always easy to separate the primary and secondary effects of a specific nutrient deficiency. Moreover, in terms of the conversion of food material into eggs, variations may occur in the numbers of eggs produced as well as in egg size and composition.

With present knowledge it is not generally possible to explain the effects of a specific nutrient limitation in terms of specific physiological mechanisms, although some general conclusions can be drawn. Where specific synthesizing mechanisms exist (e.g. lipoproteins of yolk and albumen proteins), and where specific (active?) uptake mechanisms operate (e.g. mechanisms in the oocyte for the uptake of certain yolk components), then the bird can apparently maintain the relative composition of the egg irrespective of reasonably wide fluctuations in diet amount and composition. In contrast, some minor components of the egg (in particular the vitamins and minerals) appear to enter passively as a result of the uptake mechanisms for the major components, and for these minor components egg composition tends to depend more directly on the diet.

REFERENCES

Bell, D. J. and Freeman, B. M., 1971. *The Physiology and Biochemistry of the Domestic Fowl* Vol. 3. Academic Press, London.

Calvert, C. C.,1967. Studies on hatchability of fertile eggs from hens receiving a linoleic acid deficient diet, *Poult. Sci.* **46**: 967–73.

Chaney, L. W. and Fuller, H. L., 1975. The relation of obesity to egg production in broiler breeders, *Poult. Sci.* **54**: 200–7.

Chen, P. H., Common, R. H., Nikolaiczuk, N. and MacRae, H. F., 1965. Some effects of added dietary fats on the lipid composition of hen's egg yolk, *J. Fd Sci.* **30**: 838–45.

Cherry, J. A., 1979. Adaptation in food intake after changes in dietary energy. In *Food Intake Regulation in Poultry* (ed. K. W. Boorman and B. M. Freeman), pp. 77–86. British Poultry Science, Edinburgh.

Chung, R. A., Rogler, J. C. and Stadelman, W. S., 1965. The effect of dietary cholesterol and different dietary fats on cholesterol content and lipid composition of egg yolk and various body tissues, *Poult. Sci.* **44**: 221–8.

Douglas, C. R., Harms, R. H. and Nesbeth, W. G.,1978. Performance of laying hens as influenced by length of time without feed, *Poult. Sci.* **57**:968–70.

Evans, A. J., Perry, Margaret M. and Gilbert, A. B., 1979. The demonstration of very low density lipoprotein in the basal lamina of the granulosa layer in the hen's ovarian follicle, *Biochim. biophys. Acta* **573**: 184–95.

Farrell, H. M., Buss, E. G. and Clagett, C. O., 1970. The nature of the biochemical lesion in avian renal riboflavinuria. V. Elucidation of riboflavin transport in the laying hen. *Int. J. Biochem.* **1**: 168–72.

Feeney, R. E. and Allison, R., 1969. *Evolutionary Biochemistry of Proteins*. John Wiley, New York.

Follett, B. K. and Robinson, Jane E., 1980. Photoperiod and gonadotrophin secretion in birds, *Prog. Reprod. Biol.* **5**: 39–61.

Freeman, B. M. and Vince, M. A., 1974. *Development of the Avian Embryo*. Chapman and Hall, London.

Fuller, H. L., Potter, D. K. and Kirkland, W., 1969. Effect of delayed maturity and carcass fat on reproductive performance of broiler breeder pullets, *Poult. Sci.* **48**: 801–9.

Gardner, F. A. and Young, L. L., 1972. The influence of dietary protein and energy levels on the protein and lipid content of the hen's egg, *Poult. Sci.* **51**: 994–7.

Gilbert, A. B., 1971a. The female reproductive effort. In *The Physiology and Biochemistry of the Domestic Fowl*, Vol. 3 (ed. D. J. Bell and B. M. Freeman), pp . 1153–62. Academic Press, London.

Gilbert, A. B. 1971b. The egg: its physical and chemical aspects. In *The Physiology and Biochemistry of the Domestic Fowl*, Vol. 3 (ed. D. J. Bell and B. M. Freeman), pp. 1379–99. Academic Press, London.

Gilbert, A. B., 1973. The use of a calcium restricted diet to control egg production in the domestic fowl, *4th Eur. Poult. Conf., Lond.*, pp. 69–76.

Gilbert, A. B., 1979. Female genital organs. In *Form and Function in Birds*, Vol. 1 (ed. A. R. King and J. McLelland), pp. 237–360. Academic Press, London.

Gilbert, A. B., 1980. Controlling factors in the synthesis of egg proteins. In *Protein Deposition in Animals* (ed. P. J. Buttery and D. B. Lindsay), pp. 85–106. Butterworths, London.

Gilbert, A. B., Peddie, J., Mitchell, G. G. and Teague, P. W., 1981. The egg laying response of the domestic hen to variation in dietary calcium, *Br. Poult. Sci.* **22**: 537–48.

Gilbert, A. B. and Blair, R., 1975. A comparison of the effects of two low-calcium diets on egg production in the domestic fowl, *Br. Poult. Sci.* **16**: 547–52.

Gornall, D. A. and Kuksis, A., 1973. Alterations in lipid composition of plasma lipoproteins during deposition of egg yolk, *J. Lipid Res.* **14**: 197–205.

Guenter, W., Bragg, D. B. and Kondra, P. A., 1971. Effect of dietary linoleic acid on fatty acid composition of egg yolk, liver and adipose tissue, *Poult. Sci.* **50**: 845–50.

Harms, R. H., Moreno, R. S. and Damron, B. L., 1971. Evidence for protein storage in laying hens and its utilization under nutritional stress, *Poult. Sci.* **50**: 592–5.

Hillyard, L. A., White, H. M. and Pangburn, S. A., 1972. Characterisation of apolipoproteins in chicken serum and egg yolk, *Biochemistry, Wash., D.C.* **11**: 511–8.

Hodges, R. D., 1969. pH and mineral ion levels in the blood of laying hen (*Gallus domesticus*) in relation to egg formation, *Comp. Biochem. Physiol.* **28**: 1243–57.

Holdsworth, G., Mitchell, R. H. and Finean, J. B., 1974. Transfer of very low density lipoprotein from hen plasma into egg yolk, *FEBS Lett.* **39**: 275–7.

Ingram, G. R., Cravens, W. W., Elvehjem, C. A. and Halpin, J. G., 1951a. Studies on the lysine and tryptophan requirements of the laying and breeding hen, *Poult. Sci.* **30**: 426–30.

Ingram, G. R., Cravens, W. W. Elvehjem, C. A. and Halpin, J. G., 1951b. The methionine requirement of the laying hen, *Poult. Sci.* **30**: 431–4.

Jeroch, H., 1971a. [Studies on the vitamin B_2 requirements of laying hens. (1) Requirements for egg production], *Arch. Tierernähr.* **21**: 151–60.

Jeroch, H., 1971b. [Studies on the vitamin B_2 requirements of laying hens. (2) Requirements for reproduction], *Arch. Tierernähr.* **21**: 249–56.

Jeroch, H., 1971c. [Studies on the vitamin B_2 requirements of laying hens. (3) Variations in the vitamin B_2 supply to the hens as affecting the formation of vitamin B_2 reserves in newly hatched chicks and the development of offspring fed a vitamin B_2-deficient diet, *Arch. Tierernähr.* **21**: 713–23.

Jeroch, H., 1972. [Studies on the vitamin B_2 requirements of laying hens. (4) Variations in the vitamin B_2 supply to hens as affecting the development of descendent chicks receiving graded vitamin B_2 supplements], *Arch. Tierernähr.* **22**: 97–111.

Latshaw, J. D., Ort, J. F. and Diesem, C. D., 1977. The selenium requirements of the hen and effects of a deficiency, *Poult. Sci.* **56**: 1876–81.

Lofts, B. and Murton, R. K., 1973. Reproduction in Birds. In *Avian Biology* (ed. D. S. Farner and J. R. King), Vol. 3, pp. 1–107. Academic Press, London.

Masoro, E. J., 1962. Biochemical mechanisms related to the hemeostatic regulation of hypogenesis in animals, *J. Lipid Res.* **3**: 149–64.

Menge, H., 1968. Linoleic acid requirement of the hen for reproduction. *J. Nutr.* **95**: 578–82.

Menge, H., Calvert, C. C. and Denton, C. A., 1965. Further studies of the effect of linoleic acid on reproduction in the hen, *J. Nutr.* **86**: 115–9.

Morck, T. A., 1978. Influence of maternal iron status on chick embryo survival, *Fedn Proc. Fedn. Am. Socs. exp. Biol.* **37**: 487 (Abstr.).

Morris, T. R., 1968. The effect of dietary energy level on the calorie intake of laying birds, *Br. Poult. Sci.* **9**: 285–95.

Morris, T. R. and Nalbandov, A. V., 1961. The induction of ovulation in starving pullets using mammalian and avian gonadotrophins, *Endocrinology* **68**: 687–97.

Patel, M. B. and McGinnis, J., 1977. The effect of levels of protein and vitamin B_{12} in hen diets on egg production and hatchability of eggs and on livability and growth of chicks, *Poult. Sci.* **56**: 45–53.

Perry, M. M. and Gilbert, A. B., 1979. Yolk transport in the ovarian follicle of the hen (*Gallus domesticus*): lipoprotein-like particles at the periphery of the oocyte in the rapid growth phase, *J. Cell Sci.* **39**: 257–72.

Perry, M. M., Gilbert, A. B. and Evans, A. J., 1978a. Electron-microscope observations on the ovarian follicle of the domestic fowl during the rapid growth phase, *J. Anat.* **125**: 481–97.

Perry, M. M., Gilbert, A. B. and Evans, A. J., 1978b. The structure of the germinal disc region of the hen's ovarian follicle during the rapid growth phase, *J.Anat.* **127**: 379–92.

Rogler, J. C., Parker, H. E., Andrews, F. N. and Carrick, C. W., 1961. The iodine requirements of the breeding hen, *Poult. Sci.* **40**: 1554–62.

Romanoff, A. L. and Romanoff, A. V., 1949. *The Avian Egg*. John Wiley, New York.

Roth, T. F., Cutting, J. A. and Atlas, S. B., 1976. Protein transport: a selective membrane mechanism, *J. Supramol. Struct.* **4**: 527–48.

Scott, M. L. Nesheim, M. C. and Young, R. J., 1976. *Nutrition of the Chicken*. 2nd edn. M. L. Scott and Associates, New York.

Sell, J. L., Choo, S. H. and Kondra, P. A., 1968. Fatty acid composition of egg yolk and adipose tissue as influenced by dietary fat and strain of hen, *Poult. Sci.* **47**: 1296–302.

Sonneborn, D. W. and Hansen, H. J., 1970. Vitamin B_{12} binders of chicken serum and chicken preventriculus are immunologically similar, *Science, Wash., D.C.* **158**: 591–2.

Sturkie, P. D., 1955. Absorption of egg yolk in body cavity of the hen, *Poult. Sci.* **34**: 736–7.

Taylor, T. G., Morris, T. R. and Hertelendy, F., 1962. The effect of pituitary hormones on ovulation in calcium deficient pullets, *Vet. Rec.* **74**: 123–5.

Vogtmann, H. and Clandinin, D. R., 1975. The effects of crude and refined low erucic acid rapeseed oils in diets for laying hens, *Br. Poult. Sci.* **16**: 55–61.

Wasserman, R. H., Corradino, R. A., Fullmer, C. S. and Taylor, A. N., 1974. Some aspects of vitamin D action : calcium absorption and the vitamin D-dependent calcium-binding protein, *Vitams Horm.* **32**: 299–324.

Weiss, J. F., Naber, E. C. and Johnson, R. M., 1967. Effect of dietary fat and cholesterol on the *in vitro* incorporation of acetate-^{14}C into hen liver and ovarian lipids, *J. Nutr.* **93**: 142–52.

White, H. B., Dennison, B. A., Della Fera, M. A., Whitney, C. J., McGuire, J. C., Meslar, H. W. and Sammelwitz, P. H., 1976. Biotin-binding protein from chicken egg yolk, *Biochem. J.* **157**: 395–400.

Whitehead, C. C. and Shannon, D. W. F., 1974. The control of egg production using a low-sodium diet, *Br. Poult. Sci.* **15**: 429–34.

Williams, J. B. and Sharp, P. J., 1977. A comparison of plasma progesterone and luteinizing hormone in growing hens from eight weeks of age to sexual maturity, *J. Endocr.* **75**: 447–8.

Wingfield, J. C. and Farner, D. S., 1980. Control of seasonal reproduction in temperate-zone birds, *Prog. Reprod. Biol.* **5**: 62–101.

Yukso, S. C. and Roth, T. F., 1976. Binding to specific receptors on oocyte plasma membranes by serum phosvitin-lipovitellin, *J. Supramol. Struct.* **4**: 89–97.

7 GROWTH AND FATTENING
D. B. Lindsay

Growth might be defined simply as an increase in the size of an animal, but when growth is distinguished from fattening there is an implied exclusion of size increase due to fat deposition. Thus it is convenient to define growth in terms of an increase in the amount of body protein.

A cynic might say that growth occurs in the young and fattening in the middle-aged. There is an element of truth in this since the rate of protein deposition is maximal at the earliest stages of development and has decreased substantially by the time that fat deposition has become apparent. Nevertheless, there is a significant deposition of fat simultaneously with protein in the young, and it is only because protein deposition declines markedly with age that fattening is most apparent in mature animals. This is clearly shown in Figure 7.1, which illustrates the growth of the major tissues in steers.

Since the largest amount of body protein is found in muscle, growth is dependent particularly on the development of muscle tissue. However, for full muscle development to occur, a firm supporting structure is needed (the reason for this is discussed later) and this necessitates the prior growth of the skeleton. Visible fat appears relatively late in growth. Thus there is a characteristic pattern in which skeleton, muscle and fat are successively developed, and in discussing these tissues it is convenient to follow the same sequence.

DEVELOPMENT OF THE SKELETON

A typical long bone of the mature skeleton contains a core of marrow. In the middle of the bone this is yellow and fatty; towards the extremities it is red and a site of haematopoiesis. During development, or in mature bone as a result of anaemia, this red marrow will make up a much larger part of the core. The bony surround may be cortical – a hard, compact bone typical of the shaft (diaphysis) – or cancellous (spongy) consisting of a fine network of bony spicules or trabeculae. It

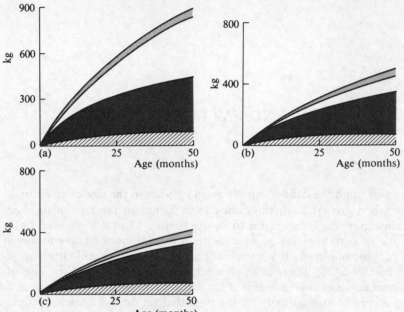

Fig. 7.1.   Growth of the tissues of cattle. Metabolically active tissue (MAT) was defined as the whole body weight, less that of fat, skeleton, skin, hooves and horn. It will contain most body protein (approximately 190 g/kg). (a), (b) and (c) represent growth at three planes of nutrition, (b) being 1.5 and (a) 2.5 times greater intake than (c), which was just above maintenance. The curves for each tissue were constructed from equations developed by Koch, Kromann and Wilson (1979) using earlier data ▨, skin; ▨ fat; ■, MAT; □, skeleton).

is in this form that bone is initially laid down. Bone is generally surrounded by periosteum – a layer of connective tissue. Periosteum is lacking at the ends of the bone, where it is covered with articular cartilage, and at one or two other sites where tendons and ligaments are inserted.

Fine structure

Bone structure differs significantly from that of cartilage. The ground substance consists of an organic matrix, osteoid, impregnated with calcium salt, mostly in ordered crystalline form. In a series of cavities (lacunae) within this are the bone cells or osteocytes. These have long cytoplasmic processes which run in fine canaliculi through which they may maintain contact with each other. Indeed, it has been suggested that they may even form a syncytium (Talmage, 1970). Osteocytes in their lacunae are frequently arranged around a larger central canal containing blood vessels, so that in section they often appear to form a series of rings. On the outer (next to the periosteum) and inner (next to the marrow) surfaces there is a continuous layer of osteogenic cells (osteoblasts) whose processes may also make contact with the osteocytes. It is important to recognize that new growth occurs only from osteoblasts. They secrete matrix, which calcifies and in which they become embedded, thereby becoming osteocytes. Growth in bone, therefore, occurs only by apposition, that is, from the surfaces. A schematized impression of the fine structure of bone is shown in Fig. 7.2. Two other features shown there are also worthy of comment.

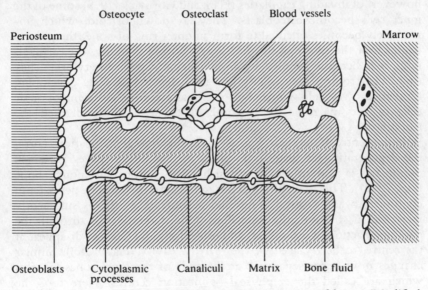

Fig. 7.2. Schematic diagram of the major constituents of bone. (Modified from Vaughan, 1980.)

The large, multinucleate cells known as osteoclasts are involved in the removal (resorption) of bone. The nutrient supply to the osteocytes is via the bone fluid. This medium surrounds the processes in the canaliculi and also the blood vessels, and reaches to the osteoblasts. It is hypertonic to blood plasma, with a higher potassium and lower ionized calcium content (Talmage, 1970).

Initial growth

It is characteristic of bone that it develops only following the replacement of a 'model' of connective tissue already present. In a few cases (mostly in those bones of the skull known as the calvaria) the method is called intramembranous and there is replacement only of the cells of a primitive connective tissue; for most bones, however, the process is called endochondral and involves the replacement of a cartilage model. It is generally considered that the method of formation is basically similar in both processes.

In endochondral ossification, a mass of mesenchymal cells, growing by repeated interstitial proliferation, and held in an intercellular cartilaginous matrix, takes on the general outline of the future bone. The outer cells form the perichondrium, the outer layer of which eventually differentiates into fibroblasts, destined to become the outer periosteal sheath. The inner layer remains relatively undifferentiated. As a result, however, of invading capillaries (Ham and Cormack, 1979) some of the inner cells become osteoblasts. They lay down osteoid, which immediately becomes calcified to form an outer ring of bone (the process begins near the centre of the diaphysis). Within this ring, the cartilaginous cells become invaded by an advancing capillary network. They first hypertrophy, then calcify and then degenerate. The developing capillaries carry cells which will eventually form the haematopoietic cells of the marrow. From some of these cells are derived the osteoclasts.

In the centre of the shaft, known as the diaphyseal ossification centre, the degenerating cartilage cells break up and leave spaces in which osteoblasts lay down a matrix which calcifies, forming spongy bone (Fig. 7.3(a)). This gradually extends to the extremities. The periosteum continues to add cortical bone, and eventually, as this is sufficiently increased in strength, the cancellous bone is remodelled through the combined action of osteoblasts and osteoclasts and tends to disappear at the centre, to be replaced by the marrow cavity (Fig. 7.3(c)). Similar changes now occur separately at the ends of the long bones, at sites which are called the epiphyseal ossification centres. Here too, the cartilage is first invaded by capillaries, hypertrophies, calcifies and then degenerates, to be replaced by cancellous bone. Some cartilage remains at the ends, to form the articular cartilage, and some remains towards the centre of the shaft, where it forms the epiphyseal plate. This acts as a centre for the continued growth in length of the bone after birth, until maturity is reached. In the rat, this plate is never completely replaced by bone and thus, in contrast to farm animals (and man), the bone continues to show some degree of growth throughout life (see Fig. 7.3(b)). In the growth from the epiphyseal disc, the chondrocytes of the cartilage proliferate, forming characteristic columns of cells. These cells compress the cells below them, on the diaphyseal side, and these hypertrophy, calcify and then degenerate, to be replaced by new cancellous bone, formed by osteoblasts. This bone eventually becomes remodelled and, particularly at the sides, merges to become cortical

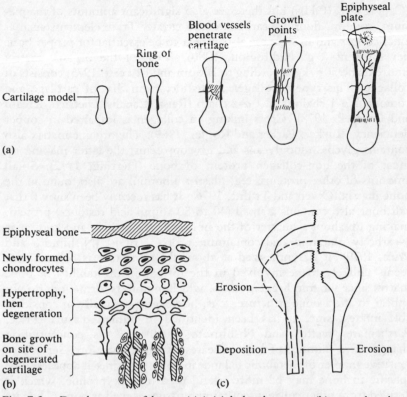

Fig. 7.3. Development of bone: (a) initial development; (b) growth subsequently, in the epiphyseal region; and (c) remodelling of the shaft of the growing bone. (Adapted from Bloom and Fawcett, 1975, and Ham and Cormack, 1979.)

bone (Fig. 7.3(c)). There is thus a continual growth in length of the bone, although the width of the epiphyseal plate of cartilage remains fairly constant. Meanwhile, along the shaft, bone is both eroded and replaced. The added bone, as discussed earlier, is formed from the layer of osteoblasts lining the periosteum. At the same time there is erosion of bone at the inner layer, to a lesser degree. Thus the bone increases in width, with an increase in the space occupied by the marrow cavity and a much smaller increase in the cross-sectional area of the cortical bone.

Structure and formation of the bone matrix

Up to 650 g/kg of the matrix in adult animals is mineral although, in severe malnutrition or with bone disease, the mineral content may be as low as 350 g/kg. Most of this mineral is crystalline hydroxyapatite

(Ca_{10} $(PO_4)_6$ $(OH)_2$) but there are also significant amounts of magnesium, sodium, fluoride, carbonate and citrate. Trace elements such as zinc, copper and manganese also appear to be essential for proper bone development (e.g. Hidiroglou, 1980). Most of the organic matrix (more than 950 g/kg according to Bloom and Fawcett, 1975) consists of collagen. This type 1 collagen is distinct from that of cartilage and contains 2 α-1 chains and 1 α-2 chain (Raisz, Canalis, Dietrich, Kream and Gworek, 1978). Cross-linking in collagen is impaired in copper deficiency (Rucker, Parker and Rogler, 1969). The organic matrix also contains glycosaminoglycans and glycoproteins, the latter making up most of the non-collagen protein of bone (Herring, 1972). Small amounts of other proteins, e.g. plasma albumin, are also found in the bone matrix (Owen and Triffitt, 1976). It has recently been shown that calf bone also contains a small (40 to 50 amino acid residues) protein, making up about a quarter of the non-collagen protein and known as γ-carboxy glutamic acid-containing protein (BGP) (Nishimoto and Price, 1979). It is synthesized at about the same rate as collagen but seems unlikely to be involved in the formation or stability of bone matrix since vitamin K antagonists, which inhibit its formation, do not appear to affect bone structure. It is, however, potentially of considerable interest since it has been identified in human plasma (Price, Parthemare, Deftos and Nishimoto, 1980) and its concentration changes in a number of bone diseases. It may, therefore, serve as a sensitive marker of metabolic balance in bone, and since it appears to be specific to bone may be more useful than hydroxyproline, which is derived from other collagen-containing tissues as well as bone. The rate of synthesis of BGP has recently been shown to be increased by 1,25-dihydroxy vitamin D_3 (Price and Baukol, 1980).

Osteoblasts have a well-developed Golgi apparatus and high (relative to osteoclasts) prolyl hydroxylase and alkaline phosphatase activity (Luben, Wong and Cohn, 1976). They secrete collagen (or procollagen which is cleaved and assembled to fibres extracellularly (Vaughan, 1980)) from one cell surface so that the fibres lie parallel to the long axis of the cell. Mineralization, the deposition of apatite which occurs at intervals on the collagen fibres, was originally thought to occur by purely chemical processes once the concentration of calcium and phosphate was above saturation. There is evidence, however, that it is actively induced by the extrusion of vesicles, probably pinched-off cytoplasmic processes from the osteoblasts, or osteocytes as some will have become (Anderson, 1969; Bernard and Pease, 1969). From these vesicles, crystal growth may develop by a process analogous to chemical 'seeding'.

Resorption of bone is still subject to much discussion. Osteoclasts are large cells, up to 50 to 100 μm across, and with as many as 50 nuclei. They are asymmetric with the nuclei found on the side away from bone while, adjacent, the plasma membrane has a 'ruffled' border, with many mitochondria near. The cells are also rich in large lysosomes and it has been suggested that they release acid hydrolases (they have much higher acid phosphatase activity than do osteoblasts (Luben *et al.*, 1976)) so that local acid production helps to solubilize bone mineral. They must also release collagenase, although the presence of this is not readily shown, partly perhaps because it is initially combined with an inhibitor (Sellers and Reynolds, 1977) and partly because it is only synthesized when needed (Vaughan, 1980). Although the rôle of osteoclasts in bone resorption is generally accepted, it is possible that other (mononucleate) cells (macrophages) are also involved. Moreover, the absorption of calcium from the matrix, in the homeostatic control of calcium, is now thought to involve osteoblasts and osteocytes (Talmage, Cooper and Park, 1970). The general view developed by Talmage and his colleagues is that there are two processes involved in resorption; the initial rapid process involves the 'packaging' of calcium by osteocytes, and transfer through the cytoplasm to osteoblasts and to the blood stream. This process is relatively rapid and is followed, when necessary, by a more prolonged process of resorption of the matrix, a process which involves osteoclasts and macrophages.

Factors affecting bone accretion and resorption

The rates of formation and breakdown of bone seem to be sensitive to more hormones than are other tissues such as muscle and adipose tissue (see below); this is probably because bone has a function as a mineral reservoir, in addition to its supportive rôle. It is at all events not surprising that it is very sensitive to changes in nutrition. Synthesis and resorption of bone continue after maturity – not only the mineral but also for the organic matrix and osteocytes. In large animals, after maturity, these changes result in no change in shape or size, but there is 'remodelling' with, in some cases, changes in strength. Extensive mobilizing of calcium, with resulting effects on the skeleton, may occur in sheep and cattle, in pregnancy and lactation; perhaps the most extreme case occurs in laying birds, when a reserve of trabecular bone is built up over part of the laying cycle to be made available during egg production.

Calcium and phosphate
An adequate intake of calcium and phosphate is required for the proper mineralization of the skeleton, both during development and for maintenance. However, Raisz *et al.* (1978) have also shown that, for rat foetal bone in culture, changes in phosphate concentration within the

physiological range (2 to 4 mmol/l) can also affect the rate of collagen synthesis. Calcium had a similar effect only when the concentration fell below 0.5 mmol/l. It seems likely that similar effects may occur in the intact animal. Thus, Table 7.1 shows the effects of phosphorus and/or calcium deficiency on skeletal growth in young lambs (Field, Suttle and Nisbet, 1975). A low phosphate intake had much more effect than a low calcium intake in limiting the growth of the skeleton; surprisingly, the effect was much less when both calcium and phosphate concentrations were low.

Table 7.1   The effect of diets low in calcium, inorganic phosphorus (Pi), or low in both on the growth of the skeleton in lambs. (The control diet contained about 4 g Ca per kg DM and 3.5 g Pi per kg. Low-Ca diets contained 0.64 to 0.68 g/kg, and low-Pi diets 1.1 to 1.3 g/kg. Animals weighed, on average, 15 kg at the start of the experiment. Only mild and temporary physical abnormalities were seen in animals on the deficient diets. Results are taken from Field *et al.* (1975)

Diets	Control	Low Pi	Low Ca	Low Pi and Ca
Food intake (kg per 16 weeks)	158	92	118	142
Body weight gain (kg per 16 weeks)	24.7	10.0	17.1	18.8
Gain in fat-free skeleton (kg per 16 weeks)	1.4	0.4	1.0	0.9

Vitamins

D_3 (cholecalciferol)

The importance of vitamin D for proper bone development has been known for some years, since a lack caused rickets in growing children or animals, and osteomalacia in adults. It is now known that, for physiological activity, D_3 is converted via 25-(OH)-D_3 to 1,25(OH)$_2$-D_3 (see, e.g. De Luca, 1980). This metabolite is known to have powerful calcium-mobilizing effects on bone, which can be demonstrated *in vitro* (e.g. Brommage and Neuman, 1979). Such effects, however, can obviously not explain the action of vitamin D in the treatment of rickets, where mineralization is defective. It has therefore been suggested that the major effect is that on intestinal absorption of calcium, and that the mineralization effect of vitamin D is indirect. Ornoy, Goodwin, Noff and Endelstein(1978), however, suggested that a further metabolite of vitamin D (24,25(OH)$_2$D$_3$) was responsible for normalizing mineral deposition in these circumstances. De Luca (1980) pointed out that 24(F)25(OH)D$_3$ was equally effective in preventing rickets, although the 24 position was not available, and this throws some doubt on the rôle of $24,25(OH)_2D_3$ as a hormone with direct effect on bone.

Vitamin A
This is also important, a lack resulting in diminished growth of the skeleton. It has been shown to have effects on the lysosomal membranes of osteoclasts (Reynolds and Dingle, 1970). Hypervitaminosis A can result in accelerated erosion of cartilage, which can lead to obliteration of the epiphyseal plate and premature termination of growth.

Vitamin C
This exerts an effect since it is required for collagen synthesis. Raisz *et al.* (1978) have observed that it is an essential additive to bone tissue in culture. It is required in the hydroxylation of proline.

Hormones
Parathyroid hormone (PTH) and calcitonin (CT)
It is likely that these hormones have several modes of action on bone.

1. There are rapid effects by which PTH increases and CT decreases the flux of calcium into blood. These effects initially involve increased entry of calcium into cells lining bone fluid (osteoblasts and osteocytes). Talmage (1978) has suggested 20 to 500 times more calcium flux occurs in this way than bone resorption.
2. PTH can increase bone resorption and decrease accretion. Raisz *et al.* (1978) have shown that PTH can inhibit collagen synthesis in cultured bone. Luben *et al.* (1976) have shown that PTH can affect isolated presumptive osteoclasts, increasing hyaluronic acid synthesis and acid phosphatase activity, while calcitonin antagonizes these effects. PTH also reduced alkaline phosphatase and prolyl hydroxylase in presumptive osteoblasts; CT had no effect on this action.
3. PTH in low doses may also have an anabolic effect (Raisz *et al.*, 1978).

Other hormones
Insulin increased the rate of collagen synthesis in cultured foetal rat bone and also stimulated the orderly deposition of new matrix; somatomedin C also stimulated collagen synthesis, whereas growth hormone produced no response (Raisz *et al.*, 1978). The well known effect of hypohysectomy in limiting normal skeletal growth, and of

growth hormone in stimulating it, may therefore be mediated by somatomedins (SM) although Raisz and his colleagues speculated that the major effect of SM may be on cartilage, whereas insulin might act directly on bone cells. These same workers could obtain no effect of thyroid hormones in bone culture, but Mundy, Shapiro, Bandeli, Canalis and Raisz (1976) found that T_4 and T_3 increased calcium release from cultured foetal rat bone. In infants, thyroid deficiency results in severe dwarfism (Vaughan, 1980). Corticosteroids also affect bone development, producing osteoporosis, although at low dosage they too may produce anabolic effects (Raisz *et al.*, 1978). Oestrogens and testosterone also have effects on skeletal growth. Both stimulating and inhibiting effects have been described, the difference perhaps depending on dose (Short, 1980). Direct effects on cultured bone have not been demonstrated, and it has therefore been argued that these hormones affect bone indirectly.

Local factors

Prostaglandins have been reported to increase bone resorption and an osteoclast activating factor (OAF), which was isolated from cultures of human leucocytes but has subsequently been demonstrated to be present in several tissues including bone, has also been described (Raisz, Mundy, Dietrich and Canalis, 1977). Bone development is known to be affected by immobilizing the limb, and by mechanical and other forms of stress, and it is possible that locally produced factors such as OAF may mediate these effects.

DEVELOPMENT OF MUSCLE

Structure of mature muscle

The basic unit of muscle is the fibre, and examination of a single muscle reveals a number of bundles of fibres, held by an outer layer of tough connective tissue, the epimysium (Fig. 7.4). The layer below this, which also separates the various bundles, is the perimysium. Between the individual muscle fibres is a further fine layer of connective tissue, the endomysium. All muscle fibres have thus closely investing them a fine layer of connective tissue, containing a network of capillaries. A fibre (Fig. 7.4(c)) is virtually one very elongated cell (the average length is about 10 to 20 mm, but human fibres more than 340 mm long have been reported). The fibre contains many nuclei (typically 100 to 200 per cell), these being found generally in the outer parts of the cell. There is a

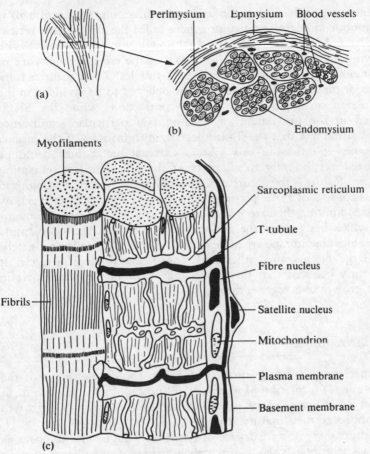

Fig. 7.4.   Structure of muscle: (a) typical flat muscle, sartorius, as found on
the medial surface of the bovine upper hind limb; (b) section of (a)
showing the various connective tissues binding the muscle fibres
(fibre bundles and spaces are not to scale); and (c) constituents of a
muscle fibre. (Adapted from Bloom and Fawcett, 1975.)

limiting cell membrane, the sarcolemma, and within it mitochondria
are found, the number varying markedly with the type of muscle.
There may also be some lipid inclusions, but Golgi apparatus, rough
endoplasmic reticulum (ribosomes) and lysosomes are much less common than in many cells. Cullen and Mastaglia (1980) reported that they
can occur in small numbers adjacent to the myonuclei. The most
striking features of the fibre, however, constituting more than half of
the cell protein, are the myofibrils. Each consists of a number of fine
protein threads, myofilaments, which are packed in groups, separated
by sarcoplasma. The greater part of these filaments consists of two

interdigitating proteins, myosin and actin. Investing the myofibrils is the smooth endoplasmic reticulum, here called the saroplasmic reticulum (SR) and intimately associated (although not continuously) with this, lying perpendicular to the long axis of the cell lies a network of membranous tubules, the transverse or T-tubules. These features fulfil two major functions. The T-tubules are believed to be involved in the transmission of impulses, to induce contraction, while the SR is involved in the movement of calcium. Of particular significance perhaps is the fact that the T-tubules are invaginations of the plasma membrane, and thus in this system external metabolites could be transferred very rapidly to all parts of the cell. The last remaining significant feature is the nature of the sarcolemma. It is now recognized that this consists of a true plasma membrane (to which the term is now restricted) limiting the sarcoplasm and, below this, a basement membrane which lies against the endomysium. Between the sarcolemma and basement membrane are to be found a number of satellite cells, cells with a large nucleus, and earlier easily confused with the fibre nuclei. It is currently believed that these cells may play an important part in muscle growth and regeneration.

Early development

In essence, there are four distinct stages in the development of the muscle cell: (1) formation of *myoblasts*; (2) fusion of myoblasts to form *myotubes*; (3) conversion of myotubes to form *myofibres*; (4) growth of myofibres to their mature size.

In culture there is some degree of synchrony, but *in vivo* myogenesis occurs asynchronously, so that in a given region of an embryo different stages may occur simultaneously. In most mammals stages 1 to 3 are characteristic of prenatal development and stage 4 of postnatal development. The number of myofibres is therefore considered to be largely fixed at birth, and this number may be determined by the number of myoblasts formed in stage 1. However, much less is known about control of this number.

Formation of myoblasts

Almost all muscle develops from embryonic cells of mesodermal origin. The first identifiable cells are myoblasts, which are spindle-shaped cells, rich in ribosomes and contain a single nucleus. Two views have been expressed as to the origin of these cells. According to one view, there are cells in the mesenchyme, not yet identifiable but committed to a myogenic future; such cells have been described as 'presumptive myoblasts'. An alternative view suggests that mesenchymal cells have potential for more than one form of differentiation, the particular route followed depending partly on the environment. In support of this view, Nathanson and Hay (1980) showed that minced embryonic muscle grown on bone matrix developed into fibroblast-like cells, whereas when they were grown on collagen there was an eventual development of muscle fibres. However, McLachlan and Wolpert (1980) who have summarized all the evidence on the subject have argued that the first view represents the process which normally occurs. From cross-transfer experiments using chick and quail somites, it has been shown that the muscle cells in the wing are derived only from the somites, with the remaining cells of different origin.

Formation of myotubes

The committed stage of myogenesis involves the fusion of myoblasts. They become aligned end-to-end and the surface membranes fuse, resulting in elongated multi-nucleated cells known as myotubes. This fusion process is rather specific. Myoblasts may fuse with each other, or with myotubes, which can also fuse with each other (Stromer, Goll, Young, Robson and Parrish, 1974). They will not, however, fuse with other cell types, except myocardial cells under certain conditions (Fischman, 1972).

Myoblasts of different animal origin, e.g. rat and chicken, may fuse although fusion between cells of the same animal origin is preferred (Yaffe, 1969). What determines myoblast fusion is still unsettled. Bischoff and Holtzer (1969) in a widely used theory of cellular differentiation have suggested that in cell replication, following several proliferative cycles there is a specific cycle, referred to by them as a 'quantal cell cycle', in which before G_1[†] there is a change, perhaps irreversible, that leads to withdrawal from the mitotic cycle, producing a cell committed to fusion. On this basis, myoblasts are characterized by having lost the ability to synthesize DNA and fusion is imminent. The evidence in favour of this concept has been reviewed by Allen, Merkel and Young (1979). This theory is not without its critics, however. O'Neill and Stockdale (1972) and Konigsberg, Sollman and Mixter (1978) have produced some evidence that environmental cues (e.g. composition of the surrounding medium) play some part in differentiation. They argue that such cues affect the length of time the myoblast remains in G_1, and that myoblasts have an intrinsic tendency

---

† Cell replication is usually shown as occurring in four stages : (S), the stage of DNA synthesis; (M) the stage of mitosis; (G_2) the period between, the post-synthetic gap; and G_1, the pre-synthetic gap, following M and before new synthesis. When mitosis is halted, the cells are said to be in G_0, that is, the cells are quiescent in the G_1 phase.

to fuse. Thus, the longer the cell remains in G_1, the greater the probability that fusion will occur.

As pointed out above, this argument although unsettled may be of more than academic interest. It has been argued (Stromer *et al.*, 1974) that were myoblasts on average able to pass through an additional proliferative cycle the number of myofibres would be doubled. On the other hand, the existence of animals with double muscling where the number of fibres is increased (although the origin of this is not known) leads to doubt about whether this would be in the best interests of animal husbandry.

What does seem reasonably sure is that the nuclei in myotubes no longer undergo mitosis, so that the number of nuclei in the myotube reflects the number of myoblasts that have fused to form that myotube. The other striking feature of myotubes is the presence of the thick and thin filaments within the cell. The presence of small amounts of contractile proteins can be observed in some spindle-shaped cells. It is claimed (see Fischman, 1972) that these cells are irreversibly committed to fusion and have already withdrawn from the mitotic cycle. On this basis it can be argued that the synthesis of the contractile protein occurs only in cells that have ceased mitosis, though there cannot be any specific or inevitable reason for this, since this does not apply to cardiac muscle. It is clear, however, that the bulk of synthesis of contractile protein begins only in the myotube.

Development of the myofibre

Myotubes are characterized by the presence of contractile protein near the periphery of the cell, with the cell contents (sarcoplasm) and nuclei positioned towards the centre. When the myotube is filled with myofibrils, the nuclei begin to migrate outwards, and eventually to lie under the sarcolemma. The development of the detailed architecture of the myofibre is known only in outline (e.g. Stromer *et al.*, 1974). There is some evidence that a system of microtubules acts as a form of cytoskeleton on which the orderly development of the sarcomeres (the individual units of the myofilament) can proceed. The SR and T-tubular systems develop apparently around the myofibrils. The SR may be developed from the nuclear envelope, while the T-tubular system may be derived from the plasmalemma.

Maturation of the myofibres

The final process of muscle maturation involves increase in length of the myofilaments, increase in the number of myofibrils per myofibre, and an increase in the mean diameter of the myofibrils (Goldspink, 1972). This stage, the main process observed in postnatal growth, is markedly affected by many external factors – it requires innervation, tonic activity and the presence of a number of hormones. In contrast there is evidence that the first three stages may proceed in the absence of all of these.

Although, as has been seen, there is good evidence that the total number of myofibres increases little, if at all, at this stage, it must not be supposed there is no change in the DNA content of the muscle. In fact, Allen *et al.* (1979) have reviewed evidence showing that of the total DNA found in muscle at maturity between 50 and 99% was accumulated postnatally. This is largely due to an increase in the number of nuclei present. In pigs up to 1 year of age, there is an eight-fold increase in nuclear number in muscle fibres which is actually greater than the increase in mean fibre volume, that is, there are a larger number of nuclei per unit volume (Stickland, Widdowson and Gold-spink, 1975). The question arises as to the origin of these additional nuclei. It is suggested that they are derived from the satellite cells, referred to earlier, which lie just outside the sarcolemma. They have been shown to have mitotic activity and it has been suggested that they are in fact modified presumptive myoblasts arrested in the G_1 phase. It is known that the number of satellite nuclei decreases steadily during growth (Goldspink, 1972) although they do not disappear completely when growth is complete, and indeed are believed to play an important part in the regeneration of muscle that can occur following injury (Nag and Foster, 1981). Why there should be an increase in the number of nuclei per myofibre is not clear, although it has been plausibly argued that a nucleus may direct or control only a limited cellular mass. There is some evidence consistent with the possibility that nuclear accretion can limit muscle growth. Moss (1968) studied muscle growth and nuclear numbers in the pectoral muscle of chickens from 0 to 27 days of age, with growth stunting by fasting from 7 to 9 days. Starved/re-fed birds had smaller muscle mass and nuclear numbers than control birds, but the mass per unit nucleus was exactly the same, suggesting that the limit to recovery in compensatory growth is set by the number of nuclei that can be produced in the re-feeding period.

Protein turnover in muscle

It has been recognized for many years that the deposition of protein in tissues represents the net effect of two processes, protein synthesis and protein degradation. Control of protein deposition may be exerted through either or both of these processes.

Protein synthesis

Excellent summaries of the processes of protein synthesis as it occurs in eucaryotic cells have been made by Pain (1978) and Pain and Clemens (1980) and the outline presented below is based on these. Protein synthesis occurs in two parts. *Transcription* is the process of formation in the nucleus of a sequence of bases coding for a particular protein as messenger RNA (mRNA). In addition to a coded sequence, mRNA contains additional bases which are not translated and at the 5' end a base sequence known as the 'cap' which may be involved in the initiation of protein synthesis, while at the 3' end there is a 'poly A' sequence which may either play some part in regulation of protein synthesis or be concerned in the turnover of mRNA itself. *Translation* is the process occurring in the cytoplasm by which the coded base sequence in mRNA is used to direct formation of one specific polypeptide. In addition to mRNA the process requires transfer RNA (tRNA) and ribosomal RNA (rRNA). The various tRNA species have a clover-leaf structure. Each has one triplet base sequence (anti-codon) which binds specifically to the complementary codon (representing a particular amino acid) on mRNA, while at the 3' end there is a site at which the specific amino acid can be bound. rRNA is associated with about 70 proteins in the form of ribosomes. There are two ribosomal subunits, described from their sedimentation rate in the centrifuge as 40S and 60S subunits. They can be combined to form an 80S subunit.

Translation involves first formation of the various amino acyl tRNA, these reactions being catalysed by a series of synthetases:

$$\text{amino acid} + \text{tRNA} + \text{ATP} = \text{aminoacyl-tRNA} + \text{AMP} + \text{Pi}$$

This process is often described as the charging of tRNA species. There are two methionyl-tRNA. In addition to one used where appropriate in polypeptide sequences (meth-tRNA$_m$), there is a second designated meth-tRNA$_f$ which acts as an initiator for all polypeptides. The *ribosomal cycle* (see Fig. 7.5(a)) involves *initiation* in which 40S, 60S ribosomes and meth-tRNA$_f$ are bound to the initiating point of mRNA; *elongation* in which the ribosome moves along the mRNA, acquiring a lengthening polypeptide chain; and *termination* in which the polypeptide and ribosome are released, the latter re-entering the cycle. Each process requires the catalytic influence of only partly-defined proteins which are given a suitably non-committal terminology. Thus, in initiation, there are eucaryotic initiation factors (eIF-1, eIF-2, etc.); in elongation, there are EF-1, EF-2; and in termination RF.

Initiation (Fig. 7.5(b))

This requires dissociation of 80S ribosomes into subunits. This probably involves eIF-3 becoming bound to the 40S subunit, while the

Process of translation in protein synthesis

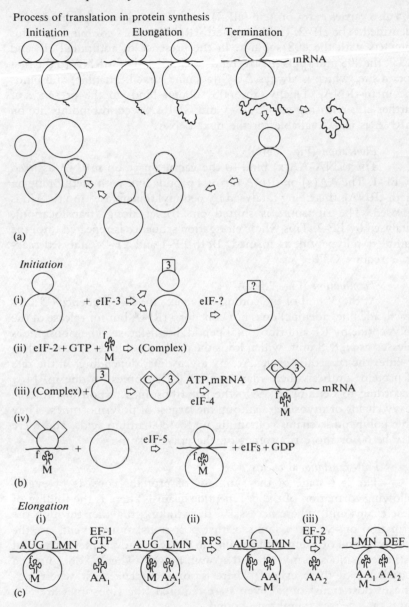

(d) *Termination*

Releasing factor (RF) + Ribosomal peptidyl transferase ⇨ Peptide + tRNA + mRNA

Fig. 7.5. Steps in the synthesis of protein in eucaryotes: ◯, 60S ribosome; ○, 40S ribosome; ⚛, tRNA; eIF, eucaryotic initiation factors; EF, elongation factors; RPS, ribosomal peptidyl synthetase; AA₁, AA₂, amino acids; AUG, first codon; LMN, DEF, subsequent codons. (Adapted from Pain, 1978, and Pain and Clemens, 1980.)

60S also carries extra protein (eIF-?) not associated with factors already identified. The eIF-2, GTP and meth-tRNA$_f$ form a complex, and this interacts with the 40S subunit. In the presence of additional eIF and ATP, the 40S unit (plus tRNA) binds at the 5' end of mRNA to the first codon site, which is always AUG (adenine, uracil, guanine) and binds the meth-tRNA$_f$. Finally, the 60S subunit binds in the presence of further eIF, releasing eIF-2, eIF-3 and GDP. A second binding site on mRNA is now available for the next tRNA.

Elongation (Fig. 7.5(c))
The tRNA-AA(x) bind to the vacant space on mRNA assisted by EF-1. The AA(x) on tRNA forms a peptide link with methionine on meth-tRNA$_f$, this being catalysed by peptidyl transferase, and tRNA$_f$ is released. The ribosome is shifted one triplet along (translocation), catalysed by EF-2. This whole elongation sequence is repeated until the complete polypeptide is formed. Both EF-1 and EF-2-catalysed reactions require GTP.

Termination (Fig. 7.5(d))
At the 3' end of the coding sequence, the last sequence (UAA–uracil, adenine, adenine) does not code for a tRNA but for release of the polypeptide by RF and ribosomal peptidyl transferase. The ribosome is released as an 80S unit, which joins the pool of 80S units and may then re-enter the ribosome cycle. At any given time, depending on the rate of protein synthesis there may be several ribosomes on one mRNA. According to Lehninger (1975) the polyribosomes responsible for the heavy chains of myosin are among the largest of polyribosomes. They have polypeptide chains containing up to 1800 amino acids, and there may be 60 or more ribosomes on the polyribosome.

Post-translational events
The last stage of the synthesis of proteins consists of events following formation of the polypeptide chains. There is the folding of these chains and, where necessary, their linking together through the formation of -S-S- crosslinks. Other post-translational events are the hydroxylation of some of the proline in collagen and the methylation of histidine residues in myosin and actin in muscle. There is only limited knowledge of these events. There is some evidence that where significant post-translational events are required, the ribosomes are to a significant degree membrane-bound.

Control of the rate of protein synthesis
The nature of the particular proteins present is determined by the mRNA present. Probably the relative proportions of these proteins are determined by the relative amounts of the mRNA, although this is

not invariably true. It is known for example (Buckingham, Caput, Cohen, Whalen and Gros, 1974) that mRNA for myosin is present in myoblasts before fusion and several hours before significant synthesis of myosin begins. Whether, when synthesis of a specific protein is increased, this is due to increased production or decreased breakdown of mRNA is not generally known. Control of the rate of protein synthesis in general, however, is not normally determined by the amount of mRNA available, but at the level of translation (Pain 1978). There are several possible sites where such control could be exerted. At present, the evidence favours events in initiation as being generally of more significance than elongation or termination (Pain and Clemens, 1980). It is possible to get some estimation of changes in the rate of initiation relative to that of elongation from changes in profiles of polysomes in tissues, that is, from the proportion of rRNA that is in polysomal form (with a series of ribosomes on mRNA) relative to that in monosomal form. There are some technical difficulties in doing this with muscle, because ribosomes tend to precipitate with myosin when preparing cell extracts (see Pain and Clemens, 1980). Nevertheless, in diabetic muscle, for example, where there is a decrease in the rate of protein synthesis, there is a decreased polysome/monosome ratio. It is to be noted that the changed polysome profile does not of itself give any indication of the rate of protein synthesis. If the rate of protein synthesis were increased in diabetes, then the observed polysome profile would indicate an increase in rate of elongation, relative to initiation. It is only because direct evidence (e.g., from incorporation of ^{14}C-amino acids into protein) shows that the rate is decreased in diabetes that it can be concluded that there is also a decline in the rate of initiation relative to elongation. Similar changes are reported to occur in muscle following starvation, hypophysectomy or treatment with large doses of glucocorticoids (see Pain and Clemens, 1980, for details). Reference to the initial steps of protein synthesis suggests several sites at which control might be exerted. One obvious one is the very first step, the charging of tRNA. This might well be expected to be determined by amino acid availability, or by reduced activity of amino acyl tRNA synthetase. From measurements in rat liver, however, (Allen, Raines and Regen, 1969) tRNA appeared to be 80 to 95% charged, even in fasting, although there was some decrease when the diet was markedly imbalanced with respect to particular amino acids. This sort of control seems even less likely to be of significance in muscle since, unlike the liver, variation in the supply of amino acids has *in general* no effect on the rate of protein synthesis.

In Ascites tumour cells in culture the rate of protein synthesis is markedly dependent on the supply of indispensable amino acids in the medium. Pain and Clemens (1980) and their colleagues have shown that in these conditions there is significantly reduced formation of the ternary complex, GTP/eIF-2/meth-tRNA$_f$ (see Fig. 7.5) and this seems to be limited by the eIF-2 available. Austin and Clemens (1981) have suggested that amino acid imbalance results in the formation of an eIF-2 phosphorylated derivative and thus makes the availability of eIF-2 limiting. Although it has been shown that in ribosome-free extracts of the muscle of rats fasted or treated with cortisone there is decreased ability to form ternary complex (Rannels, Pegg, Rannels and Jefferson, 1978; Rannels, Rannels, Pegg and Jefferson 1978), this change occurs rather slowly and is directly proportional to the rate of reduction in tissue RNA content, making it more likely that this is a response to some other change rather than a direct control mechanism.

Protein degradation

The degradation of proteins (Ballard, 1977; Meyer, Burgess and Russell, 1980) is an important component of protein turnover, but it is much less well-characterized than the process of protein synthesis. The only well-recognized system is the autophagolysosomal system. This system of organelles contains a series of peptide hydrolases only active at acid pH. The major proteolytic enzymes are the cathepsins, A, B$_1$, B$_2$, C, D and E, cathepsin D being regarded as the major endopeptidase. What are described as primary lysosomes are formed at the Golgi apparatus, or something functionally similar, and consist simply of a series of enzymes surrounded by a membrane, forming a vesicle. Other vesicles contain portions of the cellular material, such as mitochondria or endoplasmic reticulum, surrounded by a membrane (autophagic vacuoles) or extracellular material formed by pinching off of the plasma membrane (heterophagic vacuoles). These vacuoles will eventually merge with primary lysosomes, to form secondary lysosomes and the proteolytic degradation then occurs within the secondary lysosome.

It has been suggested that the lysosomal system may only be involved in cellular pathology, but Dean (1975) has shown that in the perfused liver addition of liposomes containing pepstatin, a specific inhibitor of cathepsin D, will reduce protein breakdown by 50%, which suggests that lysosomes are substantially involved in normal protein breakdown. Moreover, the extent of formation of lysosomes is found to be greatly increased by glucagon, which is known to increase protein breakdown, and this action is opposed by insulin. There is also evidence (Chua, Kao, Rannels and Morgan, 1978) that lysosomes play some part in protein degradation in the perfused rat heart since perfusion in the absence of insulin results in increased size of autophagic vacuoles in myocardial cells, as well as decreased latency[†] of cathepsin

† The term 'latency' refers to the increase in cathepsin D activity in homogenates when the lysosomal membranes are disrupted by detergents.

D, features which were reversed by concentrations of insulin which decreased the rate of protein degradation.

The involvement of lysosomes can also be used to account for the observation, now well established (see Ballard, 1977), that protein degradation is an energy-requiring process, although proteolytic reactions are exergonic. This could come about through a need for ATP-coupled reactions to drive protons into lysosomes, in order to keep the internal environment there sufficiently acidic for effective action of cathepsins. The reported inhibitory effect of ammonia on protein degradation (Seglen, 1975) in the liver might also be explained by the penetration of ammonia into lysosomes, elevation of the pH and consequent inhibition of the cathepsins.

Nevertheless, there is good evidence that the lysosomal system cannot be the only means by which protein is degraded in cells. Ballard (1977) has argued that there must be at least two systems. In particular, there are a number of proteins with much shorter half-lives than the average for the cell. In some cases these turn over much more rapidly than the organelle in which they are found. The rate of breakdown of these proteins is found to be insensitive to hormones such as insulin and glucagon and to inhibitors believed to affect the lysosomal system. Several neutral proteinases have been described (see Waterlow, Garlick and Millward, 1978). The authors point out that most of these proteinases show some degree of specificity towards particular proteins. It is interesting that a number of such proteinases has been described in muscle, where normally lysosomes are sparse. However, it cannot yet be concluded that the lysosome system is less important in protein degradation in skeletal muscle since none of the neutral proteinases in muscle have been properly characterized. Moreover, at least abnormal proteins (N-ethyl maleimide labelled) have been shown to be degraded by the lysosomal system in rat gastrocnemius (Gerard and Schneider, 1979).

It is perhaps not surprising that no single system will account generally for protein degradation. Meyer *et al.* (1980) have suggested that there are three distinct processes involving peptide cleavage.
1. *Immediate post-translational changes in newly synthesized proteins.* For all proteins, this will include the removal of the initiator amino acid (methionine); in addition there may also be removal of 'signal' peptide sequences, especially in proteins destined to be secreted from the cell.
2. *Degradation of newly synthesized protein.* In part this may be required for the correction of errors in protein synthesis (what has been called 'proof reading') but there may also be mistakes due to environmental conditions. Ballard (1977) has given several examples of this. Thus, he and his colleagues have shown that haemoglobin synthesized by reticulocytes in the absence of histidine has a much shorter half-life than that made under normal circumstances. He has suggested that this

may be explained by premature termination of the newly synthesized peptide, which is then rapidly degraded. Increased rate of protein degradation may, therefore, be a factor in conditions of nutritional imbalance. It is interesting also that in some human genetic abnormalities (certain forms of thalassaemia) an excess of α- over β-chains of haemoglobin is produced. Although the excess α-chain material is normal polypeptide, however, much is rapidly degraded, suggesting that peptide chains without the correct conformation will suffer greatly accelerated rates of degradation. There is other evidence too that some normal peptides may be rapidly degraded soon after synthesis. For example, results of Sodek (1976) suggest that only 30% of synthesized collagen of skin undergoes maturation to insoluble fibres, and Bienkowski, Cowan, McDonald and Crystal (1978) have shown that a significant fraction of collagen newly synthesized by fibroblasts is rapidly destroyed. Scornik and Botbol (1976) found that 50% of newly labelled hepatic protein was degraded within 3 h. It is interesting to find that several inhibitors of protein synthesis at the same time also reduce the rate of protein degradation. It has been argued, indeed, that the energy requirement for protein degradation is due to a requirement for simultaneous protein synthesis, perhaps for the synthesis of specific proteins; alternatively, inhibition of protein synthesis might lead to the accumulation of intermediates (such as uncharged tRNA) which could interfere with protein degradation. Whatever the explanation, it is striking that there is frequently some association between rate of protein synthesis and of degradation.

3. *Physiological degradation of the bulk of the cellular protein.*

The distinction between these three processes is not sharply defined, but will be a function of the time following synthesis during which a protein is subject to some degree of proteolysis. Immediate changes following synthesis (1 and partly 2) will perhaps be due to specific proteinases, while the longer lasting and more stable a protein is, the more likely it is that it will be degraded by the lysosomal system (i.e. 3).

Control of the rate of protein degradation

Several characteristics of proteins have been shown to result in increased susceptibility to degradation. These include: size of subunit, larger ones showing increased susceptibility; nature of the isoelectric point, those with more acidic ones also being more susceptible to degradation; number of hydrophobic groups, those with larger numbers also being more susceptible; and the degree of thermal stability, those with the least thermal stability being most susceptible. Waterlow et al. (1978) have also suggested that enzymes with regulatory functions are less stable than others. It has been argued on these and on other grounds that the first and perhaps rate-limiting step in protein degradation is loss of the normal conformation. In suitable proteins this will be assisted by a high-SH to -S-S- ratio; thus glutathione, which tends to open -S-S- links in some proteins, lowers their conformational stability. In this form it is suggested they become membrane-bound and susceptible to proteolysis. Ballard (1977) picturesquely described this membrane function as like that of an intracellular flypaper. In lysosomes, the first step is likely to be the inclusion of the proteins within a vacuole, before fusion of this with a primary lysosome, since there is little evidence that proteins can penetrate lysosomal membranes by other than a micropinocytotic process. Once inside the lysosomes, degradation may well occur as already described.

It should be noted that protein degradation is as important in embryonic as in more mature tissues. Indeed, it may even be more so, since it perhaps plays a significant part in the remodelling of tissues during growth. Thus, Vandenburgh and Kaufman (1980) have shown that embryonic chicken muscle containing myotubes and fibroblasts shows evidence of two sorts of degradation – for short-life and long-life proteins – degradation of the latter being more subject to control than the former; they were inhibited by leupeptin more than pepstatin, suggesting that cathepsin B was more important than cathepsin D.

Some factors affecting post-natal muscle growth

Hormones
Insulin
The presence of muscle wasting in diabetes suggested that insulin played an important rôle in maintenance of normal muscle and it has been proposed (e.g., Goldberg, Tischler, De Martino and Griffin, 1980) that insulin is probably the most important factor regulating protein balance in skeletal muscle. One action, the rôle in initiation of the translational component of protein synthesis, has already been discussed. Jefferson, Boyd, Flaim and Peavy (1980) have shown that this action is not general, and may be limited to fast-twitch muscle[†]; in both soleus muscle, which is mostly slow-red fibres, and cardiac muscle insulin had no effect on peptide chain initiation. In all muscles, however, insulin lack led to a reduction in RNA (by approximately 15%) which must be due mainly to a reduction in number of ribosomes, since 85 to 95% of RNA is ribosomal. In rats with chronic

[†] Skeletal muscles have generally a population of three sorts of muscle fibre: fast-twitch red (high glycolytic and high oxidative capacity); fast-twitch white (high glycolytic/slow oxidative capacity); and slow-twitch red (low glycolytic/moderate oxidative capacity). Red muscles show some metabolic characteristics in common with cardiac muscle.

diabetes (7 days after induction) there was an altered polysomal profile, which suggested that further effects on elongation or termination reactions had occurred. These changes were not reversed acutely by insulin. Insulin also has an action in stimulating the transport of some amino acids into muscle but this is presumably supportive rather than primary since, in the heart at least, when protein synthesis is accelerated by the action of insulin the intracellular concentration of amino acids actually falls.

As discussed earlier, insulin is also active in reducing the rate of protein degradation. Goldberg (1979) has shown that this action occurs in the isolated diaphragm, as well as in the cardiac muscle. Inhibition of degradation also results from the addition of glucose, although glucose has no effect on the rate of protein synthesis. Moreover, insulin and glucose together are more effective than either alone. A response similar to that obtained with glucose can also be produced by other energy-yielding substances such as ketones. Whether these effects of nutrients apply generally to skeletal muscle is not certain: the diaphragm is more akin to cardiac and red muscle. As pointed out earlier, the action of insulin in inhibiting protein degradation may operate through an effect on the lysosomal system, and there may be little effect on proteins of short half-life. In muscle this would imply that the major effect would be on actin and myosin, which have a slower turnover time than the sarcoplasmic proteins.

Growth hormone

The stunting of growth and decreased development of skeletal muscle that follow hypophysectomy suggest that growth hormone probably plays some part on protein turnover in muscle. Hypophysectomy in fact reduces protein synthesis in muscle by at least 50%, and there is a 30% reduction in protein degradation (see Goldberg *et al.*, 1980). There is also a decrease in the amount of RNA present in the tissue and thus probably in the number of ribosomes (Jefferson *et al.*, 1980). Treatment of hypophysectomized animals with growth hormone for several days restores protein synthesis almost to normal but has no effect on protein degradation. Thus growth hormone appears to affect the protein synthesis but not protein breakdown. The effect appears to be primarily on the efficiency of protein synthesis, that is on the rate of synthesis per ribosome, rather than on the number of ribosomes, and may be direct since Dreskin and Kostyo (1980) demonstrated a response in synthesis within 30 min of injection of the hormone. Some of the actions of growth hormone are now known to be mediated by a series of polypeptides, the somatomedins. These substances may have some action on muscle protein synthesis (see, e.g. Waterlow *et al.*, 1978; Young, 1980) but if the action of growth hormone discussed here is mediated in this way, it would seem necessary that they be produced locally within the muscle. Their main action in affecting growth is more likely to be through their influence on bone and cartilage development. Growth hormone is also important in the regulation of DNA synthesis in muscle and it is possible that the somatomedins play a significant part in this action (Waterlow *et al.*, 1978).

Thyroid hormones

As has been indicated growth hormone is unable to affect the reduced rate of protein degradation that occurs following hypophysectomy. This appears to be due to lack of thyroid hormones, and can be reversed after several days' treatment with thyroxin (T_4) or tri-iodothyronine (T_3). Goldberg *et al.* (1980) have shown that effects on synthesis and degradation occur with small doses of thyroid hormone, and that as the hormone dose is increased the additional response in protein synthesis progressively diminishes but the rate of protein degradation continues to be increased. Brown, Bates, Holliday and Millward (1981) have also demonstrated effects of T_3 on protein synthesis and degradation in thyroidectomized as well as hypophysectomized growing rats. Thyroidectomy resulted primarily in a fall in the amount of RNA, with no effect on the rate of synthesis per unit of RNA. However, in hypophysectomized animals, when plasma insulin concentrations were low, thyroid hormone was found to increase the efficiency of protein synthesis. It was suggested that these effects on protein synthesis could be manifested in elongation as well as initiation of the translational process of protein synthesis. However, although thyroid hormones can improve translation, Brown *et al.* (1981) pointed out that hypophysectomized rats treated only with thyroid hormone do not grow. They suggested that this is because there is no increase in DNA: as pointed out earlier this may specifically require growth hormone. It may well be that the most important effects of thyroid hormones in determining normal growth are on proteolysis, and those effects seem to involve lysosomal enzymes. Goldberg *et al.* (1980) reported that thyroidectomy reduced activity of cathepsins B and D more than threefold and similar effects were reported by Brown *et al.* (1981). Goldberg *et al.* (1980) further point out that the changes in lysosomal enzymes are found only in skeletal muscle and liver, which are the two sites at which proteolysis is affected by thyroid hormones.

Glucocorticoids

Glucocorticoids have been known for many years to restrict growth and induce muscle wasting. However, in many studies pharmacological doses have been used and, even in many so-called physiological studies, the effects have largely pertained to the response of animals to a stress. At present there is no general agreement on the action of glucocorticoids on protein balance in muscle. Waterlow *et al.* (1978) concluded that the major effect of glucocorticoids was to decrease muscle protein synthesis (and DNA synthesis) with little effect on protein degradation. However, the experiments on which this view was based involved administration of synthetic or naturally occurring glucocorticoids to normal rats, and as the authors emphasised themselves, it is difficult to interpret experiments because treatment with glucocorticoids to normal rats, and as the authors emphasized themselves, it is difficult to interpret such experiments because treatment with diaphragm muscle, was 30% greater in fed and 40% greater in fasted adrenalectomized rats than in corresponding non-adrenalectomized animals. However, the rate of protein degradation in adrenalectomized animals was similar to that in fed control animals and was 25% less than that in fasted control animals. Cortisol treatment of adrenalectomized animals resulted in a restoration of the normal rate of protein degradation. It was therefore suggested that an effect of glucocorticoids on protein degradation rate is only seen in fasted animals. Young (1980) has referred to experiments showing that growth in adrenalectomized rats was not affected by physiological doses of cortisol, and these results seem to suggest that glucocorticoids at physiological concentrations either have no effect on protein synthesis or degradation rates, or have the same effect on each. However, Young also drew attention to experiments in which N^τ-methylhistidine[†] output was compared in normal and adrenalectomized rats, and there were no marked differences between the two groups. Addition of corticosterone (100 mg/kg body weight) on the other hand did result in an increased output of N^τ-methylhistidine, and even with physiological doses (8 mg/kg) the effect was apparent (+25 to 30%). Thus, while it is possible that glucocorticoids exert effects by reducing protein synthesis and increasing protein degradation, neither effect has been firmly established to occur under normal physiological conditions. It is interesting, however, that DuBois and Almon (1980) have shown that in immobilized muscle (a procedure which results in muscular atrophy) there is a significant increase in glucocorticoid receptors, which the authors interpret to mean that there is increased sensitivity to glucocorticoids. If this is correct, examination of protein synthesis and degradation rates in these circumstances might give more positive indication of an action of glucocorticoid at normal concentrations. Booth and Seider (1979)

[†] N^τ–methylhistidine output in urine has been proposed as an index of muscle protein breakdown, since after proteolysis it cannot be re-utilized in muscle. It has been used in studies in rats and humans, and seems likely to be of value in studies in cattle, but apparently not in sheep or pigs where much may be retained for long periods in bound form (Harris and Milne, 1980)

have shown that protein synthesis declines (by 37%) within 6h of limb immobilization but it is not clear how soon the increase in glucocorticoid receptors occurs. It is unfortunate that there is no clear evidence of glucocorticoid action, because Purchas, Barton and Kirton (1980) have recently suggested that growth rates in beef cattle are inversely related to average plasma cortisol concentrations.

Sex steroids

The rôle of androgens is of obvious interest since it is well recognized that muscle growth is greater in males than females, and castration results in diminished muscle growth. The widespread use of anabolic steroids makes this topic of particular significance in the present context, although Waterlow *et al.* (1978) dismiss the effects as of no significance in the short-term regulation of muscle mass. Heitzman (1980) has pointed out that anabolic steroids increase protein deposition in ruminants and pigs, but the effects are not as consistent as in rats, horses or poultry. Both oestrogens and androgens may have anabolic affects and both may be necessary to achieve maximal growth rate. There are indications that oestrogen action may be indirect, through effects on the secretion of other hormones. This may also be true for androgens, but there is evidence that they have direct effects on muscle, since specific androgen receptors have been identified there, although the numbers are small. Vernon and Buttery (see Heitzman, 1980) have shown that, while trienbolone (a synthetic androgen) decreases both protein synthesis and degradation rates in female rats, the effect is larger on degradation rate. It has been suggested (see Heitzman, 1980) that androgens might act by competing with glucocorticoids at binding sites in muscle, or might 'down-regulate' these sites and thus reduce the rate of protein degradation. However, there is no decisive evidence that glucocorticoids act by affecting degradation of protein in muscle (see above), and there is evidence that androgen and glucocorticoid binding sites in muscle are quite distinct. An alternative view, more favoured at present, is that androgens affect thyroid function, which, as described earlier, certainly exerts significant effects on the rate of protein degradation. However, an action of this type has yet to be demonstrated. Indeed, it is not yet certain that the effect observed by Vernon and Buttery in rats applies also to farm animals. Young (1980) has suggested that the response to androgens might originate in the nucleus at the transcriptional level, but his argument is developed mainly by analogy with the action of sex hormones on tissues such as prostate, uterus and oviduct.

Effects of exercise

The ability of muscle to hypertrophy in response to exercise is readily observed in man. As mentioned above, the reverse is also true—

an immobilized muscle soon atrophies. Goldberg (1979) has shown that exercise-induced hypertrophy probably does not involve changes in muscle response to hormones. He used the technique of tenotomy in rats (section of the insertion of the gastrocnemius in the Achilles tendon). The other muscles in that limb are thereby forced to support the weight of the body and quickly hypertrophy. It was shown that this occurred in hypophysectomized and diabetic animals, and so presumably needs the presence of neither pituitary nor pancreatic hormones. Fasting or cortisol treatment can also result in weight increase in worked muscle, while other muscles are losing weight. Passive stretch (that is, immobilizing of a muscle under tension) also results in increased growth (Goldspink, 1977). It is even possible to get some growth in stretched denervated muscle, although this is less than in normal muscle. Thus, an intact nerve supply is not essential to avoid atrophy, and the major factor is clearly the work or tension maintained in a muscle.

The mechanism of hypertrophy has been the subject of dispute. Goldberg (1979) was unable to demonstrate effects on protein synthesis but claimed that the rate of protein degradation was significantly reduced. Laurent and Millward (1980), however, have criticized most of the evidence relating to changes in the rate of protein degradation, which is notoriously difficult to determine (see Waterlow *et al.*, 1978). In studies of the hypertrophy of the wing muscle of chickens subjected to a load, Laurent and Millward (1980) were able to demonstrate a marked increase in the rate of protein synthesis. This rate was substantially greater than the rate of growth and there must therefore have been an increase in the rate of proteolysis. Thus, hypertrophy resembles normal growth, in having high rates of both synthesis and degradation. Laurent and Millward argue that stretch may be the most important factor regulating normal muscle growth since the effect of tension occurs in the absence of other hormones, and in fasting when nutrient availability may be minimal. It may be that growth of bone, to which muscles are generally connected through their tendons, provides the normal tension which acts as the stimulus for growth.

Nutrient supply
Amino acids

In rat liver, the rate of protein synthesis is greatly affected by the concentration of amino acids in the perfusing medium (Jefferson and Korner, 1969). A six-fold increase above normal physiological concentrations, when the effect was maximal, resulted in a four-fold increase in rate of synthesis. Omission of a dispensable amino acid (except proline) had little effect, but omission of an indispensable one (except histidine) markedly reduced the rate of synthesis. In contrast, in rat muscle, Li and Jefferson (1978) found that increasing the input of amino acids five-fold resulted in only a 20 to 30% increase in the rate of protein synthesis with a similar response in protein degradation, and these effects were only seen in young (presumably rapidly growing) animals. Omission of particular amino acids had in general no effect on synthesis rate but the branched-chain amino acids, and leucine in particular, were found to be potent – they were in fact wholly responsible for the changes in synthesis attributable to total amino acid supply. These findings are not really understood, particularly since, as discussed earlier, the rate of protein synthesis seems to depend on the process of initiation and not the availability of aminoacyl-tRNA. However the results do suggest that, in normal circumstances, the concentration of amino acids will not determine the rate of protein synthesis in muscle.

In sheep and cattle, there is a net output of amino acids from hind limb tissue (mostly muscle) after 24 to 28 h of fasting (see Lindsay and Buttery, 1980). This probably reflects a fall in the rate of protein synthesis, although this is not known positively. Yet plasma amino acid concentrations have decreased by no more than 10%. Similarly in other adverse nutritional states, protein synthesis is generally affected. In rats, the rate varies throughout the day, being least just before a meal, and it is also reduced in animals given protein-free, or low-protein diets. Indeed, even with marginal malnutrition over several generations, there results a systematic lowering of the rate of protein synthesis in most of the body tissues. With acute malnourishment in young animals, the effect may be less in muscle than other tissues, so that growth in muscle may continue while there is an actual loss of body weight. The point about all these changes is that there is no discernible pattern in the plasma concentrations of amino acids – they may be high or low, quite independently of rate of protein synthesis; moreover the concentrations of individual amino acids may change independently of each other, so that as one falls another increases (see Waterlow *et al.*, 1978). Rate of synthesis is thus not controlled by blood plasma amino acid concentrations, but is more probably determined by the hormonal and mechanical factors discussed above.

Energy sources

The roll of nutrients such as glucose, volatile fatty acids (VFA), free fatty acids (FFA) and ketones is not at all clear, though there is much evidence from studies *in vivo* that an increase in the supply of energy-yielding nutrients improves nitrogen retention. Eskeland, Pfander and Preston (1974), for example, showed that infusion of glucose, acetate, propionate or butyrate into lambs reduced urinary nitrogen output and improved nitrogen retention. Glucose and propionate were more effective than non-glucogenic VFA. Many similar experiments have been reported in humans and rats (see Munro, 1964), but the mechanism is not understood. There is evidence from study with isolated rat tissues (see Goldberg *et al.*, 1980) that glucose inhibits protein degradation in muscle but does not affect protein synthesis. In contrast, studies in man (Sim, Wolfe, Young, Clarke and Moore, 1979) have shown that glucose infusion during fasting increases whole-body protein synthesis (estimated from glycine turnover) but has no effect on protein degradation (as estimated from N^τ-methylhistidine output). These results are not necessarily inconsistent, since protein synthesis in muscle accounts for only approximately one quarter of total body synthesis (see below), and the evidence suggested that at least one effect of glucose was on synthesis of protein in the small intestine. In growing lambs there is some association of glucose turnover with growth (see Lindsay, 1979) but this may mean no more than that both are correlated with energy intake. Glucose is such a powerful insulin secretogogue that *in vivo* it is difficult to separate effects of insulin and glucose. Lindsay (1979) has speculated that glucose turnover is maintained in fasting mainly because of a link with protein turnover (in man, the rate of glucose production in fasting may plausibly be explained by the energy needs of the brain, but this is not a satisfactory explanation in domestic animals). Such a link might be through a need for the synthesis of dispensable amino acids in peripheral tissues. Aspartate flux, for example (Lindsay, 1982), is inadequate to account for peripheral protein turnover rates. It has also been suggested (see Lindsay and Buttery, 1980) that ketones could inhibit the oxidation of leucine in muscle. There is no direct evidence that this happens but such an effect could explain why protein mobilization is limited during fasting whilst there is extensive mobilization of fat. Alternatively, fatty acids and perhaps also ketones and acetate may reduce the oxidation of glucose or of glycogen, and thereby make more glucose available for synthesis of dispensable amino acids.

DEVELOPMENT OF FAT

Structural lipids are present in all tissues, in the form of phospholipids, but deposition of lipid as an energy reserve occurs in most animals only as triacylglycerols and this is normally found only in specialized cells in white adipose tissue. Small amounts of triacylglycerols do occur normally in tissues such as liver and kidney, but substantial deposition is an indication of a pathological condition. Thus, studies of fattening, that is, the growth of fat, are concerned with the development of white adipose tissue.

Development of adipose tissue

This subject has been reviewed recently by both Leat and Cox (1980) and Hausman, Campion and Martin (1980). Adipose tissue occurs in two forms, white and brown, of which only the former is used for the storage of mobilizable lipid. Brown adipose tissue (BAT) occurs at specific sites and is most readily observed in neonates and rodents. In some species, such as the sheep, it tends to disappear as the animal matures but in others, especially in hibernating animals and rodents, it persists into adult life. BAT is currently considered to function as a source of heat through local oxidation of fatty acids, and may therefore be a significant component (in some circumstances) of non-shivering thermogenesis. The difference in colour is principally due to the presence of large amounts of cytochromes in BAT, and it also has a richer vascularity. Histologically the two types of cell are clearly distinguished at maturity (Fig. 7.6). White adipose tissue contains large cells dominated by a single vacuole of lipid, with no surrounding membrane. There is a flattened nucleus at one side. The cytoplasm contains only a few mitochondria, although ribonucleoprotein, smooth endoplasmic reticulum and Golgi apparatus can occasionally be seen in the flattened periphery. In BAT, in contrast, there is a larger cytoplasm to lipid ratio, generally multiple lipid locules, glycogen granules, and the nucleus is less flattened; most characteristically, there are numerous well developed mitochondria. In addition, unmyelinated nerve fibres are invariably found in close proximity.

There are three questions of particular interest in the histogenesis of adipose tissue. First, what are the cells from which adipose cells originate? Secondly, can BAT cells be converted into white adipose tissue, in those species in which BAT gradually disappears as the animal matures? Finally, are the number of adipose cells fixed, and if so at what stage of maturity, so that any subsequent development can only be by hypertrophy rather than hyperplasia? The main difficulty in answering these questions has been in identifying adipose cells. This is obviously easy when they are mature and filled with lipid; but before any lipid is present, the 'pre-adipocytes' show little to distinguish them from other cells of connective tissues.

There is, at present, no agreement as to the nature of the cells which ultimately give rise to adipocytes. Indeed, 20 to 30 years ago, there was still a body of opinion which doubted whether there were specific cells whose sole function was the storage (and perhaps synthesis) of fat (Le Gros Clark, 1971). It was suggested that adipocytes were fibroblasts which had accumulated an unusually large amount of lipid. Against this view, however, it is clear that fat cells appear at quite characteristic sites during embryonic development. Moreover, human skin fibroblasts in culture show no tendency to

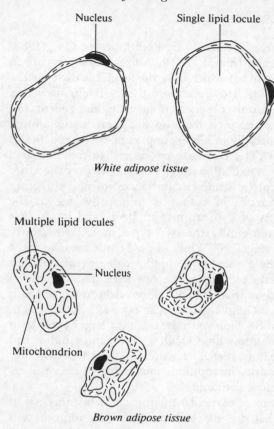

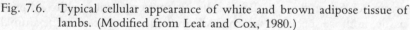

Fig. 7.6.   Typical cellular appearance of white and brown adipose tissue of lambs. (Modified from Leat and Cox, 1980.)

undergo adipose cell conversion, in contrast to fibroblast-like cells from adipose tissue (Van and Roncari, 1978). The main argument that pre-adipocytes are fibroblasts or fibroblast-like, however, is merely that the adipose cells depleted of lipid look rather similar to fibroblasts microscopically. An alternative view is that adipocytes are derived from reticulo-endothelial cells. It is certain that 'pre-adipocytes' always develop in close association with blood vessels, and it has been argued that a short distance from capillary lumen to adipocyte is essential for the efficient transport of fatty acids. The development in the embryo of adipocytes in intimate association with blood precursor cells has led to suggestions that endothelial cells, perivascular reticular cells, macrophages, or phagocyte precursors may give rise to adipocytes.

Whether white adipose tissue is derived from BAT is also not clearly resolved. In species such as the lamb, where BAT is substantially lost in the first 2 to 3 weeks of life, to be replaced by white adipose tissue, there appear at this stage to be numbers of cells with intermediate characteristics, and thus Gemmell, Bell and Alexander (1972) concluded that at these sites white adipose tissue probably was derived from BAT. Since at birth all the adipose tissue appeared characteristic of BAT, this might indicate that BAT was an invariable intermediate stage. However, Leat and Cox (1980) have pointed out that sternal (brisket) fat in the foetus near term is unilocular (that is, contained one large lipid inclusion) with sparse, poorly developed mitochondria. It is thus typical white adipose tissue, and shows no sign of having been derived from BAT. It appears that, although BAT may be transformed into white adipose tissue, white adipose tissue need not arise in this way.

The period for which hyperplasia continues in neonatal species has also proved difficult to determine. The problems have been critically examined by Kirtland and Gurr (1979). Once fat cells begin to accumulate lipid, they no longer show mitotic figures, as Bell (1909) showed with ox adipose tissue. The crucial problem, however, is for how long pre-adipocytes are able to continue cell division, and whether this is affected by the lipid loading of other adipocytes, or by nutritional conditions. There is certainly an increase in adipose cell numbers in farm livestock in early post-natal development; in pigs up to about 5 months of age; in sheep up to about 11 months; and in cattle up to 14 months (Hood, 1982). How far this represents true hyperplasia is uncertain. Kirtland and Gurr (1979) suggest that in pigs, for example, true hyperplasia, as estimated from the incorporation of ^{3}H-thymidine, may be completed much sooner than indicated by cell, counting techniques. On the other hand, there is evidence that even in mature animals there may be some capacity to increase cell numbers, although this possible hyperplasia has not as yet been verified by the ^{3}H-thymidine technique.

The overall increase in adipose cell numbers does mask the fact that adipose tissue development occurs sequentially within an animal. There is generally development first of the internal depots, such as perirenal and omental fat, then of intermuscular or subcutaneous fat and finally of intramuscular or, more accurately, of interfascicular fat. Thus, Allen (1976) has shown that in cattle at 14 months of age size distribution of adipose cells in perirenal or subcutaneous adipose tissue is roughly normally distributed about a mean of 150 μm diameter, and a range of 60 to 200 μm. In interfascicular adipose tissue, however, at this age the distribution is bivariate, with two peaks, one below 50 and one around 100 μm. This rather suggests development of a new population of cells, although, as Allen was careful to point out, it could also be due to phased periods of differentiation initially, followed by a similar pattern of filling out of cells. The same bivariate pattern was observed in subcutaneous tissue in very fat cattle.

Much of the original impetus for the study of adipose cell number developed from the work of Knittle and Hirsch (1968). They suggested that differences in food intake during suckling resulted in permanent differences in adipose cell number; that lipogenic activity was similar in large and small cells; and thus that the increased cell number might result in a permanently impressed tendency to greater fatness. Their findings have not gone without challenge (see Kirtland and Gurr, 1979), but of particular relevance in the present context is whether similar effects may be found in farm animals. In studies in pigs (see Allen, 1976) underfeeding during suckling did not result in appreciable change in adipose cell numbers if comparison was made at a constant final body weight (80 kg), although there was some difference in cell numbers in interfascicular fat if comparison was made at the same age (53 days). Moreover, large adipose cells are more lipogenically active than small adipose cells – the activity appears to be related to the cell surface area, although with very large cells there may be some decrease in activity. Thus, a greater number of adipose cells does not necessarily imply increased fatness. Hood (1982) pointed out that commercial fattening of farm livestock is primarily a matter of hypertrophy, rather than hyperplasia, and that alteration of adipose cell numbers by dietary or other means, even if it is possible, is unlikely to have any practical application.

Factors affecting the deposition of fat in adipose tissue

There are three processes at which control might be directly exerted on the extent of accumulation of fat in adipose cells: 1. the rate of deposition of long-chain fatty acids in adipose tissue; 2. the rate of synthesis of fatty acids within the cells; and 3. the rate of release of fatty acids from adipose tissue. Net change in fat stores will be the resultant sum of processes $1 + 2 - 3$.

Rate of deposition of long-chain fatty acids

Long-chain fatty acids taken up by adipose tissue could be derived either for dietary long-chain fatty acids, or from acids synthesized in other tissues from small molecules. In chickens, the liver and not adipose tissue is a major site for the synthesis of fatty acids (O'Hea and Leveille, 1969a) but in pigs (O'Hea and Leveille, 1969b) the liver accounts for less than 5% of fatty acids synthesized from glucose although much more if acetate is the substrate. However, only approximately 5% of the metabolizable energy (ME) is absorbed as acetate (see Lindsay, 1981) and thus, if glucose and acetate are the only important precursors, less than 20% of total fatty acids synthesized are made in the liver. In sheep, Ingle, Bauman and Garrigus (1972) found about 5% of fatty acids were synthesized from acetate in the liver and up to 30% in the gastrointestinal tract. However, of total lipogenesis, as estimated by incorporation of ^3H_2O into lipid, Prior (1978) found that the contribution of the liver might be rather larger, from 10 to 18% of the total fatty acid synthesized. While, therefore, extra-adipose sites may make some contribution to long-chain fatty acid synthesis, most of the long-chain fatty acids arriving at adipose tissue will be of dietary origin.

A typical pig diet is rich in carbohydrate. Even so, a pig eating 3 kg food per day may take in at least 100 g lipid per day . Ruminants are also generally held to have low-fat diets, and certainly sheep on a forage diet receive only 20 to 60 g long-chain fatty acids per day (Ulyatt and MacRae, 1974). However, the amount may be rather greater on concentrate diets and there is some evidence that the supply of long-chain fatty acids may be increased through synthesis of microbial lipid in the rumen (see Sutton, Storry and Nicholson, 1970). Thus, Sutton (1974) estimated that in dairy cows approximately 15% of ME was absorbed as lipid. Ruminants are intolerant of large amounts of fat added to their diet, because it interferes with ruminal fermentation (Devendra and Lewis, 1973). It is possible, however, to add 'protected' lipid (by coating oil droplets with formaldehyde-treated protein) (Scott, Cook and Mills, 1971) which is resistant to the action of rumen microorganisms and by this means large amounts of dietary fat may be given. Fatty acids can be absorbed by ruminants with fairly high efficiency. Hartmann, Harris and Lascelles (1966) were able to recover in the thoracic duct lymph of lactating cows nearly half of a dose of about 500 g lipid, within 24 h of administration. In ruminants the mixture of absorbed fatty acids is particularly rich in stearic acid, formed as a result of ruminal hydrogenation. The efficiency of absorption of fatty acids is in the order $18:0 < 16:0 < 18:1$ in ruminants, as in other animals (Harrison and Leat, 1975), but stearic acid is nevertheless particularly well absorbed in ruminants.

Most long-chain fatty acid is absorbed as triacylglycerols via the lymphatic system (Harrison and Leat, 1975). It is not clear at present what factors might control this, although Emery (1979) has suggested intestinal sterolgenesis may be important. Lymph in sheep is fairly rich in phospholipid, and Harrison and Leat (1975) suggested that most of the triacylglycerol transported to blood is in the form of very low density lipoprotein (VLDL). Gooden, Fraser, Bosanquet and Bickerstaffe (1979) have shown that, when corn oil is infused into the duodenum, the size of lymph lipoprotein is increased so that there is then substantial absorption of chylomicrons. Thus, the absorption of fatty acids in ruminants is very similar to that in other species. However, chylomicrons are rarely seen in ruminant plasma, even when substantial amounts of dietary lipid are fed. It may be that even under these conditions, the proportion of dietary intake as fat is substantially less than in many non-ruminants, especially in humans.

Lipoprotein lipolysis.

The first stage in the uptake of fatty acids by adipose tissue is their release by hydrolysis of lipoprotein triacylglycerol, a process which is mediated by lipoprotein lipase (LPL). This enzyme is formed in only a limited number of tissues (principally adipose tissue, muscle and mammary gland) and is active on the capillary walls (see Nilsson-Ehle, Garfinkel and Schotz, 1980) in conjunction with a small protein, apoprotein C_{ii}. In lactating cows, this activator increased with the intake of dietary fat, or with total plasma lipid (Super, Palmquist and Schanbacher, 1976). Its availability could therefore play some rôle in regulatory activity. In adipose tissue LPL activity is known to be increased by insulin and inactivated by catecholamines (Robinson, Cryer and Davies, 1975), although the opposite seems to be true in muscle. Superficially, LPL activity might be supposed always to be adequate, since FFA are released into the blood, as well as being taken up by adipose tissue. Since the mechanism of uptake is not understood, however, it is more realistic to suppose that LPL sensitivity to dietary and hormonal conditions indicates that its activity is likely to be limiting at least in some conditions. The FFA passing into the plasma will in part be taken up by the liver, and may then be presented to adipose tissue in the form of hepatic-derived lipoprotein. How significant this recycling is in farm livestock is not known, although the rate of lipoprotein formation in the sheep liver is apparently rather slow (from the negligible conversion of FFA to triglyceride: Bergman, Havel, Wolfe and Bohmer, 1971).

The last stage in the deposition of fat involves the synthesis of triacylglycerols. Emery (1979) has suggested this is an important stage of control of fat deposition in ruminants. He showed that glyceride-synthesizing activity was greater in fat than in lean type sheep, and declined from ewes to wethers to rams.

Rate of synthesis of fatty acids within adipose cells

There is compelling evidence that synthesis of fatty acids from small molecules (synthesis *de novo*) normally plays an important part in the fattening of pigs. Hood and Allen (1973) calculated from gain in body fat content, and long-chain fatty acid content of the diet, that 70 to 80% of the fatty acids in pigs must be derived from synthesis *de novo*, the greatest values being seen in breeds with a propensity to fatten. It is interesting to apply these results to a typical study of carcass deposition in pigs. In the work of Kotarbińska and Kiclanowski (1969), pigs of mean weight 80 kg were shown to be depositing about 191 g crude fat per day. Thus about 30% of the ME intake was being deposited as fat and fat synthesis *de novo* was accounting for approximately 21 to 24% of the ME intake. In comparison with this it can be calculated from a study by O'Hea and Leveille (1969b) with ^{14}C-glucose that approximately 130 g of glucose per kg was incorporated into adipose tissue. Only 4/6 of the glucose carbons appeared in the fatty acids synthesized and thus approximately 200 g of glucose per kg (13/0.66) was used for lipogenesis. Since glucose absorbed is about half of ME intake (see Lindsay, 1981) in such pigs, fat synthesis from glucose would account for approximately 10% of the ME intake. Other small molecules (lactate, VFA) would probably make some contribution to lipogenesis but it is unlikely that the total lipid synthesized would be much above 15% of the ME. These isotopic experiments, however, were made with young pigs weighing about 15 kg and it is possible that in these animals lipogenesis was less than in the more mature animals used in the studies of carcass deposition.

The results for pigs may be contrasted with those obtained in studies with sheep. It has been generally accepted for some years (see for example, Bauman, 1976) that acetate and not glucose is the major carbon source for lipogenesis in ruminants. However, from studies by Ingle *et al.* (1972) it can be calculated that only 5 to 12% of injected ^{14}C-acetate was recovered in the adipose tissue of growing or market-weight lambs. In a study by Prior (1978) in which a similar technique was used, recovery was again at best about 12%. Acetate accounts for about 25 to 30% of ME intake (see, for example, Sutton, 1974; Pethick, Lindsay, Barker and Northrop, 1981). Thus, lipogenesis from acetate might account for only approximately 3.0 to 3.5% of ME. The potential amount of lipogenesis in fattening sheep, cannot be estimated directly because of the lack of information about how much energy is absorbed as long-chain fatty acids. As already discussed, dietary fat intake is often not very high, but the amount that might be available by microbial synthesis is subject to much uncertainty. Nevertheless, it seems highly probable that lipogenesis is greater than the estimates above, and the question arises as to the cause of this discrepancy. It may be that incorporation of ^{14}C-acetate is much more than measured. However, oxidation of acetate is generally substantial. Pethick *et al.* (1981) estimated that in sheep at least 80% of the acetate supply was oxidized, and this might well have been an underestimate; thus, at most, 20% of the acetate supply might be used for lipogenesis. The proportion of ME accounted for by acetate is also unlikely to have been underestimated (it is probably in fact lower for fattening rations containing cereal concentrates). Thus it seems possible that some metabolite other than acetate may be of substantial importance as a precursor for lipogenesis. Ballard, Filsell and Jarrett (1972) indicated that glucose might play a more significant rôle in lipid synthesis in animals receiving a high-concentrate diet than in those fed a maintenance, forage diet and, more recently, the studies of Prior (1978) have suggested that lactate might play a significant rôle as a lipogenic precursor; in both cases, however, it is doubtful if the evidence suggests that these substrates have greater importance than acetate. Prior and Jacobson (1979) have shown that in vitro lactate incorporation is decreased by acetate, while acetate incorporation is actually increased by lactate. These effects were seen at physiological concentrations of lactate, and only further complicate its rôle in lipogenesis. For many years calorimetric studies (see, for example, Blaxter, 1962; Tyrrell, Reynolds and Moe, 1979) have left doubts concerning the efficiency of use of acetate for lipogenesis and these doubts do not seem to be resolved by the more fundamental studies.

The biochemical features characterizing lipogenesis in ruminants have been discussed elsewhere (see Bauman 1976 and Ch. 3). Bauman and Davis (1975) and Bauman (1976) have presented evidence suggesting that the step catalysed by acetyl-CoA carboxylase (conversion of acetyl-CoA to malonyl-CoA) may be the key regulatory step in lipogenesis in adipose tissue in fattening lambs, and this step is commonly regarded as rate-limiting in non-ruminant lipogenesis. Since the reaction is a late stage in lipogenesis, irrespective of the precursor substrate, it suggests that rate of lipogenesis is independent of the availability of a particular substrate.

In non-ruminants (although most of the evidence is derived from studies in rats) insulin markedly stimulates lipogenesis in adipose tissue and this effect is antagonized by adrenalin. A large part of the effect may occur through action on acetyl-CoA carboxylase, and pyruvic dehydrogenase (see Denton, 1975). In ruminants, Prior and Smith (1982) have suggested that the involvement of insulin in lipogenesis is much less plausibly established. It is possible that the sensitivity to insulin may be much less than in non-ruminants, but it would be surprising were the difference qualitative rather than quantitative.

Mobilizing of fatty acids from adipose tissue

Lipolysis of triacylglycerol in adipose tissue results in formation of glycerol and free (unesterified) fatty acids, this reaction being catalysed by a 'hormone-sensitive lipase'. Some of the fatty acid is promptly re-esterified. This requires α-glycerophosphate, derived from glucose, since glycerol kinase is absent, or virtually so, in adipose tissue (Bauman, 1976). Thus, free glycerol and some non-esterified fatty acids (FFA) are released into blood. FFA are predominantly derived from adipose tissues, although the liver can release FFA (Bergman *et al.*, 1971). Normally, however, the liver extracts approximately 25% of leanness in many animals (e.g., Chappel and Dunkin, 1975), but it lipoprotein (VLDL) or (in times of substantial energy deficit) as ketones and acetate. A significant amount of the FFA taken up by the liver in fed animals may also be oxidized there. The major factor controlling the utilization of FFA is the plasma concentration (although it must be admitted this conclusion is largely based on studies in fasted or underfed animals) (see Lindsay, 1975). Thus, it may be that the major factor controlling the utilization of FFA is the rate of mobilization from adipose tissue. The controlling lipase is readily stimulated by catecholamines and sympathetic nervous stimulation, and these effects are antagonized by insulin (see Siddle and Hales, 1975). It has been argued that in ruminants these responses are muted (see, for example, Bauman, 1976). However, Bassett (1970) showed that in sheep the response to catecholamines *in vivo* was of quite comparable sensitivity to that seen in non-ruminants, and he suggested that apparent insensitivity was largely a result of technical difficulties in some of the studies *in vitro*. Although insulin effects on lipolysis *in vitro* are quite modest (Bauman, 1976), *in vivo* insulin has an immediate effect in lowering FFA concentrations in sheep (e.g., Lindsay, 1961). It has also been argued that growth hormone has some lipolytic rôle (see, for example, Emery, 1979). There is much evidence that growth hormone treatment is associated with loss of adipose tissue, and encourages the development of leanness in many animals (e.g., Chappel and Dunkin, 1975), but it has been curiously difficult to demonstrate direct effects of growth hormone on the mobilization of adipose tissue.

It is also uncertain how far other metabolites have an effect on FFA mobilization. *In vitro*, the effects are often erratic (see Bauman, 1976) but *in vivo* acetate, for example, has a marked and immediate effect in lowering FFA (Lindsay, 1961). It is frequently difficult to assess such effects, since they might occur indirectly, by stimulating endocrine secretions, although for acetate this seems unlikely.

INTERACTIONS IN THE GROWTH OF SKELETAL, MUSCULAR AND ADIPOSE TISSUES

So far, some of the factors that affect the growth of particular tissues have been discussed. These tissues, however, do not grow independently of each other. In an agricultural context, what is particularly of interest is the nature of the carcass – the proportions of fat and muscle that have been laid down as an animal approaches maturity. Traditionally, a substantial covering of fat has been favoured, as is implied by the terms 'fat lamb' or 'fat cattle' for animals raised primarily for meat, but in recent years there has been increased emphasis on the production of animals with a high proportion of muscle. In this last section, some of the factors that determine the amounts of muscle or fat deposited are discussed.

Genetic differences

Breed differences are well known to affect body composition. In pigs, the Piétrain has up to 100 g/kg more muscle than the Large White of the same body weight. Lister (1976) has pointed out that in part this is a consequence of reduced voluntary food intake by Piétrains (compare Fig. 7.1); but even when Large White pigs are matched for food intake with Piétrains, they accumulate more fat. Similar compositional differences are found in sheep, in comparing for example the Suffolk and Welsh Mountain breeds, or with cattle by comparing Hereford and Charolais. In all animals, however, the pattern of growth described in the introduction to this chapter and illustrated in Fig. 7.1 is observed, that is, the approach to mature size occurs sooner in skeleton and in muscle than in fat. Those breeds with a higher proportion of lean tissue are those which take longer to reach maturity. Thus, comparison of the Piétrain and Large White of equal body weight involves comparison of animals of different physiological age, that is, of different fractional maturity and it is not surprising that the 'younger' Piétrain has a higher proportion of muscle and bone. Moreover, as discussed earlier, there is a general pattern of fat deposition. Thus, the slower maturing animals will tend to have a lower proportion of their fat in the subcutaneous depots.

Energy costs

As judged from experimental determinations (Mount, 1980a), the cost of synthesizing protein (J/J deposited) is substantially greater than the cost of synthesizing fat. For protein synthesis, efficiencies range from 0.40 to 0.70, whereas for fat they are more typically about 0.70 to 0.75. This observed difference is surprising because theoretically little difference is to be expected. Millward, Garlick and Reeds (1976) calculated that, even if fatty acids were first synthesized from carbohydrate (see Flatt, 1970, for relevant pathways), the energy cost should be approximately 0.15 J/J deposited; while for protein synthesis (assuming 4 to 5 mol of ATP used per peptide bond: see earlier in this chapter) the cost should be very similar. Thus, for both, the efficiency should be approximately 0.87 (1/1.15). There are difficulties though in determining the energy cost of protein synthesis. It is usually done through multiple regression analysis of tissue deposition in growing animals, that is, by supposing that the ME intake $(ME_i) = C + E_pP + E_FF$, where C is the energy used for maintenance, P and F are the amounts of protein and fat gained, and E_P and E_F are the efficiencies of utilization of energy for protein and fat deposition. However, what maintenance means in a growing animal is open to question, as is the assumption that the various components of the partial regression equation are independent of each other. An alternative approach has been developed by Pullar and Webster (1977) using congenitally obese and lean rats. This method, though not entirely free of assumptions (see van Es, 1980) overcomes some of the difficulties encountered with the regression technique and has still given results showing marked differences in the efficiency of protein and fat deposition ($E_P = 0.44$; $E_F = 0.77$). The explanation most favoured to account for the low apparent efficiency for protein is that the value does not take account of protein turnover. As indicated earlier, protein deposition is the net effect of two processes, synthesis and degradation. Thus, in growing pigs at approximately 25 kg weight, Edmunds, Buttery and Fisher (1980) determined that the total protein synthesized was about 250–450 g/day, whereas protein deposited was less than 100 g/day. They did point out, however, that even supposing that all the turnover was growth-related (which is almost certainly not true) it was insufficient to account for the low efficiency of protein deposition. Perhaps also to be considered is the cost of protein degradation, since as discussed earlier, it is energy-requiring, perhaps to meet the needs of lysosome formation. Close (1978) has suggested that the efficiency of protein deposition varies with food intake, so that the efficiency is least at high rates of intake, and where rates of protein deposition are greatest. This is quite probable since rate of degradation and thus of turnover is likely to increase when the rate of synthesis is high and there may be a parallel increase in the requirement for dispensable amino acids which have to be synthesized.

There are also energy costs associated with the growth of bone, although these are not usually considered. Preedy and Waterlow (1981) have shown that in young rats the rate of synthesis of bone protein is high, and may account for 15% of the rate of whole-body protein synthesis. In addition, if, as discussed earlier, mineralization occurs by vesicle formation this too is likely to have an energy requirement. These costs may be included in the 'maintenance' energy component but they could also be regarded as contributing to the energy cost of protein deposition since the rate of growth of bone, and hence development of tension in muscle, may be a factor in determining the rate of muscle growth.

Environmental temperature is another, often neglected, factor that can influence the energy costs of tissue deposition (Mount, 1980b). Apart from the fact that voluntary food intake may be affected by the external temperature, there are additional direct effects on metabolism. Below the critical temperature (which varies inversely with food intake) there is an increased maintenance energy requirement to maintain deep-body temperature, and heat generated in the deposition of nutrients is also used for this purpose. Efficiency of utilization of energy for both fat and protein deposition is increased as environmental temperature falls (Close, 1978).

Models for growth

Models have been developed which attempt to predict the expected growth rate from a known food intake (for example see Whittemore, 1976). In such models it is supposed that protein deposition is determined by the amount and quality of the protein intake up to some maximal value. The energy cost of 'maintenance' (which is partly determined by the environmental temperature) plus the energy cost of protein deposited (and the cost of synthesis) is then subtracted from the energy intake, and from the energy surplus the amount of fat that could be deposited is calculated. Perhaps the greatest difficulty in developing such models is that (as discussed above) energy cannot really be partitioned into such separate packages. Nevertheless, there is some virtue in asserting that protein deposition has priority over fat deposition. Close, Mount and Brown (1978) determined energy balance in growing pigs with varying environmental temperatures. At 'maintenance', that is, at zero energy retention, they showed that there was a net deposition of protein, with a net loss of body fat. There should therefore be some point, in terms of energy intake, at which protein is deposited but not fat. Such a point has not been defined, although it might perhaps be determined as the point at which the plasma FFA concentration reaches its nadir. The rate of protein deposition under these circumstances may of course be much less than maximal – perhaps less than half maximal.

Effects of nutrient flow

Amino acids

The absorption of amino acids during and after a meal has several consequences.

1. The major use of amino acids is for protein synthesis, and initially this occurs predominantly in tissues with a high rate

of turnover. In growing pigs (Edmunds *et al.*, 1980) only 25% of protein synthesis occurred in muscle. However, the rate of breakdown of protein is also high in tissues with a high turnover, so that over an appreciable time 75% of the protein deposited was found in muscle. Rate of synthesis, and even more perhaps the rate of breakdown, will be determined by: genetic potential; hormonal environment (which itself is determined partly by genotype and partly by absorbed nutrients); and possibly also amount and composition of the absorbed amino acids.

2. Amino acids surplus to need for protein synthesis are catabolized. The preferential use for protein synthesis arises first because the enzymes initiating catabolism have a lower affinity for their substrate (higher K_m) than those initiating synthesis. Only at a raised intracellular concentration does amino acid catabolism become significant although there does seem to be a low, minimal rate of catabolism for many amino acids. Secondly, catabolism does not occur in all tissues. For most of the amino acids, catabolism is restricted to the liver, although for the branched-chain and some of the dispensable amino acids it occurs more generally in extrahepatic tissues also (Lindsay, 1980).

3. The inflow of amino acids may initiate an endocrine response. This may be through a direct stimulus; or during absorption amino acids may stimulate production of gut hormones which then stimulate release of anabolic hormones; or amino acids taken up by the brain may have an effect on production of neurotransmitters, and this may result in a stimulus to hormonal secretion.

Carbohydrate and fatty acids

The first demand on the use of absorbed carbohydrates and fatty acids will be their catabolism to meet energy requirements. After this need is met there will be deposition of nutrients partly as glycogen but mainly as fat. Deposition of nutrients probably occurs under all circumstances even when energy intake is minimal but a net gain in tissue stores depends on the balance between deposition and mobilization. Thus for example in animals fed once daily there is a net deposition of tissue just after a meal, but a net loss in subsequent hours before the next meal. Carbohydrate may also be used in the synthesis of dispensable amino acids. Thus there is some indication that, in sheep, aspartate supply in the blood plasma may be too low to meet the needs of peripheral tissues for protein synthesis (see Lindsay, 1982) and most aspartate must be synthesized in the tissues themselves. Whether aspartate production can ever be limiting for protein synthesis, however, has not been established. Absorbed carbohydrates and fatty acids may also affect the pattern of hormone secretion and, although the mechanisms involved may be similar to those already described for amino acids, it is likely that the overall response will be rather different.

The partition of nutrients

How then might changes in dietary intake of protein or energy affect the partition of nutrient use between protein and fat deposition? Clearly, no simple answer is possible since nutritional changes which reduce the deposition of fat are likely also to reduce the deposition of protein (Fig. 7.1). This is emphasized in a recent study by Byers and Rompala (1980) involving two breeds of cattle given various levels of food intake. In this experiment protein deposition was observed to vary from 60 to 190 g/day and fat deposition from 80 to 600 g/day, but overall the two were highly significantly positively correlated. Studies with ruminants present special problems in interpretation because it is difficult to vary independently the amount of energy and protein absorbed. However, Reeds, Fuller, Cadenhead, Lobley and McDonald (1981) have made a revealing study in growing pigs and some of their results are summarised in Table 7.2. Although there was an increase in the rate of whole-body protein synthesis when additional fat, carbohydrate or protein was provided, the response was greatest with protein. However, this response was accompanied by an increase in the rate of protein breakdown whereas, with increased intake of carbohydrate and fat, protein breakdown was unaffected or slightly decreased. Thus, if anything, addition of energy-yielding nutrients was more effective than

Table 7.2   The effect of increasing fat, carbohydrate or protein above that in a basal ration on the growth of pigs. (All the values are expressed as $g/kg^{0.75}$ per day. Dietary protein is calculated as $6.25 \times$ apparently digestible dietary nitrogen. Results taken from Reeds *et al.* (1981). Values in parentheses give the measured increases in synthesis, breakdown or deposition in response to the dietary supplement; other values have been calculated from the original data

Diet	Protein synthesis	Protein breakdown	Protein deposited	Fat deposited
Basal diet containing 1.2 MJ energy, 13.4 g protein	34.2	28.0	6.2	7.5
Basal diet plus supplement of				
Fat (0.77 MJ)	37.6(+ 3.4)	25.9(−2.1)	11.7(+5.5)	16.2(+8.7)
Carbohydrate (0.42 MJ)	38.3(+ 4.1)	27.4(−0.6)	10.9(+4.7)	14.7(+7.2)
Protein (0.31 MJ, 13.8 g protein)	46.3(+12.1)	35.3(+7.3)	11.0(+4.8)	6.3(−1.2)

protein in increasing protein gain. The increased synthesis and breakdown associated with increased protein intake resulted in an increased energy cost, so that fat deposition actually fell, whereas as might be expected with increased energy intake there was a marked increase in fat deposition. Although additional dietary protein increased the proportion of gain that was channelled into body tissue protein, it did so by decreasing the efficiency of utilization of the nutrients in terms of energy deposition. If any conclusion may be reached it is that, in searching for a means of increasing protein deposition, it may be more fruitful to look for ways of reducing protein degradation than of increasing protein synthesis.

Finally, it should be noted that by altering more than one variable in the animals' environment – by, for example, changing environmental temperature as well as nutrition, so that the nutrient availability for growth remains unchanged – in pigs, at least, it is possible not only to alter the partition of nutrient use between protein and fat synthesis but also the body conformation (Weaver and Ingram, 1969).

REFERENCES

Allen, C. E., 1976. Cellularity of adipose tissue in meat animals, *Fedn Proc. Fedn Am. Socs exp. Biol.* **35**: 2302–07.

Allen, R. E., Merkel, R. A. and Young, R. B., 1979. Cellular aspects of muscle growth: myogenic cell proliferation, *J. Anim. Sci.* **49**: 115–27.

Allen, R. E., Raines, P. L. and Regen, D. M., 1969. Regulatory significance of transfer RNA charging levels. I. Measurements of charging levels in livers of chow-fed rats, fasting rats, and rats fed balanced or imbalanced mixtures of amino acids, *Biochim. biophys. Acta.* **190**: 323–36.

Anderson, H. C., 1969. Vesicles associated with calcification in the matrix of epiphyseal cartilage, *J. Cell Biol.* **41**: 59–72.

Austin, S. A. and Clemens, M. J., 1981. The regulation of protein synthesis in mammalian cells by amino acid supply, *Biosci. Rep.* **1**: 35–44.

Ballard, F. J., 1977. Intracellular protein degradation. In *Essays in Biochemistry* Vol. 13 (ed. P. N. Campbell and W. N. Aldridge), pp. 1–37. Academic Press, London.

Ballard, F. J., Filsell, O. H. and Jarrett, I. G., 1972. Effects of carbohydrate availability on lipogenesis in sheep, *Biochem. J.* **126**: 193–200.

Basset, J. M., 1970. Metabolic effects of catecholamines in sheep, *Aust. J. biol. Sci.* **23**: 903–14.

Bauman, D. E., 1976. Intermediary metabolism of adipose tissue, *Fedn Proc. Fedn Am. Socs exp. Biol.* **35**: 2308–13.

Bauman, D. E. and Davis, C. L., 1975. Regulation of lipid metabolism. In *Digestion and Metabolism in the Ruminant* (ed. I. W. McDonald and A. C. I. Warner), pp. 496–509. University of New England Publishing Unit, Armidale.

Bell, E. T., 1909. On the histogenesis of the adipose tissue of the ox, *Am. J. Anat.* **9**: 412–38.

Bergman, E. N., Havel, R. J., Wolfe, B. M. and Bohmer, T., 1971. Quantitative studies of the metabolism of chylomicron triglycerides and cholesterol by liver and extrahepatic tissues of sheep and dogs, *J. clin. Invest.* **50**: 1831–39.

Bernard, G. W. and Pease, D. C., 1969. An electron microscopic study of initial intramembranous osteogenesis, *Am. J. Anat.* **125**: 271–90.

Bienkowski, R. S., Cowan, M. J., McDonald, J. A. and Crystal, R. G., 1978. Degradation of newly synthesized collagen, *J. biol. Chem.* **253**: 4356–63.

Bischoff, R. and Holtzer, H., 1969. Mitosis and the process of differentiation of myogenic cells *in vitro J. Cell Biol.* **41**: 188–200.

Blaxter, K. L., 1962. *The Energy Metabolism of Ruminants.* Hutchinson, London.

Bloom, W. and Fawcett, D. W., 1975. *A Textbook of Histology.* 10th edn. Saunders, Philadelphia.

Booth, F. W and Seider, M. J., 1979. Early changes in skeletal muscle protein synthesis after limb immobilization of rats, *J. appl. Physiol.* **47**: 974–77.

Brommage, R. and Neuman, W. F., 1979. Mechanism of mobilization of bone mineral by 1,25 dihydroxyvitamin D_3, *Am. J. Physiol.* **237**: E113–120.

Brown, J. G., Bates, P. C., Holliday, M. A. and Millward, D.J., 1981. Thyroid hormones and muscle protein turnover. The effect of thyroid-hormone deficiency and replacement in thyroidectomized and hypophysectomized rats, *Biochem. J.* **194**: 771–82.

Buckingham, M. E., Caput, D., Cohen, A., Whaler, R. G. and Gros, F., 1974. The synthesis and stability of cytoplasmic messenger RNA during myoblast differentiation in culture, *Proc. natn. Acad. Sci. U.S.A.* **71**: 1466–70.

Byers, F. M. and Rompala, R. E.,1980. Level of energy effects on patterns and energetic efficiency of tissue deposition in small or large mature-size beef cattle. In *Energy Metabolism* (ed. L. E. Mount), pp. 141–46. Butterworth, London.

Chappel, R. J. and Dunkin, A. C., 1975. Relation of concentration of growth hormone in blood plasma to growth rate and carcass characteristics in the pig, *Anim. Prod.* **20**: 51–62.

Chua, B., Kao, R., Rannels, D. E. and Morgan, H. E., 1978. Hormonal and metabolic control of proteolysis, *Biochem. Soc. Symp.*, *No.43*, pp. 1–15.

Close, W. H., 1978. The effects of plane of nutrition and environmental temperature on the energy metabolism of the growing pig. 3. The efficiency of energy utilization for maintenance and growth, *Br. J. Nutr.* **40**: 433–8.

Close, W. H., Mount, L. E. and Brown, D., 1978. The effects of plane of nutrition and environmental temperature on the energy metabolism of the growing pig. 2. Growth rate including protein and fat deposition, *Br. J. Nutr.* **40**: 423–31.

Cullen, M. J. and Mastaglia, F. L., 1980. Morphological change in dystrophic muscle, *Br. med. Bull.* **36**: 145–52.

Devendra, C. and Lewis, D., 1973. The interaction between dietary lipids and fibre sheep. 1. A comparison of the methods used for crude fibre and acid-detergent fibre estimations, *Anim. Prod.* **17**: 275–80.

Dean, R. T., 1975. Direct evidence of importance of lysosomes in degradation of intracellular proteins, *Nature, Lond.* **257**: 414–6.

De Luca, H. F., 1980. Some new concepts emanating from a study of the metabolism and function of vitamin D, *Nutr. Res.* **38**: 169–82.

Denton, R. M., 1975. Hormonal regulation of fatty acid synthesis in adipose tissue through changes in the activities of pyruvate dehydrogenase (*EC* 1.2.4.1) and acetyl-CoA carboxylase (*EC* 6.4.1.2), *Proc. Nutr. Soc.* **34**: 217–24.

Dreskin, S. C. and Kostyo, J. L., 1980. Acute effects of growth hormone on the function of ribosomes of rat skeletal muscles, *Hormone Metab. Res.* **12**: 60–6.

DuBois, D. C. and Almon, R. R., 1980. Disuse atrophy of skeletal muscle is associated with an increase in number of glucocorticoid receptors, *Endocrinology* **107**: 1649–51.

Edmunds, B. K., Buttery, P. J. and Fisher, C., 1980. Protein and energy metabolism in the growing pig. In *Energy Metabolism* (ed. L. E. Mount), pp. 129–33. Butterworth, London.

Emery, R. S., 1979. Deposition, secretion, transport and oxidation of fat in ruminants, *J. Anim. Sci.* **48**: 1530–37.

Eskeland, B., Pfander, W. H. and Preston, R. L., 1974. Intravenous energy infusion in lambs: effects on nitrogen retention, plasma free amino acids and plasma urea nitrogen, *Br. J. Nutr.* **31**: 201–11.

Field, A. C., Suttle, N. F. and Nisbet, D. A., 1975. Effect of diets low in calcium and phosphorus on the development of growing lambs, *J. Agric. Sci., Camb.* **85**: 435–42.

Fischman, D. A., 1972. Development of striated muscle. In *The Structure and Function of Muscle* (ed. G. H. Bourne), 2nd edn, Vol. 1, 75–143. Academic Press, New York.

Flatt, J. P., 1970. Conversion of carbohydrate to fat in adipose tissue: an energy-yielding and, therefore, self-limiting process, *J. Lipid. Res.* **11**: 131–43.

Gemmell, R. T., Bell, A. W. and Alexander, G., 1972. Morphology of adipose cells in lambs at birth and during subsequent transition of brown to white adipose tissue in cold and in warm conditions, *Am. J. Anat.* **133**: 143–64.

Gerard, K. W. and Schneider, D. L., 1979. Evidence for degradation of myofibrillar proteins in lysosomes. Myofibrillar proteins derivatized by intramuscular injection of N-ethymaleimide are sequestered in lysosomes, *J. biol. Chem.* **254**: 11798–805.

Goldberg, A. L., 1979. Influence of insulin and contractile activity on muscle size and protein balance, *Diabetes* **28**: 18–24.

Goldberg, A. L., Tischler, M., De Martino, G. and Griffin, G., 1980. Hormonal regulation of protein degradation and synthesis in skeletal muscle, *Fedn Proc. Fedn Am. Socs exp. Biol.* **39**: 31–6

Goldspink, G., 1972. Postembryonic growth and differentiation of striated muscle. In *The Structure and Function of Muscle* (ed. G. H. Bourne), 2nd edn, Vol. 1, pp. 179–236. Academic Press, New York.

Goldspink, D. F., 1977. The influence of immobilization and stretch on protein turnover of rat skeletal muscle *J. Physiol., Lond.* **264**: 267–82.

Gooden, J. M., Fraser, R., Bosanquet, A. G. and Bickerstaffe, R., 1979. Size of lipoproteins in intestinal lymph of sheep and suckling lambs, *Aust. J. biol. Sci.* **32**: 533–42.

Ham, A. W. and Cormack D. H., 1979. *Histology*. 8th edn. Lippincott, Philadelphia.

Harris, C. I. and Milne, G., 1980. The occurrence of the N^τ-methylhistidine-containing dipeptide, balenine, in muscle extracts of various mammals, *Biochem. Soc. Trans.* **8**: 552.

Harrison, F. A. and Leat, W. M.F., 1975. Digestion and absorption of lipids in non-ruminant and ruminant animals: a comparison, *Proc. Nutr. Soc.* **34**: 203–10.

Hartmann, P. E., Harris, J. G. and Lascelles, A. K., 1966. The effect of oil-feeding and starvation on the composition and output of lipid in thoracic duct lymph in the lactating cow, *Aust. J. biol. Sci.* **19**: 635–44.

Hausman, G. J., Campion, D. R. and Martin, R. J., 1980. Search for the adipocyte precursor cell and factors that promote its differentiation, *J. Lipid. Res.* **21**: 657–70.

Heitzman, R. J., 1980. Manipulation of protein metabolism with special reference to anabolic agents. In *Protein Deposition in Animals* (ed. P. J. Buttery and D. B. Lindsay), pp. 193–203. Butterworth, London.

Herring, G. M., 1972. The inorganic matrix of bone. In *The Biochemistry and Physiology of Bone* (ed. G. H. Bourne), 2nd edn, pp. 127–89. Academic Press, London.

Hidiroglou, M., 1980. Zinc, copper and manganase deficiencies and the ruminant skeleton: a review, *Can. J. Anim. Sci.* **60**: 579–90.

Hood, R. L., 1982. Relationships between growth, adipose cell size, and lipid metabolism in ruminant adipose tissue, *Fedn Proc. Fedn Am. Socs exp. Biol.* **41**: 2555–61.

Hood, R. L. and Allen, C. E., 1973. Cellularity of bovine adipose tissue, *J. Lipid. Res.* **14**: 605–10.

Ingle, D. L., Bauman, D. E. and Garrigus, U. S., 1972. Lipogenesis in the ruminant: *in vivo* site of fatty acid synthesis in sheep, *J. Nutr.* **102**: 617–24.

Jefferson, L. S., Boyd, T. A., Flaim, K. E. and Peavy, D. E., 1980. Physiological control mechanisms of protein synthesis in animal cells, *Biochem. Soc. Trans.* **8**: 282–7.

Jefferson, L. S. and Korner, A., 1969. Influence of amino acid supply on ribosomes and protein synthesis of perfused rat liver, *Biochem. J.* **111**: 703–12.

Kirtland, J. and Gurr, M. I., 1979. Adipose tissue cellularity: a review. 2. The relationship between cellularity and obesity, *Int. J. Obesity* **3**: 15–55.

Knittle, J. L. and Hirsch. J., 1968. Effect of early nutrition on the development of rat epididymal fat pads: cellularity and metabolism, *J. clin. Invest.* **47**: 2091–8.

Koch, A. R., Kromann, R. P. and Wilson, T. R., 1979. Growth of body protein, fat and skeleton in steers fed on three planes of nutrition, *J. Nutr.* **109**: 426–36.

Konigsberg, I. R., Sollman, P. A. and Mixter, L. O., 1978. The duration of the terminal G_1 of fusing myoblasts, *Devl Biol.* **63**: 11–26.

Kotarbińska, M. and Kielanowski, J., 1969. Energy balance studies with growing pigs by the comparative slaughter technique. In *Energy Metabolism of Farm Animals* (ed. K. L. Blaxter., J. Kielanowski and Greta Thorbeck), pp. 299–310. Oriel Press, Newcastle upon Tyne.

Laurent, G. J. and Millward, D. J., 1980. Protein turnover during skeletal muscle hypertrophy, *Fedn Proc. Fedn Am. Socs exp. Biol.* **39**: 42–7.

Leat, W. M. F. and Cox, R. W., 1980. Fundamental aspects of adipose tissue growth. In *Growth of Animals* (ed. T. L. J. Lawrence), pp. 137–74. Butterworth, London.

Le Gros Clark, W. E., 1971. *The Tissues of the Body.* 4th edn. Oxford University Press, Oxford.

Lehninger, A. L., 1975. *Biochemistry: the Molecular Basis of Cell Structure and Function.* 2nd edn. Worth, New York.

Li, J. B. and Jefferson, L. S., 1978. Influence of amino acid availability on protein turnover in perfused skeletal muscle, *Biochim. biophys. Acta* **544**: 351–9.

Lindsay, D. B., 1961. Endocrine control of metabolism in ruminants. In *Digestive Physiology and Nutrition of the Ruminant* (ed. D. Lewis), pp. 235–41. Butterworth, London.

Lindsay, D. B., 1975. Fatty acids as energy sources, *Proc. Nutr. Soc.* **34**: 241–8.

Lindsay, D. B., 1979. Metabolism in the whole animal, *Proc. Nutr. Soc.* **38**: 295–301.

Lindsay, D. B., 1980. Amino acids as energy sources, *Proc. Nutr. Soc.* **39**: 53–9.

Lindsay, D. B., 1981. Characteristics of the metabolism of carbohydrate in ruminants compared with other animals. In *The Problem of Dark-cutting in Beef* (ed. D. E. Hood and P. V. Tarrant), pp. 101–22. Nÿhoff, The Hague.

Lindsay, D. B., 1982. Relationships between amino acid catabolism and protein anabolism in the ruminant, *Fedn Proc. Fedn Am. Socs exp. Biol.* **41**: 2550–4.

Lindsay, D. B. and Buttery, P. J., 1980. Metabolism in muscle. In *Protein Deposition in Animals* (ed. P. J. Buttery and D. B. Lindsay), pp. 125–46. Butterworth, London.

Lister, D., 1976. Effects of nutrition and genetics on the composition of the body, *Proc. Nutr. Soc.* **35**: 351–6.

Luben, R. A., Wong, Glenda L. and Cohn, D. V., 1976. Biochemical characterization with parathormone and calcitonin of isolated bone cells: provisional identification of osteoclasts and osteoblasts, *Endocrinology* **99**: 526–34.

McLachlan, J. and Wolpert, L., 1980. The spatial patterns of muscle development in chick limb. In *Development and Specialisation of Skeletal Muscle* (ed. D. F. Goldspink), pp. 1–17. Cambridge University Press, London.

Meyer, R. J., Burgess, R. J. and Russell, S. M., 1980. Factors controlling intracellular breakdown of proteins. In *Protein Deposition in Animals* (ed. P. J. Buttery and D. B. Lindsay), pp 21–49, Butterworth, London.

Millward, D. J., Garlick, P. J. and Reeds, P. J., 1976. The energy cost of growth, *Proc. Nutr. Soc.* **35**: 339–49.

Moss, F. P., 1968. The relationship between the dimensions of the fibres and the number of nuclei during restricted growth, degrowth and compensatory growth of skeletal muscle, Am. J. Anat. 122: 565–72.

Mount, L. E., 1980a. Energy Metabolism. Butterworth, London.

Mount, L. E., 1980b. Growth and the thermal environment. In Growth in Animals (ed. T. L.J. Lawrence), pp. 47–63. Butterworth, London.

Mundy, G. R., Shapiro, J. L., Bandeli, J. G. Canalis, E. M. and Raisz, L. G., 1976. Direct stimulation of bone resorption by thyroid hormones, J. clin. Invest. 58: 529–34.

Munro, H. N., 1964. General aspects of the regulation of protein metabolism by diet and hormones. In Mammalian Protein Metabolism, Vol. I (ed. H. N. Munro and J. B. Allison), pp. 381–481. Academic Press, New York.

Nag, A. C. and Foster, J. D., 1981. Myogenesis in adult mammalian skeletal muscle in vitro, J. Anat. 132: 1–18.

Nathanson, M. A. and Hay, E. D., 1980. Analysis of cartilage differentiation from skeletal muscle growth on bone matrix. 1. Ulstrastructural aspects, Devl Biol. 78: 301–31.

Nilsson-Ehle, P., Garfinkel, A. S. and Schotz, M. C., 1980. Lipolytic enzymes and plasma lipoprotein metabolism. A. Rev. Biochem. 49: 667–93.

Nishimoto, S. K. and Price, P. A., 1979. Proof that the γ-carboxyglutamic acid–containing bone protein is synthesized in calf bone. Comparative synthesis rate and effect of coumarin on synthesis, J. biol. Chem. 254: 437–41.

O'Hea, E. K. and Leveille, G. A., 1969a. Lipid biosynthesis and transport in the domestic chick (Gallus domesticus) Comp. Biochem. Physiol. 30: 149–59.

O'Hea, E. K. and Leveille, G. A., 1969b. Significance of adipose tissue and liver as sites of fatty acid synthesis in the pig and the efficiency of utilization of various substrates for lipogenesis, J. Nutr. 99: 338–44.

O'Neill, M. C. and Stockdale, F. E., 1972. A kinetic analysis of myogenesis in vitro, J. Cell Biol. 52: 52–65.

Ornoy, A., Goodwin, D., Noff, D. and Edelstein, S., 1978. 24,25-Dihydroxyvitamin D is a metabolite of vitamin D essential for bone formation, Nature, Lond. 276: 517–9.

Owen, M. and Triffitt, J. T., 1976. Extravascular albumin in bone tissue, J. Physiol. Lond. 257: 293–307.

Pain, V. M., 1978. Protein synthesis and its regulation. In Protein Turnover in Mammalian Tissues and in the Whole Body (ed. J. C. Waterlow, P. J. Garlick and D. J. Millward), pp. 15–54. North-Holland, Amsterdam.

Pain, V. M. and Clemens, M. J., 1980. Mechanism and regulation of protein biosynthesis in eukaryotic cells. In Protein Deposition in Animals (ed. P. J. Buttery and D. B. Lindsay), pp. 1–20. Butterworth, London.

Pethick, D. W., Lindsay, D. B., Barker, P. J. and Northrop, A. J., 1981. Acetate supply and utilization by the tissues of sheep in vivo, Br. J. Nutr. 46: 97–110.

Preedy, V. R. and Waterlow, J. C., 1981. Protein synthesis in the young rat – the contribution of skin and bones, J. Physiol., Lond. 317: 45–6P.

Price, P. A. and Baukol, S. A., 1980. 1,25-Dihydroxyvitamin D₃ increases synthesis of the vitamin K-dependent bone protein by osteosarcoma cells, *J. biol. Chem.* **255**: 11660–3.

Price, P. A., Parthemare, J. G., Deftos, L. J. and Nishimoto, S. K., 1980. New biochemical marker for bone metabolism. Measurement by radioimmunoassay of bone gla protein in plasma of normal subjects and patients with bone disease, *J. clin. Invest.* **66**: 878–83.

Prior, R. L., 1978. Effect of level of feed intake on lactate and acetate metabolism and lipogenesis *in vivo* in sheep, *J. Nutr.* **108**: 926–35.

Prior, R. L. and Jacobson, J. J., 1979. Lactate, pyruvate and acetate interactions during *in vitro* lipogenesis in bovine adipose tissue, *J. Anim. Sci.* **49**: 1410–6.

Prior, R. L. and Smith, S. B., 1982. Hormonal effects on partitioning of nutrients for tissue growth: role of insulin, *Fedn Proc. Fedn Am. Socs exp. Biol.* **41**: 2545–9.

Pullar, J. D. and Webster, A. J. F., 1977. The energy cost of fat and protein deposition in the rat, *Br. J. Nutr.* **37**: 355–63.

Purchas, R. W., Barton, R. A. and Kirton, A. H., 1980. Relationships of circulating cortisol levels with growth rate and meat tenderness of cattle and sheep, *Aust. J. agric. Res.* **31**: 221–32.

Raisz, L. G., Canalis, E. M., Dietrich, J. W., Kream, B. E., and Gworek, S. C., 1978. Hormonal regulation of bone formation, *Recent Prog. Horm. Res.* **34**: 335–48.

Raisz, L. G., Mundy, G. R., Dietrich, J. W. and Canalis, E. M., 1977. Hormonal regulation of mineral metabolism. In *International Review of Physiology, Endocrine Physiology*, Part II, Vol. 16 (ed. S. M. McCann), pp. 201–40. University Park Press, Baltimore.

Rannels, D. E., Pegg, A. E., Rannels, S. R. and Jefferson, L. S., 1978. Effect of starvation on initiation of protein synthesis in skeletal muscle and heart, *Am. J. Physiol.* **235**: E126–33.

Rannels, S. R., Rannels, D. E., Pegg, A. E. and Jefferson, L. S., 1978. Glucocorticoid effects on peptide-chain initiation in skeletal muscle and heart, *Am. J. Physiol.* **235**: E134–9.

Reeds, P. J., Fuller, M. F., Cadenhead. A. Lobley. G. E. and McDonald, J. D., 1981. Effects of changes in the intakes of protein and non-protein energy on whole-body protein turnover in growing pigs *Br. J. Nutr.* **45**: 539–46.

Reynolds, J. J. and Dingle, J. T., 1970. A sensitive *in vitro* method for studying the induction and inhibition of bone resorption *Calcif. Tissue Res.* **4**: 339–49.

Robinson, D. S., Cryer, A. and Davies, P., 1975. The role of clearing-factor lipase (lipoprotein lipase) in the transport of plasma triglycerides, *Proc. Nutr. Soc.* **34**: 211–5.

Rucker, R. B., Parker, H. E. and Rogler, J. C., 1969. The effects of copper on collagen cross linking, *Biochem. biophys. Res. Commun.* **34**: 28–32.

Scornik, O. A., and Botbol, Violeta, 1976. Role of changes in protein degradation in the growth of regenerating livers, *J. biol. Chem.* **251**: 2891–97.

Scott, T. W., Cook, L. J. and Mills, S. C., 1971. Protection of dietary polyunsaturated fatty acids against microbial hydrogenation in ruminants, *J. Am. Oil Chem. Soc.* **48**: 358–64.

Seglen, P. O., 1975. Protein degradation in isolated hepatocytes is inhibited by ammonia, *Biochem. biophys. Res. Commun.* **66**: 44–52.

Sellers, A. and Reynolds, J. J., 1977. Identification and partial characterization of an inhibitor of collagenase from rabbit bone, *Biochem. J.* **167**: 353–60.

Short, R. V.,1980. The hormonal control of growth at puberty . In *Growth in Animals* (ed. T. L. J. Lawrence), pp. 25–45. Butterworth, London.

Siddle, K. and Hales, C. N., 1975. Hormonal control of adipose tissue lipolysis, *Proc. Nutr. Soc.* **34**: 233–9.

Sim, A. J. W., Wolfe, B. M., Young, V. R., Clarke, D. and Moore, F. D., 1979. Glucose promotes whole-body protein synthesis from infused amino acids in fasting man. Isotopic demonstration, *Lancet* **1**: 68–72.

Sodek, J., 1976. A new approach to assessing collagen turnover using a micro-assay, *Biochem. J.* **160**: 243–6.

Stickland, N. C., Widdowson, E. M. and Goldspink, G., 1975. Effects of severe energy and protein deficiencies on the fibres and nuclei in skeletal muscle of pigs, *Br. J. Nutr.* **34**: 421–8.

Stromer, M. H., Goll, D. E., Young, R. B., Robson, R. M. and Parrish, F. C., 1974. Ultrastructural features of skeletal muscle differentiation and development, *J. Anim. Sci.* **38**: 1111–41.

Super, D. M., Palmquist, D. L. and Schanbacher, F. L., 1976. Relative activation of milk lipoprotein lipase by serum of cows fed varying amounts of fat, *J. Dairy Sci.* **59**: 1409–13.

Sutton, J. D., 1974. Energy supply from the digestive tract of cattle. In *Principles of Cattle Production* (ed. H. Swan and W. H. Broster), pp. 121–43. Butterworth, London.

Sutton, J. D., Storry, J. E. and Nicholson, J. W. G., 1970. The digestion of fatty acids in the stomach and intestines of sheep given widely different rations, *J. Dairy Res.* **37**: 97–105.

Talmage, R. V., 1970. Morphological and physiological considerations in a new concept of calcium transport in bone, *Am. J. Anat.* **129**: 467–76.

Talmage, R. V., 1978. Discussion. In *Recent Prog. Horm. Res.* **34**: 351–3.

Talmage, R. V., Cooper, C. W. and Park, H .Z., 1970. Regulation of calcium transport in bone by parathyroid hormone, *Vitams Horm.* **28**: 103–40.

Tyrrell, H. F., Reynolds. P. J. and Moe, P. W., (1979). Effect of diet on partial efficiency of acetate use for body tissue synthesis by mature cattle, *J. Anim. Sci.* **48**: 598–606.

Ulyatt, M. J. and MacRae, J. C., 1974. Quantitative digestion of fresh herbage by sheep. I. The sites of digestion of organic matter, energy, readily fermentable carbohydrate, structural carbohydrate and lipid, *J. agric. Sci., Camb.* **82**: 295–307.

Van, R. L. R. and Roncari, D. A. K., 1978. Complete differentiation of adipocyte precursors. A culture system for studying the cellular nature of adipose tissue, *Cell & Tiss. Res.* **195**: 317–29.

Vandenburgh, H. and Kaufman, S., 1980. Protein degradation in embryonic skeletal muscle, *J. biol. Chem.* **255**: 5826–33.

van Es, A. J. H., 1980. Energy costs of protein deposition. In *Protein*

Deposition in Animals (ed. P. J. Buttery and D. B. Lindsay), pp. 215–224. Butterworth, London.

Vaughan, J., 1980. Bone growth and modelling. In *Growth in Animals* (ed. T. L. J. Lawrence), pp. 83–99 Butterworth, London.

Waterlow, J. C., Garlick, P. J. and Millward, D. J., 1978. *Protein Turnover in Mammalian Tissues and in the Whole Body*. North-Holland, Amsterdam.

Weaver, M. E. and Ingram, D. L., 1969. Morphological changes in swine associated with environmental temperature, *Ecology* **50**: 710–3.

Whittemore, C. T. 1976. A study of growth responses to nutrient inputs by modelling *Proc. Nutr. Soc.* **35**: 383–91.

Yaffe, D., 1969. Cellular aspects of muscle differentiation *in vitro*, *Curr. Top. Dev. Biol.* **4**: 37–77.

Young, V. R., 1980. Hormonal control of protein metabolism with particular reference to body protein gain. In *Protein Deposition in Animals* (ed. P. J. Buttery and D. B. Lindsay), pp. 167–191. Butterworth, London.

8   MILK SECRETION AND ITS NUTRITIONAL REGULATION

J. A. F. Rook and P. C. Thomas

The possession of mammary glands and the ability to secrete milk for the nourishment of the young are unique mammalian characteristics. All of the larger domesticated farm animals are mammals but only those of the ruminant species are used for the commercial production of milk. In the technologically developed western countries, the domestic cow (*Bos taurus*) is the dominant milk-producing animal but goats (*Capra hircus*) are still used locally in small numbers. In the developing countries, species other than the cow, the buffalo (*Bubalus bubalis*), the sheep (*Ovis aries*) and the goat, may be of equal or greater importance. The horse (*Equus caballus*), the ass (*Equus osinus*), the camel (*Camelus* sp.) and the pig (*Sus scrofa*), and possibly other species, have also been milked by man to provide human food.

The dominant rôle of the cow in milk production in developed countries, and its consequent commercial importance, has meant that milk secretion has been more widely studied in the cow, and in the goat because of its convenience as a substitute experimental animal, than in other species. This chapter will be based primarily on information for the cow and goat but information for other farm animals, and where necessary other species, will be provided as appropriate.

THE CONSTITUENTS OF MILK

Milk is an extremely complex biological fluid and contains an array of different kinds of molecules. With the exception of some arctic and aquatic species, for which fat is the major milk component, the most abundant constituent of milk is water and much of the remainder is accounted for by lipid, protein and carbohydrate materials synthesized within the mammary gland. In addition, milk contains many different mineral constituents in macro- or trace-amounts, some of which, calcium, phosphorus and sulphur, for example, are secreted as components of, or in association with, the milk proteins; a variety of both water- and lipid-soluble materials transferred from blood plasma to milk; specific blood proteins, especially when there has been damage to the secretory cells; and traces, perhaps accidentally, of intermediates of biosynthesis in the mammary secretory cells.

Fat

Lipid and fatty acid composition

The lipid of cow's milk consists principally of triglyceride (970 to 980 /kg) with small amounts of diglyceride (2.5 to 4.8 g/kg), monoglyceride (0.16 to 0.38 g/kg), cholesterol ester (trace), cholesterol (2.2 to 4.1 g/kg), free fatty acids (1.0 to 4.4 g/kg) and phospholipid (2 to 10 g/kg); higher values have been reported for the proportions of diglycerides and free fatty acids but these are indicative of lipolysis prior to analysis. The milk lipids of the goat and sheep are of similar composition to those of the cow, but those of simple-stomached animals, man and the pig, for example, characteristically have higher proportions of sterols and sterol esters and consequently a lower proportion of triglycerides.

The major fatty acids of milk lipid are acids containing 16 to 18 carbon atoms and a high proportion of these acids are monounsaturated. Milk lipid, however, contains a much wider range of fatty acids than most other body lipids and includes, in particular, short-chain fatty acids in the range of 4 to 14 C atoms. The proportion of short-chain fatty acids is especially high in the milk lipid of herbivorous animals, which is also characterized by very small amounts of diunsaturated fatty acids, and the presence of trace amounts of branched-chain saturated acids and positional and configurational isomers of unsaturated acids. According to Patton and Jensen (1975), 437 different fatty acids have been identified in the milk lipid of the cow and others are still to be identified. The acids include all normal saturated fatty acids from C_2 to C_{28}, monomethyl branched-chain fatty acids from C_{16} to C_{28}, multimethyl branched-chain fatty acids from C_{16} to C_{28}, cis and trans monoenoic fatty acids from C_{10} to C_{26}, numerous cis- and polyenoic fatty acids, keto- and hydroxy-fatty acids, and cyclo-hexyl fatty acids. The uncommon acids have their origin variously in the ruminal partial hydrogenation of dietary polyunsaturated fatty acids, the intestinal digestion and assimilation of structural lipids of rumen bacteria, the substitution of methyl malonyl-CoA (derived from propionyl-CoA) for malonyl–CoA in fatty acid synthesis in the body tissues, and the metabolism of the phytol moiety of chlorophyll (Garton, 1976).

Typical values for the fatty acid composition of the milk lipid of the cow, ewe and sow are given in Table 8.1.

In natural triglycerides the glycerol moiety has the L-configuration and the primary alcohol positions are not biochemically interchangeable. According to the *sn*, stereospecific numbering, system, the C atom in the secondary alcohol group is numbered *sn-2*, and the C atoms above and below C atom *sn-2* are numbered *sn-1* and *sn-3* respectively (see Buchnea, 1978). Detailed information on the structure of milk triglycerides is available for the cow (Patton and Jensen, 1975). Butyric and hexanoic acids are esterified virtually entirely in position *sn-3*, most of the octanoic acid is in position *sn-3* although some is in *sn-2*, and with decanoic acid a higher proportion is in *sn-2*, and some is in *sn-1*. As the chain length of the fatty acid is increased further, the proportions in *sn-2* and then *sn-1* increase, and both 16:0 and 18:0 are found in greatest concentration in *sn-1*. Higher proportions of unsaturated fatty acids are present in *sn-2* than in the other positions, and *trans*-unsaturated acids are present almost entirely in positions *sn-1* and *sn-3*.

Globule membrane

The triglycerides of milk lipid are arranged physically in the form of globules and each globule is surrounded by a membrane. The evidence from the electron microscopic studies of Wooding (1977) is that, at the moment of secretion, the globule is surrounded immediately by a 'thin dense line'. From its location, this is probably a phospholipid monolayer or a phospholipid–cholesterol monolayer and limited analytical data support this conclusion. Circumferential to this line is a zone of dense material whose composition is unknown and enclosing the dense material is a membrane with the ultrastructural characteristics of a normal, phospholipid bilayer-type, biological membrane. The initial structure persists for only a short while and matures to one where 70% of the surface area is covered by the 'thin dense line' and the other membrane components are condensed into plaques, or subsequently blebs, of dense material covered by a bilayer-type membrane.

Protein

Protein is a component of the milks of all species but the number and kinds of proteins vary. Caseins are usually the major components but there are inter-species differences in the composition of the caseins and their amounts, and variations between species in the whey (non-casein) proteins. In addition, between individuals within a species there are

Table 8.1 Typical values for the principal fatty acids of milk lipids (g/kg)

Species	Acids														
	4:0	6:0	8:0	10:0	12:0	14:0	15:0	16:0	16:1	18:0	18:1	18:2	18:3
Cow[†]	33	16	13	30	31	95	6	263	23	146	288	24	0
Ewe[‡]	33	38	56	66	13	130	–	182	28	131	104	45	49
Sow[†]	–	–	–	0–7	Trace–5	40	Trace–8	329	113	35	352	119	0–7

[†] Jenness, 1974.
[‡] Yousef and Ashton, 1967.

Table 8.2   The proteins of cow's milk

Protein fraction	Genetic variants	Comment
α_{s_1}–Caseins	A, B, C, D	Major component contains 8 and minor component 9 phoshphorylated residues
α_{s_2}–Caseins	A, D	Components contain 10, 11, 12 or 13 phosphorylated residues
κ–Caseins	A, B	Components containing 0 to 5 carbohydrate chains
β–Caseins	A^1, A^2, A^3, B, D, E, C	
γ–Caseins (γ_1-, γ_2-, γ_3-)	A^1, A^2, A^3, B	
	A, A, B	
	A, B	
β–Lactoglobulin	A, B, C, D, Dr	
α–Lactalbumin	A, B	Several minor proteins, some glycoproteins
Immunoglobulins, IgGi, IgG2, IgA, IgM		Heterogeneous
Protose peptones; components 3, 5, 8 fast, 8 slow		Possibly heterogeneous
Bovine serum albumin		Heterogeneous

genetic variations, associated with minor changes in amino acid composition and sequence, in the composition of the individual caseins and of the non-casein proteins synthesized within the mammary gland. The various protein constituents of cow's milk are shown in Table 8.2.

Caseins

These are a group of milk-specific proteins, usually but not invariably characterized by serine-bound phosphate, a high proline content, few or no cysteine residues and a low solubility at pH 4.0 to 5.0. They are present largely in the form of micellar complexes with calcium and inorganic phosphate.

In cows' milk, there are five families of caseins, α_{s_1}-, α_{s_2}-, β-, κ-, and γ-, and the first four of these families are each coded by a single gene. Within each family there are genetic variants of the major component or components and within the α_{s_1}-, α_{s_2}- and κ-casein groups additional minor components. The primary structures of the genetic variants of α_{s_1}-casein and β-casein are known and the various γ-caseins are identical with fragments of β-caseins. The amino acid sequences of the κ-caseins are also known but the location and structures of the carbohydrate moieties in the carbohydrate—containing components are uncertain. κ-Caseins differ from the other caseins by having a phenylalanine-methionine bond which is readily hydrolysed in the presence of chymosin (rennin) and some other proteases. The hydrolysis destroys the ability of the κ-casein to stabilize other caseins against precipitation by Ca^{2+} and converts it into insoluble para-κ-casein and a soluble caseino-macropeptide.

α_{s_0}-Casein, a minor constituent, has a composition and sequence of amino acids identical with that of α_{s_1}-casein, except there is a phosphoseryl residue at position 41 in the sequence instead of a seryl residue. The α_{s_2}-caseins have a different kind of polypeptide chain to that of α_{s_1}-casein, and the components of the group differ in the number of phosphorylated residues.

κ-Casein has been shown to be present in the milks of many other species, the sheep, the goat, the pig and man included, and in those species has properties similar to that of bovine κ-casein. Apart from bovine milk, however, the characterization of other caseins is incomplete; α_s-casein has been shown to be present with certainty only in the milks of ruminants. Most of the non-bovine milk proteins are homologous with the recognized families of those of *Bos taurus*, α_{s_1}-caseins, α_{s_2}-caseins, β-caseins, κ-caseins, β-lactoglobulins and α-lactalbumins.

The primary function of the caseins is assumed to be nutritional. They contain well balanced proportions of the essential amino acids, except that cystine is low but whey proteins are rich in that amino acid. Caseins are readily attacked by proteases and their presence, mainly in the form of micelles, increases the ability of the milk to carry minerals which are constituents of the micelles.

Non-casein (whey) proteins

In bovine milk, these proteins include β-lactoglobulin, α-lactalbumin, proteose-peptones, and, normally, trace amounts of serum albumin and immunoglobulins. The primary structures of the genetic variants of β-lactoglobulin have been tentatively established. β-Lactoglobulin Dr (Droughtmaster) has the same amino acid composition as the A variant but contains additional carbohydrate residues. The primary structures of the B variant of α-lactalbumin, the only variant in milk from western cattle, and of the A variant, present with B in milk from African Fulani and African and Indian Zebu cattle, have also been determined. The proteose-peptone fraction is a heterogeneous mixture of heat-stable polypeptides which are soluble at pH 4.6 but insoluble in trichloroacetic acid (120g/l), and some represent the C-terminal portions of β-casein.

β-Lactoglobulin is a major component of the whey proteins of cows' milk and an equivalent protein is present in sows' milk, but it may be absent from the milks of non-ruminant artiodactyls and has been shown to be absent from human milk. There are also large, between-species differences in the numbers and types of other whey proteins, the milks of rodents having only a few components, those of carnivores many. α-Lactalbumin, however, has been found in the milks of a great many species and presumably is present in all milks that contain lactose, since it is a modifier protein, which causes a structural change in galactosyl transferase such that it catalyses the transfer of galactose to glucose in the synthesis of lactose. The rôle of β-lactoglobulin is uncertain but it may play a part in the regulation of phosphorus metabolism in the mammary gland.

Carbohydrates

Lactose (O-β-D-galactopyranosyl-(1-4)-α-D-glucopyranose) is the distinctive and usually predominant carbohydrate of most milks. There have been reports that it may be absent from the milks of certain sea mammals (Otanoides), but it has now been shown to be present in low concentration in the milk of the Northern fur seal and also in the milk of certain monotremes. Milks also contain, normally in low concentration, monosaccharides, including glucose and galactose, and neutral and acid oligosaccharides in addition to peptide and protein-bound carbohydrates, but, in certain species and at particular stages of lactation, oligosaccharides may be present in substantial amounts.

Salts

The principal cations of milks are sodium, potassium, calcium and magnesium, and the principal anions phosphate, chloride and citrate. They are present as ions and as unionized or weakly ionized salts, and some are in part covalently bound to other constituents. The sodium, potassium and chloride are present almost wholly in a soluble form whereas only one-third of the calcium, one-half of the phosphorus and two-thirds of the magnesium are soluble. Typical values for the concentrations (g/l) of these constituents in bovine milk are: calcium, 1.25; magnesium, 0.12; sodium, 0.58; potassium, 1.38; chloride, 1.03; Phosphorus, 0.96; and citric acid, 1.75 (Jenness, 1974).

THE MECHANISMS OF MILK SYNTHESIS AND SECRETION

The mammary gland

There are inter-species differences in the number, location and shape of mammary glands, in the distribution of secretory tissue within the glands and in the proportion of fibrous connective tissue. The secretory tissue, however, invariably consists of epithelial cells grouped to form alveoli with fine exit ducts and these in turn are grouped together to from lobules, each with a main duct. The lobular ducts merge into a lactiferous sinus or in many species (the ruminants, for example) into a cistern formed by a fusion of sinuses (Figs. 8.1 and 8.2).

Synthesis of milk constituents, which is a continuous process, occurs within the alveolar cells from materials extracted from blood plasma, and the synthesized constituents are transferred to the alveolar lumen in association with the other constituents of milk, which include water and the mineral elements, derived directly from blood plasma. The epithelium of the teat and duct system is generally impermeable to milk constituents, including ions and lactose, but permeable to water. In the later stages of pregnancy, however, and following the abrupt cessation of milking, engorgement of the gland with milk may lead to a passage of water-soluble materials from milk to blood plasma via the intercellular junctions.

On secretion, milk becomes distributed between the alveolar lumen, the ducts and the sinuses (or cisterns) in proportions which vary from species to species. A loss of milk from the cistern is prevented by a teat 'sphincter', which in the cow surrounds the streak canal at the tip of the teat. Only milk within a sinus or cistern may be removed by sucking or milking and the transfer of milk from the alveolar fine duct system is dependent on a process of contraction of the alveoli known as 'milk

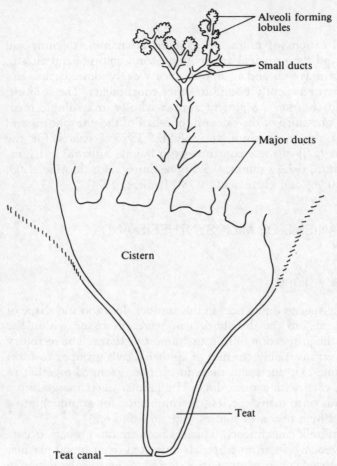

Fig. 8.1.   Schematic representation of the arrangement of the secretory portions (alveoli) and secretory ducts in the mammary gland of the
goat.

ejection'. This is achieved through contractile myoepithelial cells
present in the secretory tissue. These may be stimulated to contract by
the rapid mechanical manipulation of mammary tissue during the acts
of sucking and milking, and this explains the ability to obtain normal
yields of milk from denervated udders in some goats and cows. The
cells are also induced to contract by oxytocin, which is released from
the neurohypophysis on the nervous stimulation resulting from suckling or milking or associated activities, and in the sow this mechanism
is predominant. In ruminants, nervous stimulation causes a multiple
release of oxytocin, whereas in the sow there is a single and brief
ejection phase. Differences in the pattern of oxytocin release may relate

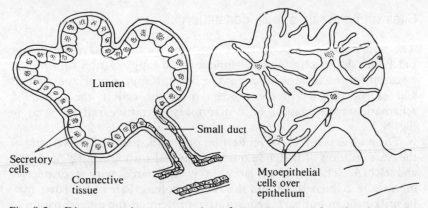

Fig. 8.2. Diagrammatic representation of a cross-section of an alveolus, and a surface view.

to differences between species in the length and frequency of the sucking episodes, which in the natural state vary from hourly in the pig and approximately 4-hourly in ruminants, to once-daily in the rabbit, for example.

On contraction of the myoepithelial cells, milk is expressed from the alveolar fine-duct system through the larger ducts into the cisterns and teats of the gland. From there it may be removed by sucking or milking but some milk, in the cow 10 to 20% of the original volume, is invariably retained in the secretory tissue. This milk, which is not removed by the usual milking process but may in part be removed by further natural stimulation or the intravenous injection of oxytocin, is known as 'residual milk'. On the movement of milk through the fine-duct system, in the cow and probably most ruminants clustering of fat globules restricts their passage relative to the aqueous phase, and the fat content of milk expressed from the gland increases progressively throughout a milking. The residual milk is rich in fat and may contain 30 to 50% of the milk fat originally present in the udder. The amount of residual milk varies with the amount of milk in the udder at the beginning of milking and, therefore, since milk secretion is a continuous process, with the interval between milkings. When two intervals are of different length, the volume of milk, and to a greater extent the amount of fat removed from the gland during the short interval, is more than that secreted during that interval, and the opposite is the case during the long interval; the fat content of milk removed after a short interval tends to be high and that after a long interval low.

Effects due to clustering of fat globules have not been observed in the sow.

Sites of synthesis of milk constituents

The subcellular components of the secretory cell have distinctive biochemical and physiological functions, an appreciation of which is essential for the understanding of the biosynthesis of milk constituents and of the transfer of constituents from the cell to the lumen. A schematic representation of a mammary secretory cell is given in Fig. 8.3.

The *nucleus* is the site of replication of genetic material (DNA) and of the transcription of the code on that material through mRNA, rRNA and tRNA. The onset of lactation is associated with a distinctive increase in cellular RNA and in soluble protein. Part of the latter may be milk protein but part is constitutive protein, as the differentiation of cytomembranes and the Golgi components which takes place in pregnancy continues during the first days of lactation.

The particle-free supernatant, the *cytosol* (cytoplasm less the mitochondrial and microsomal fractions), is the site of formation of key intermediates and cofactors necessary for the initial steps of the synthesis of milk constituents. It contains the enzymes of the Embden-Meyerhof glycolytic pathway (in several species multiple forms of hexokinase have been demonstrated and certain forms may be bound to mitochondrial particles), of the pentose phosphate pathway, and for the conversion of glucose-6-phosphate to UDP-galactose, the initial step of lactose synthesis. The enzymes for fatty acid synthesis (acetyl-CoA synthetase, acetyl-CoA carboxylase, ATP-citrate lyase and fatty acid synthetase) and linked activities (NAD-malate dehydrogenase, NADP-malate dehydrogenase and NADP-isocitrate dehycrogenase), and for triglyceride and phospholipid synthesis (glycerokinase, glycerophosphate dehydrogenase, fatty acyl-CoA synthetase and phosphotidate phosphohydrolase) are also present.

The primary rôle of *mitochondria* in the secretory cells, in common with other cells, is the transfer of energy from oxidized substrates to the terminal high-energy bond of ATP, the form of energy used in biosynthesis. With the onset of lactation, the number of mitochondria in the secretory cells is greatly increased. Additionally, mitochondria are important for the supply of carbon chains for the synthesis of non-essential amino acids, and the selective permeability of the mitochondrial membrane (malate, citrate, 3-hydroxybutyrate, aspartate and glutamate may be transferred but other anions are excluded) gives it a rôle in the regulation of cell metabolism.

The *microsomal* fraction includes the Golgi apparatus, the rough and smooth membranes of the endoplasmic reticulum, and the lateral and basal cell membranes. At parturition, there is marked hypertrophy of the endoplasmic reticulum, and the Golgi apparatus and the endoplasmic reticulum becomes highly granulated. Polypeptide synthesis for

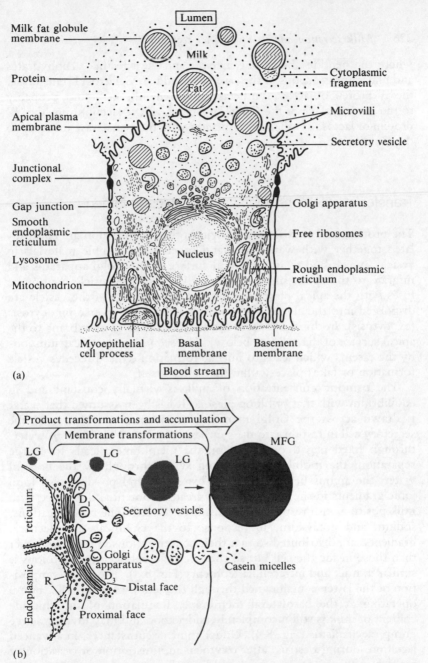

Fig. 8.3. Diagrammatic representation of: (a) a cross-section of a cell in the secretory epithelium of a lactating mammary gland; and (b) of the flow of membranes, and the transformation and accumulation of constituents, in the lactating secretory cell (D_1, D_2, D_3, dictyosomes; LG, lipid globule; MFG, milk fat globule; R, ribosomes). (From Larson, 1979.)

where the peptide chains polymerize, and the specific carbohydrates and phosphorus groups of the caseins are added. Galactosyl transferase, the 'A' protein of lactose synthetase, is also membrane bound, probably to the inner surface of the Golgi apparatus, and α-lactalbumin, the 'B' protein of lactose synthetase, associates with the transferase on entry to the Golgi region.

Transfer of milk constituents to the alveolar lumen

The proteins and lactose formed within the Golgi region are encapsulated together with water, ions and other water-soluble materials in vesicles which bud from the apical surface of the Golgi apparatus and migrate to the apical surface of the cell. There the vesicle membrane fuses with the apical plasmalemma and the contents of the vesicle are disgorged into the alveolar lumen by a process of reverse pinocytosis (exocytosis). In this way, there is a transfer of Golgi membrane to the apical surface of the cell (see below). The sequestration of calcium ions by the caseins which leads to micelle formation either precedes vesicle formation or takes place within the vesicle itself.

The osmotic concentration of milk is virtually constant and in equilibrium with that of blood plasma. It has been assumed that water is drawn across the Golgi membrane and apical membrane of the secretory cell in response to the synthesis of lactose. The flow of water, through fixed negative charges on the membranes, leads to charge separation, the mobile cations being swept through by the flow of water, the anions being repelled. This effect, and possibly also local ionic gradients in the surface layers, creates a potential difference with milk positive with respect to the inside of the cell. The mobile cations, sodium and potassium, in response to the chemical and electrical gradients, are distributed so that their concentrations in milk are lower than those inside the cell but so that the ratio between the two ions is similar in milk and intracellular contents (Fig. 8.4). The ionic composition of the latter is maintained through the action of a Na^+/K^+ pump operating at the basolateral membrane. Regulation of the chloride content of milk is still incompletely understood and may involve active pump mechanisms (Fig. 8.4). Under some circumstances, in advanced lactation, during oestrus, after oxytocin administration or cessation of regular milking, or in pathological conditions such as mastitis, the chloride concentration in milk may be elevated in association with an increased concentration of sodium and reduced concentrations of lactose and potassium. These effects arise through 'leakage' in the tight junctions between the mammary cells and represent a paracellular route of entry of constituents from blood plasma to milk (Fig. 8.4). The

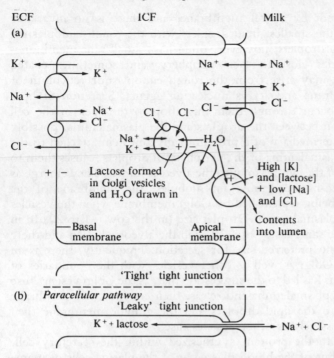

Fig. 8.4. (a) A schematic representation of the movements of ions, lactose
                and water between extracellular fluid (ECF), intracellular fluid
                (ICF) and milk. The directions of electrical potential differences
                are indicated by plus and minus signs.
           (b) A schematic representation of the paracellular movement of ions
                through leaky tight junctions between the mammary cells.
                (From Peaker, 1977.)

milk protein (casein, β-lactoglobulin and α-lactalbumin) formation
occurs under the control of polyribosomes bound to the membranes of
the endoplasmic reticulum, and the polypeptides are transported
through the lumina of the endoplasmic reticulum to the Golgi region
effects on the composition of milk tend to be most marked when the
volume of milk being secreted is low.

Synthesis of milk constituents and milk secretion can begin before
parturition but copious milk secretion is associated with a rapid rise in
the milk concentration of citrate. The citrate is derived from that
formed in the cytosol of the secretory cells but appears to be concentrated in the Golgi vesicles, possibly through an association with
calcium prior to its secretion.

The site of lipid droplet formation is still uncertain but it may be the
cisternae of the rough endoplasmic reticulum. Droplets within the cell
are surrounded only by the single dense line (identified by electron

microscopy), not by a unit membrane, and there is no invariable association of the smallest lipid droplets with the rough endoplasmic reticulum. The droplets, however, often have small unit membrane-bounded vesicles close to their periphery, and sometimes coated vesicles which may arise from the rough endoplasmic reticulum or basal plasmalemma and act as nucleating agents. Secretion of lipid droplets may occur through their migration to the apex of the cell where attraction between the droplets and the plasmalemma, possibly through the intermediary of a protein or glycoprotein attached to the inside of the plasmalemma or the periphery of droplets, causes them to be drawn out of the cytoplasm into the alveolar lumen. They emerge as unit membrane-bounded milk fat globules, the membrane of the plasmalemma being replenished by Golgi membrane when the vesicles fuse with the plasmalemma. Droplet size (in the cow 0.1 to 20 μm in diameter) is the same inside the cell as in the alveolar lumen and there appears to be no preferred size for secretion. Frequently, there is an association of Golgi as well as other vesicles with the boundaries of droplets and this has led to the suggestion that, as the Golgi vesicles fuse with the apical plasmalemma and release their contents, the membrane is transferred to the lipid droplets and the globule membrane then extends progressively as other vesicles fuse.

In addition to the proteins synthesized within the secretory cell, immunoglobulins of the blood plasma or of the plasma cells of mammary tissue are transported across the mammary epithelium into milk. Transfer is through the secretory cell by a selective mechanism dependent on specific receptor sites on the basal membrane, and is regulated by the concentrations of oestrogen and progesterone in blood such that it is enhanced in late pregnancy.

Regulation of mammary development and lactation

The hormonal requirements for the growth and development of an actively lactating gland have been studied most extensively in the rat and mouse but there is much detailed information on sheep and goats. Experiments with endocrinectomized animals have shown that administration of oestrogen, progesterone, adrenal steroids, prolactin and growth hormone, in appropriate combination and sequence, will induce the development of an atrophic duct system into a fully lactating gland, but in the pregnant animal there are firm indications that placental lactogens may substitute for certain of these hormones, in particular prolactin or growth hormone, depending on species.

The most rapid phase of development of lobular alveolar tissue is in mid-pregnancy but there is a progressive increase in cytoplasmic volume throughout pregnancy. At parturition there is a distinct increase in cytoplasmic membranes and in rough endoplasmic reticulum, and Golgi vesicles containing casein micelles begin to appear in the apical cytoplasm. Differentiation of enzymes may take place earlier in lactation but secretion is dependent on the structural changes within the cell. Development of the rough endoplasmic reticulum and Golgi membranes is induced by glucocorticoids whereas the formation of Golgi vesicles may be dependent on secretion of prolactin.

Lipid synthesis and secretion commences before that of lactose and protein and precedes parturition, but cannot take place until the cell membranes have developed. Lactose synthesis is linked to that of protein, because of its dependence on the continuous synthesis and transfer of α-lactalbumin (the B protein of lactose synthetase) to the Golgi region, but the mechanisms which initiate and regulate protein synthesis and composition are not well described. The existence of genetic variants of the major milk proteins has been taken as evidence of the expected control at the DNA level and it is assumed that both feed-back inhibition (where the action of the initial enzyme of a pathway is inhibited by accumulation of product) and repression inhibition (where enzyme formation is inhibited) operate.

The hormonal trigger mechanism that determines the onset of copious milk secretion at the end of pregnancy has not been firmly resolved. During pregnancy, milk secretion is inhibited by the high ratio of progesterone to oestrogen in blood plasma which inhibits pituitary secretion of prolactin, and by the high concentrations of progesterone and oestrogen which promote the growth of mammary tissue but make it insensitive to the action of prolactin. At parturition there is a distinct fall in progesterone secretion and a rise in the secretion of prolactin and adrenal corticoids, and the withdrawal of progesterone has been suggested as the most likely lactogenic trigger, a mechanism that may be common to all species.

The minimum range of hormones required to maintain lactation at a high level varies between species. In the rabbit, for example, prolactin alone is sufficient but, in the cow, sheep and goat, prolactin, growth hormone, thyroxine, parathyroid hormone, adrenal corticoids and oxytocin are necessary, and growth hormone may have a greater importance than prolactin. Milk secretion is also dependent on other hormones such as insulin and glucagon, which are important because of their effects on the partition of substrate metabolism between the mammary gland and body tissues.

Present evidence indicates that the secretion of some of the key hormones regulating milk secretion, and possibly the number and sensitivity of the receptor sites for the hormones in 'target' tissues, varies according to a prescribed lactational pattern. In early lactation, cows tend to partition dietary nutrients towards milk secretion and there is often mobilization of adipose tissue to provide energy to there are lactational changes in the blood plasma concentrations of hormones (Bines and Hart, 1978). In cows, levels of growth hormone, a lipogenic hormone, are high and those of insulin, an anabolic hormone, are low in early lactation, and in late lactation the pattern is reversed. Responses in milk secretion to changes in diet can thus be expected to be modified by the animal's stage of lactation and hormonal status. The position is complex, however, because the plasma concentrations of the hormones are themselves modulated by the level of nutrition and the type of diet. In ruminants, for example, growth hormone levels have been negatively correlated, and insulin levels positively correlated, with dietary energy intake (see Trenkle, 1978), and there is some evidence that growth hormone levels may be increased by the infusion of protein (casein) into the abomasum and possibly by the absorption of amino acids in the small intestine; in ruminants and in man intravenous injections of arginine have stimulated growth hormone release. For insulin, in ruminants levels are increased by starchy cereal diets and may be responding to changes in the composition of the mixture of short-chain fatty acids formed in the rumen or in the amount of glucogenic substrates absorbed in the small intestine, and in non-ruminants the intestinal absorption of glucogenic materials is of established importance.

Metabolic pathways for the synthesis of milk constituents

Lipid

Fatty acids incorporated into milk lipids may be derived directly from the fatty acids of plasma constituents or synthesized *de novo* in the gland.

The major pathway for synthesis *de novo*, the malonyl pathway, has two basic reactions: (1) the carboxylation of acetyl-CoA to malonyl-CoA, which is catalysed by acetyl-CoA carboxylase

$$CH_3COSCoA + HCO_3^- + ATP \longrightarrow$$
$$CH_2(COOH)COSCoA + ADP + Pi \quad [1]$$

and (2) condensation of a primer fatty acyl-CoA molecule with successive molecules of malonyl-CoA, the chain length being extended by increments of two carbon units, which is catalysed by a group of enzymes known collectively as fatty acid synthetase

$$CH_3COSCoA + nCH_2(COOH)COSCoA + 2nNADPH \longrightarrow$$
$$CH_3CH_2(CH_2CH_2)_{n-1}CH_2COOH + nCO_2$$
$$+ 2nNADP + (n+1)CoA + (n-1)H_2O \quad [2]$$

The limiting step is [1] and acetyl-CoA carboxylase is inhibited by longer-chain fatty acids, by their CoA esters and by malonyl-CoA.

In most tissues, including mammary tissue of non-herbivorous animals such as the sow, acetyl-CoA is the normal primer molecule but in ruminant mammary tissue butyryl-CoA, which may be synthesized from acetate or formed directly from 3-hydroxybutyrate, may also act as the primer molecule. With diets associated with a very high ruminal production of propionic acid, propionate may be incompletely metabolized in the liver and enter the peripheral circulation, and may then act as the primer molecule to give fatty acids with an odd number of carbon atoms.

In non-herbivorous animals the primary source of acetyl-CoA is glucose, which is catabolized oxidatively in the cytosol, through the Embden-Meyerhof and pentose phosphate pathways, to pyruvate, which then enters the mitochondria where it is oxidized to acetyl-CoA. The acetyl-CoA has then to be transported to the cytosol, the main site of fatty acid synthesis. Permeability of the mitochondrial membrane to acetyl-CoA is low and transfer is primarily by the citrate-cleavage pathway. Acetyl-CoA condenses with oxaloacetate to form citrate, under the action of citrate synthetase which is present exclusively in the mitochondria. The citrate is translocated across the mitochondrial membrane to the cytosol where it is cleaved by ATP-citrate lyase, located solely in the cytosol, with the release of acetyl-CoA.

The activity of ATP-citrate lyase in ruminant mammary tissue, however, is low and the acyl-CoA for fatty acid synthesis is derived within the cytosol by the activation of the short-chain fatty acids or during the synthesis of butyrate from acetate or 3-hydroxybutyrate. An acyl-CoA synthetase has been located predominantly in the cytosolic fraction of ruminant mammary tissue, which is active towards acetate and propionate but not butyrate; the activity towards 3-hydroxybutyrate has not been determined. The activity of the enzyme is greater in sheep than in rat mammary tissue.

Fatty acid synthetase is a multi-enzyme complex with seven subunits (acetyl transacylase, malonyl transacylase, β-ketothioester synthetase, β-ketothioester reductase, β-hydroxyacylthioester dehydrase, enoyl-thioester reductase and acylthioester hydrolase) and the properties of the enzyme in mammary tissue are similar to that of the enzyme in other tissues. In most non-mammary tissues the product of fatty acid synthesis is unesterified palmitic acid and a palmitoyl thioesterase is closely associated with the fatty acid synthetase complex. The palmitic acid synthesized may be converted to stearic acid by chain elongation in the mitochondria or microsomes. The main product of fatty acid synthesis is similarly palmitic acid in non-lactating mammary tissue but at parturition there is a massive increase in fatty acid synthesizing activity and a production of shorter-chain fatty acids: the pattern of support milk synthesis; as lactation advances, past the peak in yield, the responsiveness of milk secretion to increased dietary allowances declines and there is a progressively increasing partition of nutrients towards the synthesis of adipose tissues. In parallel with these effects, short-chain fatty acids produced is characteristic for the species (Table 8.1). This change is under hormonal control and in some species, at least, is induced by prolactin. The reasons for the shortening of the chain length are not fully understood but it is probably due to the presence of specific acylthioester hydrolases, which give rise to the characteristic patterns of fatty acid release. A discrete, medium-chain acyl hydrolase has recently been identified and characterized in rabbit, rat and mouse lactating mammary tissue, but in ruminant mammary tissue the enzyme appears to form an integral part of the fatty acid synthetase complex (Dils, 1980).

In addition to the malonyl pathway, a minor pathway has been identified in several species of mammary tissue which, by a reversal of β-oxidation, allows the synthesis of butyrate from acetyl-CoA.

The differentiation of mammary tissue at parturition is also associated with the development of desaturase activity within the microsomes; in the cow and goat the desaturase is highly specific for the conversion of stearic to oleic acid and shows only limited activity

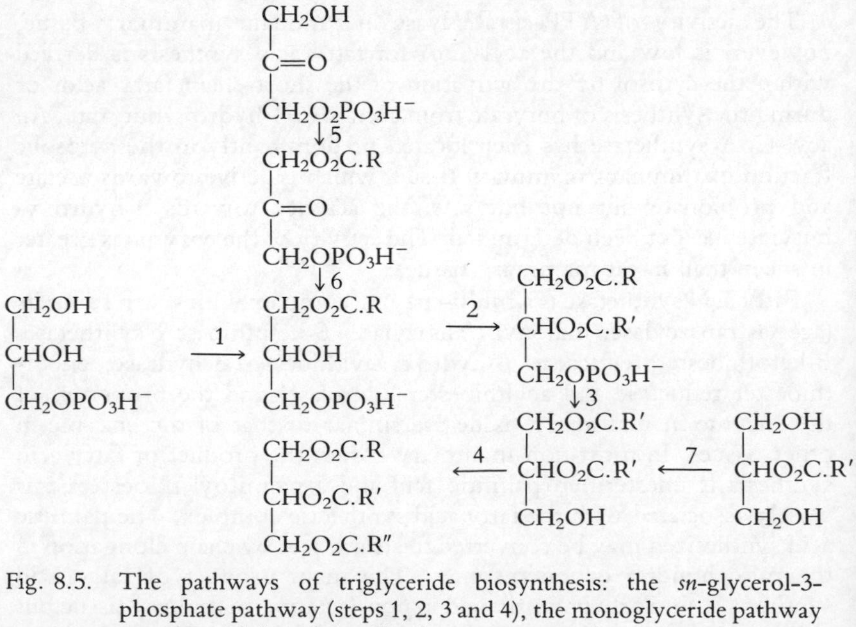

Fig. 8.5.   The pathways of triglyceride biosynthesis: the *sn*-glycerol-3-phosphate pathway (steps 1, 2, 3 and 4), the monoglyceride pathway (steps 7 and 4) and the dihydroxyacetone pathway (steps 5, 6, 2, 3 and 4). (From Moore and Christie, 1979.)

towards palmitic acid, whereas in the sow there is extensive conversion of palmitic to palmitoleic acid.

There are three main pathways for the biosynthesis of triglycerides (Fig. 8.5) but the principal pathway in mammary tissues is the *sn*-glycerol-3-phosphate route. The glycerol-3-phosphate is derived either from the phosphorylation of glycerol released during the hydrolysis of plasma lipids or by glycolysis via the triose phosphates; glycerolkinase activity is increased substantially at parturition. Fatty acids are converted to acyl-CoA esters prior to incorporation into glycerides under the action of acyl-CoA synthetase, the nature and location of which in mammary tissues are as yet not well defined. The positional distribution of the fatty acids is probably determined by the specificities of the acyltransferases, found predominantly in the endoplasmic reticulum, and required for esterification at each position but it may also be affected by the existence of alternative pathways of triglyceride synthesis.

The phospholipids of milk are probably synthesized *de novo* by the phosphatidic pathway (Fig. 8.5) whereas the cholesterol may be of dietary origin, or synthesized elsewhere within the body or within the mammary gland; cholesterol esters are synthesized within the mammary gland.

Proteins

The milk proteins are synthesized from amino acids by the same processes as have been described more generally for protein synthesis (Fig. 8.6). The genetic coding information on the DNA template in the nucleus is transcribed by the synthesis of mRNA, which is then

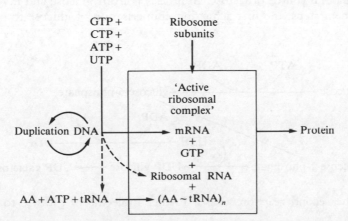

Fig. 8.6. The overall pathway of protein biosynthesis (AA, amino acid). (From Larson, 1965.)

transferred to the ribosomes where it associates with rRNA. Individual which form a codon in the long strands of mRNA, are successively recognized by the corresponding nucleotide triplets (anticodons) of the tRNA amino acid complexes, leading in the presence of mRNA to an alignment of amino acids sufficiently close for peptide bond formation. In lactation the secretory cell makes use of the coded information for milk protein synthesis and the derepression of the appropriate part of the genome is under hormonal control.

The carbohydrate moieties of the caseins are probably synthesized and added to the amino acid chains in the Golgi apparatus. This is also the site of addition of phosphate to the hydroxyl groups of serine and threonine. The phosphorylating kinase 'recognizes' seryl and threonine residues in specific sequences of amino acids, and genetic variation in these sequences causes modification of the extent of phosphorylation and of the quaternary structure of the micelle. Occasional misreading of the sequences may also account for the synthesis of the minor caseins of milk. The amino acid sequences 'recognized' for phosphorylation of serine are -serine[†]-X-glutamic acid- followed by -serine[†]-Y-serine(P)-X-glutamic acid (where X and Y are any amino acids and the phosphorylation is of the serine[†] residue); in α_{s_0}-casein, an additional phosphate is incorporated in the sequence -serine-lysine-aspartic acid-. It has been concluded that the kinase fails to distinguish between the aspartyl residue and the usual glutamyl residue but the efficiency of incorporation is reduced and only approximately one molecule in eight is phosphorylated.

Lactose

With the exception of a few plants, the mammary gland is the only natural source of lactose. Synthesis is from glucose and involves two main steps, the first achieving epimerisation of glucose to galactose:

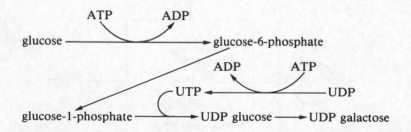

and the second reaction with a further molecule of glucose to give lactose:

$$\text{UDP galactose} + \text{glucose} \longrightarrow \text{lactose} + \text{UDP}.$$

The enzyme catalysing the second reaction is referred to as lactose synthetase but the reaction is a galactosyl transfer catalysed by the enzyme galactosyl transferase (the A protein of lactose synthetase). The normal acceptor in the reaction is N-acetylglucosamine and the product N-acetyl-lactosamine but in the presence of α-lactalbumin (the B protein of lactose synthetase) the specificity of the enzyme is modified, and glucose becomes the preferred acceptor and lactose the product. amino acids on activation (formation of CoA derivatives) combine with their specific tRNA and the sequence of groups of three nucleotides,

Lactose may act as a substrate for glycosyl transferases and give rise to the oligosaccharides usually present in milks in low concentration.

The supply of energy and reducing equivalents

The synthesis of milk constituents from their precursors requires a supply of intermediates and cofactors, the most important of which are energy in the form of ATP and reducing equivalents in the form of NADPH. The biochemical pathways which provide these requirements have been referred to as 'satellite' pathways and their relationship to the synthetic pathways is outlined in Fig. 8.7.

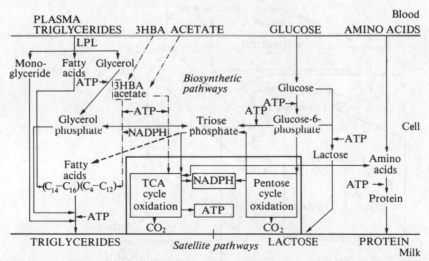

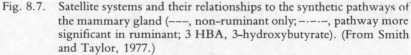

Fig. 8.7. Satellite systems and their relationships to the synthetic pathways of the mammary gland (– – –, non-ruminant only; – · – · –, pathway more significant in ruminant; 3 HBA, 3-hydroxybutyrate). (From Smith and Taylor, 1977.)

The major source of ATP is the oxidation of materials in the tricarboxylic acid cycle and related pathways with the associated phosphorylation of ADP resulting from the transfer of hydrogen from NADH along the mitochondrial cytochrome system. In theory, any of the major substrates could act as a source of oxidizable material but under normal conditions glucose and acetate would be expected to be of greatest importance. Species differences in the details of the pathways are not well established but in ruminants a low activity of pyruvate dehydrogenase may restrict glucose oxidation by the tricarboxylic acid cycle. Also, in comparison with the non-ruminant mammary gland, there is a considerable activity of fructose-biphosphatase which, through the recombination of triose phosphates to produce glucose-6-phosphate, allows 'recycling' so that the whole of the glucose molecule may be oxidized to carbon dioxide in the pentose phosphate cycle. This offers the capability for glucose sparing when this is required by limitations in the supply of substrates.

Reducing equivalents from the oxidation of substrates in the tricarboxylic acid cycle are not available for fatty acid synthesis within the

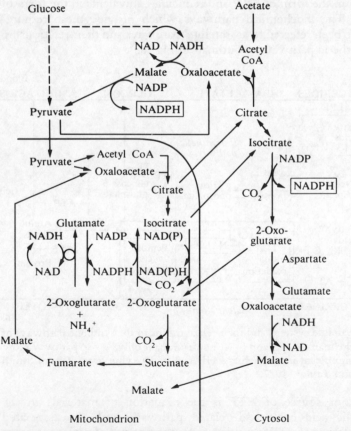

Fig. 8.8. Pathways of NADPH regeneration. (From Smith and Taylor, 1977.)

cytosol, since they are produced within the mitochondria and the mitochondrial membrane is impermeable to the nicotinamide co-enzymes. A major source of NADPH for fatty acid synthesis is thought to be the oxidation of glucose by the pentose phosphate pathway within the cytosol, which produces NADPH specifically. There are, however, alternative pathways (Fig. 8.8). The oxidation of glucose to pyruvate produces NADH which may be used for the formation of NADPH by an oxaloacetate-malate shunt, dependent on the coupled operation of NAD-malate dehydrogenase and NADP-malate dehydrogenase. This requires the production of oxaloacetate within the cytosol through the cleavage of citrate in the formation of acetyl-CoA for fatty acid synthesis. In ruminant mammary tissue, however, the low activity of ATP-citrate lyase reduces the importance of this pathway. A third source of cytosolic NADPH is the dehydrogenation of isocitrate to 2-oxoglutarate, which may be linked with a reduction of 2-oxoglutarate back to isocitrate in the mitochondria. This is an important pathway for ruminant mammary tissue in which there is a much higher activity of isocitrate dehydrogenase, malate dehydrogenase and glutamate dehydrogenase than in non-ruminant mammary tissue. There are also important species differences between non-ruminants in the importance of the various pathways: in the pig, as compared with the rat, the activity of isocitrate dehydrogenase is high and that of NADP-malate dehydrogenase low.

THE PRECURSORS OF MILK CONSTITUENTS

Methods for the identification and measurement of uptake of milk precursors

Techniques involving the incubation of preparations of mammary tissues (homogenates, tissue slices and isolated mammary cells) have been used to identify precursors and intermediates of milk synthesis but there is always the possibility that the metabolism of the tissue is altered when it is isolated. The techniques are, therefore, better suited to the qualitative study of metabolic pathways and their control than to the study of the quantitative relationships between substrate supply and milk synthesis. The techniques that have proved of most value in the study of the physiology of the relationship between substrate supply and milk secretion are measurements *in vivo* of arteriovenous differences across a gland and the transfer of radioactivity from plasma precursors to milk constituents, or a combination of the two, and, to a lesser extent, the use of the isolated perfused udder. These techniques and their limitations will be described briefly but this description will be preceded by a short account of blood supply to the gland.

Blood supply

As mammary glands are skin structures, their blood and nerve supply is that of the skin tissues from which they derived. The glands of different species are located in different parts of the body: cows, sheep and goats have inguinal mammary glands and these have the blood and nerve supply of the inguinum, whereas pigs have mammary glands that extend along the abdomen and have therefore a multiple blood and nerve supply (Fig. 8.9).

The main arterial supply to the mammary glands of ruminants is the pudic artery. Venous drainage from the area of the glands is by the caudal epigastric vein which drains into the external pudic vein. The direction of flow is normally under the control of valves but, during the development of the udder and the onset of lactation, blood flow into the inguinal area increases substantially, the epigastric vein is dilated and the valves can become incompetent. Some of the mammary blood then flows forward into the caudal superficial epigastric vein (the 'milk vein'). Progressively, valves of the external pudic vein may also become incompetent and that allows blood from the abdomen to pass into the 'milk vein'.

In the pig, mammary arteries are derived chiefly from the epigastric artery and venous drainage is into the superficial epigastric veins which lie lateral to the glands.

Developing mammary tissue acquires a rich blood supply. In the dog, cat and goat, each alveolus is surrounded by a network of 5 to 10 capillaries, each section approximately 50 μm long and 10 to 15 μm apart, and there is a separate capillary network for each lobule and its associated ductule supported by one to three arterioles and venules. Vascular shunts and lymphatics are absent from the secretory tissue itself and excess tissue fluid enters the fine lymphatics that surround the lobules. All the arteries and arterioles have a network of sympathetic nerves and, in the conscious animal, mild stress or disturbance affects blood flow.

Arteriovenous-difference technique

This provides a measure of the uptake of a constituent from blood as it passes through a gland, as reflected in the change of concentration, and requires the simultaneous sampling of the arterial supply and venous drainage under stable conditions. Stress must be minimized in the taking of samples, as it causes a reduction in mammary blood flow, and increases in blood plasma concentrations of glucose and lactic acid due to a release of adrenalin, and care must be taken to ensure that the samples are representative of the total blood flow.

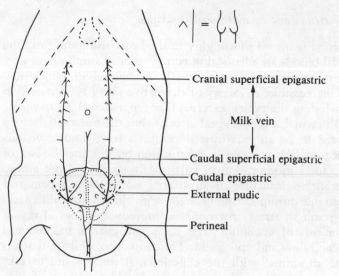

Cranial superficial epigastric

Milk vein

Caudal superficial epigastric

Caudal epigastric

External pudic

Perineal

(a)

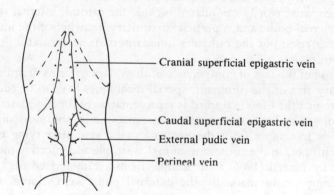

Cranial superficial epigastric vein

Caudal superficial epigastric vein

External pudic vein

Perineal vein

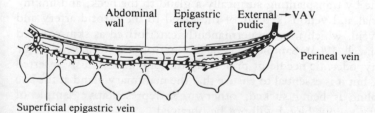

Abdominal wall   Epigastric artery   External pudic →VAV

Perineal vein

Superficial epigastric vein

(b)

Fig. 8.9. (a) The superficial abdominal veins of the cow: the positions and directions of valves are shown (all the veins are accompanied by arteries);

(b) The superficial abdominal veins of the female piglet, which drain the mammary gland in the adult, and dissection of the mammary glands of a lactating sow. (From Linzell, 1974.)

Arterial blood is mixed thoroughly in the heart and lungs, and the various arterial bloods are identical in composition. Samples need not, therefore, be taken from the mammary arteries themselves, which may be small and inaccessible. A variety of alternative sites has been used in ruminants including the radial, external iliac (approached *per rectum* or *per vaginum*), brachial and coccygeal arteries, but the most satisfactory site has proved to be an exteriorized carotid artery; jugular venous blood has frequently been used in substitution but the metabolism of head tissues causes modification of particularly lactic acid and amino acid concentrations. Puncture of an arterial wall produces pain and imposing restraint during sampling, even with the use of mild anaesthesia, may result in stress. Anaesthesia, moreover, is not always a satisfactory means of avoiding stress as in the goat it has reduced mammary blood flow and milk yield. The most successful approach is to familiarize an animal with the experimental routine and to take samples from previously catheterized vessels. The arteries of pigs readily go into spasm and may be difficult to cannulate but vessels that have been satisfactorily cannulated include the carotid, internal saphenous, external pudic and superficial mammary branches of the internal thoracic arteries; but the catheters, once inserted, need careful protection from piglets.

Because of the loss of competence of the valves of veins draining the mammary area of the ruminant, special techniques have to be adopted to ensure that the blood sampled is representative of the blood draining the whole of a gland. In animals under anaesthesia, the most suitable method is to sample from the external pudic vein after tying off all other veins but, in the conscious animal, a simple and effective method devised by Linzell (1966) is to sample from a catheterized milk vein while compressing manually the external pudic vein. Some of the problems of sampling mammary arterial and venous blood may be overcome by transplanting surgically a gland to the neck, and linking the arterial and venous sytems of the gland to the carotid artery and jugular vein, which may be permanently exteriorized as skin-covered loops (Linzell, 1963). Samples may be drawn from the 'milk vein' of the pig by hypodermic needle or preferably through a previously inserted catheter, but it is essential to ensure that the mammary gland at the site of sampling is being sucked, otherwise a representative sample of mammary venous blood will not be obtained.

The errors attached to many early estimates of arteriovenous differences were high, ± 20% (Barry, 1964), but much smaller errors have been achieved in subsequent work (see Linzell, 1974) and, for most of the recognized precursors, an uptake in excess of experimental error has been established. As the ratio of blood flow to volume of milk secreted during full lactation is about 500:1, the method cannot, however, be applied to constituents of the plasma, for example plasma protein, present in high concentration. The rate of lymph drainage from the mammary gland is not sufficient to affect the validity of the arteriovenous-difference method.

The quantitative use of arteriovenous-difference data requires a knowledge also of mammary blood flow which, in the conscious animal, has been measured by a variety of techniques including thermodilution, indicator dilution, the use of an electromagnetic flowmeter and several methods based on the Fick principle, which allow the calculation of blood flow from the rate of diffusion of materials from blood to tissue or *vice versa*. Several of the methods require the collection of a representative sample of venous blood and the precautions outlined for the determination of arteriovenous differences must be adopted.

Isolated perfused udder

Techniques, which have been most widely applied to the goat and guinea pig have been devised for the surgical removal of the gland and the maintenance of secretory activity for a period of 12 to 24 h by perfusion with blood or a semi-synthetic perfusate, and the response to the inclusion of a substrate in, or its elimination from, the perfusate provides evidence for its rôle in milk secretion. Under the most successful conditions, the isolated udder yields only approximately half of the volume of secretion before removal but the technique has proved valuable, especially when used in conjunction with isotopically labelled substrates.

Use of isotopes

The labelling of constituents of the blood plasma by injecting a tracer amount of a slightly modified material, usually an isotope, allows the identification and measurement of their appearance in milk. The method has been used to study the cellular site and stage of synthesis at which ions are bound or incorporated into larger molecules and to investigate the permeability of mammary membranes to water-soluble constituents, but its prime rôle has been the identification of the precursors of the major synthesized materials in milk. The interpretation of results requires caution as there may be a transfer of label by exchange reactions in the mammary gland without net synthesis, or the labelled compound may be transformed into a second compound elsewhere within the body and that compound then used for milk synthesis. This latter difficulty may be overcome by the use of the isolated perfused udder or by giving labelled material into one gland only and comparing the specific activities of constituents in the milk of the gland with those of other glands.

Table 8.3 Arteriovenous differences across the mammary glands of conscious lactating animals (from Linzell, 1974)

	Goat						Cow						Pig					
	A			E			A			E			A			E		
	Mean	s.e.	No.	Mean	s.e.	No.	Mean	s.e.	No.	Mean	s.e.	No.	Mean	s.e.	No.	Mean	s.e.	No.
Blood																		
O_2, vols/l	118.5	8	38	0.45	0.01	38	143.7	2.4	19	0.29	0.01	19	129	6	6	0.33	0.06	6
Glucose (mg/l)	455	15	34	0.33	0.01	34	495	13	29	0.25	0.01	29	66	13	13	0.30	0.01	13
Acetate (mg/l)	89	6	34	0.63	0.02	34	90.7	5.6	28	0.56	0.02	28	19.0	0.2	11	0.45	0.02	11
Lactate (mg/l)	71.3	3	11	0.28	0.03	11	82	6.1	30	0.10	0.03	30	125	7.5	11	0.15	0.02	11
Plasma (mg/l)																		
3-Hydroxybutyrate	58	4.7	9	0.57	0.03	9	53	6.2	23	0.40	0.04	23	12.4	0.4	11	0.15	0.01	11
Acetoacetate	2.5	0.5	4	0.08	0.08	4	5.5	0.11	8	0.34	0.13	8	5.8	0.3	7	0.02	0.04	7
Triglycerides	219	25	10	0.40	0.05	10	90.4	6.9	20	0.58	0.02	20	319	1	11	0.22		11
Free fatty acids	87	4	18	0.03	0.04	18	79.8	7.5	25	0.04	0.05	25	4.2	1	6	−0.02	0.10	6
Phospholipids	1600	190	8	0.04	0.03	8	800	190	11	0	0.05	11	553	6	10	0.05	0.01	10
Cholesterol	370	40	7	−0.05	0.06	7	230	40	5	0	0.01	5	172	6.5	10	0.01	0.02	10
Cholesterol esters	1000	170	7	0.02	0.04	7	1830	170	11	0.01	0.03	11	240	23	3	0.15	0.08	3
Free glycerol	3.4	0.6	6	0.07	0.05	6												
Methionine	2.7	0.2	10	0.72	0.09	10	2.5	0.2	10	0.57	0.05	10	8.1	0.7	10	0.37	0.01	10
Phenylalanine	7.0	0.5	10	0.63	0.05	10	7.2	0.2	11	0.43	0.03	11	21.1	0.8	12	0.32	0.01	12
Leucine	20.7	0.8	10	0.63	0.05	10	21.8	1.1	11	0.44	0.01	11	42.8	1.6	12	0.33	0.02	12
Threonine	9.6	0.6	10	0.60	0.02	10	9.8	0.5	11	0.34	0.01	11	26.9	0.9	12	0.23	0.01	12
Lysine	21.3	1.9	10	0.49	0.06	10	12.4	0.5	11	0.59	0.01	11	42.2	2.0	12	0.26	0.01	12
Arginine	25.3	1.1	10	0.48	0.07	10	12.9	0.7	11	0.47	0.04	11	40.8	1.8	12	0.27	0.01	12
Isoleucine	17.9	0.8	10	0.47	0.05	10	17.3	0.6	11	0.45	0.01	11	30.1	0.8	12	0.31	0.01	12
Histidine	10.4	1.2	10	0.42	0.05	10	9.8	0.3	11	0.27	0.02	11	24.1	0.14	12	0.25	0.01	12
Valine	27.9	1.1	10	0.37	0.05	10	30.7	1.4	11	0.27	0.02	11	49.0	2.0	12	0.26	0.01	12

Plasma (mg/l)	Goat A Mean	s.e.	No.	Goat E Mean	s.e.	No.	Cow A Mean	s.e.	No.	Cow E Mean	s.e.	No.	Pig A Mean	s.e.	No.	Pig E Mean	s.e.	No.
Glutamate	19.3	1.1	10	0.58	0.04	10	9.4	0.3	11	0.56	0.05	4 0.55	62.4	2.2	12	0.39	0.02	12
Tyrosine	9.5	0.7	10	0.39	0.05	10	7.2	0.3	11	0.45	0.05	4 0.50	25.8	0.9	12	0.25	0.02	12
Asparagine	8.9	0.7	10	0.37	0.07	10	4.2	0.5	7	–	–	– 0.31	6.2	0.8	5	0.01	0.09	5
Proline	25.9	1.9	10	0.36	0.06	10	8.1	1.1	7	–	–	– 0.26	44.6	1.9	10	0.31	0.03	9
Ornithine	11.1	1.4	10	0.36	0.07	10	9.3	0.4	10	0.42	0.04	4 0.52	19.0	2.3	5	0.16	0.08	5
Aspartate	2.8	0.3	10	0.33	0.07	10	1.5	0.1	11	0.50	0.09	4 0.23	4.4	0.3	11	0.13	0.02	11
Alanine	16.6	1	10	0.25	0.04	10	16.1	0.6	11	0.19	0.04	4 0.05	36.5	2.1	12	0.09	0.01	12
Glutamine	37.4	2.7	10	0.23	0.05	10	26.3	2.3	7	–	–	0.23	64.0	12.1	4	0.09	0.04	4
Glycine	68.5	7.8	10	0.05	0.02	10	17.9	0.7	11	0.10	0.02	4 0.08	51.4	2.1	12	0	0.01	12
Citrulline	19.3	1.8	10	0.03	0.06	10	12.4	0.7	11	0.12	0.03	4 0.07	–	–	–	–	–	–
Serine	14.1	1.2	10	0	–	10	8.9	0.7	11	0.31	0.04	4 0.20	16.6	1.2	4	0.22	0.03	4

The extraction coefficient (E) is the arteriovenous difference expressed as a proportion of arterial concentration (A). Data for the goat are taken from animals in Linzell's laboratory. For the cow, the details are taken from Hartmann and Lascelles (1964), Verbeke and Peeters (1964), Kronfeld, Raggi and Ramberg (1968), and Bickerstaffe, Annison and Linzell (1974); and for the pig, from Spincer, Rook and Towers (1969), and Linzell, Mepham, Annison and West (1969). The second value for E for amino acids in the cow is from Verbeke and Peeters (1964), who give only mean A and arteriovenous-difference values.

MILK PRECURSORS

A compilation of data on arteriovenous differences across the lactating mammary glands of the goat, cow and pig has been provided by Linzell (1974) (Table 8.3). Average values for the goat for extraction rate and uptake by the gland are given in Fig. 8.10 and the utilization of the various precursors for the synthesis of milk in the three species is represented schematically in Fig. 8.11.

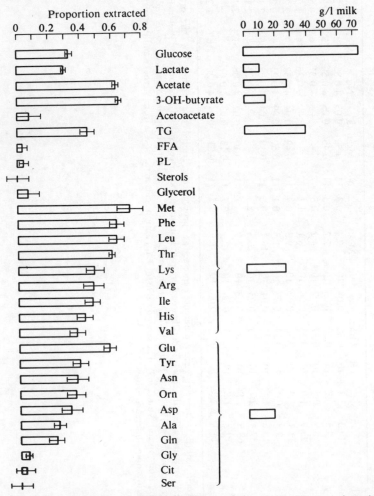

Fig. 8.10.   Summary by Linzell (1974) of the extraction rate (arteriovenous difference as a proportion of the arterial concentration) for the main precursors of milk in the goat in relation to their incorporation into milk constituents (bars indicate s.e.) TG, triglyceride; FFA, free fatty acid; PL, phospholipid; cit, citrate).

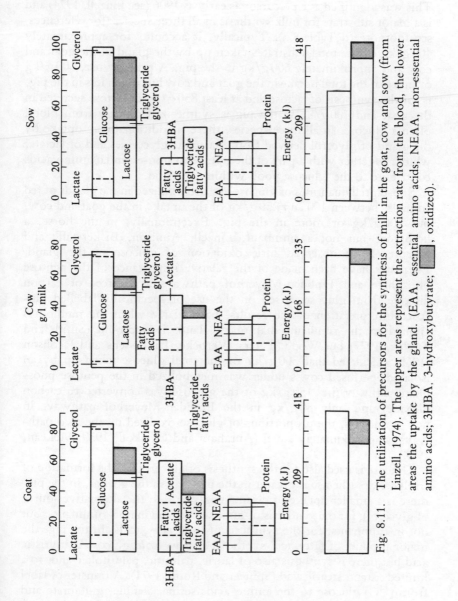

Fig. 8.11. The utilization of precursors for the synthesis of milk in the goat, cow and sow (from Linzell, 1974). The upper areas represent the extraction rate from the blood, the lower areas the uptake by the gland. (EAA, essential amino acids; NEAA, non-essential amino acids; 3HBA, 3-hydroxybutyrate; oxidized).

Glucose

This was identified as a precursor as early as 1906 (see Linzell, 1974) and is a major substrate for milk synthesis in all three species (for references, see footnote to Table 8.3). Typically, it accounts for approximately 400 g/kg of the total substrates taken up by the gland in the goat and cow and approximately 600 g/kg in the pig. A primary use, 600 g/kg or more of the total uptake in the goat and cow but much less in the pig, is for the synthesis of lactose and at least 850 g/kg of lactose secreted in the goat and 700 g/kg in the pig is synthesized directly from blood plasma glucose. In all three species, there is additionally an uptake by the gland of glycerol derived from plasma triglycerides and of lactate, which, together with a part of the uptake of non-essential amino acids contribute to the 'glucose pool' within the gland.

Substantial quantities of glucose are also oxidized in the glands of fed animals, between 100 and 250 g/kg of the uptake in the goat and cow, but 300 g/kg or more in the pig. Exceptionally, in the horse, a herbivore but not a ruminant, Linzell, Annison, Bickerstaffe and Jeffcott (1972) observed little oxidation of glucose in the gland. Estimates have been made of the relative importance of the pentose phosphate and Embden-Meyerhof pathways as sources of carbon dioxide from glucose, based on the use of specifically labelled glucose. Interpretation of the results, particularly when the method is applied to the ruminant mammary gland, is uncertain (Smith and Taylor, 1977) but Wood, Peters, Verbeke, Lauryssens and Jacobson (1965) calculated that 300 g/kg of the total glucose taken up by an isolated, perfused cow's udder was metabolized in the pentose phosphate pathway (i.e. 150 g/kg of the glucose was converted to carbon dioxide) and only 80 g/kg in the Embden-Meyerhof pathway. In non-ruminants, the proportions of glucose oxidized by the two pathways is approximately equal (Abraham and Chaikoff, 1959; McLean, 1964).

Glucose is used also for the synthesis of glycerol for the formation of triglycerides (the use is greater in the pig than in the goat as, in the pig, there is a smaller uptake of plasma triglycerides, the alternative source of glycerol); for the synthesis of milk citrate; and in non-ruminants, but not in ruminants, for the synthesis of milk fatty acids. In the pig, the major product of fatty acid synthesis *de novo* from glucose is myristic acid but there is synthesis also of lauric, palmitic, palmitoleic and, to a limited extent, stearic acid (Spincer and Rook, 1971). A transfer of label from [14C] glucose to the amino acids serine, alanine, glutamate and aspartate of milk proteins in the goat (Mepham and Linzell, 1966) and to casein in the isolated perfused pig gland has also been observed, and at least part of this transfer probably reflects net synthesis (see below).

Amino acids

The earliest experiments with isotopically labelled amino acids demonstrated a substantial transfer of radioactivity to casein but initial arteriovenous-difference studies gave a discrepancy between the uptake of amino acids by a gland and the output in milk protein, and an unidentified plasma protein was postulated as a significant alternative source (see Barry, 1961). There is now ample evidence, however, that the mammary uptake of amino acids supplies sufficient carbon and nitrogen to account for the output of those elements in the milk proteins (caseins, β-lactoglobulin and α-lactalbumin) but there are differences between individual amino acids and between species in the extent to which the uptake of an amino acid balances its output. The uptake of essential amino acids is, without exception, equal to or in excess of the output in milk but the relationship between uptake and output for non-essential amino acids is more variable from time to time, from animal to animal and from species to species; there is isotopic evidence for interconversions between amino acids and for the net synthesis of non-essential amino acids from glucose and acetate (Clark, Spires and Davis, 1978; Mepham, 1979). In the goat, cow and sheep, the ratio of mammary gland uptake to milk protein output is close to unity for methionine, histidine, phenylalanine and tyrosine, and, on the basis of evidence from the guinea-pig, the same may be true for tryptophan (see Mepham, Peters and Davis, 1976). This implies that these amino acids are almost exclusively incorporated into milk protein. On the other hand, the uptakes of ornithine and citrulline, amino acids not present in milk protein, and of arginine, threonine, lysine, valine, leucine and isoleucine, are in excess of that required for milk protein synthesis. There is isotopic evidence that there is metabolism of ornithine to proline and glutamate, of citrulline to proline and arginine, and of arginine to proline, glutamate and ornithine, and that threonine, lysine and the branched-chain amino acids are partly deaminated and oxidized to carbon dioxide. The oxidation appears to be an important feature of the metabolism of this group of amino acids and in experiments with perfused guinea-pig glands (Mepham, Peters and Alexandrov, 1979) oxidation was increased when protein synthesis was restricted through the supply of those essential amino acids which are quantitatively incorporated into milk protein.

Fatty acids

The earliest feeding experiments indicated that whilst milk fat secretion in the goat and cow was not dependent on a dietary supply of fat, with usual diets a proportion of the fatty acids of milk fat originated in the fatty acids of dietary constituents. The conclusion drawn from the first arteriovenous-difference studies, however, was that the precursor involved in this transfer was blood phospholipids but this has not been confirmed. Isotopic and arteriovenous studies in several species have now clearly identified the triglycerides of plasma chylomicra and lipoproteins as a primary source of the longer-chain fatty acids and as a partial source of the glycerol of milk fat.

Bickerstaffe (1971) reported an uptake of triglycerides by the mammary gland of the cow from all blood plasma lipoprotein fractions but there is much contrary evidence for a preferential uptake from chylomicra and low-density lipoproteins. Separation of the plasma lipid fractions by ultracentrifugal techniques has demonstrated significant arterio-mammary venous differences in the triglyceride components of the chylomicra and low-density (1005 to 1019 kg/m^3) lipoproteins in lactating, but not in non-lactating goats (Barry, Bartley, Linzell and Robinson, 1963). Infusion, into the mammary arteries of lactating goats, of labelled chylomicra prepared from the intestinal lymph of a goat given a duodenal infusion of [^{14}C] glyceryl tripalmitate and [^{3}H] palmitic acid confirmed uptake of fatty acids from the chylomicra and low-density β-lipoproteins (930 to 1006 kg/m^3) but not from β- or α-lipoprotein fractions of higher density; the triglycerides taken up had a similar specific radioactivity to that of the fractions from which they were derived (West, Bickerstaffe, Annison and Linzell, 1972). Glascock and his colleagues (Glascock, Welch, Bishop, Davies, Wright and Noble, 1966) have, in the cow (a species in which chylomicra are present in low concentration), identified specifically uptake from triglyceride present in the lipoprotein fraction (< 1050 kg/m^3) precipitable with dextran sulphate, and primarily from the fraction of density < 1039 kg/m^3.

The principal fatty acids of blood plasma triglycerides are palmitic, stearic and oleic acids, but, depending on diet, significant proportions of shorter(lauric and myristic)- and longer(C_{20} and C_{22})-chain fatty acids, and in non-ruminants of linoleic acid may also be present. The content of linoleic acid in the triglycerides of ruminant blood plasma is normally low, because of the extensive hydrogenation of dietary unsaturated fatty acids in the rumen, but the feeding of lipids rich in polyunsaturated fatty acids and protected from hydrogenation gives a substantial increase. Fatty acids that are present in plasma triglycerides are transferred to milk fat but the efficiency of transfer varies, and saturated acids may, in part, be reduced to the corresponding monounsaturated fatty acids under the action of microsomal desaturase.

In cattle, there appears to be a preferential uptake of plasma triglycerides containing a high concentration of stearic acid and a low concentration of oleic acid (West *et al.*, 1972), or a low concentration of linoleic acid (Moore, Steele and Noble, 1969), observations which may be explained partly by differences in the fatty acid composition of the triglycerides of the various lipoprotein fractions (Stead and Welch, 1975). Mammary lipoprotein lipase, the enzyme concerned with the hydrolysis of plasma triglycerides may, however, be specific in its action. The presence of C_{20} and C_{22} polyunsaturated acids in plasma triglycerides inhibits uptake of all fatty acids (Storry, Hall, Tuckley and Millard, 1969a).

Although in well fed cows and goats there is no arteriovenous difference in the plasma free fatty acid fraction, experiments with labelled fatty acids have demonstrated an uptake of fatty acids that is offset by a partial release into the plasma of the fatty acids of the hydrolysed lipoprotein triglycerides. There is also a specific increase in the oleic acid content of venous blood due to desaturation of stearic acid, probably under the action of a desaturase present in the cells of the capillary endothelium. When the arterial concentration of free fatty acids is elevated, however, above approximately 300 μmol/l according to Kronfeld (1965), as occurs during starvation or during the physiological undernutrition of early lactation, the relative rates of uptake and release are altered and there is net uptake of free fatty acids which are used for triglyceride synthesis and, through oxidation, as a source of energy (Linzell, 1967a and b). During the early period of a fast, endogenous fat in the udder may also be used for milk fat synthesis as there is then a distinct shrinkage of udder volume (Annison, Linzell and West, 1968).

In herbivorous animals (ruminants, horse and rabbit) there is additionally a substantial uptake of short-chain fatty acids, primarily acetate, but also in ruminants 3-hydroxybutyrate, and there is even a small uptake of acetate in the pig. In the fed goat and cow 300 to 500 g/kg of the acetate taken up and approximately 250 g/kg of the 3-hydroxybutyrate taken up is oxidized but the remainder is used primarily for fatty acid synthesis. The acids synthesized range from C_4 to C_{16} in the goat and cow, with possibly small amounts of stearic acid. Palmitic acid is invariably a major product, but there are distinctive species differences in the composition of the shorter-chain fatty acids. In the cow the proportions of capric, lauric and especially myristic acids are high, whereas in the goat the proportions of capric and myristic acids are high and that of lauric acid much lower. By comparison, in the rabbit there are especially high proportions of caprylic and capric acids and an unusually low proportion of myristic acid. Ruminant milk fat is also distinguished by a high molar content of butyric acid, approximately 50 g/kg of which is derived from 3-hydroxybutyrate, 3-Hydroxybutyrate is also incorporated into other fatty acids synthesized *de novo* but in amounts diminishing with increase in chain length. This is consistent with the contribution of 3-hydroxybutyrate to a C_4 unit, which subsequently condenses sequentially with one or more C_2 units, and only a small cleavage of 3-hydroxybutyrate to C_2 units. Although the proportions in milk fat of fatty acids synthesized *de novo* or derived from the constituent fatty acids of plasma lipids varies with diet and physiological state, typically all of the fatty acids from caproic to lauric, most of the myristic acid and at least half of the palmitic acid are synthesized in the gland (Bines and Brown, 1968; Palmquist, Davis, Brown and Sachan, 1969).

Transport across the basal membrane of the cell

Little is known of the mechanisms of transport of glucose, acetate and amino acids specifically across the basal membrane of the secretory cell. A simple passive process for the transport of glucose is improbable as the extraction of glucose is efficient down to comparatively low concentrations of glucose in arterial blood. The mechanism is sensitive to insulin in the non-ruminant but not in the ruminant. Numerous systems have been described for the transport of amino acids across cell membranes but those operating in mammary tissue have yet to be established. The deep infolding of the basal membrane may promote transport by increasing surface area and one suggestion is that extracellular components could be taken up in pinocytotic vesicles (see Mepham, 1977). There is, however, evidence that the enzymes of at least one amino acid transport system, the γ-glutamyl-transpeptidase cycle, are present in mammary cell membranes (Baumrucker, 1979). This transport system, which has been extensively studied in kidney tissue, is of a low-specificity, high-capacity type and might be well suited to the transport of the large quantities of amino acids required for milk protein synthesis; however, its quantitative importance in the gland has yet to be ascertained. Experiments with explants from mice in mid-pregnancy and with slices of lactating guinea-pig mammary gland have shown that insulin stimulates amino acid uptake by mammary tissue.

The mechanism of uptake of plasma triglycerides by the mammary gland is similar to that for adipose tissue and dependent on prior hydrolysis through the action of lipoprotein lipase. Evidence in support is the release of lipoprotein lipase (Barry *et al.*, 1963) and fatty acids (Annison, Linzell, Fazakerly and Nichols, 1967) into the venous blood, and the distinctive increase in lipoprotein lipase activity of mammary tissue coincident with lactation (Robinson, 1963). Full confirmation has been provided by electron microscopic and histochemical studies (Schoefl and French, 1968). Lipoprotein lipase activity is confined to the capillaries and hydrolysis occurs in chylomicra that are attached to the endothelial surface of the capillaries. The endothelial cells engulf the large fat particles by the formation of vesicles. The evidence for non-ruminants is that there is an initial hydrolysis at the luminal surface specifically of the acyl ester bond at position *sn*-1, and a further partial hydrolysis of the diglyceride to monoglyceride. The mixture of monoglyceride and diglyceride is transported in microvesicles across the endothelial cell, and continuing hydrolysis of diglyceride results in a release of monoglycerides and fatty acids into the subendothelial space, where there is partial hydrolysis of the monoglycerides. The fatty acids, monoglycerides and part of the glycerol are transported into the secretory cell and used in milk fat synthesis. A more extensive luminal hydrolysis may occur in ruminants as in the lactating goat there is only a small incorporation of 2-monoglycerides into milk triglycerides.

THE ROLE OF SUBSTRATE SUPPLY IN THE REGULATION OF MILK SECRETION

The rate of milk secretion by an animal is determined by a number of factors. These include the total weight of mammary tissue, the number of secretory cells in that tissue and the synthetic activity of the secretory cells. At a cellular level the maximum rates of reaction are determined by the amounts and activities of the enzymes present but under physiological conditions the rates are usually regulated by the concentrations of substrates, products and sometimes cofactors. Biological syntheses are accomplished through a sequence of reactions but often the substrates of the intermediate enzymes are removed as rapidly as they are formed and the rate of the whole sequence depends on the concentrations of the initial substrates, the cofactors for the initial step and the final product. As products of milk synthesis are removed continuously from the sites of synthesis under normal milking or sucking conditions, the concentrations of materials used as milk precursors or sources of cofactors within the intracellular fluid of the secretory cell could be major factors regulating milk synthesis, through a direct mass-action effect or possibly through an induction of enzyme activity. The concentrations of metabolites within the secretory cell will be dependent on the concentrations of precursors in arterial blood, but the relationship will be modified by blood flow through the gland and by the permeability of the capillary wall and other membranes that separate the arterial blood from the intracellular fluid of the secretory cell.

To add further complexity, the weight of mammary tissue, its content of secretory cells, the amount and activity of enzymes in those cells, the arterial concentration of substrates and the efficiency of extraction of substrates by the gland may all potentially alter in response to a change in endocrine status induced by a change of dietary substrate (nutrient) supply, and the time-course of the effects may be much longer than those due to the direct effect of an increase in substrate supply to the gland.

Without exception in the experimental studies that have been undertaken so far, detailed information on the amount of active secretory tissue, on blood flow and on endocrine status was not available, and the interpretation of results must be largely in terms of the superficial relationship between arterial concentration of substrate and the daily rate of synthesis and secretion of milk and its constituents. Furthermore, milk secretion has been characterized usually only in gross terms, of the yields of water, fat, lactose and protein, and of the individual fatty acids of the milk fat.

Lactose synthesis and secretion, and milk volume

Unequivocal evidence for the importance of glucose for lactose synthesis and milk secretion was provided by the experiments of Hardwick, Linzell and Price (1961). Using isolated goat's udders perfused with a simplified medium adequate in energy, amino acids and minerals, they examined the influence on milk secretion of the withdrawal from the perfusate of glucose and acetate separately. The withdrawal of glucose produced an abrupt inhibition of both lactose and milk secretion whereas the withdrawal of acetate produced a more progressive reduction in the synthesis and secretion of all milk constituents and especially fat (see below). The depression of milk secretion on the withdrawal of glucose appeared to be due to the dependence of water secretion on the synthesis and secretion of lactose. On the re-introduction of glucose into the perfusate the first milk removed from the udder was rich in protein and fat, suggesting that synthesis of those constituents had continued until their accumulation in the small amounts of milk within the alveoli inhibited their further synthesis.

Studies *in vivo* with cows and goats in which plasma glucose concentration was depressed by intravenous infusion of insulin (for references, see Rook and Hopwood, 1970), or intraruminal infusion of butyric acid (Storry and Rook, 1962), have shown little effect on lactose secretion or milk volume of variations in plasma glucose concentration within the normal range of 0.4 to 0.8 g/l, but an approximately linear relationship within the range of 0.1 to 0.3 g/l (Fig. 8.12). In insulin-treated goats, in fasted goats, in normally fed goats with a low plasma glucose concentration, intravenous infusion

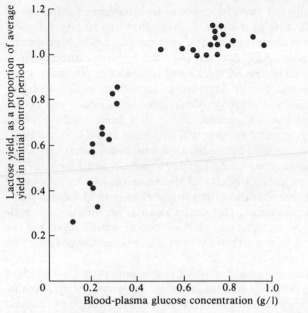

Fig. 8.12. The relationship between lactose yield and blood plasma glucose concentration in goats in which plasma glucose concentration was modified by intravenous infusion of insulin. (From Rook and Hopwood, 1970.)

of glucose increased milk and lactose secretion, an effect obtained within 1 h. When the infusion was made into the artery of one gland autotransplanted to the neck, that gland responded before the control gland *in situ*, indicating a direct effect on mammary tissue (Linzell, 1967b).

The above observations are consistent with a direct precursor (glucose) concentration to product (lactose) yield relationship but other results have indicated that under certain conditions blood flow through the udder may also limit glucose uptake. Stress, and in some animals a reduction in plasma glucose concentration induced by insulin administration, may cause sympathetic activity which depresses blood flow through vasoconstriction (Linzell, 1967b).

Some of the results of Linzell (1967b) suggested that milk and lactose secretion may be affected also by variation in plasma glucose concentration within the normal physiological range of values, but the experimental techniques that he adopted included short-interval milking with the aid of oxytocin and that technique has since been found to increase the rate of secretion in otherwise untreated goats (Linzell and Peaker, 1971). In experiments lasting several days, Fisher and Elliot (1966) obtained increases in the rate of secretion of lactose and milk in normally-fed cows in response to intravenous infusions of glucose (0.75 kg/day) or propionate (0.56 kg/day, an unphysiological treatment), but there are several other experiments in which propionic acid (in amounts up to 1.5 kg/day) has been infused intraruminally into fed cows over periods of several weeks and increases in plasma glucose concentration observed but no increase in lactose or milk yield (see Rook, Balch and Johnson, 1965). Moreover, with goats and cows, intra-abomasal infusions of glucose have also been without effect (Clark, Spires, Derrig and Bennink, 1977; Farhan and Thomas, 1977) and, although responses have been obtained with cows given very large intra-abomasal infusions, up to 2.8 kg/day (Frobish and Davis, 1977), these may be due to indirect effects of the infusion (see the abomasal infusion of protein, below) rather than to the change in glucose supply. The indications are, therefore, that under normal physiological conditions glucose supply and plasma glucose concentration may not be important regulators of the rate of synthesis and secretion of lactose or of milk volume.

Intraruminal infusions of acetic acid (in amounts up to 2.0 kg/day) over several weeks in cows in mid-lactation have consistently maintained the yield of milk and of milk lactose, fat and protein or reduced their rates of lactational decline, in association with a distinct increase in the plasma concentration of acetate (see Rook *et al.*, 1965). The responses are progressive, however, and develop over a period of 10 days or more. Intravascular infusions of acetate have no effect on milk secretion in lactating goats fasted for 24 h (Linzell, 1967b) but succinate infused intravenously into the cow (Rook, Storry and Wheelock, 1965) or goat (Rook and Hopwood, 1970) causes a rapid fall in milk secretion, with little alteration of composition, and a possible interpretation of this effect is that oxidation of acetate is inhibited.

The experimental evidence does not support a direct relationship between plasma acetate concentration and the rate of milk secretion; such a relationship is in fact unlikely as acetate concentration may vary 10-fold in the cow during a feeding cycle whereas, under normal husbandry conditions, the rate of milk secretion is remarkably constant. The probability is that the responses of the gland to acetate supply are modulated by hormonal factors or are dependent on a hormonal control of secretion unrelated to the direct supply of acetate to the gland. The mechanism may in some way be related to the rôle of acetate in ATP production as, in contrast to the effects of variations in glucose supply, the yields of all the main milk constituents are modified. During the physiological undernutrition of early lactation, or during fasting, the uptake of free fatty acids by the gland will provide an alternative source of C_2 units for oxidation, as may those amino acids oxidized in the gland, but in the ruminant the ability of the mammary gland to utilize glucose in this way must be restricted.

There is little information for species other than the cow and goat, but in a single study in the sow (Reynolds and Rook, 1977) insulin infused intravenously depressed plasma glucose concentration and the yields of water and lactose but had no significant effect on the yield of protein. Intravenous infusion of glucose did not alter blood plasma glucose concentration but nevertheless increased the yields of lactose, protein and water, a response which may be related to the sensitivity of sow (non-ruminant) mammary tissue to insulin. The mammary gland of the lactating rat utilizes glucose extensively as a substrate for oxidation, as does the sow; additionally, ketone bodies may also be used but there is then inhibition of glucose uptake, attributable to inhibition of glycolysis at the phosphofructokinase step by a high concentration of citrate arising from ketone body metabolism (Williamson, McKeown and Ilic, 1975). Chronic insulin administration in rats produces an increased yield of milk with lowered fat, raised lactose and unchanged protein contents (Raskin, Raskin and Baldwin, 1973).

Protein synthesis and secretion

In quantitative terms, milk protein synthesis dominates the use of amino acids in the mammary gland but the regulation of protein synthesis through amino acid supply also has significance to the milk non-protein constituents since their formation is dependent on the synthesis of enzyme proteins and, for lactose, α-lactalbumin.

The almost quantitative incorporation into milk protein in most species of certain of the amino acids (methionine, histidine, phenylalanine, tyrosine and tryptophan) taken up from the blood plasma by the mammary gland, and the high extraction rate from blood plasma of some of those acids (Table 8.1), has been taken as circumstantial evidence that the supply of one or more of the acids may be limiting for milk protein synthesis. Studies with the isolated perfused gland of the guinea-pig have shown that, when the supply and uptake of one of this group of amino acids is restricted, there is a simultaneous marked reduction in the uptake of other acids in the group, whereas that of the amino acids oxidized extensively in the gland is much less affected (Mepham *et al.*, 1979).

Linzell and Mepham (1974) studied the effects of infusion of essential amino acids for a period of approximately 2 h into the arterial supply of a single mammary gland transplanted to the neck of the goat. This technique allows the substrate concentration to be maintained at a higher level for the infused gland than for the untransplanted gland, which may be used as a control. The infusate contained all of the essential amino acids and glutamic acid and tyrosine, which also have a high extraction rate. The response in arterial concentrations of the acids was variable but in one goat there were marked elevations in the mammary arterial concentrations of most of the acids and an associated increase in arteriovenous differences, and in milk yield and protein yield of the infused gland. From a detailed consideration of their results, the authors concluded that the amino acid most probably limiting milk protein synthesis in the goat was methionine, threonine or tryptophan.

However, the first limiting amino acid in a particular circumstance will presumably depend on the composition of the amino acid supply to the gland and, in turn, that must be influenced by the composition of the amino acids absorbed from the intestine. Relative to milk protein the mixture of essential amino acids absorbed between the duodenum and ileum is often especially deficient in methionine although the proportions of all amino acids, excepting arginine, threonine and possibly isoleucine, are generally low.

In cows and goats intra-abomasal infusions of casein have increased milk protein yield partly through an effect on milk protein content and partly through an effect on milk yield itself (see Gow, Ranawana, Kellaway and McDowell, 1979). These responses were initially taken to indicate that milk protein synthesis and/or milk yield is limited by the supply of individual amino acid or acids to the mammary gland. However, in experiments with cows given intra-abomasal infusions of single amino acids or amino acid mixtures, responses in milk secretion have generally been smaller than those obtained with casein and often mainly in milk protein content rather than in milk yield. In the most extensive series of experiments so far conducted, Schwab, Satter and Clay (1976) obtained equal responses in milk protein yield to the infusion of casein or a mixture of 10 essential amino acids but no single amino acid gave a response of more than 16% of the total response observed, although 43% was obtained with a mixture of lysine and methionine, the two most limiting amino acids with the diet used. Clark (1975) suggested that the mechanism of the casein effect on milk yield and protein yield could involve a hormonal, possibly growth hormone, response to the entry of protein to the abomasum or to the absorption of a complementary mixture of amino acids from the small intestine. Initial studies indicated that blood plasma growth hormone levels in goats were indeed raised by abomasal infusions of casein but subsequent experiments have failed to confirm the result (see Gow *et al.*, 1979).

The short-term infusion of non-essential amino acids into an auto-transplanted gland in the goat (Mepham and Linzell, 1974) in some instances resulted in an increased arteriovenous difference in response to an elevated arterial concentration but there was then a depression of glucose uptake and no change in milk protein synthesis. In long-term experiments with cows receiving diets adequate in protein, where the dietary supply of essential amino acids was theoretically in excess of requirement, Halfpenny, Rook and Smith (1969) found that propionic acid infused intraruminally increased milk protein yield in association with a specific increase in the concentrations of glutamic acid and alanine in the blood. They proposed that variations in diet leading to an increased proportion of propionic acid in the rumen increased milk protein yield through effects on the supply of certain non-essential amino acids, glutamic acid in particular, which contribute to a glutamic acid 'pool' within the mammary gland. A simple precursor-product relationship, as may operate for certain of the essential amino acids, is unlikely, however, as the increase in milk protein secretion in response to propionic acid infusion or dietary change occurs slowly over a period of 10 days or so, and the effects may be indirect and possibly endocrinological in origin. Propionic acid infusion via its effects on insulin secretion should enhance the general uptake of amino acids into muscle and there would be an associated release of alanine and glutamine into the circulation (Bergman and Heitmann, 1978). Without special precautions during blood plasma analysis, glutamine is determined as glutamate, which might account for the changes in plasma amino acid composition observed by Halfpenny *et al.* (1969).

Urea diffuses freely between blood plasma and milk and the concentration of urea, and therefore of non-protein nitrogen, in milk is closely dependent on that of blood plasma.

Fat synthesis and secretion

Lipid substrates

Some of the earliest investigations of the effect of diet on milk fat secretion indicated that the composition of dietary fat influences the fatty acid composition of plasma triglycerides and thereby milk fat composition. The rôle of the composition of the fatty acids of plasma triglycerides and their concentration in the regulation of milk fat secretion has been examined more fully by studying responses to the infusion into the jugular vein of emulsified oils which are used readily for milk fat formation. Initial studies in the cow were of the effects of intravenous infusion of cottonseed oil, which is rich in linoleic acid (Tove and Mochrie, 1963; Storry and Rook, 1964). These demonstrated clearly that the concentration and fatty acid composition of plasma triglycerides are important determinants of milk fat secretion. The infusion caused a massive increase in the output in milk fat of linoleic acid, which in cows' milk is present normally only in small amounts, and there was a partial compensating reduction in the rate of secretion of other C_{18} acids and of minor components of the C_{14}, C_{15} and C_{16} fatty acid series, and a net increase in the secretion of milk triglycerides. There was little effect on the rate of secretion of palmitic acid or of the short-chain (C_4 to C_{12}) fatty acids. Corresponding results have been obtained with an infusion of soya bean oil, which is similar in composition to cottonseed oil (Storry *et al.*, 1969a), and it appears that the size and composition of the pool of preformed fatty acids used for milk fat synthesis is influenced directly by the supply of plasma triglycerides. Under the conditions used in the infusion experiments, increased incorporation of preformed fatty acids into milk fat did not depress the synthesis of fatty acids *de novo*. However, a possible inhibition of acetyl-CoA carboxylase, a rate limiting step in the *de novo* synthesis of fatty acids, by an increased mammary uptake of long-chain fatty acids has been suggested to explain the effect of dietary fat additions on milk fat secretion (Moore and Steele, 1968).

The effects of intravenous infusion of a wide range of simple and other triglycerides have now been determined in the cow (Storry *et al.*, 1969a; Storry, Tuckley and Hall, 1969b) and sow (Witter, Spincer, Rook and Towers, 1970). The infusion in the cow of tripropionin and tributyrin does not increase the secretion in milk fat of the corresponding fatty acid, but triglycerides containing fatty acids of six or more C atoms (C_6, C_8, C_9, C_{10}, C_{12}, C_{14}, $C_{18:1}$) give an increased milk output of the corresponding fatty acid, the size of the response increasing with chain length. There is also an increased secretion of fatty acids containing an odd number of C atoms up to C_{15} with infusions of tripropionin and tripelargonin, and of acids containing an even number of C atoms up to C_{16} with tricaproin and possibly also tricaprylin, suggesting chain elongation within the mammary gland; other evidence in support of chain elongation is, however, lacking. With the exception of triolein, infusion of the triglycerides appears to cause a specific reduction in the secretion of oleic acid, possibly because of inhibition of desaturase activity. Mammary desaturase activity is inhibited by normal C_{18} unsaturated fatty acids (Bickerstaffe and Annison, 1971). Triglycerides below trilaurin have a variable effect on milk fat secretion but there is a consistent increase with triglycerides containing the longer-chain fatty acids.

Fatty acids with less than 12 C atoms are normally present only in trace amounts in the plasma triglycerides, as the shorter-chain fatty acids of the diet are absorbed from the digestive tract via the portal system and oxidized extensively in the liver. With emulsions infused into the jugular vein there is a rapid metabolism of the shorter-chain fatty acids of infused triglycerides and little change in the fatty acid composition of plasma triglycerides, and this is the primary cause of the poor response in milk fat secretion; but the possibility that there is a less efficient uptake of the shorter-chain fatty acids of plasma triglycerides cannot be excluded. Infusion of cod-liver oil, which contains a high proportion of polyunsaturated C_{20} and C_{22} acids, depresses the secretion of C_{14} to C_{18}

fatty acids, but not C_4 to C_{12} and, although the polyunsaturated C_{20} and C_{22} fatty acids reach a high concentration in the plasma triglycerides, their concentrations in milk fat remain extremely low. It appears that there is an inhibition of lipoprotein lipase and a reduction in the uptake of fatty acids by the gland but, additionally, there may be a specific discrimination against the uptake of the polyunsaturated C_{20} and C_{22} fatty acids. Cyclopropene fatty acids such as sterculic acid, which are not normally present in the diet or plasma triglycerides, depress mammary uptake of fatty acids from plasma triglycerides and inhibit mammary desaturase activity (Cook, Scott, Mills, Fogerty and Johnson, 1976).

Comparable studies with the sow have suffered from the disadvantage that measurement of milk yield is difficult and imprecise, and interpretation of results has depended solely on changes in milk fat composition. Nevertheless, similar conclusions have been drawn except that, in the sow, specific depression of oleic acid content by infused triglycerides containing fatty acids of 6 to 14 C atoms, and chain elongation, have not been observed. The range of triglycerides infused has been extended to include tripalmitin and tristearin, in spite of physiological problems associated with their use, and in response to the infusion of tripalmitin there is an increase not only in palmitic acid content but also in palmitoleic acid content of milk fat: this observation is consistent with extensive desaturation in the sow mammary gland of palmitic to palmitoleic acid.

Circumstantial evidence for the rôle of natural variations in plasma triglyceride concentration in the regulation of the uptake of the component fatty acids by the mammary gland and their incorporation into milk triglycerides has been provided by many observations with cattle: from studies in which plasma triglyceride concentration and the secretion in milk fat of the longer-chain fatty acids have been increased by the inclusion in the diet of supplementary fat; by the characteristically high output of long-chain fatty acids in milk fat during early lactation when milk yield is sustained, in part, by an extensive mobilization of adipose tissue triglyceride; and by the reduced output of milk fat and its longer-chain fatty acids in association with a reduced plasma triglyceride concentration during the feeding of high-concentrate low-roughage diets, the intraruminal infusion of propionic acid, or the intravenous infusion of glucose (see Ch. 14). A close correlation between plasma triglyceride concentration and the secretion in milk fat of the longer-chain fatty acids is not always evident, however, but the explanation may be one of technique. Sampling and analysis for the determination of plasma triglyceride concentration may in many instances be too infrequent to allow an accurate assessment of the mean concentration or, in studies where only total triglyceride concentration has been measured, there may not have been a close relationship between the concentration of total triglycerides and that of the fractions of importance for milk fat synthesis. A positive curvilinear relationship between the concentration of plasma unesterified fatty acids, within the range of 38 to 47 mg/l, and the yield of total milk fatty acids has been observed but it is unlikely that this is a direct, causal relationship (Moore   et al., 1969); as indicated previously, net utilization of unesterified fatty acids is evident only at high plasma concentrations.

Non-lipid substrates

Glucose in the simple-stomached animal, and acetate and 3-hydroxybutyrate in the ruminant, are unquestionably used for synthesis *de novo* of fatty acids of milk fat but direct evidence that use is regulated by their plasma concentrations is lacking. Withdrawal of acetate from the perfusate of an isolated perfused goat's udder preferentially depresses milk fat secretion (Hardwick et al., 1961). Also, in numerous studies, the plasma concentrations of acetate and/or 3-hydroxybutyrate have been related to the rate of secretion of the short-chain fatty acids of milk fat. These studies include experiments in which secretion of the short-chain acids has been depressed by diets lacking in physical fibrousness which had depressed the milk fat content. Substantial increases in the plasma concentration of 3-hydroxybutyrate, in response to its intravenous infusion, have not, however, been associated with a consistent increase in milk fat secretion, either in normal cows or in cows in which milk fat content had been depressed by diet (Storry and Rook, 1965).
in response to its intravenous infusion, have not, however, been associated with a consistent increase in milk fat secretion, either in normal cows or in cows in which milk fat content had been depressed by diet (Storry and Rook, 1965).

Intraruminal infusion of acetic and butyric acids, or intravenous infusion of acetate into cows in which milk fat secretion has been depressed, does not give a complete recovery of the normal rate of secretion of the short-chain acids, even in circumstances where the plasma concentrations of acetate and 3-hydroxybutyrate are raised above normal; whereas, in contrast, intravenous infusion of triglyceride, or feeding protected fat (Storry, Brumby, Hall and Johnson, 1974), may do. When cows are transferred from milk fat-depressing diets to normal diets, milk fat secretion increases progressively over a period of 3 weeks but recovery of blood composition is complete in 7 to 10 days (Storry and Sutton, 1969), and the reduction in fatty acid synthesis and milk fat secretion appears to be associated with changes in the metabolism of the mammary gland that are only slowly reversible.

The time-course of possible responses to increases in the plasma concentration of precursors of milk fat is difficult to assess with certainty as there is an interval of several hours between the synthesis of triglyceride and its appearance as globular fat within the lumen of the alveolus, and the large amount of residual fat within the udder masks for some time any change in the rate of secretion or composition of the newly formed fat. Distinct responses in milk fat yield and composition have been observed within 12 h of intravenous infusion of triglyceride and 1 to 2 days of intraruminal infusion of acetic or butyric acids, or intravenous infusion of acetate. Because of technical difficulties, it is not yet known whether the variations in plasma composition throughout the interval between meals modify milk fat secretion.

COMPETITION BETWEEN MAMMARY AND OTHER TISSUES

The composition and amount of substrates that enter the peripheral circulation and become available for use by the mammary gland differ profoundly from the products of digestion absorbed from the gut. This is due in part to the extensive metabolism of some absorbed materials during transfer across the gut wall and, for those materials absorbed into the portal blood, within the liver, but there is a continuous turnover of body tissues, and, depending on endocrine balance and nutrient supply, there may be substantial net depletion or net repletion of constituents of major tissues such as adipose tissue, muscle and liver (see Ch. 3). The endocrine balance in early lactation, and in particular the increased secretion of growth hormone, favours the use of nutrients for milk secretion and a net depletion of other tissues, but with advances in lactation, especially in association with pregnancy, endocrine factors promote an increasing use of nutrients by other tissues. These endocrine effects may be modulated by diet and, although the details of the endocrine mechanisms, and of the nutritional-endocrine interactions, are as yet poorly understood, there are a few documented examples of the effect of diet on the partition of the use of nutrients in the lactating animal.

Diets containing a high proportion of starchy concentrates and a low proportion of forage, especially forage in a ground form, which favour the production of propionic acid in the rumen, depress milk fat secretion in the lactating ruminant, and a component of that depression is a reduced uptake and secretion in milk fat of the long-chain fatty acids of plasma triglycerides. McClymont and Vallance (1962) suggested that an increased supply of glucogenic material, propionic acid or glucose itself, possibly through a stimulation of insulin release, promotes lipogenesis in adipose tissue (lipogenesis in the ruminant mammary gland is insensitive to insulin) and reduces triglyceride mobilization, and therefore unesterified fatty acid release and plasma triglyceride concentration. A comprehensive study of the effects of low-roughage diets on milk fat secretion (Annison, Bickerstaffe and Linzell, 1974) has confirmed that there is a substantial increase in glucose entry rate, a reduced entry rate of plasma palmitate (a typical plasma unesterified fatty acid), a slight fall in circulating plasma triglycerides and a distinct fall in their extraction rate by the udder. High activities in adipose tissue enzymes involved in fatty acid and triglyceride synthesis, and possibly low activities in mammary tissue, have been reported for animals receiving milk fat-depressing diets (Baldwin, Lim, Cheng, Cabrera and Ronning, 1969), and Walker and Elliot (1973) have confirmed that low-roughage diets stimulate insulin secretion. Both glucose and propionic acid have been considered as agents promoting insulin release but the regulation of the hormone is poorly understood and the rôle of the glucogenic precursors is uncertain. Present evidence suggests that release of the hormone may be stimulated by neural factors, or through the activity of the gut hormones secretin and cholecystokinin-pancreozymin in particular, and may only in part be related to the supply of glucogenic and other substrates. Infusions of propionic acid into the rumen have consistently depressed milk fat secretion (see Rook *et al.*, 1965) but much smaller and variable effects have been obtained with propionic acid infused intravenously or intra-abomasally, although it should be recognized that both are unphysiological treatments (Fisher and Elliot, 1966; Frobish and Davis, 1977). Likewise, results with glucose infusions are not without contradictions; intravenous administration has reduced fat secretion (Fisher and Elliot, 1966) as have intra-abomasal infusions at moderate levels (see Ranawana and Kellaway, 1977), but in cows given infusions containing up to 2.8 kg glucose per day, a level providing a duodenal entry of glucose above that which could be achieved by normal dietary means, Frobish and Davis (1977) observed only a small depression in milk fat yield. Alternative mechanisms to explain the effects of low-roughage diets on milk fat synthesis and energy partition have also been considered. Recently, it has been proposed that milk fat synthesis may be inhibited by an accumulation of methylmalonate which could arise from an increased ruminal production of propionic acid coupled with a decreased production of vitamin B_{12} but evidence in support of the idea is contradictory (see Elliot, Barton and Williams, 1979). Annison (1973) has also discussed the possibility that the high level of *trans* fatty acids present within the plasma triglycerides in animals given low-roughage diets may inhibit fatty acid uptake by the mammary gland.

In addition to the effect on milk fat secretion, in the early part of lactation diets which favour a high ruminal production of propionic acid can restrict milk yield; at that stage of lactation the release of unesterified fatty acids from the adipose tissue may be important in maintaining the energy supply to the mammary gland. Diets deficient in protein also depress milk yield and at fixed levels of energy intake there is presumably redirection of energy substrates towards adipose tissue synthesis. In early lactation this effect may once again restrict the release of unesterified fatty acids so that the direct effects of dietary protein deficiency on milk secretion are reinforced by the lack of energy supply (see Ørskov, Grubb and Kay, 1977).

References

Abraham, S. and Chaikoff, I. L., 1959. Glycolytic pathways and lipogenesis in mammary glands of lactating and non-lactating normal rats, *J. biol. Chem.* **234**: 2246–53.

Annison, E. F., 1973. Studies on the low milk fat syndrome in the cow induced by low roughage diets. In *Production Disease in Farm Animals* (ed. J. M. Payne, K. G. Hibbit and B. F. Sansom), pp. 115–21. Baillière Tindall, London.

Annison, E. F., Bickerstaffe, R. and Linzell, J. L., 1974. Glucose and fatty acid metabolism in cows producing milk of low fat content, *J. agric. Sci., Camb.* **82**: 87–95.

Annison, E. F., Linzell, J. L., Fazakerly, S. and Nichols, B. W., 1967. The oxidation and utilization of palmitate, stearate, oleate and acetate by the mammary gland of the fed goat in relation to their overall metabolism, and the role of plasma phospholipid and neutral lipids in milk fat synthesis, *Biochem. J.* **102**: 637–47.

Annison, E. F., Linzell, J. L. and West, C. E., 1968. Mammary and whole animal metabolism of glucose and fatty acids in fasting lactating goats, *J. Physiol., Lond.* **197**: 445–59.

Baldwin, R. L., Lim, H. J., Cheng, W., Cabrera, R. and Ronning, R. 1969. Enzyme and metabolite levels in mammary and abdominal adipose tissue of lactating dairy cows, *J. Dairy Sci.* **52**: 183–87.

Barry, J. M., 1961. Protein metabolism. In *Milk: the Mammary Gland and its Secretion* (ed. S. K. Kon and A. T. Cowie), Vol. 1, pp. 389–419. Academic Press, New York.

Barry, J. M., 1964. A quantitative balance between substrates and metabolic products of the mammary gland, *Biol. Rev.* **39**: 194–213.

Barry, J. M., Bartley, W., Linzell, J. L. and Robinson, D. S., 1963. The uptake from the blood of triglyceride fatty acids of chylomicra and low-density lipoproteins by the mammary gland of the goat, *Biochem. J.* **89**: 6–11.

Baumrucker, C. R., 1979. γ-Glutamyl transpeptidase of bovine milk membranes: distribution and characterisation, *J. Dairy Sci.* **62**: 253–8.

Bergman, E. N. and Heitmann, R. N., 1978. Metabolism of amino acids by the gut, liver, kidneys and peripheral tissues, *Fedn Proc. Fedn Am. Socs exp. Biol.* **37**: 1228–32.

Bickerstaffe, R., 1971. Uptake and metabolism of fat in the lactating mammary gland. In *Lactation* (ed. I. R. Falconer), pp. 317–32. Butterworth, London.

Bickerstaffe, R. and Annison, E. F., 1971. Triglyceride synthesis in goat and sow mammary tissue, *Int. J. Biochem.* **2**: 153–62.

Bickerstaffe, R., Annison, E. F. and Linzell, J. L., 1974. The metabolism of glucose, acetate, lipids and amino acids in lactating dairy cows, *J. agric. Sci., Camb.* **82**: 71–85.

Bines, J. A. and Brown, R. E., 1968. Incorporation of carbon from acetate and butyrate into milk components, *J. Dairy Sci.* **51**: 698–705.

Bines, J. A. and Hart, I. C., 1978. Hormonal regulation of the partition of energy between milk and body tissue in adult cattle, *Proc. Nutr. Soc.* **37**: 281–7.

Buchnea, D., 1978. Stereospecific synthesis of enantiomeric acylglycerols. In *Handbook of Lipid Research*, Vol. 1 (ed. A. Kuksis), pp. 223–87. Plenum Press, New York.

Clark, J. H., 1975. Lactational responses to postruminal administration of proteins and amino acids, *J. Dairy Sci.* **58**: 1178–97.

Clark, J. H., Spires, H. R. and Davis, C. L., 1978. Uptake and metabolism of nitrogenous components by the lactating mammary gland, *Fedn Proc. Fedn Am. Socs exp. Biol.* **37**: 1233–8.

Clark, J. H., Spires, H. R., Derrig, R. G. and Bennink, M. R., 1977. Milk production, nitrogen utilization and glucose synthesis in lactating cows infused postruminally with sodium caseinate and glucose, *J. Nutr.* **107**: 631–44.

Cook, L. J., Scott, T. W., Mills, S. C., Fogerty, A. C. and Johnson, A. R., 1976. Effects of protected cyclopropene fatty acids on the composition of ruminant milk fat, *Lipids* **11**: 705–11.

Dils, R. R., 1980. Biochemical and hormonal control of milk fat synthesis, *Rep. Hannah Res. Inst., 1979*, pp. 55–62

Elliot, J. M., Barton, E. P. and Williams, J. A., 1979. Milk fat as related to vitamin B_{12} status, *J. Dairy Sci.* **62**: 642–5.

Farhan, S. M. A. and Thomas, P. C., 1977. The effect of intra-abomasal infusions of glucose or casein on milk secretion in Saanen goats receiving a low-protein diet, *Proc. Nutr. Soc.* **36**: 57A(Abstr.).

Fisher, L. J. and Elliot, J. M., 1966. Effect of intravenous infusion of propionate or glucose on bovine milk composition, *J. Dairy Sci.* **49**: 826–9.

Frobish, R. A. and Davis, C. L., 1977. Effects of abomasal infusions of glucose and propionate on milk yield and composition, *J. Dairy Sci.* **60**: 204–9.

Garton, G A., 1976. The occurrence and origin of branched-chain fatty acids in bacterial, avian and mammalian lipids, *Rep. Rowett Res. Inst., 1975*, **31**: 124–35.

Glascock, R. F., Welch, V. A., Bishop. C., Davies, T., Wright, E. W. and Noble, R. C., 1966. An investigation of serum lipoproteins and their contribution to milk fat in the dairy cow, *Biochem. J.* **98**: 149–56.

Gow, Christine B., Ranawana, S. S. E., Kellaway, R. C. and McDowell, G. H., 1979. Responses to post-ruminal infusions of casein and arginine, and to dietary protein supplements in lactating goats, *Br. J.*

Nutr. **41**: 371–82.

Halfpenny, A. F., Rook, J. A. F. and Smith, G. H., 1969. Variations with energy nutrition in the concentrations of amino acids of the blood plasma in the dairy cow, *Br. J. Nutr.* **23**: 547–57.

Hardwick, D. C., Linzell, J. L. and Price, S. M., 1961. The effect of glucose and acetate on milk secretion by the perfused goat udder, *Biochem. J.* **80**: 37–45.

Hartmann, P. E., 1966. The uptake of L-lactate and D-glucose by the mammary gland of the cow, *Aust. J. biol Sci.* **19**: 495–7.

Hartmann, P. E. and Lascelles, A. K., 1964. The uptake of plasma lipid and some non-lipid constituents by the mammary gland of the cow, *Aust. J. biol. Sci.* **17**: 935–44.

Jenness, R., 1974. The composition of milk. In *Lactation,* Vol. III (ed. B. L. Larson, and V. R. Smith), pp. 3–107. Academic Press, New York.

Kronfeld, D. S., 1965. Plasma non-esterified fatty acid concentrations in the dairy cow: responses to nutritional and hormonal stimuli, and significance in ketosis, *Vet. Rec.* **77**: 30–5.

Kronfeld, D. S., Raggi, F. and Ramberg, C. F., 1968. Mammary blood flow and ketone body metabolism in normal fasted and ketotic cows, *Am. J. Physiol.* **215**: 218–27.

Larson, B. L., 1965. Biosynthesis of the milk proteins, *J. Dairy Sci.* **48**: 133–9.

Larson, B. L., 1979. Biosynthesis and secretion of milk proteins: a review, *J. Dairy Res.* **46**: 161–74.

Linzell, J. L., 1963. Some effects of denervating and transplanting mammary glands, *Q.Jl exp. Physiol.* **45**: 34–60.

Linzell, J. L., 1966. Measurement of venous flow by continuous thermodilution and its application to measurement of mammary blood flow in the goat, *Circulation Res.* **18**: 745–54.

Linzell, J. L., 1967a. The effect of very frequent milking and of oxytocin on the yield and composition of milk in fed and fasted goats, *J. Physiol., Lond.* **190**: 333–46.

Linzell, J. L., 1967b. The effect of infusions of glucose, acetate and amino acids on hourly milk yield in fed, fasted and insulin treated goats, *J. Physiol., Lond.* **190**: 347–57.

Linzell, J. L., 1974. Mammary blood flow and substrate uptake. In *Lactation,* Vol. 1 (ed. B. L. Larson and V. R. Smith), pp. 143–225. Academic Press, New York.

Linzell, J. L., Annison, E. F., Bickerstaffe, R. and Jeffcott, L. B., 1972. Mammary and whole-body metabolism of glucose, acetate and palmitate in the lactating horse, *Proc. Nutr. Soc.* **31**: 72–3A (Abstr.).

Linzell, J. L. and Mepham, T. B., 1974. Effects of intramammary arterial infusion of essential amino acids in the lactating goat, *J. Dairy Res.* **41**: 101–9.

Linzell, J. L., Mepham, T. B., Annison, E. F. and West, C. E., 1969. Mammary metabolism in lactating sows: arteriovenous differences of milk precursors and the mammary metabolism of [^{14}C] glucose and [^{14}C] acetate, *Br. J. Nutr.* **23**: 319–33.

Linzell, J. L. and Peaker, M., 1971. The effects of oxytocin and milk removal on milk secretion in the goat, *J. Physiol., Lond.* **216**: 717–34.

McClymont, G. L. and Vallance, S., 1962. Depression of blood glycerides and milk-fat synthesis by glucose infusion, *Proc. Nutr. Soc.* **21**: xli–ii(Abstr.).

McLean, P., 1964. Interrelationships of carbohydrate and fat metabolism in the involuting mammary gland, *Biochem. J.* **90**: 271–8.

Mepham, T. B., 1977. Synthesis and secretion of milk proteins. In *Comparative Aspects of Lactation* (ed. M. Peaker), pp. 57–75. Academic Press, London.

Mepham, T.B., 1979. Nitrogen metabolism in the mammary gland. In *Protein Metabolism in the Ruminant* (ed. P. J. Buttery), pp. 4.1–5.1. Agricultural Research Council, London.

Mepham, T. B. and Linzell, J. L., 1966. A quantitative assessment of the contribution of individual amino acids to the synthesis of milk proteins by the goat, *Biochem. J.* **101**: 76–83.

Mepham, T. B. and Linzell, J. L., 1974. Effects of intramammary arterial infusion of non-essential amino acids and glucose in the lactating goat, *J. Dairy Res.* **41**: 111–21.

Mepham, T. B., Peters, R. A. and Alexandrov, S., 1979. Effects of restriction of amino acid supply to the isolated perfused guinea-pig mammary gland, *J. Dairy Res.* **46**: 69–73

Mepham, T. B., Peters, A. R. and Davis, S. R., 1976. Uptake and metabolism of tryptophan by the isolated perfused guinea-pig mammary gland, *Biochem. J.* **158**: 659–62.

Moore, J. H. and Christie, W. W., 1979. Lipid metabolism in the mammary gland of ruminant animals, *Prog. Lipid Res.* **17**: 347–95.

Moore, J. H. and Steele, W., 1968. Dietary fat and milk fat secretion in the cow, *Proc. Nutr. Soc.* **27**: 66–70.

Moore, J. H., Steele, W. and Noble, R. C., 1969. The relationship between the dietary fatty acids, plasma lipid composition and milk fat secretion in the cow, *J. Dairy Res.* **36**: 383–92.

Ørskov, E. F., Grubb, D. A. and Kay, R. N. B., 1977. Effect of postruminal glucose or protein supplementation on milk yield and composition in Friesian cows in early lactation and negative energy balance, *Br. J. Nutr.* **38**: 397–405.

Palmquist, D. L., Davis, C. L., Brown, R. E. and Sachan, D. S., 1969. Availability and metabolism of various substrates in ruminants. V. Entry rate into the body and incorporation into milk fat of D(−) β-hydroxybutyrate, *J. Dairy Sci.* **52**: 633–8.

Patton, S. and Jensen, R. G., 1975. Lipid metabolism and membrane functions of the mammary gland. In *Progress in the Chemistry of Fats and Other Lipids* (ed. R. T. Holman), Vol. 14, pp. 163–279. Pergamon Press, Oxford.

Peaker, M., 1977. The aqueous phase of milk: ion and water transport. In *Comparative Aspects of Lactation* (ed. M. Peaker), pp. 113–34. Academic Press, London.

Ranawana, S. S. E. and Kellaway, R. C., 1977. Responses to postruminal infusions of glucose and casein in lactating goats, *Br. J. Nutr.* **37**: 395–402.

Raskin, R. L., Raskin, M. and Baldwin, R. L., 1973. Effects of chronic insulin and cortisol administration on lactational performance and mammary metabolism in rats, *J. Dairy Sci.* **56**: 1033–41.

Reynolds, L. and Rook, J. A. F. 1977. Intravenous infusion of glucose and insulin in relation to milk secretion in the sow, *Br. J. Nutr.* **37**: 45–53.

Robinson, D. S., 1963. Changes in the lipolytic activity of the guinea-pig mammary gland at parturition, *J. Lipid Res.* **4**: 21–3.

Rook, J. A. F., Balch, C. C. and Johnson, V. W., 1965. Further observations on the effects of intraruminal infusions of volatile fatty acids and of lactic acid on the yield and composition of the milk of the cow, *Br. J. Nutr.* **19**: 93–9.

Rook, J. A. F. and Hopwood, J. B., 1970. The effects of intravenous infusion of insulin and of sodium succinate on milk secretion in the goat, *J. Dairy Res.* **37**: 193–8.

Rook, J. A. F., Storry, J. E. and Wheelock, J. V., 1965. Plasma glucose and acetate and milk secretion in the ruminant, *J. Dairy Sci.* **48**: 745–7.

Schoefl, G. I. and French, J. E., 1968. Vascular permeability to particulate fat: morphological observations on vessels of lactating mammary gland and lung, *Proc. R. Soc. Ser. B.* **169**: 153–65.

Schwab, C. G., Satter, L. D. and Clay, A. B., 1976. Responses of lactating dairy cows to abomasal infusions of amino acids, *J. Dairy Sci.* **59**: 1254–70.

Smith, G. H. S. and Taylor, D. J., 1977. Mammary energy metabolism. In *Comparative Aspects of Lactation* (ed. M. Peaker), pp. 95–109. Academic Press, London.

Spincer, J. and Rook, J. A. F., 1971. The metabolism of [U-^{14}C] glucose, [1-^{14}C] palmitic acid and [1-^{14}C] stearic acid by the lactating mammary gland of the sow, *J. Dairy Res.* **38**: 315–22.

Spincer, J., Rook, J. A. F. and Towers, K. G., 1969. The uptake of plasma constituents by the mammary gland of the sow, *Biochem. J.* **111**: 727–32.

Stead, D. and Welch, V. A., 1975. Lipid composition of bovine serum lipoproteins, *J. Dairy Sci.* **58**: 123–7.

Storry, J. E., Brumby, P. E., Hall, A. J. and Johnson, V. W., 1974. Responses in rumen fermentation and milk-fat secretion in cows receiving low-roughage diets supplemented with protected tallow, *J. Dairy Res.* **41**: 165–73.

Storry, J. E., Hall, A. J., Tuckley, N. and Millard, D., 1969a. The effects of intravenous infusions of cod-liver and soya-bean oils on the secretion of milk fat in the cow, *Br. J. Nutr.* **23**: 173–80.

Storry, J. E. and Rook, J. A. F., 1962. Effects of large intraruminal additions of volatile fatty acids on the secretion of milk constituents, *16th int. Dairy Congr., Copenh.*, Vol. A, pp. 64–70.

Storry, J. E. and Rook, J. A. F., 1964. Plasma triglycerides and milk-fat synthesis, *Biochem. J.* **91**: 27–9C.

Storry, J. E. and Rook, J. A. F., 1965. Effect in the cow of intravenous infusions of volatile fatty acids and of lactic acid on the secretion of the component fatty acids of the milk fat and on the composition of the blood, *Biochem. J.* **96**: 210–7.

Storry, J. E. and Sutton, J. D., 1969. The effect of change from low-roughage to high-roughage diets on rumen fermentation, blood composition and milk-fat secretion in the cow, *Br. J. Nutr.* **23**: 511–21.

Storry, J. E., Tuckley, B. and Hall, A. J., 1969b. The effect of intravenous infusions of triglycerides on the secretion of milk fat in the cow, *Br. J. Nutr.* **24**: 269–78.

Tove, S. B. and Mochrie, R. D., 1963. Effect of dietary and injected fat on the fatty acid composition of bovine depot fat and milk fat, *J. Dairy Sci.* **46**: 686–9.

Trenkle, A., 1978. Relation of hormonal variations to nutritional studies and metabolism of ruminants, *J. Dairy Sci.* **61**: 281–93.

Verbeke, R. and Peters, G., 1964. Uptake of free plasma amino acids by the lactating cow's udder and amino acid composition of udder lymph, *Biochem. J.* **94**: 183–9.

Walker, C. K. and Elliot, J. M., 1973. Effect of roughage restriction on serum insulin in the dairy cow, *J. Dairy Sci.* **56**: 375–7.

West, C. E., Bickerstaffe, R., Annison, E. F. and Linzell, J. L., 1972. Studies on the mode of uptake of blood triglycerides by the mammary gland of the lactating goat. The uptake and incorporation into milk fat and mammary lymph of labelled glycerol, fatty acids and triglycerides, *Biochem. J.* **126**: 477–90.

Williamson, D. H., McKeown, S. R. and Ilic, Vera, 1975. Metabolic interactions of glucose, acetoacetate and insulin in mammary gland slices of lactating rats, *Biochem. J.* **150**: 145–52.

Witter, R. C., Spincer, J., Rook, J. A. F. and Towers, K. G., 1970. The effects of intravenous infusions of triglycerides on the composition of milk fat in the sow, *Br. J. Nutr.* **24**: 269–78.

Wood, H. G., Peeters, G. J., Verbeke, R., Lauryssens, H. and Jacobson, B., 1965. Estimation of the pentose cycle in the perfused cow's udder, *Biochem. J.* **96**: 607–15.

Wooding, F. B. P., 1977. Comparative mammary fine structure. In *Comparative Aspects of Lactation* (ed. M. Peaker), pp. 1–14. Academic Press, London.

Yousef, I. M. K. and Ashton, W. M., 1967. A study of the composition of Clun Forest ewe's milk. III. Ewe's milk fat: a preliminary study, *J. agric. Sci., Camb.* **68**: 103–7.

9   NUTRITIONAL IMBALANCES

J. A. F. Rook

Numerous disorders endemic to man and his domestic animals have been shown to be nutritional in origin. A simple dietary deficiency of an essential nutrient is comparatively rare under natural circumstances and most commonly a 'deficiency state' is accentuated or 'conditioned' by the dietary supply of some other nutrient or nutrients. The aetiology of several disorders of cattle and sheep, historically termed metabolic disorders, for a long time remained obscure. Initially, they were attributed to hormonal or neural responses to abnormal intakes of dietary constituents or to environmental stress, or else to specific defects of metabolism in affected animals. Individual differences in susceptibility to the diseases are common but no evidence has been adduced for any primary defect of metabolism. Present indications are that the disorders are associated with an imbalance in the dietary supply of major nutrients, usually exacerbated by a high demand for specific nutrients for productive purposes, and they are now sometimes referred to as 'production diseases' (Payne, 1977).

Partition of nutrients

Within the body there is competition between the tissues for the various nutrients. In terms of priority of demand, three broad categories may be identified that are most readily applicable to the use of energy-producing materials but with suitable qualifications may be applied also to other nutrients. First, there is a utilization of nutrients in the maintenance of the structural and functional integrity of the organism (there is a constant turnover of most tissue components), in processes essential to life (including heat production) and in productive work. Secondly, there is synthesis of materials associated with growth, foetal development and lactation. Thirdly, there is storage of nutrients absorbed in excess of requirement as, for example, the storage of surplus energy in the form of adipose tissue.

The requirements for processes within the first category *must* be met, either from dietary sources or through mobilization of body stores. The rates of accretion of materials in the second category are sensitive to nutrient supply but there is a physiological upper limit determined by genetic characteristics. In animals that are underfed, body stores of nutrients may be catabolized and used for accretion of the materials but provision of additional food leads to a reduced catabolism and ultimately to a storage of nutrients. For each successive increment of additional food, there is a progressively smaller increment in the rates of accretion of body materials (the Law of Diminishing Returns).

Among the various synthetic processes within the second category, there is a partition of nutrients approximately in proportion to the metabolic rates of the tissues (Child, 1920). The competition in the growing pregnant animal has been represented schematically by Hammond (1944) (Fig. 9.1). Synthesis of certain tissues and fluids, nervous

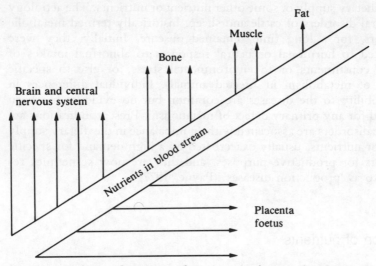

Fig. 9.1. Priority of partition of nutrients in the growing, pregnant animal. (After Hammond, 1944.)

and associated tissues, foetal tissues and milk, for example, may be maintained not only through mobilization of nutrient stores but at the expense of growth of other tissues or as a consequence of their catabolism. For some nutrients, the major minerals for example, accretion in foetal tissues and secretion in milk may be governed largely by the rates of synthesis of other materials and continue in spite of a deficient supply.

A short-term, cyclical pattern of net depletion and net repletion of body stores is thus characteristic for animals subjected to intermittent feeding. For some nutrients a similar, but much longer-term pattern is apparent throughout a reproductive cycle, whereby nutrient stores may be mobilized during late pregnancy or during early lactation when milk secretion is at a peak, and replenished when secretion has declined or during the interval between lactations. Many metabolic disorders appear to arise through a failure of these homeostatic mechanisms to accommodate a high production requirement, or to adapt quickly enough to a rapid *change* of requirement, at a time when the uptake of a nutrient from the diet may be restricted.

In this chapter, the aetiology of the classical metabolic disorders, ketosis, parturient paresis and hypomagnesaemic tetany, and other disorders that have been described more recently, acidosis, ammonia toxicity and amino acid imbalance, are considered within the conceptual framework of nutritional imbalance. An imbalance in diet composition or amount also contributes to many other disorders, as diverse as the 'fat-cow syndrome' (Morrow, 1976), abomasal displacement (Whitlock, 1973), the 'low milk-fat syndrome' (p. 579), and hypoglycaemia in the piglet: a general account of metabolic diseases in farm animals has been published (Payne, 1977). Bloat was originally classed as a metabolic disorder but its aetiology is distinctly different from that of the other disorders.

KETOSIS

Both the cow and the sheep are subject to ketosis. The clinical condition occurs most commonly in high-yielding cows in the 3rd to the 6th week of lactation when yield is at a peak ('bovine ketosis') and in ewes in late pregnancy carrying two or more lambs ('pregnancy toxaemia', 'twin lamb disease'). The clinical signs are dullness or nervousness (more common in pregnancy toxaemia) and, in the cow, loss of appetite and body condition, and a sudden fall in milk yield. Spontaneous recovery is usual in the cow as the fall in milk yield reduces nutrient demand, but in the sheep pregnancy toxaemia may be fatal unless the foetus is aborted, as the viable foetus maintains its requirements for nutrients. In bovine ketosis there is uncertainty as to whether inappetence immediately precedes or follows the onset of the disorder, whereas pregnancy toxaemia is normally precipitated by a sudden fall in food intake caused either by a lack of food or by stress interfering with normal feeding behaviour. Cows that become over-fat during pregnancy, the 'fat-cow syndrome', are more likely to develop ketosis (Morrow, 1976).

Cows in early lactation and multi-foetate ewes when deprived of food show biochemical characteristics in many respects similar to but not identical with those of the spontaneous disorders.

Biochemical characteristics

The concentrations in whole blood of glucose and citrate are decreased, and of 3-hydroxybutyrate, acetoacetate, acetone and free fatty acids increased, and the changes are usually more pronounced in pregnancy toxaemia than in bovine ketosis (Table 9.1). The ratio of 3-hydroxybutyrate to acetoacetate is also decreased in contrast to the increase observed during ketosis in non-herbivorous animals. Liver stores are depleted of glycogen and there is deposition of fat.

Table 9.1 The concentrations (mmol/l) of constituents of the whole blood of normal and ketotic lactating dairy cows (Baird, 1977)

	Normal	Ketotic
Glucose	2.72	2.00
3-hydroxybutyrate	0.42	3.98
Acetoacetate	0.04	0.92
Citrate	0.14	0.05
Free fatty acids[†]	0.17	1.02

[†] mmol/l blood plasma.

The cause of the characteristic clinical signs is uncertain. There may be a combination of effects due to acidosis (3-hydroxybutyric acid and acetoacetic acid are comparatively strong acids), *very* high concentrations of acetone which depress central nervous activity, hypoglycaemia (glucose is essential for the metabolism of nervous tissues such as brain), or possibly anhydraemia. Ketotic animals lose water which may account for the rapid loss of body condition.

The demand for glucose

The biochemical changes are consistent with a lack of glucose and its precursors. There are obligatory demands for glucose in pregnancy for the metabolism of the foetus and associated tissues, and in lactation for milk lactose synthesis (each litre of milk contains the equivalent of approximately 50 g of glucose), which increase substantially the overall glucose demand. Multiple births are much more common in the ewe than in the cow and, in lactation in the ewe, the limitation on milk removal imposed by the sucking of the lamb restricts the development of milk yield and gives a flatter lactation curve than for the cow; as between species, the demand for glucose is relatively higher for the sheep in late pregnancy and for the cow in early lactation.

The amount of glucose absorbed directly from the gut of the ruminant is low and much of the required glucose is synthesized within the liver (and kidney) from propionate, lactate, glucogenic amino acids and glycerol. Some estimates of portal and hepatic production rates for these metabolites in a lactating cow when fed or deprived of food for 48 h are given in Table 9.2. The importance of propionate for hepatic

Table 9.2   Portal and hepatic output (+) and uptake (−) (mmol per min) of key gluconeogenic and ketogenic metabolites in a lactating cow in the fed state and after deprivation of food for 48 h (Baird, 1977)

Metabolite	Fed		Deprived of food for 48 h	
	Portal	Hepatic	Portal	Hepatic
Glucose	+0.2	+5.5	−0.3	+2.9
Propionate	+6.6	−6.1	+0.3	−0.3
Lactate	+1.4	−2.4	+1.9	−2.5
Glycerol	−0.1	−0.2	−0.1	−0.5
Serine + threonine	+0.35	−0.54	−0.03	−0.31
Alanine	+0.53	−0.70	−0.08	−0.30
Glutamine	−0.61	−0.32	+0.18	−0.55
Asparagine	+0.23	−0.14	−0.04	−0.05
Aspartate	−0.06	−0.13	+0.06	−0.18
Glutamate	−0.08	+0.41	−0.10	+0.10
Acetate	+19.4	+6.1	+0.3	+0.8
3-hydroxybutyrate	+2.6	+3.3	−0.5	+5.1
Acetoacetate	+0.6	−0.9	−0.2	+1.0
Butyrate	+1.5	−1.0	0	0

gluconeogenesis is reflected in the probable presence in herbivorous livers of a specific propionyl-CoA synthetase. The net portal production of lactate may result from absorption of lactic acid from the rumen, glycolysis in the gut wall or, probably quantitatively the most important, propionate metabolism, although butyrate has been shown to inhibit partially the activation of propionate in gut tissue (Ash and Baird, 1973). Bergmann (1977) has calculated, for the fed sheep, that the maximum contributions to glucose turnover from the various substrates are > 40% for propionate, 15% for lactate, 35% for glucogenic amino acids and > 10% for glycerol. Any reduction in the supply of glucogenic materials from the gut depresses hepatic glucose production, which becomes increasingly dependent on a supply of lactic acid from anaerobic glycolysis in other tissues, glycerol from triglyceride catabolism and, more particularly, glucogenic amino acids from the breakdown of muscle protein (Ballard, Filsell and Jarrett, 1976).

Alternative energy substrates

An increase in the demand specifically for glucose, or a reduction in the supply of glucogenic materials, requires the provision of alternative substrates as an energy source. In the fed state, there is a substantial entry into portal blood of acetate, 3-hydroxybutyrate, acetoacetate and butyrate, in addition to an uptake from the gut of ketogenic amino acids and triglyceride fatty acids. There is also a continuous release of endogenous substrates and the rate of this release is dramatically increased as food intake is reduced. The primary endogenous substrates are the free fatty acids released during the catabolism of adipose tissue triglycerides but a proportion of these are partially oxidized in the liver to ketone bodies or in the liver and other tissues to acetate, and these substrates are in turn released to be utilized in other tissues.

Even in the fed animal, endogenously-produced acetate may account for 40% to 50% of the blood-acetate entry rate (Annison and Armstrong, 1970). Several tissues are a source of acetate but usually, as with the lactating mammary gland and the head, there is no net production. In the liver, however, at least in lactating ruminants, there is net production of acetate (Baird, Symonds and Ash, 1975), of the order of 0.75 mmol per min in ewes in early lactation (Costa, McIntosh and Snoswell, 1976). The acetate is probably derived from acetyl-CoA produced by oxidation of free fatty acids, and the activities in ruminant liver of acetyl-CoA hydrolase and acetylcarnitine hydrolase are consistent with the observed rates of hepatic acetate production *in vivo*.

Ketone-body production is a normal consequence of free fatty acid metabolism in the liver but in ketosis the proportion of free fatty acid uptake that is accounted for increases markedly, from less than 30 to up to 80% in the sheep (Katz and Bergman, 1969). The ketone bodies are formed via acetoacetyl-CoA, a normal intermediate in their oxidation, and from acetyl-CoA, as shown below.

All the enzymes of the pathway are found in the liver of ruminants; the presence of hydroxymethylglutaryl-CoA synthase was demonstrated by Baird, Hibbitt and Lee (1970). Acetoacetate is the parent

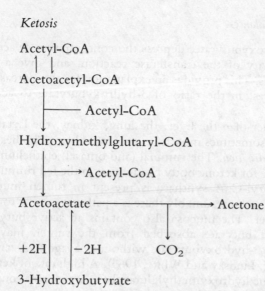

Acetyl-CoA

Acetoacetyl-CoA

——— Acetyl-CoA

Hydroxymethylglutaryl-CoA

——→ Acetyl-CoA

Acetoacetate ————————————→ Acetone

+2H   −2H CO_2

3-Hydroxybutyrate

ketone body but is reversibly reduced to 3-hydroxybutyrate under the action of 3-hydroxybutyrate dehydrogenase, which is widely distributed in body tissues. Acetoacetate is unstable and spontaneously produces acetone and carbon dioxide. The acetone is poorly utilized and is lost in urine and breath.

Acetoacetyl-CoA deacylase has also been demonstrated in ruminant liver (Baird *et al.*, 1970) and there may be a direct conversion of acetoacetyl-CoA to acetoacetate. It has been generally assumed, however, that liver cannot utilize ketone bodies due to a low activity or absence of 3-oxo-acid-CoA transferase. This enzyme has now been detected in high activity in ruminant and other mammalian livers (Zammit, 1980) and it has been proposed that the rôle of the enzyme is to produce a substrate cycle between acetoacetyl-CoA and acetoacetate, as follows (Zammit, Beis and Newsholme, 1979).

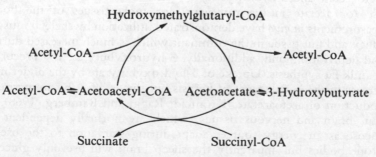

Hydroxymethylglutaryl-CoA

Acetyl-CoA   Acetyl-CoA

Acetyl-CoA ⇌ Acetoacetyl-CoA   Acetoacetate ⇌ 3-Hydroxybutyrate

Succinate   Succinyl-CoA

Although the net direction of flux would always be towards the production of acetoacetate and 3-hydroxybutyrate, the cycle could offer a mechanism for the fine regulation of ketone body production. A low NAD/NADH ratio in the mitochondria of the liver would promote the production of 3-hydroxybutyrate, depress the concentration of aceto-acetate and the activity of the transferase reaction, and give a net increase in ketogenesis. This provides an explanation for the increase in ketotic non-herbivores, in the ratio of 3-hydroxybutyrate to aceto-acetate in the blood.

Several tissues other than the liver, the lung, kidney, the lactating mammary gland and sometimes muscle, interconvert ketone bodies but there is always *net utilization*. The ruminal (and omasal) epithelium is, however, a major site for ketone body production in the fed ruminant. Hydroxymethylglutaryl-CoA synthase is present in rumen mucosa (Ash and Baird, 1973) and presumably there is a pathway similar to that described for the liver. The mucosa also contains an active butyryl-CoA synthetase and butyrate absorbed from the rumen may be converted directly to 3-hydroxybutyrate without cleavage to 2-carbon units (Annison, Leng, Lindsay and White, 1963). A high rate of ketone body formation by the hydroxymethylglutaryl-CoA pathway coupled with a direct formation of 3-hydroxybutyrate from butyrate may account for the very high ratio of 3-hydroxybutyrate to acetoacetate in the blood of the fed ruminant. Theoretically, acetate absorbed from the rumen is a source of ketone bodies but it appears not to make a quantitatively important contribution. Of the circulating 3-hydroxybutyrate, in the fed sheep 78 to 94% was produced from absorbed butyrate but, within 3 to 4 days of fasting, all the ketone bodies were produced from plasma free fatty acids (Leng and West, 1969).

Utilization of ketone bodies

Acetoacetate and 3-hydroxybutyrate are alternative substrates to glu-cose (or acetate in the ruminant) for most tissues of the body. Measurements *in vivo* have demonstrated utilization by skeletal muscle, kidney and gut tissue in the ruminant which is much increased during food deprivation, and, additionally, 3-hydroxybutyrate is a precursor for milk fat synthesis. Uptake of 3-hydroxybutyrate by the udder may increase in the initial stages of ketosis but this is offset by an increased production of acetoacetate (Kronfeld, Raggi and Ramberg, 1968). In man, brain and nervous tissues, which are normally dependent on glucose as an energy source, adapt during starvation to the use of ketone bodies but apparently the sheep brain will use only glucose, even under hypoglycaemic, hyperketonaemic conditions (Lindsay and Setchell, 1976).

Bergmann and Kon (1964) have shown that, in both normal and ketotic sheep, peripheral tissues utilize ketone bodies in direct proportion to their plasma concentration up to a value of 200 mg (expressed as acetone) per l. Above that entry rate there is little further increase in utilization but no evidence of inhibition except possibly in animals *in extremis*, and a small increase in the production of ketone bodies leads to a disproportionate increase in their blood concentration. The hyperketonaemia, therefore, appears to be a consequence of over-production of ketone bodies, not underutilization.

The aetiology of ketosis

The predisposing conditions for ketosis in the ruminant are a high requirement for glucose and therefore gluconeogenesis, and a high overall demand for energy-supplying nutrients that cannot be met fully from dietary sources. The preferential use of glucogenic materials for glucose synthesis leads to an increased oxidation of alternative sub-strates, principally acetate and 3-hydroxybutyrate of dietary origin, and free fatty acids from adipose tissue. Any reduction of food intake, a primary factor in pregnancy toxaemia but possibly a secondary factor in bovine ketosis, produces the normal physiological response of an enhanced release of free fatty acids. The fatty acids may be oxidized directly by peripheral tissues but in the liver, a major site for their utilization, there are several alternative uses: they may be partially oxidized to acetate or to ketone bodies, or incorporated into tri-glycerides. Characteristically, in ketosis the production of ketone bod-ies is increased as is deposition of triglyceride in the liver, presumably because synthesis of triglycerides exceeds the capacity for their secre-tion from the liver: in excessively fat animals massive triglyceride deposition in the liver, which restricts gluconeogenesis, results in the pathological condition known as 'fat-cow syndrome' (Reid, Roberts and Manston, 1979).

Krebs (1966) postulated that, because of the high requirement for gluconeogenesis, there would be an excessive drain on oxaloacetate and its precursors and this would limit condensation of oxaloacetate with acetyl-CoA. As a consequence, oxidation of acetyl-CoA would be limited and its use would be diverted to ketone body production. Reduced concentrations in the liver of intermediates of the tricarboxy-lic acid cycle and the glycolytic pathway that are involved in glu-coneogenesis, and a substantial fall in the liver content of glycogen, have been reported (Table 9.3).

Further evidence in support of this thesis is the therapeutic effect of the administration of glucocorticoids and glucose, both of which give increases in the hepatic concentrations of glycogen and of gluconeoge-nic intermediates of the tricarboxylic acid cycle (Baird and Heitzman,

Table 9.3   Hepatic concentrations (mmol/kg wet tissue) of
intermediates of gluconeogenesis, ketone bodies
and glycogen measured *in vivo* in normal and
ketotic lactating cows (Baird, 1977)

	Normal	Ketotic
Hydroxybutyrate + acetoacetate	0.72	3.18
Citrate	0.34	0.11
Malate	0.60	0.59
Oxaloacetate (concentration $\times 10^2$)	0.49	0.24
Phosphoenolypyruvate	0.08	0.06
Glycogen (as glucose equivalents)	143	40

1971; Treacher, Baird and Young, 1976). Glucocorticoids increase the
supply of glucogenic amino acids to the liver, and both glucocorticoids
and glucose may, at least in the cow, decrease the activity of phosphoenolpyruvate carboxykinase. That could restrict the use of carbon
skeletons for glucose synthesis, increase the utilization of acetyl–CoA
within the cycle and therefore reduce ketone body production (Heitzman, Herriman and Mallinson, 1972).

Although a lack of tricarboxylic acid intermediates may be a
contributory factor, it is unlikely that that alone is responsible for the
massive diversion of fatty acid catabolism to ketone body production,
as the capacity of the liver for the utilization of acetyl–CoA through the
tricarboxylic acid cycle under normal conditions is small in relation to
the total utilization of free fatty acids in ketosis. There is, moreover,
evidence in the rat that the partition of fatty acid use as between
oxidation and ketogenesis is under strict dietary and hormonal control,
and that the critical regulation step may be early in the oxidative
sequence, probably the acylcarnitine-transferase reaction (McGarry,
Meier and Foster, 1973). Other aspects of intermediate metabolism that
could be of importance are the rate of esterification of free fatty acid and
the redox state of subcellular compartments, which affects the equilibrium between acetoacetate and 3-hydroxybutyrate, but the importance
of these factors has not been fully investigated. There is the further
possibility that the balance between hepatic production of acetate and
ketone bodies may be affected. This balance may be regulated by the
availability of carnitine (see Baird, 1977) but there is no evidence for a
ketogenic rôle for carnitine in the ruminant (Erfle, Fisher and Sauer,
1971).

Consideration has been given to the possibility that there is a
primary hormonal cause. The hormonal status of early lactation or of
advanced pregnancy that gives milk secretion or the growth of the
foetus precedence over other metabolic demands must be seen as a
primary factor responsible for the exceptional release of free fatty acids

from adipose tissue. Secondarily, however, there may be an abnormal alteration in the hormonal regulation of the use of fatty acids in the liver which may initiate some of the above projected changes in intermediate metabolism. The hormonal changes associated with the development of pregnancy toxaemia and bovine ketosis, except for the expected reduction in insulin secretion associated with hypoglycaemia, have not been adequately described. Abnormal secretion rates of several hormones, adrenocorticotrophin (Robertson, Lennon, Bailey and Mixner, 1957), thyroxin (Kellog, Balok and Miller, 1971), insulin (Kronfeld, 1965) and glucagon (Brockman and Johnson, 1977), for example, have been suggested from time to time but the evidence remains equivocal.

PARTURIENT PARESIS

Parturient paresis ('milk fever') is primarily a disease of cattle which occurs usually immediately prior to, or within 2 to 3 days of, parturition. Similar conditions have been observed, but with lower frequency, in goats and also in sheep in late pregnancy. Clinically, there are changes in muscular tone which range from fine muscular tremors to paresis, recumbency and coma. Some cows fail to respond to treatment and exhibit a chronic condition; they remain recumbent and eventually die.

Biochemical characteristics

The most characteristic change is a fall in blood serum calcium concentration, a change which is observed in most cows at parturition but is exaggerated in disordered animals. The bound and ionized fractions of the calcium are affected. There are associated changes in other blood minerals which include falls in the blood serum concentrations of phosphorus and its fractions, and frequently potassium, and a rise in that of magnesium. Blood glucose concentration and pH may also be increased. Typical values for the composition of the blood of normal and affected animals are given in Table 9.4.

The cause of the clinical signs has not been firmly established. Calcium of the soft tissue is important for the transmission of impulses from nerve to muscle but the expected effect of a depression in ionic calcium concentration would be increased hypersensitivity, not paralysis. Kowalczyk and Mayer (1972) have proposed that hypocalcaemia alters the permeability of the cell membrane to potassium and sodium,

Table 9.4 Mean values for the composition of the blood plasma of normal and parturient hypocalcaemic cows (Blum, Ramberg, Johnson and Kronfeld, 1972)

Constituent	Normal	Hypocalcaemic
Total Ca (mmol/l)	2.3	1.6 (1.1)[†]
Ionized Ca (mmol/l)	0.8	0.6 (0.5)[†]
P (mg/l)	47[‡]	25
Mg (mg/l)	18[‡]	24
Glucose (mg/l)	670[‡]	700

[†] Values for paretic animals.
[‡] Values 13 to 2 days before parturition.

causing a reduction in the potential difference across the membrane and paralysis of muscular contractions. Prolonged hypocalcaemia could thus cause muscle degeneration and give rise to a chronic, irreversible condition. Increases have been observed in the concentrations of glutamic oxaloacetic transaminase and bilirubin in the serum, and in the secretion of myoglobin in the urine, which are indicative of muscle degeneration, and these changes have been proposed as a guide to prognosis (Jönsson and Pehrson, 1969).

Calcium and phosphorus demand and supply

There are several indications that the disorder arises from a primary imbalance between demand and supply for calcium and phosphorus. Parturient hypocalcaemia and the associated hypophosphataemia coincide with a sharp increase in the demand for calcium and phosphorus, due to the rapid transition from meeting the needs of the foetus at term to meeting the requirements for secretion of colostrum, which in the cow is especially rich in calcium and phosphorus. Mean values, reported by Rook and Campling (1965), for the colostrum of British Friesian heifers were 1.67 g calcium and 1.70 g phosphorus per 1, as compared with values of 1.10 and 0.85 g/l for normal milk. The most direct demonstration of the importance of the colostral loss of calcium as a factor in the aetiology of the disorder is that removal of the udder prevents the usual fall in serum calcium concentration at parturition (Niedermeier, Smith and Whitehair, 1949). Mild hypophosphataemia, however, may still be observed, indicating that other factors are involved.

Comparisons have revealed differences between species in the trends in serum calcium concentration during pregnancy and early lactation that can be related to the extent and rapidity of changes in the

Table 9.5 Estimates of calcium accretion by the foetus and calcium secretion in colostrum and milk, in the cow, sow and woman (the pre-partum values are from Simkiss, 1967)

Days *pre*(−) or *post*(+) *partum*	−60	−30	−15	−5	−1	+1	+2	+3
Cow								
g Ca/day	3.2	7.8	–	–	9.8	15.3	18.8	20.0
mg Ca/kg per h	0.27	0.65	–	–	0.82	1.28		
Sow								
g Ca/day	0.4	1.8	4.0	7.2	9.8	3.5		
mg Ca/kg per h	0.06	0.30	0.66	1.20	1.63	0.58		
Woman								
g Ca/day	0.10	0.15	–	–	0.30	0.006		
mg Ca/kg per h	0.06	0.09	–	–	0.18	0.004		

requirement for calcium (Table 9.5). Parturient hypocalcaemia has not been reported in the sow, in which the foetal drain of calcium increases substantially but progressively throughout the last month of pregnancy to a peak at parturition, to be followed by a much reduced demand for secretion of calcium in the colostrum. The sow's colostrum has a low content of calcium; a typical figure is 0.5 g/l as compared with a value of 2.2 g/l for normal milks (Lucas, 1962). In woman, although the foetal drain of calcium shows the expected increase throughout pregnancy, it is still comparatively low at term; both human colostrum and normal milk have a low calcium concentration (0.30 to 0.35 g/l), and the volume of secretion may remain low for the first 2 days after delivery. Slightly lower than normal values for serum calcium concentration may be observed towards the end of pregnancy but delivery is usually followed by a distinct increase in concentration.

Breed, age and individuality of the cow all influence the severity of parturient hypocalcaemia and the incidence of 'milk fever'. The incidence is higher in Channel Island cows than in British Friesian or Shorthorn cows and in older than in younger animals (Leech, Davis, Macrae and Withers, 1960; Mullen, 1975). There are related differences for both breed and age in the loss of calcium (and phosphorus) in colostrum (Table 9.6) but this is probably only one of several influential factors. Although milk-yielding ability is of importance – beef breeds, the cows of which give little milk, are not normally susceptible to the disorder – high-yielding dairy cows are not invariably more prone to parturient hypocalcaemia than low-yielding cows. The amount of exchangeable calcium in the skeleton and the rate of exchange are also reduced with age (Hansard, Comar and Davis, 1954). Other factors which influence the mobilization of the calcium and phosphorus of

Table 9.6   Influence of age of cow on the blood plasma calcium and inorganic phosphate concentrations at parturition, and on the loss of calcium and phosphorus in milk (Payne, 1977)

Age (years)	No. of cows	Plasma Ca (mg/1)	Plasma P (mg/l)	Secretion in milk during first 24 h of lactation (g)	
				Ca	P
2	17	97	43	6.8	7.3
3	5	90	36	11.7	11.5
4	7	84	36	15.6	18.4
5	13	78	28	21.8	17.7
6–7	9	72	23	16.3	17.3
8–14	14	69	23	19.3	18.8

bone are also crucial. The incidence of the disorder is reduced when the diet offered *pre partum* has a low ratio of calcium to phosphorus (Table 9.7) or a low alkali–alkalinity and total alkalinity (Table 9.8), or when a massive dose of vitamin D_3 is given intravenously in the last 8 days of gestation (Manston and Payne, 1964): the vitamin D analogue, 1-α-hydroxycholecalciferol, is most effective when administered between 24 and 120 h before calving (Davies, Allen, Hoare, Pott, Riley, Sansom, Stenton and Vagg, 1978). The ratio of calcium to phosphorus in cows' colostrum is approximately unity whereas that of bone is 2:1, and the need to meet the demand for phosphorus imposes a greater stress than that for calcium, although it has been suggested (Symonds and Treacher, 1967) that part of the intracellular phosphorus may also be available to meet these needs. The mobilization of bone mineral, however, is sensitive to the nutritional status for calcium and not that for phosphorus (S. M. Briggs and J. A. F. Rook, unpublished results), and within the context of the aetiology of the disorder calcium kinetics are of major importance.

Calcium kinetics

Cows are able to maintain milk secretion and good mineralization of bone on diets that barely meet the maintenance requirements for calcium, as measured using tracer techniques with cows receiving usual amounts of dietary calcium. This demonstrates clearly the ability of the cow, long-term, to maintain calcium homeostasis through the regulation of the secretion of calcium into the gut. Irrespective of dietary calcium supply, however, cows usually mobilize bone mineral and are in negative calcium balance in early lactation, and often for much of the lactation, and there is a complementary repletion of bone mineral and therefore positive calcium balance in later lactation and in the dry

Table 9.7 Influence of the dietary calcium to phosphorus ratio on the occurrence of 'milk fever', and on blood serum concentrations of calcium and phosphorus in Jersey cows that had completed at least three lactations (Boda and Cole, 1954)

Ca:P ratio in diet offered *pre partum*[†]	Incidence of 'milk fever' (%)	Serum concentrations (mg/l)							
		Day 1 *post partum*				Day 4 *post partum*			
		Ca	s.e.	P	s.e.	Ca	s.e.	P	s.e.
1:3.3	0	95.3	11.2	49.9	12.6	101.8	10.1	45.1	9.8
1:1	15	86.8	12.8	44.3	14.3	96.8	9.9	44.7	12.9
5.9:1	26	88.9	10.3	42.6	9.1	98.7	10.8	52.2	7.8
6:1	36	—				—			

[†] All cows received a normal ration *post partum*.

Table 9.8 The influence of the 'alkalinity' of the diet on the occurrence postpartum of hypocalcaemia and 'milk fever' (Ender and Dishington, 1970)

Diet	Period	Daily dietary intake of				Average serum Ca concentration during the first 2 days *post partum* (mg/l)	No. of cows showing signs of milk fever
		Ca (g)	P (g)	Alkali-alkalinity (meq)[†]	Alkalinity (meq)[‡]		
'Alkaline'	12 to 5 weeks *pre partum*	140	26	+2968	+9776		
	Weeks 1 and 2 *pre partum*	140	28	+2994	+10173		
	Post-partum	156	58	+3518	+12331	62	4/10
'Acid'	12 to 5 weeks *pre partum*	140	26	+2968	+9776		
	Weeks 1 and 2 *pre partum*	144	26	−228	+8595		
	Post-partum	152	51	+252	+9922	76	0/8

† (Na + K) − (S + Cl).
‡ (Na + K + Ca + Mg) − (S + Cl + P).

period. From some studies, but not all, there is evidence that cows prone to parturient hypocalcaemia tend to be in negative calcium balance towards the end of pregnancy also. Ramberg, Mayer, Kronfeld, Phang and Berman (1970), working with cows receiving high intakes of calcium and exhibiting hypocalcaemia, found that calcium balance declined prior to parturition and after the onset of lactation but remained positive until approximately 2 weeks after parturition.

The short-term interpretation of balance measurements, however, is uncertain and is complicated further at parturition as, at that time, partial or complete anorexia, and a consequent fall in calcium intake, is a common feature (Moodie and Robertson, 1961). Moreover, a transient reduction in appetite is a consistent sign associated with subclinical hypocalcaemia, and the indications are that a constant supply of calcium from the gut is critical for the maintenance of homeostasis during the period of adjustment to the increased requirement of calcium for milk secretion (Mayer, Ramberg and Kronfeld, 1969). Continuity in supply appears to be more important than the general level, as a sharp reduction in calcium intake to a low level, from several days *pre partum*, produced severe hypocalcaemia within 24 h, but this was corrected in 1 to 2 days and there was no subsequent development of parturient hypocalcaemia (Goings, Jacobson and Littledike, 1971).

Measurements using ^{45}Ca have failed to demonstrate significant changes in the coefficient of absorption of dietary calcium, the endogenous calcium secretion or the exchangeable calcium pool size at 2 weeks before parturition, but following parturition the dietary intake, and therefore the average net absorption of calcium, increased (Sansom, 1969). Bone calcium accretion rate was, however, reduced at 2 weeks *post partum* but by 2 months *post partum* had regained the precalving level. A more rapid turnover of blood plasma calcium consistent with an increased outflow of calcium into milk (Ramberg *et al.*, 1970), and a more rapid response in the return of blood calcium to normal after the infusion of ethylenediaminetetra-acetic acid (Payne, 1964), have also been observed in lactating, as opposed to non–lactating, cows but the most critical changes in calcium metabolism may be evident only during a short period at or around parturition.

Sequential studies of calcium kinetics during late pregnancy and early lactation have been made by Ramberg *et al.* (1970). Their results for seven cows, three of which exhibited minimum plasma calcium concentrations of 55 to 61 mg/l soon after parturition, were obtained using a combination of nutritional balance and ^{45}Ca tracer techniques and analysed using a compartmental model. They are presented in a simplified form in Fig. 9.2. The outflow of calcium into milk at the onset of lactation was accompanied by a reduction in the pool size for calcium in the plasma and other soft tissue and fluid compartments, a decreased transport of calcium into bone and a major increase in

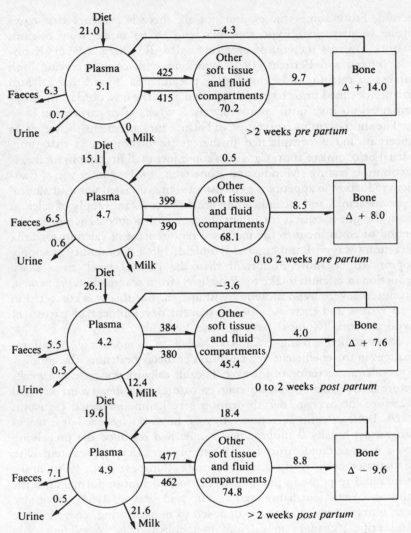

Fig. 9.2   Changes in calcium metabolism in the cow immediately *pre* and
post partum. Values are compartment masses (g) for soft tissues and
fluids, increments for bone, or rates (g/day) of transport or loss.
(After Ramberg *et al.*, 1970.)

calcium absorption from the gut. The decreased transport into bone
probably reflected the cessation of the outflow into foetal bone which at
parturition was, in one instance (Symonds, Manston, Payne and
Sansom, 1966), found to be approximately 5 g/day. The total exchangeable calcium immediately following parturition was reduced by
an average of 20 g (equivalent to the colostral output of calcium for
2 days), coincidentally with a fall in plasma calcium concentration.

The mobilization of bone calcium did not increase until 2 weeks after parturition, but the dietary intake of calcium of the cows under study was high (70 g/day) and cows with smaller intakes of calcium may show an earlier response.

The aetiology of parturient hypocalcaemia

The failure of some cows to adjust satisfactorily to the increased demands for calcium for milk secretion appears to be due to an inability to increase rapidly enough the uptake of calcium from the gut and, in animals that have previously received a surfcit of dietary calcium, the resorption of calcium from bone. Dryerre and Greig (1925) at this early date suggested that the disorder was due to a deficient production of parathyroid hormone, now known to be important not only for calcium resorption from the bone but also for calcium absorption from the gut, but there is recent evidence that there is no lack of parathyroid response to hypocalcaemia in paretic cows (Mayer, Ramberg, Kronfeld, Buckle, Sherwood, Aurbach and Potts, 1969) (Fig. 9.3).

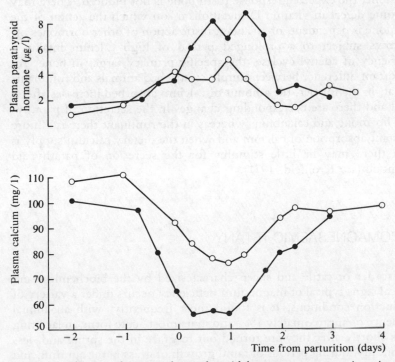

Fig. 9.3. Plasma calcium and parathyroid hormone concentrations in non-paretic parturient cows. Cow o showed only mild hypocalcaemia, cow ● severe hypocalcaemia but paresis was not observed. (After Mayer *et al.*, 1969.)

One factor that may have an adverse influence on the absorption of calcium at parturition is plasma oestrogen activity, which increases from approximately 30 days *pre partum* to a sharp peak at parturition and then falls away rapidly (Saba, 1964). High concentrations of oestrogen cause gut stasis, depress the appetite and, therefore, calcium intake and absorption (Payne, 1968), and this action may be exacerbated by a fall in plasma calcium concentration. Oestrogen has also been shown to decrease the proportion of plasma calcium that is diffusible (Bach and Messervy, 1969), and this action may be important to the onset of clinical signs. Bone resorption also is depressed in mice and men but a similar effect in ruminants would not account for the long delay in response in bone absorption observed by Mayer *et al.* (1969). Hypomagnesaemia may limit bone resorption of calcium (Allen and Sansom 1980).

Since the discovery of the hormone calcitonin, which depresses bone resorption, there has been speculation as to its possible rôle in the occurrence of parturient hypocalcaemia, but if there is one it has yet to be elucidated. The most probable explanation for a delay in response in bone resorption is that, whilst there is an efficient release of parathyroid hormone, the expected response from bone is not induced. There may be some defect in vitamin D metabolism, on which the action of the hormone is dependent, or an antagonistic action of other hormones or, in cows subject to a prolonged period of high calcium intake, a deficiency of adenyl cyclase, the specific primary target in bone. An important difference between simple-stomached animals and ruminants is that, in the former, the amount of calcium absorbed increases after a meal and there are corresponding changes in the secretion of parathyroid hormone and calcitonin, whereas in the ruminant there is a more constant absorption of calcium and when the dietary calcium supply is high there may be little stimulus for the secretion of parathyroid hormone (see Kronfeld, 1971).

HYPOMAGNESAEMIC TETANY

A disorder of cattle and sheep characterized by the biochemical and clinical signs typical of magnesium deficiency occurs under a variety of production conditions. It is found most frequently, with an annual incidence of approximately 1%, and in its most acute form, in lactating cows shortly after they are turned out to graze in the spring and, less commonly, during periods of rapid growth of grass in the autumn, and has been referred to variously as 'grass tetany', 'grass staggers' and 'lactation tetany'. A more chronic form is found in beef cattle during the winter months, in stall-fed and out-wintered animals, and in calves sucking their dams in beef herds or those reared for veal. The disorder occurs in both lowland and hill flocks of sheep, most frequently when they are on improved grassland but also on poor or restricted diets.

Biochemical and clinical signs

A constant feature is a low concentration of magnesium in the blood plasma, of 5 to 10 mg/l or less as compared with a more typical value of 20 to 35 mg/l, linked frequently with a low plasma calcium concentration of between 40 and 70 mg/l. Clinical signs are of a progressively developing hyper-irritability of the nervous system, terminating in spasticity and a violent tonic-clonic convulsion of the musculature. Although a low plasma magnesium concentration appears essential for the occurence of clinical signs, animals with a low concentration do not always show the distinctive signs, and some other factors, such as environmental or other stress, may be required to elicit them; there is recent evidence for a better correlation between low concentrations of magnesium in the cerebrospinal fluid and the occurence of tetany.

The aetiology of the disease was originally obscure but there is now good evidence that all forms of the disorder arise when the amount of magnesium absorbed (including that reabsorbed) from the gut fails to meet the requirements for tissue formation, milk secretion and secretions into the gut. A restricted uptake of magnesium from the gut may be a consequence of a low dry-matter intake, a low dietary concentration of magnesium, poor absorption, or a combination of any or all of these factors.

Experimentally induced magnesium deficiency in farm animals

Artificial, partially purified diets low in magnesium have been devised for most classes of farm livestock and used for the study of magnesium deficiency. On the withdrawal of virtually all of the magnesium from the diet, there is invariably a reduction in the excretion of magnesium in the faeces (excretion of endogenous faecal magnesium continues), a virtual cessation of excretion of magnesium in the urine and a fall in blood-plasma magnesium concentration. Magnesium is excreted in the kidney by a filtration-reabsorption mechanism and appears in the urine only when the magnesium load filtered by the glomeruli exceeds that reabsorbed by the tubules. There is a rectilinear relationship between the plasma concentration and urinary excretion of magnesium but possibly this relationship may be modified by dietary factors such as a high potassium intake; the threshold value for the excretion of magnesium in the urine is a plasma concentration of between 15 and 20 mg/l (Storry and Rook, 1963; Chicco, 1968).

The rapidity and extent of the fall in the plasma magnesium concentration varies with age, production state and, from animal to animal, variations that are attributable to differences in the production requiruent for magnesium and the ability to make use of body stores of magnesium for productive purposes. Similar effects of age and production state and individuality (Fig. 9.4) are observed in the naturally occuring disorders but with natural diets there are the additional factors of differences in the supply of magnesium and its absorption from the gut, and possibly in the endogenous faecal loss of magnesium. To explain the observed differences in the occurrence and severity of hypomagnesaemia, account must be taken of each of these factors.

Magnesium requirement

Magnesium is an essential component of biological materials and during growth or the secretion of milk there is an obligatory uptake of magnesium. Soft tissues vary in their content of magnesium, from 0.6 to 1.3 g/kg of the dry matter, and only a small depression in magnesium content is evident during magnesium deficiency. At a growth rate of 0.5 kg/day in the young calf, the daily requirement for magnesium for soft tissue growth alone is approximately 0.1 g magnesium.

Milk may vary in magnesium content from 0.07 to 0.18 g/l and the concentration appears to be independent of the dietary supply of magnesium.

The concentration of magnesium in the skeleton is substantially higher (1.5 g/kg fresh skeleton) than for soft tissue but, during magnesium deficiency, bone minerals may be deposited with a reduced magnesium content and magnesium already present may be released from the skeleton. This release, dependent on an exchange of minerals at the bone surface, may be substantial in the young calf, where the ratio of bone crystal surface to volume is high, but negligible in the fully mature adult in which there is extensive recrystallization and hydration of bone mineral, and the skeleton has a high proportion of compact bone and a restricted blood supply (Blaxter, 1956).

Hormonal effects on magnesium metabolism have been demonstrated (Care, 1967) but, with one exception, there is no indication that, during magnesium deficiency, hormonal responses directly modify the uptake or release of magnesium in soft tissue or bone; Martens and Rayssiguier (1979) have claimed that the adrenergic response to stress causes a shift of magnesium from the plasma to the tissues. A fall in

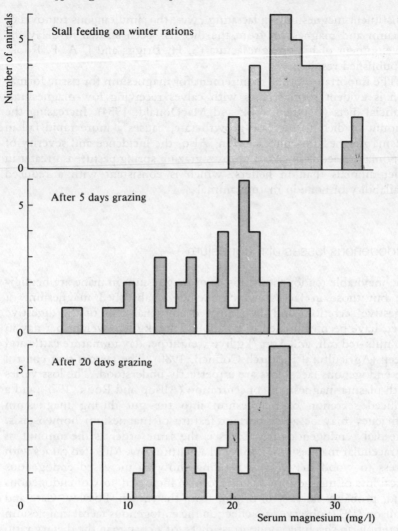

Fig. 9.4. Changes in blood-plasma magnesium concentration in a group of cows transferred from winter-stall diets to spring grazing. Values are grouped in units of 1 mg/l; □, cows given therapeutic treatment when the plasma concentration fell to 7 mg/l and withdrawn from experiment. (After Bartlett, Brown, Foot, Head, Line, Rook, Rowland and Zundel, 1957.)

magnesium concentration of extracellular fluid tends to decrease the solubility of calcium in body fluids and that effect may explain the hypocalcaemia frequently observed in association with hypomagnesaemia. Undernutrition, or any other factor that results in the catabolism of soft tissue or bone, will inevitably cause a release of the constituent magnesium: in lactating ewes, the simultaneous removal of calcium and magnesium from the diet has been shown to delay the development of hypomagnesaemia (S. H. Briggs and J. A. F. Rook, unpublished results).

The importance of the requirement for magnesium for tissue formation is evident from studies with calves receiving low-magnesium, artificial diets (Blaxter, Rook and MacDonald, 1954). Increasing the amount of diet, to increase growth rate, causes a more rapid fall in plasma magnesium concentration. Also, the incidence and severity of hypomagnesaemia in lactating cows grazing spring pasture is greater in older animals than in heifers, which is consistent with a reduced availability of bone in mature animals.

Endogenous losses of magnesium

The inevitable (endogenous) losses of magnesium in urine are negligible but those in faeces, which include unabsorbed magnesium of digestive secretions and desquamated epithelial cells of the digestive tract, have been estimated to be about 2 mg/kg live weight per day in the milk-fed calf, and 3 mg/kg live weight per day in mature cattle and sheep (Agricultural Research Council, 1980). The factors that control the endogenous faecal loss are imperfectly understood. The loss varies with plasma magnesium concentration (Allsop and Rook, 1979) and a reduced secretion of magnesium into the gut during magnesium deficiency may be an important feature of magnesium homeostasis. The daily endogenous faecal loss is the same order as the amount of extracellular magnesium, 2 to 3 g in a mature cow. Milk-fed calves with access to wood shavings as bedding show an increased endogenous faecal loss of magnesium arising from an increased flow of endogenous fluid, probably salivary in origin, from the rumen. Powley, Care and Johnson (1977) observed no effect on the endogenous faecal magnesium excretion, in sheep receiving grass diets, of a change in the dietary ratio of potassium to sodium from 21 to 2.

Absorption of magnesium

For many years it was assumed that the absorption of magnesium in the ruminant occurred mainly from the small intestine, as is the case in simple-stomached animals. There is now good evidence, however, that the major site for magnesium absorption is the stomach. The first evidence for absorption from the stomach region, indicating a net uptake of dietary magnesium of 250 to 380 g/kg in sheep and 130 to 720 g/kg in cattle, was obtained in experiments designed to measure the flow of materials, by reference to a suitable marker substance in animals fitted with re-entrant cannulae at the proximal duodenum and terminal ileum (see, for example, Rogers and van't Klooster, 1969; Grace and MacRae, 1972; Møller and Hvelplund, 1977).

Confirmation was obtained in experiments in which solutions of magnesium salts were infused at various sites along the tract, and absorption was assessed by responses in plasma magnesium concentration and urinary magnesium excretion (Strachan and Rook, 1975), changes in magnesium to dietary marker ratio at points along the tract (Tomas and Potter, 1976a; Horn and Smith, 1978) or by labelling of the magnesium with ^{28}Mg (Smith and Horn, 1976): invariably, appreciable absorption prior to the duodenum was demonstrated. The abomasum has been excluded as an important site for magnesium absorption (Pfeffer and Rahman, 1974) and the evidence for absorption from the reticulo-rumen is equivocal (Care and van't Klooster, 1965; Tomas and Potter, 1976b; Field and Munro, 1977; Horn and Smith, 1978). The major site is probably the omasum in cattle and the reticulo-rumen in sheep (Edrise, 1979; Fitt, Hutton and Armstrong, 1979).

Transfer of magnesium across the wall of the omasum or reticulo-rumen may be dependent partly on the trans-epithelial flux of water but there is also an active transport mechanism (Martens, Harmeyer and Michael, 1978), possibly of limited capacity (Field and Munro, 1977). Net absorption of magnesium is depressed at high plasma magnesium concentrations (Allsop and Rook, 1979), whereas uptake of magnesium prior to the duodenum is facilitated by a high sodium to potassium ratio in rumen liquor (Edrise, 1979; MacGregor and Armstrong, 1979), possibly through a change in the electric potential across the gut wall. That observation may explain the frequently reported effect of a high dietary concentration of potassium on the coefficient of absorption of magnesium and the occurrence of hypomagnesaemia (see, for example, Newton, Fontenot, Tucker and Polan, 1972). The corresponding effect of heavy dressings of nitrogenous fertilizer, which increase substantially the nitrogen content of swards and, as a consequence, the concentration of ammonia in the rumen liquor of grazing animals (Head and Rook, 1955), may similarly be related to an influence of ammonium ion concentration on absorption from the stomach.

Absorption is enhanced by a low rumen pH, an effect that may explain the increase in coefficient of absorption when the diet is supplemented with readily digestible carbohydrates (Madsen, Lentz, Miller, Lowrey-Harnden and Hansard, 1976), and the low coefficient of absorption for dried grass and fresh grass diets (Smith and Horn, 1976). Absorption will also be affected by the extent to which the magnesium of rumen liquor is bound to bacteria or other particulate matter (Fitt,

Hutton and Otto, 1974) or is present as insoluble inorganic complexes, both of which will be influenced by pH.

Although the stomach may be the prime site for magnesium absorption in the ruminant, there is undoubtedly absorption from certain regions of the small intestine but for most diets there is net secretion. There is, however, a small but significant net uptake of magnesium from the large intestine and its importance may increase when absorption from the stomach is low (Tomas and Potter, 1976a). The capacity for absorption from the large intestine may be highest in the young animal (Smith, 1962).

Magnesium intake

Values for the coefficient of apparent absorption of magnesium reported for diets consisting solely of roughage and succulent foods are mainly between 0.05 and 0.30, and the lower values may be more common with diets of grass rich in nitrogen or potash and cut early in the season. These values are to be compared with a range of 0.10 to 0.40 for diets containing both forage and concentrated foods (Rook and Storry, 1962). If, however, the coefficient of true absorption is calculated assuming a constant value for the endogenous faecal loss of magnesium, the ranges of values for the two groups are much closer ARC, 1980). In many circumstances, therefore, the most critical factor in the aetiology of 'grass tetany' may be an unusually low intake of magnesium.

The first growth of herbage in the spring, especially on swards that have received a heavy dressing of potassium or nitrogenous fertilizer, may have an exceptionally low content of magnesium. Values as low as 1g/kg of the dry matter have been reported, as compared with more typical values for herbage of 1.5 to 2.5g/kg. The herbage dry matter and the dry matter voluntarily consumed by the grazing animal can also be low (Ladrat, Larvor and Brochart, 1959) but, because of the high metabolizable energy content of the dry matter, satisfactory milk yields can nevertheless be sustained.

A very low magnesium content of herbage, caused by a progressive leaching of minerals, and a low dry-matter intake may also be critical factors for the development of hypomagnesaemia in store cattle grazed on winter forage. In the veal calf reared on whole milk diets, the intake of magnesium may be marginal but the primary causal factors are the high requirement for growth in the rapidly growing animal, and a decline in the coefficient of apparent absorption for magnesium from a very high value of 0.70 or more in the first few weeks of life to a value of 0.3 to 0.5.

IMBALANCES IN THE DIET COMPOSITION OF RUMINANTS

The symbiotic association between the microbes of the reticulo-rumen and the host animal allows only a limited regulation by the host (through the secretion of saliva, exchanges across the reticulo-rumen wall and passage of materials to the omasum) of the physiological conditions within the reticulo-rumen. The amount and quality of the food are, therefore, major factors governing the composition and activities of the microbial population and an imbalanced diet, particularly when introduced abruptly, may induce a fermentation within the reticulo-rumen prejudicial to the host animal. Two examples of this type of nutritional imbalance are acidosis and ammonia toxicity.

Acidosis

This disorder is found in both cattle and sheep and is the result of an excessive, and often abrupt, ingestion of foods rich in readily fermentable carbohydrates, such as cereal grains, root crops, fruits or similar materials. The acidosis is a consequence of an excessive ruminal production of lactic acid. The clinical signs are variable and depend on whether there is accumulation of lactic acid in the gastro-intestinal tract, which causes rumen stasis, dehydration and epithelial damage; or a rapid entry of lactic acid into body fluids, which results in hypotension and respiratory failure, and may prove fatal (Huber, 1976).

Dietary carbohydrates are fermented by the glycolytic pathway, in which pyruvate is a central intermediate. Pyruvate may be dissimilated in a variety of ways to produce acetate and butyrate, or propionate either by the methylmalonate pathway or by the acrylate pathway, in which lactate is an intermediate. A diversion of metabolism through the acrylate pathway probably arises when, through a rapid fermentation of carbohydrate, the rate of production of pyruvate exceeds the rate of its conversion to volatile fatty acids by other pathways; the pyruvate may act as a hydrogen acceptor for the re-oxidation of reduced pyridine nucleotide (NADH) generated by the glycolytic pathway. A change of rumen pH may be important in limiting the metabolism of pyruvate to volatile fatty acids, either because key enzymes are pH sensitive or because, at a pH below 5.5, carbon dioxide fixation, essential to the synthesis of propionate via succinate, will be inhibited by the very low concentration of bicarbonate ion (Hopgood, 1965). The pK_a of carbonic acid is 6.1.

Diets that produce acute acidosis are associated with characteristic changes in microbial population. Gram-negative organisms decrease and are replaced by Gram-positive organisms, and at a pH below 5 protozoa disappear. The introduction of such diets is frequently accompanied by a rapid increase in the numbers of acid-producing cocci (*Streptococcus bovis*), which would cause an initial lowering of pH but, as the pH falls, Gram-positive rods (lactobacilli) begin to dominate. There is an associated increase in organisms that ferment lactic acid but, where the change of diet is abrupt, the rate of multiplication may not be rapid enough to limit the accumulation of lactic acid (Dirkson, 1970).

Lactic acid has a pK_a of 3.8 and within the normal pH range of the rumen is almost completely dissociated. In the absence of neutralization, its production causes an extreme fall in pH. At a pH below 5.0, motility of the reticulo-rumen is affected and eventually stasis ensues. The site of action of the hydrogen ion is probably receptors in the duodenum and the mechanism of inhibition may depend on release of the intestinal hormone, secretin, known to inhibit the motor activities of the fore-stomach (Bruce and Huber, 1973). Accumulation of lactic acid in the rumen increases the osmolality of rumen liquor (Table 9.9), which becomes hypertonic instead of hypotonic to blood plasma, and causes a net transfer of water to the rumen, dehydration and a watery diarrhoea. Lactic acid may also have a corrosive effect on the gastro-intestinal epithelium (Ahrens, 1967).

Table 9.9   The contribution of lactic acid and other
osmotically active constituents to rumen
osmolality (mosmol) in normal and acidotic sheep
(Huber, 1971), as adapted by Huber (1976)

Constituent	Control	Acidotic
Lactic acid	0.08	89.2
Na^+	88.0	50.0
K^+	42.0	26.0
Cl^-	30.8	21.0
Rumen osmolality	255.0	402.0

Lactic acid produced during fermentation is a racemic mixture but there is no evidence for preferential absorption of either isomer. On absorption, which occurs more rapidly from the small intestine than the fore-stomach (Dunlop, Hammond and Stevens, 1964), the L-isomer is metabolized rapidly, whereas the D-isomer is metabolized only slowly and accumulates (Braide and Dunlop, 1969). Metabolism of the L-isomer generates bicarbonate but the combined absorption of the isomers progressively depletes the alkali reserve, bicarbonate decreases, and blood carbon dioxide increases (Table 9.10) and suppresses the respiratory centre, and there is an associated hypotension. Signs of

Table 9.10 Physiological effects of acidosis induced by intra-ruminal glucose infusion in sheep (Juhász and Szegedi, 1968, as adapted by Huber, 1976)

Time from start of infusion (h)	Blood pressure (kPa)	Pulse rate (per min)	Respiration rate (per min)	Blood pH	CO_2 (mmol/l)	HCO_3^- (mmol/l)	HCO_3^-/ CO_2	Lactic acid (g/l)
0	14.7	65	26	7.52	1.44	36	25.0	0.22
16	12.7	130	86	7.31	2.07	32	15.5	1.35
23	2.7–8.0	180	20	7.24	2.67	17	6.4	1.68
24[†]	–	–	–	7.08	–	–	–	–

† Dead.

acute toxicity are probably dependent on a high rate of absorption of lactic acid but the factors that favour rapid absorption are not known. Loss of reticulo-rumen motility and stasis do, however, limit absorption (Ahrens, 1967; Dunlop and Stefaniak, 1965). Toxic factors, possibly of microbial origin, could also be involved in the pathogenesis and elevated histamine levels may be responsible for laminitis.

Ammonia toxicity

Ammonia is a central intermediate in the degradation of nitrogenous materials in the rumen and their resynthesis into microbial protein. It is a product of the hydrolysis and deamination of proteins, and of a variety of non-protein nitrogenous compounds, including amino acids and urea, and is a preferred source of nitrogen for many rumen bacteria and essential for the growth of some. The factors controlling the production and the utilization of ammonia differ and, when production exceeds utilization, ammonia accumulates in the reticulo-rumen. A high concentration of ammonia in rumen liquor is not itself toxic but is associated with a high concentration of ammonia in blood. This may cause impairment of brain function and produce progressively clinical signs of hypertension, increased respiration rate, tetanic spasms, coma and death. Sub-lethal concentrations, however, do not produce permanent effects (Dang and Visek, 1964).

Accumulation of ammonia (including both unionized NH_3 and ionic NH_4^+) in the reticulo-rumen occurs when substantial amounts of a highly degradable protein (e.g. casein), a non-protein nitrogen source such as urea that is readily converted to ammonia, or ammonia itself (in the form of ammoniated molasses, for example) is introduced into the rumen or the diet. The susceptibility of dietary proteins to degradation in the rumen is determined partly by their solubility and also possibly by their molecular structure. Microbial cell growth requires a source of energy (ATP) which, within the reticulo-rumen, is obtained by anaerobic fermentation. When energy is in surplus, cell growth *in vitro* (Satter and Slyter, 1974) and duodenal flow of microbial protein in sheep *in vivo* (Okorie, Buttery and Lewis, 1977) increase with ammonia concentration up to a maximum concentration of 4.5 mmol/l, and higher concentrations are not inhibitory. Miller (1973) has reported experiments with lambs in which the flow of microbial protein to the abomasum was greatest at a rumen ammonia concentration of approximately 17 mmol/l. The inclusion with a nitrogen source of carbohydrate materials that are readily fermentable will, therefore, tend to prevent an excessive accumulation of ammonia. Certain amino acids, peptides and branched-chain fatty acids are essential for some rumen organisms in pure culture and it is possible that, under particular dietary conditions, a lack of those nutrients in rumen liquor may restrict ammonia utilization. With diets containing large amounts of non-protein nitrogen, the sulphur intake may limit cell growth.

Ammonia is absorbed into the veins draining the reticulo-rumen and the intestine (Chalupa, 1972), and into peritoneal fluid (Chalmers, Jaffray and White, 1971), but it has been questioned (Smith, 1975) whether, under the normal, slightly acid (pH 6.5 or less) conditions of rumen liquor, such absorption is substantial. The pK_a of ammonia is 9.02 at 37°C (Jacquez, Poppell and Jeltsch, 1959) and at pH 6.5 approximately 3 g/kg of the ammonia is in the form of NH_3, but there is a tenfold increase from pH 6.5 to 7.5 (Lewis and Buttery, 1973). Assuming that tissue membranes are permeable only to the lipid-soluble NH_3, and not to NH_4^+, substantial absorption of ammonia in circumstances of toxicity could be explained in terms of simple diffusion only if rumen liquor were to become alkaline. Evidence for active transport of ammonia has, however, been provided for other tissues (Lund, Brosnan and Eggleston, 1970).

The site of absorption of ammonia was for long assumed to be the reticulo-rumen itself (Lewis, Hill and Annison, 1957) but a major site would now appear to be the omasum (Hogan and Weston, 1967). It was also assumed that the route of absorption was into the hepatic portal blood and that there was metabolism of ammonia in the liver up to a threshold amount, and when this was exceeded ammonia entered the peripheral circulation. Chalmers *et al.* (1971) have suggested that ammonia could pass directly to peripheral blood via the peritoneal fluid and the thoracic lymph, and that toxicity could arise without overloading the liver, but the magnitude of this route is uncertain. In the early work of Lewis *et al.* (1957) an increase in jugular blood ammonia was observed only when rumen ammonia was above 60 mmol/l at a pH assumed to be between 6.0 and 6.5, and a corresponding value of 100 mmol/l has been obtained when rumen liquor was maintained at pH 6.0, but Chalmers *et al.* (1971) have reported a progressive rise in jugular blood ammonia concentration with a rise in rumen ammonia concentration, and no indication of a threshold value.

Feeding diets rich in protein (Morris and Payne, 1970), in contrast to high-nitrogen diets rich in urea, increases the ability of animals to metabolize ammonia, due, it has been suggested, to the former diets and not the latter causing the induction of urea-cycle enzymes. High ornithine levels in the liver of animals receiving urea-rich diets may, however, allow the urea cycle to operate close to its maximum rate (Chalupa, Clark, Opliger and Lavker, 1970). Animals are able, to a limited extent, to store ammonia in a non-toxic form as glutamine and, in comparison with other species, the ruminant spleen has an exceptionally high glutamine synthetase activity (Buttery, 1970).

Ammonia toxicity is not always associated with a change in blood pH but any rise would enhance transport of the ammonia into cells. There is invariably, however, hyperventilation and a reduction in total plasma CO_2. High concentrations of ammonia modify the activity of the tricarboxylic-acid cycle, and variable responses in plasma glucose levels have been observed (see Leonard, Buttery and Lewis, 1977) and some evidence provided for an interference with gluconeogenesis. The suggestion has been made that oxidation of isocitrate to 2-oxoglutarate is depressed by ammonia (Katanuma, Okada and Nishi, 1967) and a depletion of brain 2-oxoglutarate, due to the formation of glutamate and glutamine, could be responsible for the neurological effects (Bessman and Bessman, 1955). Other explanations offered for the primary toxic effect are a depletion of acetyl choline (Ulshafer, 1958) or a substitution of NH_4^+ for potassium ion at neuronal membranes, causing depolarization (Lund *et al.*, 1970); such an effect would be reversible. Soar, Buttery and Lewis (1973) observed a reduction in blood potassium on the withdrawal of an intravenous infusion of ammonium acetate at a toxic level, and Juhász, Szegedi and Keresztes (1975) suggested that high blood-ammonia concentrations promote a release of potassium from cells by diffusion.

It has been postulated that, even at sub-lethal levels, the effects of ammonia on intermediary metabolism may reduce the efficiency of energy transactions due to a stimulation of respiration (Buttery and Annison, 1971).

AMINO ACID IMBALANCE

Amino acid *deficiency* is a condition in which the dietary supply of one or more of the essential amino acids is less than that required for the efficient utilization of other amino acids and other nutrients. Diets are unlikely to be devoid of an essential amino acid but may be deficient in one or more. The acid for which the dietary supply provides the lowest proportion of the theoretical requirement is referred to as the first-limiting amino acid (lysine in Fig. 9.5(b)), that for which the dietary supply provides the second lowest proportion of the requirement as the second-limiting amino acid (threonine in Fig. 9.5(c)) and so on. Deficiency is therefore judged against a control diet adequate in the supply of all essential amino acids as represented in Fig. 9.5(a).

The idealized profile of dietary amino acids represented in Fig. 9.5(a), in which all essential (and non-essential) amino acids are supplied in amounts equal to theoretical requirements, does not exist in practice and some imbalance in the supply of amino acids

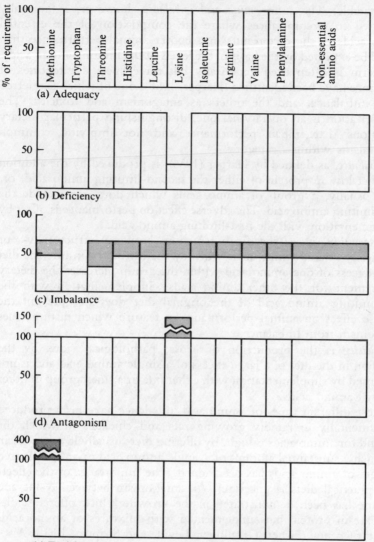

Fig. 9.5.   Diagrammatic representation of: (a) idealized amino acid-adequate diet in which all amino acids are present in amounts sufficient to satisfy but not exceed requirements; (b) idealized amino acid-deficient diet, in which one amino acid, lysine, is limiting; (c) amino acid imbalance induced by addition of all amino acids except tryptophan to a protein-deficient diet in which tryptophan is the first-limiting and threonine the second-limiting amino acid; (d) amino acid antagonism induced by addition of lysine to an adequate diet which increases the requirement for arginine; and (e) toxicity induced by addition of a large excess of methionine (□ represents amino acid(s) added). (Adapted from Austic, 1978.)

is inevitable. The term *amino acid imbalance*, however, is normally restricted to circumstances where the composition of the essential amino acids in the diet results in a poorer animal performance than would be expected on the basis of the levels of the limiting amino acids. The term is often used generically but three specific categories of imbalance have been identified (Harper, 1956), one of which is referred to as imbalance, and the others as antagonism and toxicity. The categorization is an operational one, distinguishing particular dietary conditions that impair performance and not implying common mechanisms within a category.

Imbalance, as defined by Harper (1956), is produced by the addition to a diet low in protein of either the second-limiting amino acid, or, more usually, a group of amino acids which does not include the first-limiting amino acid. The adverse effect on performance is offset by supplementation with the first-limiting amino acid.

Antagonism is a specific interaction between structurally- or chemically-related amino acids whereby the introduction into the diet of an excess of one amino acid within the group increases the dietary requirement for the other amino acids. Supplementation with the first-limiting amino acid of the original diet does not prevent the adverse effect on animal performance, a feature which distinguishes antagonism from imbalance.

Toxicity is the production of gross, pathological signs by the inclusion in the diet of a large excess of a single amino acid and is not prevented by supplementation with either one or a small group of other essential amino acids.

These different types of amino acid imbalance have been produced experimentally in rapidly growing rats and chickens in which the demand for amino acids is high, by offering diets usually low in protein to which a substantial amount of a single amino acid or an unbalanced mixture of amino acids has been added. The importance of the effects with practical diets is uncertain. An antagonism between lysine and arginine has been demonstrated in the growing chick offered a diet adequate in protein but supplemented with mixtures of amino acids devoid of lysine (Fisher, Griminger, Leville and Shapiro, 1960). Also, increases in the relative dietary requirement for maximum growth of specific amino acids have been observed as the protein content of the diet has been increased, and this relationship may have its origin in amino acid interactions (see, for example, Wethli, Morris and Shresta, 1975). In the ruminant, any imbalance of amino acids in the diet will be modified by microbial degradation and synthesis within the rumen; the amino acid composition of microbial protein does not itself match tissue requirement.

The ease with which the various conditions may be produced experimentally has, however, encouraged a search for mechanisms. In amino acid *deficiency* the restricted dietary supply reduces the concentration of the limiting amino acid or acids in blood plasma and tissues. As a consequence, the concentrations of the limiting amino acids at intracellular sites of protein synthesis, and hence the rate of protein synthesis itself, are reduced. There are similarities between amino acid deficiency and imbalance but an important distinction is that in imbalance, for certain amino acids, the normal relationship between dietary supply and plasma concentration is altered because of an interaction between amino acids. Theoretically, interaction could occur in a variety of ways: through the rôle of the amino acids in the regulation of appetite; through competition for transport during absorption from the intestine, during reabsorption in the kidney or during entry into the cells or tissues; through common or interacting pathways of amino acid catabolism; and through their use for protein synthesis (or release during protein degradation) or for the synthesis of essential metabolites, or in the formation of toxic materials. The extent to which these various mechanisms are involved in the different forms of imbalance is by no means resolved but some of the primary mechanisms have been identified.

Imbalance

The addition to a low-protein diet of essential amino acids other than the first-limiting amino acid depresses food intake and growth, and causes a reduction in the plasma concentration of the first-limiting amino acid and a marked increase in the concentrations of the supplementary amino acids (see Kumta and Harper, 1962; Leung, Rogers and Harper, 1968); partial or even complete adaptation, if the imbalance is slight, is normally observed. It was at first assumed that the supplementary acids induced an increased catabolism of the first-limiting amino acid, as in the early experiments the direct effect on amino acid utilization was invariably confounded with the depression in live-weight gain caused by the reduction in food intake. This interpretation was questioned by Fisher *et al.* (1960), who demonstrated that the effect on growth was largely offset if food intake was maintained, either by force-feeding or stimulation of appetite. Experimental studies in which the amino acid imbalance was slight have now shown that amino acid imbalance increases the efficiency of utilization of the first-limiting amino acid and thus allows the use of some of the supplementary amino acids for protein synthesis. There is a preferential uptake of the first-limiting amino acid into certain proteins, especially those of the liver, and in partial compensation a release of the amino acid through muscle protein catabolism. In comparisons between animals receiving the same amount of food, imbalance does not depress nitrogen retention and sometimes causes an increase; very slight imbalances which do not depress food intake for several days may produce initially a small, transient increase in growth rate associated with a small increase in food intake.

The pathological effects of amino acid imbalance appear, therefore, in many, but possibly not all, instances to be a direct consequence of a reduction in food intake, which results in a decrease in growth rate and also in nitrogen retention, an effect which may be partially offset by a change of body composition towards a higher nitrogen content (see Boorman, 1981). In the rat, it has been shown that sites within the brain that regulate food intake are sensitive to an alteration in the proportions of amino acids in the blood plasma. The particular sites that have been identified are the anterior prepyriform cortex and the medial amygdala, and there may also be sites within the hypothalamus sensitive to an increase in plasma amino acid concentration (Rogers and Leung, 1973). Blood plasma concentrations of ammonia or other amino acid metabolites may also serve as indicators of dietary amino acid imbalance.

The response to an amino acid imbalance in the blood plasma is such that an animal will consume a protein-free diet in preference to an imbalanced diet, even though consumption of the protein-free diet necessarily has adverse consequences whereas, if the imbalanced diet were to be consumed, the animal would grow normally and show no ill-effects (Leung *et al.*, 1968).

Antagonism

The addition of certain, specific amino acids to diets with a balanced amino acid composition but low in protein content also depresses growth and food intake but the basis of the effect is an antagonism within a group of amino acids. Several specific antagonisms have been reported but all do not conform to the classical definition. The two that have been most fully studied are the effect of excess lysine on the requirement for arginine (Boorman and Fisher, 1966; Jones, Wolters and Burnett, 1966; Smith and Lewis, 1966) and of an excess of one of three branched-chain amino acids, leucine, isoleucine and valine, on the requirement for the other two, leucine being particularly marked in its action (Spolter and Harper, 1961; D'Mello and Lewis, 1970).

The effect on food intake has been seen as a main factor (Harper, Benevenga and Wohlhueter, 1970). The possibility has been considered that the amino acid in excess (agent) causes a depletion of the other amino acid (or acids) within the group, to the extent that it becomes the first-limiting amino acid (Lewis, 1965) and produces a condition identical with that of imbalance. Dietary excess of lysine in the chick, however, depletes the arginine pool within hours but does not affect food intake for several days. Moreover, there is an effect on growth which precedes that on food intake, and a dietary excess of lysine may therefore depress growth directly, and factors other than a reduction in food intake in response to an imbalance in plasma amino acid concentrations are involved (see Austic, 1978).

The basic amino acids share common sites for transport across cell membranes and, although there is no evidence that an excessive intake of lysine limits the absorption of arginine from the gut, high plasma concentrations of lysine do impair the reabsorption of arginine in the kidney tubules and cause an increase in excretion. Excess lysine probably also depresses glycine amidino-transferase activity in the liver and restricts creatine formation from arginine but enhances the activity of kidney arginase, and increases the degradation of arginine to ornithine and urea (see Fig. 9.6) (Austic and Nesheim, 1971). (Phenylalanine, tyrosine, histidine, leucine and ornithine also increase arginase

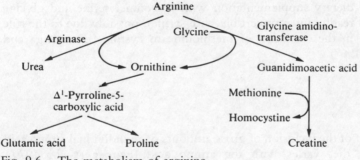

Fig. 9.6. The metabolism of arginine.

activity and the apparent arginine requirement, whereas threonine and glycine have the opposite effect.) This effect on arginase activity appears to be an important component of the effect of lysine-arginine antagonism on growth. High dietary intakes of the cations, sodium and potassium, alleviate lysine-arginine antagonism whereas a high intake of the anion, chloride, exacerbates it, effects which derive from a change in the activity of hepatic lysine-α-ketoglutarate reductase, an enzyme that catalyses an initial step in lysine catabolism. Physiologically, lysine and arginine are cations.

Antagonism between the branched-chain amino acids was considered to be due to alterations in the activities of branched-chain amino acid transferase (L-leucine: 2-oxo-glutarate aminotransferase) in muscle and α-ketoisocaproic acid dehydrogenase (2-oxoisocaproate: lipoate oxidoreductase) in liver, enzymes involved in the catabolism of all three branched-chain amino acids; it was assumed that one amino acid in excess induced an increased catabolism of all three acids (Harper *et al.*,

1970). Evidence for increased catabolism of the unsupplemented acids is, however, equivocal. Increased catabolism may occur only when a single amino acid is added in considerable excess, and even then the increased catabolism may be small in relation to the observed alterations in plasma amino acid concentrations and has not been linked closely with changes of activity in catabolic enzymes. Competition for transport among the branched-chain amino acids appears to be a less important factor than for the basic amino acids, and the most probable explanation for the observed interaction between the branched-chain amino acids, at least when the dietary imbalance is slight, is that there is some tissue redistribution of the unsupplemented acids (Smith and Austic, 1978).

An interaction between arginine, glycine and methionine has been described by Keshavarz and Fuller (1971), which probably relates to their interacting rôle in the production of creatine (Fig. 9.6). Excess methionine also depresses plasma and tissue threonine concentrations and increases threonine-serine dehydrase activity, effects which are offset by dietary supplementation with threonine, serine and glycine (which is readily interconvertible with serine), possibly due to the rôle of serine in the oxidation of methionine to cystine (Benevenga and Harper, 1967).

Toxicity

The effect of the inclusion of gross amounts of an individual amino acid within a diet varies with the amino acid (Harper *et al.*, 1970). Threonine, even in very large amounts (50g/kg of the dry matter of the diet), is tolerated well and causes only a moderate depression of food intake and growth. Tyrosine, however, when ingested in large amounts by young growing rats given a low-protein diet, not only depresses severely food intake and growth but causes severe eye and paw lesions, and in great excess is lethal. Methionine is the most toxic and in amounts exceeding 20 g/kg of the dry matter of the diet may produce severe histopathological changes. The toxic effects responsible for the pathological changes are probably due to the structural and metabolic features of the individual amino acids.

REFERENCES

Agricultural Research Council, 1980. *The Nutrient Requirements of Ruminant Livestock*. Commonwealth Agricultural Bureaux, Slough.

Ahrens, F. A., 1967. Histamine, lactic acid and hypertonicity as factors in the development of rumenitis in cattle, *Am. J. vet. Res.* **28**: 1335–42.

Allen, W. M. and Sansom, B. F., 1980. Metabolic disorders of the dairy cow. In *Feeding Strategies for Dairy Cows* (ed. W. H. Broster, C. L. Johnson and J. C. Taylor), pp. 14.1–12. Agricultural Research Council, London.

Allsop, T. F. and Rook, J. A. F., 1979. The effect of diet and blood-plasma magnesium concentration on the endogenous faecal loss of magnesium in sheep, *J. agric. Sci., Camb.* **92**: 403–8.

Annison, E. F. and Armstrong, D. G., 1970. Volatile fatty acid metabolism and energy supply. In *Physiology of Digestion and Metabolism in the Ruminant* (ed. A. T., Phillipson), pp. 422–37. Oriel Press, Newcastle upon Tyne.

Annison, E. F., Leng, R. A., Lindsay, D. B. and White, R. R., 1963. The metabolism of acetic acid, propionic acid and butyric acid in sheep, *Biochem. J.* **88**: 248–52.

Ash, R. and Baird, G. D., 1973. Activation of volatile fatty acids in bovine liver and rumen epithelium, *Biochem. J.* **136**: 311–9.

Austic, R. E., 1978. Nutritional interactions of amino acids, *Feedstuffs, Lond.* **50**(24): 24–6.

Austic, R. E. and Nesheim, M. C., 1971. Arginine and creatine interrelationships in the chick, *Poultry Sci.* **51**: 1098–105.

Bach, S. J. and Messervy, A., 1969. Observations on the diffusible calcium fraction in the serum of the cow during oestrus and during parturition, *Vet. Rec.* **84**: 210–3.

Baird, G. D., 1977. Aspects of ruminant intermediary metabolism in relation to ketosis, *Biochem. Soc. Trans.* **5**: 819–27.

Baird, G. D. and Heitzman, R. J., 1971. Mode of action of a glucocorticoid on bovine intermediary metabolism, *Biochim. biophys. Acta* **252**: 184–98.

Baird, G. D., Hibbitt, K. G. and Lee, J., 1970. Enzymes involved in acetoacetate formation in various bovine tissues, *Biochem. J.* **117**: 703–9.

Baird, G. D., Symonds, H. W. and Ash, R., 1975. Some observations on metabolite production and utilization *in vivo* by the gut and liver of adult dairy cows, *J. agric. Sci., Camb.* **85**: 281–96.

Ballard, F. J., Filsell, O. H. and Jarrett, I. G., 1976. Amino acid uptake and output by the sheep hind limb, *Metabolism* **25**: 415–8.

Bartlett, S., Brown, B. B., Foot, A. S., Head, M. J., Line, C., Rook, J. A. F., Rowland, S. J. and Zundel, G., 1957. Field investigations into hypomagnesaemia in dairy cattle, with particular reference to changes in the concentration of blood constituents during the early grazing period, *J. agric. Sci., Camb.* **49**: 291–300.

Benevenga, N. J. and Harper, A. E., 1967. Alleviation of methionine and homocystine toxicity in the rat, *J. Nutr.* **93**: 44–52.

Bergmann, E. N., 1977. Glucose metabolism in ruminants. In *Proc. 3rd int. Conf. Prod. Diseases Fm Anim.* (ed. P. W. M., Van Adrichem). pp. 25–9. Centre for Agricultural Publishing and Documentation, Wageningen.

Bergmann, E. N. and Kon, K., 1964. Acetoacetate turnover and oxidation rates in ovine pregnancy ketosis, *Am. J. Physiol.* **206**: 449–52.

Bessman, S. P. and Bessman, A. N., 1955. The cerebral and peripheral uptake of ammonia in liver disease with an hypothesis for the mechanism of hepatic coma, *J. clin. Invest.* **34**: 622–8.

Blaxter, K. L., 1956. The magnesium content of bone in hypomagnesaemic disorders of livestock. In *Ciba Symp. Bone Struct. Metab.* (ed. G. E. W. Wolstenholme and Cecilia M. O'Connor), pp. 117–34. Churchill, London.

Blaxter, K. L., Rook, J. A. F. and MacDonald, A. M., 1954. Experimental magnesium deficiency in calves. 1. Clinical and pathological observations, *J. comp. Path. Ther.* **64**: 157–75.

Blum, J. W., Ramberg, C. F., Johnson, K. G. and Kronfeld, D. S., 1972. Calcium (ionized and total), magnesium, phosphorus and glucose in plasma from parturient cows, *Am. J. vet Res.* **33**: 51–6.

Boda, J. M. and Cole, H. H., 1954. The influence of dietary calcium and phosphorus on the incidence of milk fever in dairy cattle, *J. Dairy Sci.* **37**: 360–72.

Boorman, K. N., 1981. Regulation of protein and amino acid intake. In *Food Intake Regulation in Poultry* (ed. K. N. Boorman and B. M. Freeman). British Poultry Science Ltd, Edinburgh.

Boorman, K. N. and Fisher, H., 1966. The arginine–lysine interaction in the chick, *Br. Poult. Sci.* **7**: 39–44.

Braide, V. B. C. and Dunlop, R. H., 1969. Pharmacologic differences between sodium D-lactate and sodium L-lactate in sheep, *Am. J. vet. Res.* **30**: 1281–8.

Brockman, R. P. and Johnson, Marilyn R., 1977. Evidence of a role for glucagon in regulating glucose and β-hydroxybutyrate metabolism in sheep, *Can. J. Anim. Sci.* **57**: 177–80.

Bruce, L. A. and Huber, T. L., 1973. Inhibitory effect of acid in the intestine on rumen motility in sheep, *J. Anim. Sci.* **37**: 164–8.

Buttery, P. J., 1970. Glutamine synthetase activity in the ruminant spleen, *Biochim. biophys. Acta* **198**: 616–7.

Buttery, P. J. and Annison, E. F., 1971. Considerations of the efficiency of amino acid and protein metabolism in animals. In the *Biological Efficiency of Protein Production* (ed. J. G., Watkin-Jones), pp. 141–172. Cambridge University Press, Cambridge.

Care, A. D., 1967. Magnesium homeostasis in ruminants, *WldRev. Nutr. Diet.* **8**: 127–42.

Care, A. D. and van't Klooster, A. T., 1965. *In vivo* transport of magnesium and other cations across the wall of the gastro-intestinal tract of sheep, *J. Physiol., Lond.* **177**: 174–91.

Chalmers, M. L., Jaffray, A. E. and White, F., 1971. Movement of ammonia following intraruminal administration of urea or casein, *Proc. Nutr. Soc.* **30**: 7–17.

Chalupa, W., 1972. Metabolic aspects of non-protein nitrogen utilization in ruminant animals, *Fedn Proc. Fedn Am. Socs exp. Biol.* **31**: 1152–64.

Chalupa, W., Clark, J., Opliger, Pamela and Lavker, R., 1970. Detoxication of ammonia in sheep fed soy protein or urea, *J. Nutr.* **100**: 170–6.

Chicco, C. F., 1968. Some nutritional aspects of dietary magnesium in ruminants and poultry, *Diss. Abstr. Ser. B* **29**: 1B

Child, C. M., 1920. Some considerations concerning the nature and origin of physiological gradients, *Biol. Bull. mar. biol. Lab., Woods Hole* **39**: 147–87.

Costa, N. D., McIntosh, G. H. and Snoswell, A. M., 1976. Production of endogenous acetate by the liver in lactating ewes, *Aust. J. biol. Sci.* **29**: 33–42.

Dang, H. C. and Visek, W. J., 1964. Some effects of urease administration on laboratory animals, *Am. J. Physiol.* **206**: 731–7.

Davies, D. C., Allen, W. M., Hoare, M. N., Pott, J. M., Riley, C. J., Sansom, B. F., Stenton, J. R. and Vagg, M. J., 1978. A field trial of 1α-hydroxycholecalciferol(1α-OH D₃) in the prevention of milk fever, *Vet. Rec.* **102**: 440–2.

Dirkson, G., 1970. Acidosis. In *Physiology of Digestion and Metabolism in the Ruminant* (ed. A. T. Phillipson), pp. 612–25. Oriel Press, Newcastle upon Tyne.

D'Mello, J. P. F. and Lewis, D., 1970. Amino acid interactions in chick nutrition. 2. Interrelationships between leucine, isoleucine and valine, *Br. Poult. Sci.* **11**: 313–23.

Dryerre, H. and Greig, J. R., 1925. Milk fever: its possible association with derangements in the internal secretions, *Vet. Rec. (New Ser.)* **5**: 225–31.

Dunlop, R. H., Hammond, P. B. and Stevens, C. H., 1964. D-Lactate in bovine blood following carbohydrate engorgement, *Fedn Proc. Fedn Am. Socs exp. Biol.* **23**: 262(Abstr.).

Dunlop, R. H. and Stefaniak, B. M., 1965. Absorption of lactic acid isomers from ovine intestinal loops. In *Proc. Rumen Function Conf., Chicago, Ill.*, p. 21.

Edrise, B. M., 1979. Magnesium absorption by the ruminant. *Ph. D. Thesis, Univ. Reading.*

Ender, F. and Dishington, I. W., 1970. Etiology and prevention of paresis puerperalis in dairy cows. In *Parturient Hypocalcaemia* (ed. J. J. B. Anderson), pp. 71–9. Academic Press, New York.

Erfle, J. D., Fisher, L. J. and Sauer, F., 1971. Effect of infusion of carnitine and glucose on blood glucose, ketones, and free fatty acids of ketotic cows, *J. Dairy Sci.* **54**: 673–80.

Field A. C. and Munro, C. S., 1977. The effect of site and quantity on the extent of absorption of Mg infused into the gastro-intestinal tract of the sheep, *J. agric. Sci., Camb.* **89**: 365–71.

Fisher, H., Griminger, P., Leville, G. A. and Shapiro, R., 1960. Quantitative aspects of lysine deficiency and amino acid imbalance, *J. Nutr.* **71**: 213–20.

Fitt, T. J., Hutton, K. and Armstrong, D. G., 1979. Site of absorption of magnesium from the ovine tract, *Proc. Nutr. Soc.* **38**: 65A (Abstr.).

Fitt, T. J., Hutton, K. and Otto, W. R., 1974. Relative affinities of isolated cell walls of rumen bacteria for calcium and magnesium ions, *Proc. Nutr. Soc.* **33**: 106A(Abstr.).

Goings, R. L., Jacobson, N. L. and Littledike, E. T., 1971. Responses of cows to a very low calcium intake at parturition, *J. Dairy Sci.* **54**: 791–2.

Grace, N. D. and MacRae, J. C., 1972. Influence of feeding regimen and protein supplementation on the sites of net absorption of magnesium in sheep, *Br. J. Nutr.* **27**: 51–5.

Hammond, J., 1944. Physiological factors affecting birth weight, *Proc. Nutr. Soc.* **2**: 8–14.

Hansard, S. L., Comar, C. L. and Davis, G. K., 1954. Effects of age upon the physiological behaviour of calcium in cattle, *Am. J. Physiol.* **177**: 383–9.

Harper, A. E., 1956. Amino acid imbalances, toxicities and antagonisms, *Nutr. Rev.* **14**: 225–7.

Harper, A. E., Benevenga, N. J. and Wohlhueter, R. M., 1970. Effects of ingestion of disproportionate amounts of amino acids, *Physiol. Rev.* **50**: 428–558.

Head, M. J. and Rook, J. A. F., 1955. Hypomagnesaemia in dairy cattle and its possible relationship to ruminal ammonia production, *Nature, Lond.* **176**: 262–3.

Heitzman, R. J., Herriman, I. D. and Mallinson, C. B., 1972. Some effects of glucocorticoids on the subcellular distribution of the activities of citrate synthase and phosphoenolpyruvate carboxykinase in livers of rats and cows, *FEBS Lett.* **20**: 19–21.

Hogan, J. P. and Weston, R. H., 1967. The digestion of chopped and ground roughages by sheep. II. The digestion of nitrogen and some carbohydrate fractions in the stomach and intestines, *Aust. J. agric. Res.* **18**: 803–19.

Hopgood, M. F., 1965. Isolation and metabolism of cellulolytic ruminococci, *Ph. D. Thesis, Univ. Adelaide.*

Horn, J. P. and Smith, R. H., 1978. Absorption of magnesium by the young steer, *Br. J. Nutr.* **40**: 473–84.

Huber, T. L., 1971. Effect of acute indigestion on compartmental water volumes and osmolality in sheep, *Am. J. vet. Res.* **32**: 887–90.

Huber, T. L., 1976. Physiology of systemic lactic acidosis. In *Buffers in Ruminant Physiology and Metabolism* (ed. M. S. Weinberg and Sheffner), pp. 96–103. Port City Press, Baltimore, Md.

Jacquez, J. A., Poppell, J. W. and Jeltsch, R., 1959. Solubility of ammonia in human plasma, *J. appl. Physiol.* **14**: 255–8.

Jones, J. D., Wolters, R. and Burnett, P. C., 1966. Lysine-arginine-electrolyte relationships in the rat, *J. Nutr.* **89**: 171–88.

Jönsson, G. and Pehrson, B., 1969. Studies on the denner syndrome in dairy cows, *Zentbl. VetMed. Ser. A* **16**: 757–84.

Juhász, B. and Szegedi, B., 1968. Pathogenesis of rumen overload in sheep, *Acta vet. hung.* **18**: 63–80.

Juhász, B., Szegedi, B. and Keresztes, M., 1975. The effect of dietary nitrogen level on electrolyte and water metabolism in sheep. In *Tracer Studies on Non-protein Nitrogen for Ruminants*, Vol. 2, pp. 123–132. International Atomic Energy Authority, Vienna.

Katanuma, N., Okada, M. and Nishi, Y., 1967. Regulation of the urea cycle and TCA cycle by ammonia. In *Advances in Enzyme Regulation* (ed. G. Weber), Vol. 4, pp 317–36. Pergamon Press, Oxford.

Katz, M. L. and Bergman, E. N., 1969. Hepatic and portal metabolism of glucose, free fatty acids, and ketone bodies in the sheep, *Am. J. Physiol.* **216**: 953–60.

Kellog, D. W., Balok, C. J. and Miller, D. D., 1971. Method for experimental induction of ketosis utilizing the interaction of low energy intake and thyroxine, *J. Dairy Sci.* **54**: 1499–1504.

Keshavarz, K. and Fuller, H. L., 1971. Relationship of arginine and methionine in the nutrition of the chick and the significance of creatine biosynthesis in their interaction, *J. Nutr.* **101**: 217–22.

Kowalczyk, D. F. and Mayer, G. P., 1972. Cation concentration in skeletal muscle of paretic and nonparetic cows, *Am. J. vet. Res.* **33**: 751–7.

Krebs, H. A., 1966. Bovine ketosis, *Vet. Rec.* **78**: 187–91.

Kronfeld, D. S., 1965. Growth hormone-induced ketosis in the cow, *J. Dairy Sci.* **48**: 342–6.

Kronfeld, D. S., 1971. Parturient hypocalcaemia in dairy cows, *Adv. Vet. Sci. & Comp. Med.* **15**: 133–57.

Kronfeld, D. S., Raggi, F. and Ramberg, C. F., 1968. Mammary blood flow and ketone body metabolism in normal, fasted and ketotic cows, *Am. J. Physiol.* **215**: 218–27.

Kumta, U. S. and Harper, A. E., 1962. Amino acid balance and imbalance. IX. Effect of amino acid imbalance on blood amino acid pattern, *Proc. Soc. exp. Biol. Med.* **110**: 512–7.

Ladrat, J., Larvor, P. and Brochart, M., 1959. [Research into some cases of grass tetany] *ReclMéd. vét. Éc. Alfort* **135**: 903–36.

Leech, F. B., Davis, M. E., Macrae, W. D. and Withers, F. W., 1960. *Disease Wastage and Husbandry in the British Dairy Herd. Survey 1957–1958.* Her Majesty's Stationery Office, London.

Leng, R. A. and West, C. E., 1969. Contribution of acetate, butyrate, palmitate, stearate and oleate to ketone body synthesis in sheep, *Res. vet. Sci.* **10**: 57–63.

Leonard, M. C., Buttery, P. J. and Lewis, D., 1977. The effects on glucose metabolism of feeding a high-urea diet to sheep, *Br. J. Nutr.* **38**: 455–62.

Leung, P. M.-B., Rogers, Q. R. and Harper, A. E., 1968. Effect of amino acid imbalance on dietary choice in the rat, *J. Nutr.* **95**: 483–92.

Lewis, D., 1965. The concept of agent and target in amino acid interactions, *Proc. Nutr. Soc.* **24**: 196–202.

Lewis, D. and Buttery, P. J., 1973. Ammonia toxicity in ruminants. In *Production Disease in Farm Animals* (ed. J. M. Payne, K. G. Hibbitt and B. F. Sansom), pp. 201–11. Baillière Tindall, London.

Lewis, D., Hill, K. J. and Annison, E. F., 1957. Studies on the portal blood of sheep. 1. Absorption of ammonia from the rumen of the sheep, *Biochem. J.* **66**: 587–92.

Lindsay, D. B. and Setchell, B. P., 1976. The oxidation of glucose, ketone bodies and acetate by the brain of normal and ketonaemic sheep, *J. Physiol., Lond.* **259**: 801–23.

Lucas, I. A. M., 1962. Aspects of the nutrition of young pigs. In *Nutrition of Pigs and Poultry* (ed. J. T. Morgan and D. Lewis), pp. 238–54. Butterworth, London.

Lund, Patricia, Brosnan, J. T. and Eggleston, K. V., 1970. The regulation of ammonia metabolism in mammalian tissues. In *Essays in Cell*

Metabolism (ed. W. Bartley, H. L. Kornberg and J. R. Quale), pp. 167–88. Wiley, London.

McGarry, J. D., Meier, J. M. and Foster, D. W., 1973. The effects of starvation and refeeding on carbohydrate and lipid metabolism *in vivo* and in the perfused rat liver, *J. biol. Chem.* **248**: 270–88.

MacGregor, R. C. and Armstrong, D. G., 1979. The effect of increasing potassium intake on absorption of magnesium, *Proc. Nutr. Soc.* **38**: 66A (Abstr.).

Madsen, F. C., Lentz, D. E., Miller, J. K., Lowrey-Harnden, D. and Hansard, S. L., 1976. Dietary carbohydrate effects upon magnesium metabolism in sheep, *J. Anim. Sci.* **42**: 1316–22.

Manston, R. and Payne, J. M., 1964. Mineral imbalance in pregnant "milk-fever-prone" cows and the value and possible toxic effects of treatment with vitamin D_3 and dihydrotachysterol, *Br. vet. J.* **120**: 167–77.

Martens, H., Harmeyer, J. and Michael, H., 1978. Magnesium transport by isolated rumen epithelium of sheep, *Res. vet. Sci.* **24**: 161–8.

Martens, H. and Rayssiguier, Y., 1979. Magnesium metabolism and hypomagnesaemia. In *Digestive Physiology and Metabolism in Ruminants* (ed. Y. Ruckebusch and P. Thivend), pp. 447–68. MTP Press, Lancaster.

Mayer, G. P., Ramberg, C. F. and Kronfeld, D. S., 1969. Calcium homeostasis in the cow, *Clin. Orthop.*, No. 62,: pp. 79–94.

Mayer, G. P., Ramberg, C. F., Kronfeld, D. S., Buckle, R. M., Sherwood, L. M., Aurbach, G. D. and Potts, J. T., 1969. Plasma parathyroid hormone concentration in hypocalcemic parturient cows, *Am. J. vet. Res.* **30**: 1587–97.

Miller, E. L., 1973. Evaluation of foods as sources of nitrogen and amino acids, *Proc. Nutr. Soc.* **32**: 79–84.

Møller, P. D. and Hvelplund, T., 1977. [Investigations into mineral metabolism in the gastro-intestinal tract of cattle.] *Beretn. St. Husdyrbrugs fors.*, No. 451.

Moodie, E. W. and Robertson, A., 1961. Dietary intake of the parturient cow, *Res. vet. Sci.* **2**: 217–26.

Morris, J. G. and Payne, E., 1970. Ammonia and urea toxicoses in sheep and their relation to dietary nitrogen intake, *J. agric. Sci., Camb.* **74**: 259–71.

Morrow, D. A., 1976. Fat cow syndrome, *J. Dairy Sci.* **59**: 1625–9.

Mullen, P. A., 1975. Clinical and biochemical responses to the treatment of milk fever, *Vet. Rec.* **97**: 87–92.

Newton, G. L., Fontenot, J. P., Tucker, R. E. and Polan, C. E., 1972. Effects of high dietary potassium intake on the metabolism of magnesium by sheep, *J. Anim. Sci.* **35**: 440–5.

Niedermeier, R. P., Smith, V. R. and Whitehair, C. K., 1949. Parturient paresis. III. A study of various blood constituents at parturition in mastectomized cows, *J. Dairy Sci.* **32**: 927–34.

Okorie, A. U., Buttery, P. J. and Lewis, D., 1977. Ammonia concentration and protein synthesis in the rumen, *Proc. Nutr. Soc.* **36**: 38A(Abstr.).

Payne, J. M., 1964. The responses of cows to experimentally induced hypocalcaemia, *Vet. Rec.* **76**: 77–81.

Payne, J. M., 1968. Milk fever, *Outl. Agric.* **5**: 266–72.

Payne, J. M., 1977. *Metabolic Diseases in Farm Animals*. Heineman Medical, London.

Pfeffer, E. and Rahman, K. A., 1974. Investigation of the location of magnesium absorption in ruminants. 2, *Z. Tierphysiol. Tierernähr. Futtermittelk.* **33**: 209–10.

Powley, G., Care, A. D. and Johnson, C. L., 1977. Comparison of the daily endogenous faecal magnesium excretion from sheep eating grass with high sodium or high potassium concentrations, *Res. vet. Sci.* **23**: 43–6.

Ramberg, C. F., Mayer, G. P., Kronfeld, D. S., Phang, J. M. and Berman, M., 1970. Calcium kinetics in cows during late pregnancy, parturition and early lactation, *Am. J. Physiol.* **219**: 1166–77.

Reid, I. M., Roberts, C. J. and Manston, R., 1979. Fatty liver and infertility in high-yielding dairy cows, *Vet. Rec.* **104**: 75–6.

Robertson, W. G., Lennon, H. D., Bailey, W. W. and Mixner, J. P., 1957. Interrelationships among plasma 17-hydroxycorticosteroid levels, plasma protein bound iodine levels and ketosis in dairy cattle, *J. Dairy Sci.* **40**: 732–8.

Rogers, Q. R. and Leung, P. M.-B., 1973. The influence of amino acids on the neuroregulation of food intake, *Fedn Proc. Fedn Am. Socs exp. Biol.* **32**: 1709–19.

Rogers, P. A. M. and van't Klooster, A. T., 1969. Observations on the digestion and absorption of food along the gastro-intestinal tract of fistulated cows. 3. The fate of sodium, potassium, calcium, magnesium and phosphorus in the digesta, *Meded. LandbHoogesch. Wageningen, No. 69–11,* pp. 26–39.

Rook, J. A. F. and Campling, R. C., 1965. Effect of stage and number of lactation on the yield and composition of cow's milk, *J. Dairy Res.* **32**: 45–55.

Rook, J. A. F. and Storry, J. E., 1962. Magnesium in the nutrition of farm animals, *Nutr. Abstr. Rev.* **32**: 1055–77.

Saba, N., 1964. Oestrogenic activity in plasma of pregnant cows, *J. Endocr.* **29**: 205–6.

Sansom, B. F., 1969. Calcium metabolism of cows at parturition and during milk production, *J. agric. Sci., Camb.* **72**: 455–8.

Satter, L. D. and Slyter, L. L., 1974. Effect of ammonia concentration on rumen microbial production in vitro, *Br. J. Nutr.* **32**: 199–208.

Simkiss, K., 1967. *Calcium in Reproductive Physiology*. Chapman and Hall, London.

Smith, R. H., 1962. Net exchange of certain inorganic ions and water in the alimentary tract of the milk-fed calf, *Biochem. J.* **83**: 151–63.

Smith, R. H., 1975. Nitrogen metabolism in the rumen and the composition and nutritive value of nitrogen compounds entering the duodenum. In *Digestion and Metablism in the Ruminant* (ed. I. W. McDonald and A. C. I. Warner), pp. 399–415. University of New England Publishing Unit, Armidale.

Smith, T. K. and Austic, R. E., 1978. The branched-chain amino acid antagonism in chicks, *J. Nutr.* **108**: 1180–91.

Smith, R. H. and Horn, J. P., 1976. Absorption of magnesium labelled with ^{28}Mg, from the stomach of the young steer. In *Nuclear Techniques in Animal Production and Health, Symp. IAEA/FAO, Vienna*, pp. 253–60.

Smith, G. H. and Lewis, D., 1966. Arginine in poultry nutrition. 3. Agent and target in amino acid interactions, *Br. J. Nutr.* **20**: 621–31.

Soar, J. B., Buttery, P. J. and Lewis, D., 1973. Ammonia toxicity in sheep, *Proc. Nutr. Soc.* **32**: 77–8A(Abstr.).

Spolter, P. D. and Harper, A. E., 1961. Leucine-isoleucine antagonism in the rat, *Am. J. Physiol.* **200**: 513–8.

Storry, J. E. and Rook, J. A. F., 1963. Magnesium metabolism in the dairy cow. V. Experimental observations with a purified diet low in magnesium, *J. agric. Sci., Camb.* **61**: 167–71.

Strachan, N. H. and Rook, J. A. F., 1975. Site of magnesium absorption in sheep, *Proc. Nutr. Soc.* **34**: 11–2A(Abstr.).

Symonds, H. W., Manston, R., Payne, J. M. and Sansom, B. F., 1966. Changes in the calcium and phosphorous requirements of the dairy cow at parturition with particular reference to the amounts supplied to the foetus *in utero, Br. vet. J.* **122**: 196–200.

Symonds, H. W. and Treacher, R. J., 1967. The experimental induction of hypophosphataemia in goats using anion exchange columns, *J. Physiol., Lond.* **193**: 619–29.

Tomas, F. M. and Potter, B. J., 1976a. Interaction between sites of magnesium absorption in the digestive tract of the sheep, *Aust. J. agric. Res.* **27**: 437–46.

Tomas, F. M. and Potter, B. J., 1976b. The site of magnesium absorption from the ruminant stomach, *Br. J. Nutr.* **36**: 37–45.

Treacher, R. J., Baird, G. D. and Young, J. L., 1976. Anti-ketogenic effect of glucose in the lactating cow deprived of food, *Biochem. J.* **158**: 127–34.

Ulshafer, T. R., 1958. The measurement of charges in acetylcholine level (ACR) in rat brain following ammonium ion intoxication and its probable bearing on the problem of hepatic coma, *J. Lab. clin. Med.* **52**: 718–23.

Wethli, E., Morris, T. R. and Shresta, T. P., 1975. The effect of feeding high levels of low-quality proteins to growing chickens, *Br. J. Nutr.* **34**: 363–73.

Whitlock, R. H., 1973. Abomasal displacement: a disorder of throughput. In *Production Disease in Farm Animals* (ed. J. M. Payne, K. G. Hibbitt and B. F. Sansom), pp. 230–1. Baillière Tindall, London.

Zammit, V. A., 1980. The maximum activities and intracellular distribution of enzymes involved in ketogenesis and its regulation in livers of ruminants, *Biochem. Soc. Trans.* **8**: 543–4.

Zammit, V. A., Beis, A. and Newsholme, E. A., 1979. The role of 3-oxo acid-CoA transferase in the regulation of ketogenesis in the liver, *FEBS Lett.* **103**: 212–5.

10 MICRONUTRIENTS AS REGULATORS OF METABOLISM

N. F. Suttle

HISTORICAL PERSPECTIVE

At the beginning of the 20th century it was becoming evident that simplified diets comprised of the four then known nutrients – carbohydrate, protein, fat and salts – did not allow animals to thrive (Hopkins, 1906). Crude extracts of complete foods were found to provide certain missing factors and it was not long before the first, present in certain fats, was identified and termed vitamin A. The discovery of new vitamins became a regular occurrence and the recognition of vitamin K as an essential antihaemorrhagic factor in 1935 brought the total of essential organic micronutrients to 11 (McCollum, 1957). The elucidation of specific biochemical and physiological rôles for the vitamins proved much more difficult and the main rôle of vitamin A has only recently been discovered (De Luca, 1978). The identification of essential inorganic micronutrients proceeded at a less frenetic pace and is almost certainly incomplete: seven (Cu, Mn, Zn, Co, Mo, Se and Cr) were identified between 1930 and 1959 (Underwood, 1977) and, after a quiescent period, five more were identified in the early 1970s (Sn, Ni, V, F and Si) (Mertz, 1974). Limits to the purity of diet and environment have yet to be reached which will allow the discovery of further essential elements. Biochemical rôles for the essential elements, both old and new, are still being discovered and our understanding of the complex interactions between micronutrients is still in its infancy. It is therefore important to realize from the outset that micronutrient science is young and relatively underdeveloped.

MICRONUTRIENTS AS BIOLOGICAL ACTIVISTS

Micronutrients attain their biological potency in four different ways, through associations with coenzymes, enzymes, metalloproteins and hormones. The B vitamins commonly act as assistants (*cofactors* or *coenzymes*) to the prime movers (*enzymes*) of a biochemical transformation by providing a temporary respository for the functional unit which is being moved or modified. Thus biotin facilitates the action of pyruvate- and acetylcoenzyme-A-decarboxylases by acting as a carrier for carbon dioxide. Many of the B vitamins themselves require modification (e.g. phosphorylation) before they can function as coenzymes. In some instances the B vitamin is merely the active unit (*prosthetic group*) within the coenzyme: such a relationship exists between pantothenic acid and coenzyme-A.

Trace elements generally gain essentiality through their presence in proteins with catalytic properties (*metalloenzymes*). They sometimes promote enzyme activity by forming a vital locus in the enzyme molecule, as manganese does in pyruvate decarboxylase, facilitating the binding of enzyme and substrate by aligning reactive sites. The contrasting relationships between three micronutrients and enzyme function is illustrated in Fig. 10.1. Removal of the metal from

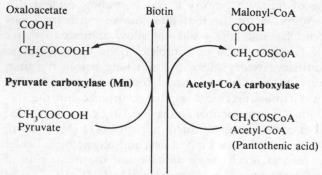

Fig. 10.1.   The contrasting rôles of biotin as coenzyme, manganese as metalloenzyme (in pyruvate carboxylase) and pantothenic acid as prosthetic group (in coenzyme-A) in the biochemical process of carboxylation (both reactions also require ATP).

enzymes such as pyruvate carboxylase by chelation leaves an *apoenzyme* which is catalytically inert because it cannot link with its substrate. There are other metalloenzymes in which the metal is responsible for the subsequent reactivity of the enzyme-substrate complex. The zinc-containing digestive enzyme carboxypeptidase comes into this category: apocarboxypeptidase will combine with substrate to give a catalytically inert complex, i.e. there is substrate inhibition of activity. Studies of the reactivity of carboxypeptidase as apo- or holo-enzyme with alternative cofactors (cobalt and nickel), and with various substrates and inhibitors, have revealed the potential complexity of metalloenzyme function (Vallee, 1964 and 1974). Some apoenzymes require the activating metal to be incorporated at synthesis (e.g. copper in apocaeruloplasmin to give ferroxidase activity (Holtzman and Gaumnitz, 1970)) whereas others can be readily reactivated *in vitro* by exposure to the cofactor (e.g. carboxypeptidase).

The reactivity of metal-protein complexes sometimes allows them to perform independent metabolic functions unassociated with enzyme activity. These can take the form of reactions in which the *metalloprotein* moves with a complexed ion or molecule, thus performing a transport function. A classical example is afforded by the rôle of iron in haemoglobin, which transports oxygen between the lungs and the tissues. Fe is part of the prosthetic haem group of this conjugated protein. Metalloproteins also function in absorptive and storage rôles.

Some of the fat-soluble vitamins are now regarded as dietary precursors of metabolites with hormone-like properties (Morton, 1974). The calciferols (vitamin D) only become metabolically active after a two-stage hydroxylation process, begun in the liver and completed in the kidney. The latter process is under endocrine control and yields a 1,25-dihydroxycholecalciferol $(1,25(OH)_2C)$ which influences the synthesis of calcium-binding protein in the intestinal mucosa (Fraser, 1975). The aldehyde of vitamin A (retinol) combines with the protein opsin to yield the light-sensitive rhodopsin on which the visual cycle depends. The hormonal activity of thyroxine, the iodinated amino acid tyrosine, provides a solitary example of direct trace-element involvement in endocrine function.

SCOPE OF REGULATORY ACTIVITIES

The range of metabolic rôles for a particular micronutrient commonly depends on three factors: the number of 'activists' of which it is whole or part, the number of biochemical transformations which each activist can assist and the distribution of these active forms in the body.

The B vitamins are restricted by their very nature to a single coenzyme activity but gain breadth of activity in some instances by performing functions which are useful to a wide range of enzymes (Table 10.1). Thus nicotinic acid and riboflavin, as NAD or NADP and as FMN or FAD, respectively, assist in a vast array of reactions

Table 10.1   The coenzyme forms and functions of the B vitamins

B vitamin	Coenzyme form	Function
Thiamine (B$_1$)	Thiamine pyrophosphate	Aerobic decarboxylation Transfer of aldehyde group
Riboflavin (B$_2$)	Flavin mononucleotide (FMN)	
	Flavin adenine dinucleotide (FAD)	Transfer of H$^+$ + e$^-$
Niacin (Nicotinic acid)	Nicotinamide adenine dinucleotide (NAD)	
	Nicotinamide adenine dinucleotide phosphate (NADP)	Transfer of H$^+$ + e$^-$, glycolysis, etc.
Pyridoxine (B$_6$)	Pyridoxal phosphate	Transamination Decarboxylation Racemisation
Pantothenic acid	Coenzyme-A	Transfer of acyl groups
		Aerobic degradation and synthesis of fatty acids
Biotin	Biotin	Transfer of CO$_2$
Folic Acid	Tetrahydrofolic acid	Transfer of methyl groups
Vitamin B$_{12}$	5-Deoxyadenosyl cobalamin	Isomerisation of methylmalonyl-CoA to succinyl-CoA
	Methylcobalamin	Transfer of methyl groups

involving oxidation/reduction and electron transfer. Similarly, pantothenic acid is involved in all the reactions requiring coenzyme-A. Nutritional deficiencies of these multireactive vitamins produce rapid and drastic signs of deficiency, usually terminating in death. On the other hand, coenzyme B$_{12}$ (5-deoxyadenosyl cobalamin) is involved only in the isomerization of methylmalonate and succinate (Fig. 10.2). Futhermore, a small change in the ligand, creating methyl cobalamin, produces a coenzyme with a totally different but equally specific function, that of methylating homocysteine to give methionine (Fig. 10.2). The symptoms of B$_{12}$ deficiency, loss of weight, neurological disorders and anaemia, are slow to develop. Another vitamin of limited activity is the fat-soluble vitamin K. Its only known function is to

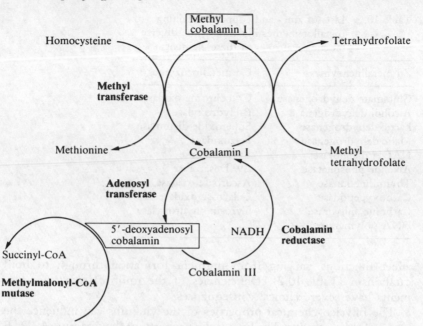

Fig. 10.2. Analogues of vitamin B$_{12}$ (cobalamin) which act as coenzymes in the metabolism of succinate (5'-deoxyadenosyl cobalamin) and methionine (methyl cobalamin I); the latter is also involved in the metabolism of folate.

facilitate, by mechanisms are yet unknown, the carboxylation of the four protein factors necessary for thrombin formation (Suttie and Jackson, 1977). The only physiological effect of vitamin K deficiency is therefore an impaired clotting mechanism.

The trace elements are restricted in their activities in so far as the enzymes with which they are associated form specific structural relationships or bonds with their substrates. Thus the molybdenum-containing flavoprotein, xanthine oxidase, which catalyses the conversion of hypoxanthine and xanthine to uric acid, has no other known catalytic activity than that of an aldehyde oxidase. Mo deficiency is rarely encountered and is difficult to induce experimentally except in the chick, which may have a particularly high requirement for Mo and xanthine oxidase in being exclusively dependent on the uric acid pathway for nitrogen excretion. Some elements, however, have widespread metabolic activity because they are associated with many different enzymes. Zn is foremost in this respect, being associated with at least 10 different enzymes (Table 10.2), affecting such diverse functions as protein digestion, respiration and bone mineralization. Similarly, Cu is an essential part of 9 different enzymes whose activities

Table 10.2   Lists of zinc- and copper-containing
metalloenzymes illustrating the diverse
biochemical rôles of these elements

Zn metalloenzymes	Cu metalloenzymes
Glutamate dehydrogenase	Cytochrome oxidase
Alcohol dehydrogenase	β-Hydroxylase
Lactic dehydrogenase	Superoxide dismutase
Malic dehydrogenase	Ferroxidase
NADH diaphorase	Lysyl oxidase
Alkaline phosphatase	Δ9, Desaturase
Thymidine kinase	Ascorbate oxidase
Carboxypeptidase	Galactose oxidase
Carbonic anhydrase	Tyrosine hydroxylase
DNA polymerase	

affect functions varying from pigment formation through to lipid catabolism (Table 10.2). Deficiencies of the multireactive trace elements have severe clinical consequences.

The physico-chemical properties of the vitamins can influence the scope of their activity. The lipophylic property of the vitamins A, D, E and K influences their distribution in a number of ways. They are associated with the chylomicrons of the lymphatic system immediately after absorption, which is assisted by the detergent activity of bile salts. Subsequently they may be transported as lipoproteins or as complexes with α-globulins to the lipid-containing cell membranes, where some of their metabolic rôles are played. By contrast, the low molecular weight and water solubility of B vitamins ensures their ubiquitous presence throughout the body. Their activities are therefore restricted primarily by the distribution of the less mobile and higher molecular weight enzymes with which they are associated: these are often confined to the cell nucleus, mitochondria or microsomes.

The trace element-containing enzymes may be confined in their activity by their localization in particular cells or organs, e.g. Zn-containing carbonic anhydrase in the erythrocyte and procarboxypeptidase in the pancreas. On the other hand, the involvement of Zn in DNA and RNA polymerase and thymidine kinase activity places it in a crucial position with regard to the multiplication and development of every living cell (Chesters, 1974).

Many of the biochemical and physiological rôles of the micronutrients are recent discoveries; for example, the rôles of Cu in superoxide dismutase (Fridovich, 1972) and selenium in glutathione peroxidase (GSHPx) (Flohé, Gunzler and Shock, 1973) were both established in the last decade. In some cases the early recognition of visible localized lesions in the deficiency state, such as those of the skin (scurvy) in vitamin C deficiency and those of the eye (xerophthalmia) in vitamin A deficiency, has proved unhelpful in identifying specific biochemical lesions underlying these particular deficiencies. It would therefore be a simpler and safer exercise to enumerate those metabolic and developmental processes which did not depend in some way on micronutrients than to attempt to define fully the scope of their regulatory rôles.

THE EXTENT OF MICRONUTRIENT INTERACTIONS

It is to be expected that highly reactive substances such as the micronutrients are also highly interactive: the outcome of these interactions is often antagonistic rather than synergistic, and potentially harmful to the animal. The mechanisms of interaction can be classified into four broad types.

Related properties

The biochemical and physiological properties of an element or an organic molecule depend upon its chemical structure and micronutrients of similar structure are likely to interact because their properties overlap. Interactions between trace elements from the transition series in the periodic table have been predicted from similarities in the energy content and special arrangement of their orbital electrons (Matrone, 1974). Thus cadmium is able to induce a deficiency of Zn, its neighbour in group II, and similar antagonisms occur between tungsten and Mo in group VI, and between silver and Cu in group XI. Physico-chemical similarities may allow the antagonist to associate with common binding groups on carrier proteins for example, the stronger affinity constants of the heavier element in each pair allowing it to inhibit competitively absorption of the lighter element. Interactions of this type occur between anions as well as cations and are believed to be responsible for the inhibition of MoO_4^{2-} absorption by the similar tetrahedral SO_4^{2-} anion in the small intestine (Mason and Cardin, 1977). Interactions between vitamins do not fall into this category because they differ vastly in chemical structure from each other but vitamin function may be impaired by physiologically useless analogues. Pyridoxine deficiency may be induced by deoxypyridoxine, and thiamine deficiency by amprolium supplementation of the diet (Morgan, 1974).

Related functions

Micronutrients with dissimilar properties can interact with each other along a common metabolic pathway. The generation of methyl cobalamin for example involves the demethylation of methyl tetrahydrofolic acid (Fig. 10.2). The latter accumulates in the plasma during vitamin B_{12} deficiency at the expense of tetrahydrofolic acid, which acts as a coenzyme – along with pyridoxal phosphate – to an important amino acid conversion, that of serine to glycine (Herbert and Das, 1976). Thus the potential for a three-way vitamin interaction arises. Other examples of the related functions of vitamins are cited by Sauberlich (1980).

The scope for such interactions is not confined to the vitamins. For example, deficiencies of Se and vitamin E have clinical features in common and each can ameliorate two clinical signs (exudative diathesis and muscular dystrophy) of the alternate deficiency in chicks. The mutual substitutiveness of vitamin E and Se arises because they both have anti-oxidant functions that influence the stability of biological membranes. Vitamin E may contribute to the structural integrity of the membrane whilst Se limits the attack of hydroperoxides upon it (through their destruction via GSHPx) (Diplock, 1974). Intriguing differences exist, however, in that a third condition, encephalomalacia, is responsive only to vitamin E in avian species. Scott (1962) concluded that vitamin E had at least three distinct functions in the animal of which only two were shared by Se. Recent evidence, that pyridoxal phosphate may add to its pluralistic rôle by facilitating the incorporation of Se from selenomethionine into the enzyme GSHPx (Yasumoto, Iwami and Yoshida, 1979), merely confirms that the interplay of micronutrient functions is complex and far from completely understood.

Interactions may also occur because the function performed by the micronutrient is not completely specific. Thus vitamin D stimulates the absorption of phosphorus, Co and lead, as well as Ca (Smith, De Luca, Tanaka and Mahaffey, 1978; Masuhara and Migicovsky, 1963).

Metabolic dependencies

The metabolism of some micronutrients is dependent upon others, giving obvious scope for nutritional interactions. The transport of Fe^{3+} bound to transferrin in plasma is dependent on the activity of the Cu-enzyme, ferroxidase (Frieden, 1971). A dietary deficiency of Cu can therefore prevent mobilization of Fe from the liver stores and its incorporation into haemoglobin giving rise to anaemia (Lee, Ragan,

Nacht and Cartwright, 1969). A dietary deficiency of Zn may have a similar effect on the transport of vitamin A by limiting the synthesis of retinol-binding protein (Smith, Brown and Cassidy, 1977). There has been some debate on the possibility that folate deficiency interferes with the absorption of other micronutrients by inducing morphological changes in the mucosa of the small intestine, but an impairment of thiamine deficiency has been established (Howard, Wagner and Schender, 1974).

Mutual incompatibilities

Situations can arise in which it is physico-chemically impossible for two or three nutrients to remain in solution in a physiological fluid; as a result of their interation, the micronutrients become insoluble and lose their capacity for biological activity. Examples are provided by the formation of insoluble copper selenides in chicks on diets high in Cu and Se (Hill, 1974), and unabsorbable copper thiomolybdates in sheep on diets rich in Mo and sulphur (Dick, Dewey and Gawthorne, 1975; Grace and Suttle, 1978); both of these interactions are located in the gut.

REGULATION OF MICRONUTRIENT METABOLISM

The metabolism of highly active and interactive substances such as the micronutrients is as important as their regulatory activity. Normal growth and development are insured against the vagaries of dietary composition and changes in the animal's basic requirements by a variety of processes which provide a relatively constant micronutrient milieu for metabolic activity. These *homeostatic mechanisms* are important not only for ensuring that each micronutrient fulfils its physiological function but also that it does not accumulate in sufficient amounts for its reactivity to be toxic to other metabolic processes. The cumulative effects of homeostatic activity are reflected by non-linearity in responses within the body to changes in micronutrient input: the curvilinear responses in plasma Zn in sheep and Cu in pigs given various intakes of Zn and Cu can be used as examples (Fig. 10.3). Some authors have gone so far as to suggest that evidence for homeostatic control is indeed evidence of the essentiality of a micronutrient (Cotzias, 1964). The general involvement of homeostatic mechanisms in micronutrient metabolism is reflected in a great variability in their absorption and

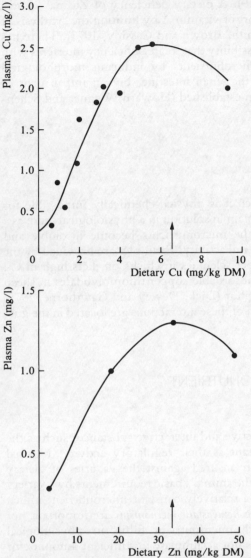

Fig 10.3.   Non-linear relationships between biochemical parameters and micronutrient intake, as illustrated by the changes in blood plasma concentration of copper in piglets (Okonkwo, Ku, Miller, Keahey and Ullrey, 1979) and zinc in lambs (Ott, Smith, Stob, Parker, Harrington and Beeson, 1965) in response to alterations in the dietary content of the elements. The arrows indicate the point below which homeostatic control begins to fail and there is transition from the depletion to the deficiency state.

retention compared with that of the major nutrients comprising the energy and protein portions of the diet. The nature of homeostatic control, however, varies widely both within and between the principal micronutrient groups.

Trace elements

The regulation of trace element metabolism in the face of wide variations in intake is illustrated in Fig. 10.4, using data from an experiment with rats (Weigand and Kirchgessner, 1978). The coefficient of Zn absorption decreases linearly from 1.0 on a ZN-deficient diet to 0.37 on a diet providing about six times more than the Zn requirement. At the same time, the proportion of the absorbed Zn excreted via the faeces increases from 0.05 to 0.46. Urinary excretion, however, makes

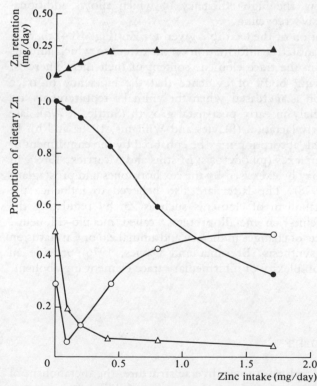

Fig. 10.4. Changes in the proportion of dietary zinc absorbed (●), in absorbed Zn excreted in faeces (○) and in urine (△), and in the amount of Zn retained (▲), in rats given a wide range of Zn intakes. (After Weigand and Kichgessner, 1978.)

no contribution to the preservation of stable Zn balance at the higher Zn intakes.

There are considerable variations between elements, between species and within species in the manner in which homeostasis is attained. Whereas Fe retention is regulated predominantly by absorptive control mechanisms in all species (Underwood, 1977), Mn retention is regulated primarily by the level of gastro-intestinal secretion, at least in the bovine (Sansom, Vagg and Taylor, 1973). Urinary excretion plays little or no part in the regulation of heavy-metal metabolism, presumably because of the protein-bound state in which they are transported. However, those elements that circulate in anionic forms, such as iodine, Mo and Se, are often excreted predominantly in the urine and, in simple-stomached species in particular, control of urinary excretion provides the principle mechanism for controlling the retention of these elements. In ruminants, both I (Miller, Swanson, Spalding, Lyke and Hall, 1974) and Mo (Suttle and Grace, 1978) are secreted prior to the sites of absorption, the high efficiency of which allows additional control via extensive recycling.

With the exception of the example given for Zn (Fig. 10.4) there is relatively little quantitative information on the extent to which animals adapt to changes in the trace element content of their diet. There is, however, a growing body of evidence that the efficiency of trace element absorption is increased when the animal's requirements are at their peak, namely in early post-natal growth (Suttle, 1979b), late pregnancy and early lactation (Davies and Williams, 1976a and b). In the suckling animal, absorption may be enhanced by the engulfment of metal-protein complexes (pinocytosis: Mistilis and Mearrick, 1969). In later life control may be exercised by the sex hormones and prostaglandins (Cousins, 1978). The latter are also believed to influence the intermediary metabolism of elements such as Zn by regulating the synthesis of cysteine-rich metalloproteins, called metallo-thioneins. The multiple effects of changes in dietary and animal Zn or Cu status on metallo-thionein synthesis (Bremner and Davies, 1976) provide an insight into the complexity of intermediary trace element metabolism.

Fat-soluble vitamins

As might be expected from their diverse structure, the metabolism of the fat-soluble vitamins is subject to an array of different regulatory processes. With the seco-steroid vitamin D, the parathyroids are known to exert hormonal control over its final conversion to the biologically active form $1,25(OH)_2C$ in the kidney via a hydroxyl-

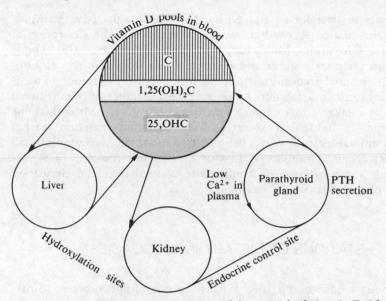

Fig. 10.5. A schematic representation of the control of vitamin D (cholecalciferol) (C) metabolism. Control is exercised by the parathyroid
gland, under the influence of the ionic calcium in the blood plasma;
parathyroid hormone (PTH) governs the rate of the second hydroxylation in the kidney which yields the potent, hormone-like,
form of the vitamin, 1,25-dihydroxycholecalciferol ($1,25(OH)_2C$).

ase enzyme. The prior hydroxylation to 25-hydroxycholecalciferol
(25,OHC) in the liver is poorly regulated so that plasma levels of
25,OHC reflect vitamin D intake and the plasma serves as a store from
which small amounts of $1,25(OH)_2C$ can be formed as needed (Fraser,
1975)(Fig. 10.5).

With vitamin A, the primary regulatory mechanism is the hepatic
storage of the vitamin. The rat is capable of storing 100 years' supply of
this micronutrient and in cattle the rate of mobilization of vitamin A
from the liver is governed by the size of the initial store (Dam and
Søndergaard, 1964). The excretion of the fat-soluble vitamins occurs
principally via the bile but there is little evidence on the extent to which
the regulation of excretion and absorption contribute to vitamin
homeostasis.

Water-soluble vitamins

The B vitamins are exceptional in that their metabolism appears to be
poorly regulated. Absorption generally occurs by the non-saturable
uncontrolled process of passive diffusion (cf. pyridoxine: Middleton,

1977; niacin: Henderson and Gross, 1979) although active transport processes may be invoked at low concentrations in the absorption of thiamine (Hoyumpa, Middleton, Wilson and Schenker, 1975). The B vitamins are poorly stored and any excess of absorption over requirement is excreted predominantly in the urine. Urinary excretion of the B vitamins or their metabolites is therefore a good indicator of nutritional status at intakes above requirement level. However, when thiamine deficiency is induced in sheep, urinary thiamine excretion reaches minimum values some weeks before blood thiamine concentrations fall (Evans, Evans, Humphreys, Lewin, Davies and Axford, 1975), indicating some measure of homeostatic control over the circulating levels of this particular B vitamin.

MANIFESTATIONS OF DIETARY INADEQUACIES

The body's homeostatic mechanisms are not omnicompetent. Situations arise in which the diet provides so little of a trace element, vitamin or pro-vitamin that synthesis of the bio-active form is less than catabolism and, in time, a functional deficiency may develop with visible signs of malaise. The interplay between constituents of the diet or digesta and the involvement of homeostatic mechanisms is such that it is often impossible to predict from dietary composition alone whether a particular nutritional regime will cause ill-health. In consequence, there has been considerable confusion about the precise levels of dietary requirements for micronutrients and the biochemical criteria of deficiency, which has not been helped by somewhat arbitrary terminology. A number of unarguable steps can, however, be identified along the path that leads to the nutritionally diseased state and they are illustrated in Fig. 10.6.

Terminology

Depletion
When excretion exceeds absorption, trace element concentrations in the body fall and the animal is depleted (Fig. 10.6, D_1). *Depletion* is accelerated by growth and is a relative term describing the failure of the diet to maintain an animal's initial trace-element status, which may be more than adequate. A similar phenomenon occurs with the vitamins although it may be more difficult to measure the excretory degradation products (output) and the extent of conversions of pro-vitamin to vitamin and coenzyme (input).

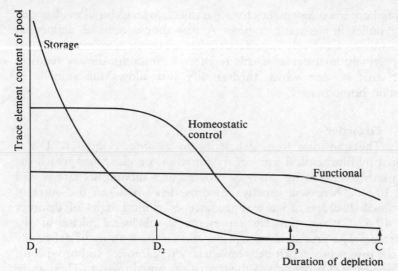

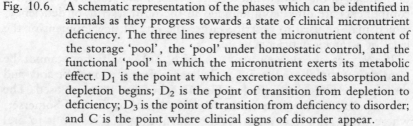

Fig. 10.6.   A schematic representation of the phases which can be identified in animals as they progress towards a state of clinical micronutrient deficiency. The three lines represent the micronutrient content of the storage 'pool', the 'pool' under homeostatic control, and the functional 'pool' in which the micronutrient exerts its metabolic effect. D_1 is the point at which excretion exceeds absorption and depletion begins; D_2 is the point of transition from depletion to deficiency; D_3 is the point of transition from deficiency to disorder; and C is the point where clinical signs of disorder appear.

Those body pools which are first to be reduced in size when animals, previously on a *luxus* intake of micronutrient, are depleted constitute *stores* (Fig. 10.6) or *reserves*, which are mobilized to meet the gap between input and output. The liver is a common store for both trace elements (e.g. Cu and Fe) and vitamins (e.g. A and B_{12}). Micronutrients can accumulate during *luxus* intakes in pools which are not readily mobilized i.e. in *sinks* rather than stores (e.g. trace elements in the inorganic matrix of bone). Pools in which the micronutrient turns over slowly can make a significant contribution to the supply of micronutrient if the rate of depletion is slow.

Deficiency
The transition from a state of depletion to one of deficiency (Fig. 10.6, D_2) is marked by biochemical signs that the homeostatic mechanisms are no longer maintaining a constant micronutrient milieu for physiological activity. In the example given in Fig. 10.3 this point would be marked by a drop in plasma Zn below 1 mg/l in the lamb. The onset of deficiency in the animal can thus be defined by reference to

accepted criteria of normality for a parameter which shows evidence of being under homeostatic control. A diet should only be defined as deficient retrospectively in so far as it has created a deficient animal, or prospectively in so far as it fails to meet a minimum dietary requirement: that is, one which theoretically just allows the animals to maintain homeostasis.

Disorder

The transition from deficiency to disorder (Fig. 10.6, D_3) is marked by biochemical signs of dysfunction, i.e. functions which the micronutrient normally catalyses proceed at a suboptimal rate *in vivo* (Fig. 10.6). There will usually be some delay between the onset of functional disorder and the appearance of clinical signs of disorder (Fig. 10.6, C) and this lag represents a subclinical phase of the syndrome. The precise onset will depend on the *intensity* of deficiency (i.e. the instaneous deficit between dietary requirement and provision), the *duration* of that deficit and the size of the initial reserve. These three components are often compounded in the term *severity* of deficiency, which may be used to describe either the rate of development or the level of a *chronic* deficiency state.

If reserves are non-existent (as with Zn), or if they cannot be translocated rapidly to the site of challenge, the effects may be *acute* and the separate phases indicated in Fig. 10.6 become superimposed. The latter condition may arise on the Mo-rich 'teart' pastures of Somerset, where cattle rapidly develop severe diarrhoea which responds to oral Cu treatment, although liver and blood Cu concentrations can be normal. This syndrome is variously described as 'molybdenum toxicity' or *induced* (as opposed to *simple*) Cu-deficiency, but such distinctions are arbitrary in that almost all micronutrients are so bound-up in interactions which are continuously rather than discontinuously variable that the term simple deficiency only applies to one which occurs with an antagonist-free diet. In the case of Cu in ruminant nutrition, this would be a diet free of Mo and S, and therefore nutritionally incomplete.

Factors affecting the onset of functional disorder

A dietary deficiency does not invariably lead to a functional disorder and the factors which predispose the animal to disorder are several-fold.

Functional activity

The rate at which biochemical transformations proceed is not a constant throughout the life of an animal and micronutrient deficiencies are most likely to produce functional disorders when the relevant reaction rates are maximal. Thus the unborn lamb is uniquely vulnerable to demyelination in the Cu-responsive condition known as swayback because of a spurt in the deposition of myelin in late foetal development (Patterson, Sweasey and Herbert, 1971). Similarly, the Cu-deficient chick is particularly vulnerable to aortic rupture because the Cu-dependent process of elastin maturation in the aorta undergoes an explosion of growth shortly after hatching (Hill, Starcher and Matrone, 1964). The presence of Zn deficiency for a small phase of foetal development can cause widespread congenital deformities in rats (Apgar, 1972).

Functional challenge

Body functions may also be subjected to discontinuous demands due to changes in the environment, including changes of diet. Lambs reared on barley-rich diets develop soft body fats containing high proportions of branched-chain fatty acids. It is thought that the B_{12}-dependent pathway of propionate to succinate (Fig. 10.2) may be overloaded on diets yielding abundant propionate in the rumen and that fatty acids are diverted along alternative pathways (Duncan and Garton, 1978). The addition of methionine to the diet of rats can induce growth retardation which is responsive to pyridoxine (Cerecedo, Foy and De Renzo, 1948); one of the functions of this vitamin is that of coenzyme to cystathionase and other enzymes involved in methionine metabolism.

Functional alternatives

A drop in the activity of a micronutrient-dependent function may be counterbalanced in tissues by the development of alternative pathways and three contrasting examples can be given. Although pyridoxine deficiency causes a reduction in the *in vitro* transamination of methionine in rat liver homogenates, *in vivo* transamination may not be rate limited, due possibly to a shift in metabolism to the trans-sulphuration pathway (Everet, Mitchell and Benevenga, 1979). A superoxide dismutase deficiency may be compensated for by the spontaneous dismutation of the superoxide ion (Fee and Valentine, 1977). In Mn-deficient chicks, Mg substitutes for Mn in the pyruvate carboxylase molecule with little or no loss of biochemical potency (Scrutton, 1971).

Functional reserves

A reduction in the amount of micronutrient present in the body in a functional form is not necessarily associated with a reduced rate of reaction even if there are no alternative pathways. Some enzymes are present in excess of the minimum amount needed. For example, it has been estimated that there is far more cytochrome oxidase present in tissues than is actually needed for the terminal electron transfer in the respiratory chain (Smith, Osborne-White and O'Dell, 1976).

Integrating example

Factors leading to the development of an outbreak of Se- and vitamin E-responsive acute myopathy in cattle when they were turned out to graze in spring illustrate well the interplay of factors which lead to the development of a functional disorder (McMurray and McEldowney, 1977). The in-wintering ration of the cattle was low in Se, leading to a run down in any initial reserve, and GSHPx activities were low prior to turnout although no clinical disease was then evident: this may have been due to the activity of functional alternatives, since work with rats has shown that in Se-deficient animals the activity of the enzyme glutathione-S-transferase (which can perform the same function as GSHPx) increases as the latter decreases (Lawrence, Parkhill and Burk, 1978). The alternative pathway may eventually have been overloaded by the following factors that combined to induce a functional and clinical disorder. The act of turnout led to a sudden increase in muscular activity thus raising the metabolic activity of the tissue ultimately affected. The new diet, grass, was thought to be relatively rich in long-chain fatty acids, which may have been metabolized to form potentially-toxic hydroperoxides in the tissues, giving an increased functional challenge. The acute myopathy which developed was preventable by administering vitamin E, although plasma tocopherol concentrations increased after turnout, emphasizing that nutritional deficits *per se* were not responsible for the onset of disorder.

Criteria for functional disorder

The treatment and prevention of micronutrient deficiencies requires the prior recognition of an existing or impending state of functional deficiency: a number of criteria can be applied although some have major disadvantages.

Clinical signs

The use of clinical signs as sole diagnostic criteria of deficiency is of limited use because they often reflect the outcome of a chain of metabolic events. A functional deficiency of any micronutrient involved along the chain may produce the same clinical signs of disorder. Deficiencies of riboflavin, biotin, folic acid and Mn can each produce a 'parrot-beak' deformity in the chick embryo (Crouch and Ferguson, 1975), presumably due to separate interferences in the normal development of the mandible. It is also possible for other factors to produce clinical signs which resemble those of micronutrient deficiencies. For example, molasses toxicity produces brain lesions in cattle which are indistinguishable from those of thiamin deficiency because both disorders are associated with impaired gluconeogenesis (Edwin, Markson, Shreeve, Jackman and Carroll, 1979). A spinal abscess can give rise to swayback-like incoordination of the hind limbs in lambs by physically rather than biochemically obstructing the passage of nerve impulses. Specific clinical signs of micronutrient disorder, such as the night blindness of vitamin A deficiency, the enlarged thyroid gland of I deficiency and the muscular paralysis of Se/vitamin E deficiencies are therefore somewhat rare.

Some micronutrient deficiencies can be associated with a number of clinical conditions of which only one may appear in a particular outbreak. Growth retardation in lambs attributable to Cu deficiency can occur on farms where swayback is not a problem (Whitelaw, Armstrong, Evans and Fawcett, 1979) because the dietary deficiency is imposed after birth, when the central nervous system is fully myelinated. Liver necrosis is a feature of Se/vitamin E deficiency in a number of species but not the chick. In avian species the plasma membranes of the capillary walls are particularly sensitive to deficiency, and exudative diathesis progresses to a fatal condition before liver necrosis has time to develop (Scott, Noguchi and Combs, 1974).

Another problem about reliance on clinical signs is that their appearance may be delayed or prevented by an earlier consequence of deficiency, namely loss of food intake. Anorexia is an early result of many micronutrient deficiencies: growth rates and the general level of metabolic activity are subsequently reduced and the demand placed on micronutrient-dependent transformations is also reduced. The control of appetite may indeed be an important defence mechanism against the ravages of a micronutrient deficiency.

Clinical signs of micronutrient deficiency are generally slow to develop but the sudden death of an animal does not rule-out the possibility of micronutrient involvement. The sudden deaths of chicks with fatty livers and kidneys (FLK syndrome), which became prevalent in the early 1960s, has only recently been attributed with certainty to a dietary biotin deficiency: the biochemical lesion is a sudden failure in glucose metabolism (Balnave, Cumming and Sutherland, 1977). There is a suggestion that some sudden deaths in bucket-fed calves immediately after feeding may be due to acute heart failure which is Se responsive (Cawley and Bradley, 1978). In both cases, subclinical deficiencies may develop into acute conditions in the face of a sudden metabolic challenge of nutritional origin.

Biochemical potential

In the quest for alternatives to clinical criteria for the diagnosis of micronutrient deficiencies, attention was initially given to those parameters that showed the most immediate response to dietary inadequacy, (Fig. 10.6) i.e. changes in body reserves (e.g. B_{12} and Cu in liver) and circulating levels (e.g. vitamins in blood). These criteria of depletion and deficiency often exaggerate the incidence of a current functional disorder and the use of functional enzyme or coenzyme tests as criteria has, therefore, been advocated; these tests also have their limitations. In experimental Cu deficiency in cattle, for example, concentrations of the Cu-dependent enzymes monamine oxidase, ferroxidase and cytochrome oxidase were little better in predicting the onset of growth retardation than the conventional signs of depletion and deficiency (Mills, Dalgarno and Wenham, 1976). These disappointing results may be due to the fact that measurements of micronutrient-dependent activity *in vitro* measures functional potential, and does not necessarily indicate that a particular process has become rate-limiting.

Evidence of biochemical dysfunction

Because of the problems presented by functional alternatives and functional reserves, the measurement of consequences of dysfunction is likely to prove more reliable than the measurement of functional potential in predicting the imminence of a disorder responsive to a micronutrient. Vitamin B_{12}-deficient sheep excrete excess amounts of methylmalonic acid (MMA) and formiminoglutamic acid (FIGLU) in the urine, and these are early signs of functional inadequacies of cobalamin and methylcobalamin respectively (Fig. 10.2 and Gawthorne, 1968). The excretion of both MMA (Millar and Lorentz, 1979) and FIGLU (Russel, Whitelaw, Moberly and Fawcett, 1975) in urine has been found to be correlated with Co-responsiveness in lambs. Because these criteria monitor dysfunctions in different metabolic pathways, they might not give the same result, notably if the diet provides a propionate rather than a cyst(e)ine challenge (e.g. cereal *v.* grass diets). Criteria of dysfunction may be found for other microelement disorders: for example, elevated liver ferritin as a consequence of impaired Fe metabolism in Cu deficiency, and increased tissue peroxide concentrations as a consequence of Se deficiency. Excretory by-products of dysfunction would be preferred, however, so as to avoid the need for surgical procedures for procuring samples.

An alternative approach in the assessment of degree of functional deficiency is to measure the functional response to repletion. An example is afforded by the measurement of transketolase activity in thiamin deficiency. Thiamin pyrophosphate (TPP) acts as a coenzyme for transketolase in the pentose phosphate pathway of glucose utilization in the erythrocyte. Addition of TPP to a blood haemolysate stimulates transketolase activity in inverse proportion to the initial thiamin status of the erythrocytes (the 'TPP effect'), and in ruminants responses correlate well with histological criteria of the thiamin-responsive disorder, cerebro cortico–necrosis (Edwin *et al.*, 1979). A by-product of dysfunction, namely elevated pyruvic acid concentrations in the blood, has also been used to monitor thiamin deficiency (Pill, 1967) but it has disadvantages in that it is non-specific and elevated in a variety of micronutrient deficiencies in which intermediary energy metabolism is impaired, e.g. those of vitamin B_{12} (MacPherson and Moon, 1974) and biotin (Balnave *et al.*, 1977).

Evidence of physiological dysfunction

There are instances in which a physiological process rather than a single biochemical step can be shown to be defective in deficient animals. The onset of myopathy in Se/vitamin E deficient animals is accompanied by the escape of intracellular enzymes such as aspartate transaminase and creatine phosphokinase through the damaged myofibrillar membrane: increased levels of these enzymes in the plasma are therefore helpful in the diagnosis of muscular dystrophy.

The use of phagocytic-killing capacity as an index of functional Se deficiency in the rat (Serfass and Ganther, 1975) and bovine (Boyne and Arthur, 1979) is also of interest in this context. The respiratory burst, which is an essential part of the process whereby phagocytes kill engulfed bacteria (Johnston and Lehmeyer, 1977) generates toxic radicals which are potentially dangerous to the phagocytes themselves (Fig. 10.7). The Se-enzyme, GSHPx, normally protects the phagocyte from peroxide damage, but in the deficient animal this protection may

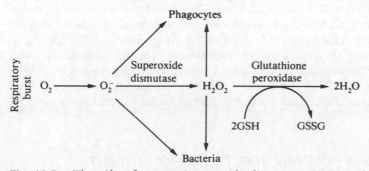

Fig. 10.7. The rôle of copper (superoxide dismutase, SOD) and selenium (glutathione peroxidase, GSHPx) enzymes in the protection of phagocytes from the damaging cytotoxic effects of the respiratory burst products, O_2^- and H_2O_2, which are essential to convey bactericidal properties to the phagocyte.

be inadequate, giving rise to a lower killing capacity. The Cu-containing enzyme, superoxide dismutase, is involved in disposing of another respiratory burst by-product (Fig. 10.7) and a deficiency of Cu has the same outcome as Se deficiency in cattle and sheep in impairing killing capacity (D. Jones and N. F. Suttle, unpublished). Two important principles are involved in such techniques: one is the concept of a biochemical challenge (brought about in this instance by artificially stimulating the respiratory burst by exposing phagocytes to *Candida albicans*) and the other is the use of an intact cell system of short biological half-life as a target tissue. The metabolic properties of the phagocyte may have a rôle to play in the early diagnosis of other micronutrient deficiencies, and in elucidating that important but elusive parameter, the *first limiting function*, in the development of a disorder.

Criteria unrelated to function

Those parameters which reflect an absence of homeostatic control through a linear relationship to intakes around the required level are difficult to interpret and of questionable diagnostic use. Three biochemical parameters of deficiency in various degrees of common usage come into this category, plasma vitamin B_{12}, whole blood GSHPx and plasma 25,OHC concentrations. These parameters, unlike those shown in Fig. 10.3, are linearly related to Co, Se and vitamin D intakes, respectively, over a wide range above the nutritional requirement (Fig. 10.8) and are depleted when intakes fall. The respective pools should, therefore, be regarded in part as stores reflecting past uptake of the micronutrient. The arbitrary subdivision of a population of GSHPx values into four tiers labelled 'deficient', 'marginally deficient', 'marginal' and 'adequate', without reference to function or clinical criteria in the population (Anderson, Berrett and Patterson, 1979), is physiologically misleading. By careful correlation with clinical parameters, plasma B_{12} levels have been subdivided to indicate varying degrees of inadequacy (Andrews and Stephenson, 1966) but it is noteworthy that, in a recent experiment, plasma vitamin B_{12} was relatively poorly correlated with Co-responsiveness in lambs (Millar and Lorentz, 1979). Parameters which reflect nutritional history rather than current functional adequacy should be interpreted with caution!

DIET AS A CONTRIBUTOR TO MICRONUTRIENT INADEQUACIES

The reasons why a particular diet does not meet the micronutrient requirements of an animal are not always obvious; they may, for

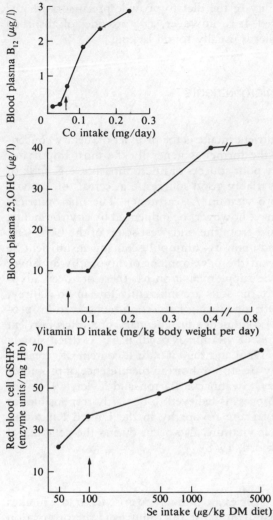

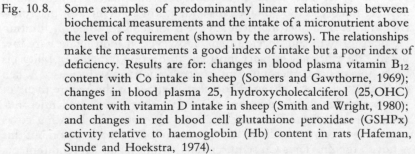

Fig. 10.8. Some examples of predominantly linear relationships between biochemical measurements and the intake of a micronutrient above the level of requirement (shown by the arrows). The relationships make the measurements a good index of intake but a poor index of deficiency. Results are for: changes in blood plasma vitamin B_{12} content with Co intake in sheep (Somers and Gawthorne, 1969); changes in blood plasma 25, hydroxycholecalciferol (25,OHC) content with vitamin D intake in sheep (Smith and Wright, 1980); and changes in red blood cell glutathione peroxidase (GSHPx) activity relative to haemoglobin (Hb) content in rats (Hafeman, Sunde and Hoekstra, 1974).

example, involve the ability of the diet to provide precursors for the reaction which is catalysed. It is, however, as a provider of absorbed micronutrients that the diet is usually found lacking.

Diet as a provider of micronutrients

Concentration

Although micronutrient intake is the product of dietary concentration and food intake, the former is generally the most important. Some foods are invariably poor sources of micronutrients, e.g. milk of Fe and Cu; others are invariably good sources, e.g. cereals of many B vitamins and grass of pro-vitamin A (carotene). The micronutrient composition of the diet may, however, be influenced by environmental factors. For example, maize from the mid-west states of the USA (and complete pig rations based upon it) commonly contains insufficient Se (10 to 50 μg/kg) to prevent the development of myopathy and liver necrosis in pigs; routine Se supplementation has therefore been advocated in those areas where the soils are inherently low in Se (Ullrey, 1974). Losses of micronutrients during harvesting, conservation, processing and storage can also influence the adequacy of a micronutrient source. Considerable losses of vitamin E occur if hay is dried slowly (Thafvelin and Oksanen, 1966) and the vitamin E content of cereals is greatly reduced when they are stored moist in the presence of propionic acid (Allen, Parr, Bradley, Swannack, Barton and Tyler, 1974). Increased use of the latter process is believed to be partly responsible for the increased incidence of acute myopathy in the United Kingdom. Losses of all the fat-soluble vitamins also occur during the pelleting of a concentrate ration (Pickford, 1968).

Food intake

Micronutrient deficiencies are unlikely to arise from low intakes of food *per se*. The demand for most micronutrients for production declines rapidly as food intake falls and, at low food intakes, macronutrient rather than micronutrient supply is more likely to be the limiting factor to growth and development. However, if food intakes are low because the efficiency of macronutrient absorption (i.e. 'digestibility') is high, the desired micronutrient concentration must increase. When food allowances are changed to meet changes in the requirement of macronutrients for production, they may alter the desired micronutrient concentration. The increased food allowance for lactating cows more than meets the additional requirement of Cu for lactation but this is not so for Zn. Thus Cu requirements diminish and Zn requirements increase during lactation (Agricultural Research Council, 1980).

Absorption

Micronutrients are useless until they are absorbed from the alimentary tract and some dietary inadequacies can be attributed to impaired absorption. The micronutrient may be present in the diet in forms which resist the animal's digestive and absorptive processes, i.e. the poor absorption is primarily an attribute of the food, which provides micronutrient of low *availability*.

Maize is a particularly poor source of niacin because the large concentrations present are there in a bound and unabsorbable form. Poor availability can result from interactions between dietary constituents. For example, cereals and some vegetable protein sources (e.g. soya beans) contain phytate which combines with Zn, Cu, Fe and Mn to form insoluble phytates, particularly when the diet is rich in Ca (Davies, 1979). Pigs and poultry are likely to develop clinical Zn-deficiency (parakeratosis) unless such diets are supplemented with Zn. The Zn deficiency may be cumulative because the digestive enzyme capable of hydrolysing phytate, alkaline phosphatase, is Zn-dependent and reduced in activity during Zn deficiency (Davies and Flett, 1978). The absorption of pyridoxal phosphate is facilitated by the same enzyme (Middleton, 1979) and may therefore be impaired in Zn deficiency.

A further example of the marked effects of antagonists on absorption is afforded by the Cu × Mo × S interaction in ruminants. The absorption of Cu is reduced by a factor of 2 to 4 as Mo and S concentrations are increased within the normal range for these elements in herbage (Fig. 10.9) (Suttle, 1978b). Such increases in the concentrations of Mo and S in improved hill-pastures are believed to have been responsible for the induction of Cu deficiency in lambs (Whitelaw *et al.*, 1979).

The absorption of thiamin is subject to interference from an unusual enzyme-based antagonism. Thiamin can be destroyed in the diet or in the gut by thiaminases produced by microbes, fungi or bracken (Edwin *et al.*, 1979). The catalytically useless analogues, which are produced by the thiaminases, may aggravate the deficiency by competing with the thiamin which escapes degradation at both the gut and tissue levels. Thus thiamin-responsive conditions occur in ruminants although synthesis by the rumen microflora would normally be expected to meet all the host's needs for thiamin and the other B vitamins.

Diet as provider of substrates and 'metabolites'

The diet can determine the extent of a micronutrient deficiency by affecting the amount of substrate or 'metabolite' that is available to a

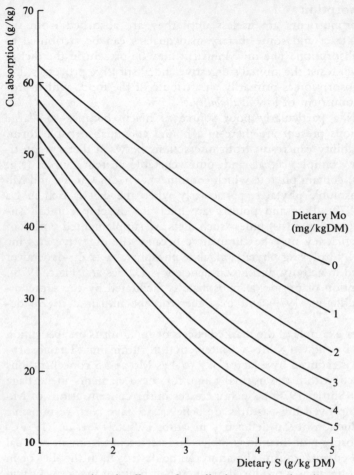

Fig. 10.9.   Predicted effects of small changes in the dietary contents of molybdenum and sulphur on the true absorption (g/kg of dietary intake) of copper in ewes given semi-purified diets (Suttle, 1978b).

micronutrient-controlled process. An extreme example of the latter is afforded by the influence of dietary Ca supply on vitamin D requirement. If the dietary supply of Ca is abundant, the physiological effect of low vitamin D intakes on Ca absorption may not become a limiting factor to the rate of Ca accretion in bone. Similarly, the provision of glucose precursors can ameliorate the biotin-responsive FLK syndrome in chicks by overcoming the consequences of impaired gluconeogenesis (Balnave *et al.*, 1977). The wheat-based diets which predispose towards FLK syndrome are presumably poor sources of glucose precursors. The importance of diet as a source of substrates is illustrated by two examples. Diets which provide energy for the milk-fed ruminant as carbohydrate rather than fat increase the requirement for thiamin (Benevenga, Baldwin and Ronning, 1966) and possibly other vitamins involved in intermediary energy metabolism. Diets rich in polyunsaturated fatty acids yield increased amounts of hydroperoxides that can damage cell membranes and aggravate Se- or vitamin E-deficiencies.

MANIPULATION OF MICRONUTRIENT METABOLISM

The practical problem of bridging the gap between dietary supply of and requirement for a given micronutrient has generally been tackled crudely through the use of multi-element or multi-vitamin supplements in the diet with generous margins of safety. Given a choice, the clinician will opt for a multi-vitamin preparation for parenteral use in farm animals. These approaches have been fostered by ease of access to supplies of micronutrients and their low cost relative to that of the remainder of the diet or the market value of the animal. It would, however, appear to be unsound in principle and potentially counterproductive in practice to administer such highly active and interactive compounds unless there is a proven nutritional deficit. Indeed, an increased awareness of the toxicological properties of micronutrients is already leading to a more rigid legal framework controlling their use in animal foodstuffs. In the absence of reliable diagnostic aids, response to therapy is often the best diagnosis available and specific therapy allows specific diagnosis.

The reversal of a nutritional deficiency will have rapid effects upon many biochemical parameters because the animal's homeostatic mechanisms will be adapted to make the most of the available micronutrient supply. One would expect a mirror image of the pattern of depletion, at least for the functional and homeostatic 'pools' illustrated in Fig. 10.6. These 'pools' would therefore be expected to return rapidly to normal before stores are repleted. Restoration of biochemical function for micronutrients with a coenzyme function is generally rapid but, where enzyme functions are involved, recovery may be limited by the rate at which a holoenzyme can be synthesized *de novo*. The restoration of physiological function may be further constrained by the rate at which additional mitochondrial material or new cells can be elaborated (Dallman, 1967). Clinical signs will be the last to respond and rates of remission will depend on the turnover of the affected cell or tissue. The rapid turnover of enterocytes in the intestinal mucosa allows Cu-deficient, scouring cattle to respond within 48 h to the oral administration of Cu (Mills *et al.*, 1976), whereas the central nervous system lesions in lambs with swayback may be irreparable because development of the myelin sheath is largely completed before birth. The rapidity of repletion should be borne in mind when attempts are made to characterize a particular micronutrient deficiency in the field; it should be matched by rapidity of analysis and interpretation if the measures for prevention and treatment are to have a contemporary relevance.

Manipulation of an animal's micronutrient metabolism is achieved most successfully by working with rather than against the homeostatic mechanisms. The dietary route of supplementation will be ineffective in building up tissue reserves when the primary control is over the efficiency of absorption. In these circumstances dietary supplements, such as those of Fe, will be predominantly excreted in the faeces. One way of circumventing the absorptive barrier is to supply the micronutrient in a slow-release form which does not give rise to high concentrations at the sites of absorption. This approach has hitherto been confined to the trace-element supplementation of ruminants in which large particles of high density ('heavy bullets') have been successfully used in the treatment of Co(Dewey, Lee and Marston, 1969) and Se(Kuchel and Buckley, 1969) deficiencies. The 'bullets' lodge in the reticulum and slowly release their micronutrient constituent until they become coated or totally eroded. Recent discoveries that particles of small size and high density, such as cupric oxide 'needles', lodge in the abomasum of ruminants and provide a slow release of Cu (Dewey, 1979; Suttle, 1979a) indicate that the slow-release method of oral supplementation may be applicable to the non-ruminant animal.

Parenteral supplementation can be an appropriate route of administration for micronutrients which are well stored and poorly excreted, i.e. the fat- but not the water-soluble vitamins, Cu but not Zn. The ability of organic chemists to produce slight modifications to naturally occurring molecules (analogues) has led to new developments in parenteral treatments. The introduction of CN or OH in place of the 5-deoxyadenosyl radical in cobalamin produces biologically active molecules that have been used in the treatment of vitamin B_{12} deficiency. They may not, however, be as potent as the natural coenzyme (Smith and Marston, 1970; Millar and Lorentz, 1979). The use of analogues of vitamin D in the treatment of milk fever, on the other hand, seems to offer advantages over the natural vitamin D_3. The normal process of hydroxylation can be by-passed in part (Fig. 10.5) by administering a 1α-OHC analogue, which only requires to be hydroxylated in the liver (Davies, Allen, Hoare, Pott, Riley, Sansom, Stenton and Vagg, 1978), or wholly by administering the $1,25(OH)_2C$ (Gast, Horst, Jorgensen and DeLuca, 1979). Both treatments have been shown to elicit the rapid increase in Ca absorption which is needed to meet the sudden increase in demand for Ca with the onset of lactation: administration of the unhydroxylated vitamin is less successful in this regard.

Some economy in the use of micronutrient supplements might be made by identifying those animals within a population that are the most or least in need of therapy. Susceptibility to Fe- and Zn-deficiency is highest in the young, rapidly growing animal because of the large contribution of the requirement for growth relative to that for maintenance (Suttle, 1979b). If the nutritional deficiency is marginal and there is a storage capacity for the micronutrient, then the oldest animals in the population, i.e. those with maximum exposure to the deficient regime, may be in the greatest need of supplementation (Suttle, Field, Nicolson, Mathieson, Prescott, Scott and Johnson, 1980). Supplementation might therefore be usefully restricted to those animals in the most need in such situations.

Advantage may also be taken of peaks in the physiological efficiency of micronutrient metabolism. There is evidence, at least in rats, that Cu and Zn are well absorbed during pregnancy and early lactation (Davies and Williams, 1976a and b). In cattle, parenteral Cu appears to be quantitatively transferred from mother to foetus during late pregnancy (Suttle *et al.*, 1980) and the oral administration of Cu in late pregnancy should be an effective way of raising the Cu status of calves (MacPherson, Voss and Dixon, 1979). Similarly, the oral administration of Fe-dextran can be as effective as the intramuscular route in treating piglet anaemia because the efficiency of Fe absorption in the neonate is high (B. F. Sansom, personal communication).

Although much has been written about variations in the micronutrient status of animals from a given population, little attention has been given to the heritability of such differences in farm animals. Differences in the susceptibility of different breeds of sheep to Cu deficiency and Cu toxicity (Wiener and Field, 1970) suggest that Cu metabolism is partly under genetic control. These observations led to attempts to manipulate genotype within a breed by appropriate selection methods, with the result that blood Cu concentrations in selected animals have been moved significantly above and below the mean for unselected animals (G. Wiener, unpublished results). These findings point clearly to the possibility of breeding animals which make optimum use of a limited dietary supply of micronutrients.

Manipulation of plant genotypes has concentrated on parameters of immediate productive value (e.g. DM yield) to the possible detriment of micronutrient composition. Differences in the biological availability of Cu (Patil, Jones and Huges, 1969) and Co (Jones, 1970) have been reported among grass cultivars and, again, this opens up the possibility of providing animals with a more utilizable dietary supply of micronutrients.

MICRONUTRIENT TOXICOLOGY

Failure of an animal's homeostatic mechanisms to deal with an excessive supply of a micronutrient can result in the malfunction of certain body processes, and terminate in clinical and fatal disorders. Of the three major micronutrient classes, trace elements are generally the most likely and water-soluble vitamins the least likely to cause toxicity, but within these classes there are wide variations. Among the essential trace elements, Cu is extremely toxic while Mn and Co are tolerated at dietary concentrations of 1 g/kg DM or more. Among the fat-soluble vitamins, E and K are virtually non-toxic but A and D have deleterious effects on health at high dose rates.

Toxicoses may be rapid (*acute*) or slow (*chronic*) in their rate of development. Acute toxicoses of dietary origin are concentration-dependent and characterized by the rapid development of lesions at sites first exposed to the toxicant. Thus, gastro-intestinal haemorrhage is a general sign of acute heavy-metal toxicity. Chronic toxicoses of dietary origin are time- as well as concentration- dependent. They are characterized by poor correlations with dietary concentration *per se*; prior accumulation of the toxic micronutrient in selected tissues (not necessarily those to show the first signs of malfunction); and the gradual development of specific lesions such as pancreatic acinar cell atrophy in Zn toxicity (Aughey, Grant, Furman and Dryden, 1977) and centrilobular necrosis of the liver in Cu toxicity (Ishmael, Gopinath and Howell, 1971).

The advent of clinical signs and physiological malfunction may not be adequate criteria of chronic toxicity. At earlier stages in the accumulation of a toxic heavy metal, for example, there can be signs that the metabolism of other elements has been impaired, e.g. the fall in plasma Cu seen in animals given diets rich in Zn (Bremner, 1979). Using parallel arguments to those considered in relation to dietary inadequacies it is suggested that there are at least two stages in the development of abnormalities, accumulation and disorder.

Accumulation

The rate at which a dietary micronutrient accumulates in the tissues to chronically toxic levels will be influenced by many of the dietary and physiological factors whose effects on micronutrient retention were discussed earlier. The pre-ruminant and pregnant ovine are both relatively susceptible to Zn toxicity (Davies, Soliman, Corrigall and Flett, 1977; Campbell and Mills, 1979), possibly due to the high efficiency of Zn absorption at those stages of development. Similarly, the milk-fed calf is particularly susceptible to Cu toxicity (Shand and Lewis, 1957). The influence of dietary factors is illustrated by the effects of Mo and S on susceptibility to Cu poisoning. Cu poisoning is prevalent in sheep given cereal-based diets that are naturally low in these two antagonists. Addition of Mo and S can reduce the absorption (Fig. 10.9) and hepatic accumulation of Cu, and thus afford complete protection from toxicity (Suttle, 1977). Excepting the milk-fed calf, cattle are much less susceptible to Cu poisoning than sheep, and the difference may be attributable to the ability of the bovine to excrete increasing amounts of Cu endogenously (and therefore accumulate less) as its liver Cu stores rise (Suttle, 1978a; McDonald, Mills, Dalgarno and Simpson, 1979). The general tolerance of animals towards Mn and Co may be explained by the very low efficiency of absorption of these elements (around 10 g/kg) and their consequently slow accumulation in the tissues.

Disorder

The transition to a state of disorder is characterized by the appearance of physiological dysfunction and commences with a subclinical phase. This phase can be marked by early histological evidence of cellular abnormalities in target organs e.g. karyomelaly in the liver parenchymal cells in Cu poisoning (Suttle, 1977), with accompanying biochemical evidence of cell damage in the form of elevated blood plasma levels of normally intracellular enzymes (Ishmael *et al.*, 1971). Tissue damage can be extensive before overt clinical signs of this particular disorder, i.e. the haemolytic crisis, appear. Other subclinical signs of toxicity include the deranged metabolism of other elements in heavy-metal toxicity, and the accumulation of metal-binding proteins, metallothioneins, at sites such as the gut mucosa, liver and kidney (Bremner, 1979).

The parenteral administration of micronutrients can lead to the early (acute) development of disorder, probably because the nutrient is presented for transport in a more reactive state than that of the absorbed nutrient. Parenteral administration of the trace elements is frequently associated with local inflammatory reactions (e.g. to Fe-dextran and Cu-chelates). The risk of chronic disorder will be influenced by the storage capacity for the micronutrient and also the current micronutrient status of animal and diet. The form in which the micronutrient is administered can also influence its toxicity; for example, Cu methionate is less toxic to sheep than Cu Ca ethylenediaminetetra-acetate (Ishmael, Howell, Treeby and Bramley, 1977), but such forms may be less effective in performing their intended function in protecting against Cu deficiency (N. F. Suttle, unpublished results).

Although the clinical and pathological signs of micronutrient excess are often striking, there are few instances in which the pathogenesis of toxicity is known. Notable exceptions are provided by vitamins A and D. Vitamin D becomes harmful because extrapolation of its normal rôle leads to widespread tissue calcification (Payne, 1963). One of the consequences of vitamin A toxicity is an increased clotting time of blood, which is believed to result from an interference with the absorption of vitamin K (Dam and Søndergaard, 1964); others, such as the abnormal development of skin, keratin and bone, are of obscure aetiology.

As mechanisms for the toxic effects of micronutrients become established and early subclinical signs of dysfunction recognized, the need for precise control on the supply of micronutrients to allow them to perform their diverse essential rôles will be emphasized.

REFERENCES

Agricultural Research Council, 1980. Trace elements. In *The Nutrient Requirements of Ruminant Livestock*, pp. 221–67. Commonwealth Agricultural Bureaux, Slough.

Allen, W. M., Parr, M. R., Bradley, R., Swannack, K., Barton, C. R. Q. and Tyler, R., 1974. Loss of vitamin E in stored cereals in relation to a myopathy in yearling cattle, *Vet. Rec.* **94**: 373–5.

Anderson, P. H., Berrett, S. and Patterson, D. S. P., 1979. The biological selenium status of livestock in Britain as indicated by sheep erythrocyte glutathione peroxidase activity, *Vet. Rec.* **104**: 235–8.

Andrews, E. D. and Stephenson, B. J., 1966. Vitamin B_{12} in the blood of grazing cobalt-deficient sheep, *N. Z. Jl agric. Res.* **9**: 491–507.

Apgar, J., 1972. Effect of zinc deprivation from days 12, 15 or 18 gestation on parturition in the rat, *J. Nutr.* **102**: 343–8.

Aughey, E., Grant, L., Furman, B. L. and Dryden, W. F., 1977. The effects of oral zinc supplementation in the mouse. *J. Comp. Pathol.* **87**: 1–15.

Balnave, D. Cumming, R. B. and Sutherland, T. M., 1977. A biochemical explanation for the fatty liver and kidney syndrome of broilers: its alleviation by the short-term use of dietary fat, *Br. J. Nutr.* **38**: 319–28.

Benevenga, N. J., Baldwin, R. L. and Ronning, M., 1966. Alterations in the liver enzyme activities and blood and urine metabolite levels during the onset of thiamine deficiency in the dairy calf, *J. Nutr.* **90**: 131–40.

Boyne, R. and Arthur, J. R., 1979. Alterations in neutrophil function in selenium-deficient cattle, *J. Comp. Pathol.* **89**: 151–58.

Bremner, I., 1979. The toxicity of cadmium, zinc and molybdenum and their effects on copper metabolism, *Proc. Nutr. Soc.* **38**: 235–42.

Bremner, I. and Davies, N. T., 1976. Studies on the appearance of a hepatic copper-binding protein in normal and zinc deficient rats, *Br. J. Nutr.* **360**: 101–12.

Campbell, J. K. and Mills, C. F., 1979. The toxicity of zinc to pregnant sheep, *Environ. Res.* **20**: 1–13.

Cawley, G. D. and Bradley, R., 1978. Sudden death in calves associated with acute mycocardial degeneration and selenium deficiency, *Vet. Rec.* **103**: 239–40.

Cerecedo, L. R., Foy, J. R. and De Renzo, E. C., 1948. Protein intake and vitamin B_6 deficiency in the rat. II. The effect of supplementing a low-protein, pyridoxine-deficient diet with cystine or methionine, *Archs Biochem.* **17**: 397–402.

Chesters, J. K., 1974. Biochemical functions of zinc with emphasis on nucleic acid metabolism and cell division. In *Trace Element Metabolism in Animals-2* (ed. W. G. Hoekstra, J. W. Suttie, H. E. Ganther and W. Mertz), pp. 39–50. University Park Press, Baltimore.

Cotzias, G. C., 1964. Transport, homeostasis and specificity in trace metal metabolism. In *Proc. 6th int. Congr. Nutr., Edinb.* (ed. D. P. Cuthbertson, C. F. Mills and R. Passmore), pp. 252–69. Livingstone, Edinburgh.

Cousins, R. J., 1978. Synthesis and degradation of hepatic zinc thionein and its role in zinc metabolism. In *Proc. 3rd int. Symp. Trace Element Metab. Man Anim.* (ed. M. Kichgessner), pp. 57–63. Arbeitskreis Tierernahrung, Weihenstephan.

Crouch, J. R. and Ferguson, T. M., 1975. Nutrition and embryonic development in the domestic fowl, *Proc. Nutr. Soc.* **34**: 1–3.

Dallman, P. R., 1967. Cytochrome oxidase repair during treatment of copper deficiency in relation to mitochondrial turnover, *J. clin. Invest.* **46**: 1819–27.

Dam, H. P. and Søndergaard, E., 1964. In *Nutrition – a Comprehensive Treatise. Vol. II, Vitamins, Nutrient Requirements and Food Selection* (ed. G H. Beaton and E. W. McHenry), pp. 2–107.

Davies, N. T., 1979. Anti-nutrient factors affecting mineral utilisation, *Proc. Nutr. Soc.* **38**: 121–8.

Davies, D. C., Allen, W. M., Hoare, M. N., Pott, J. M., Riley, C. J., Sansom, B. F., Stenton, J. R. and Vagg, M. J., 1978. A field trial of 1 α-hydroxycholecalciferol (1 α-OH D_3) in the prevention of milk fever, *Vet. Rec.* **102**: 440–2.

Davies, N. T. and Flett, A. A., 1978. The similarity between alkaline phosphatase (E.C. 3.1.3.1) and phytase (3.1.3.8) activities in rat intestine and their importance in phytate-induced zinc deficiency, *Br. J. Nutr.* **39**: 307–16.

Davies, N. T., Soliman, H. S., Corrigall, W. and Flett, A., 1977. The susceptibility of suckling lambs to zinc toxicity, *Br. J. Nutr.* **38**: 153–6.

Davies, N. T. and Williams R. B., 1976a. The effects of pregnancy on uptake and distribution of copper in the rat, *Proc. Nutr. Soc.* **35**: 4A (Abstr.).

Davies, N. T. and Williams, R. B., 1976b. Zinc absorption in pregnancy and lactation, *Proc. Nutr. Soc.* **35**: 5A (Abstr.).

De Luca, L. M., 1978. The direct involvement of vitamin A in glycosyl transfer reactions of mammalian membranes, *Vitams Horm.* **35**: 1–30.

Dewey, D. W., 1979. An effective method for the administration of trace amounts of copper to ruminants, *Search, Sydney* **8**: 326–7.

Dewey, D. W., Lee, H. J. and Marston, H. R., 1969. Efficacy of cobalt pellets for providing cobalt for penned sheep, *Aust. J. agric. Res.* **20**: 1109–16.

Dick, A. T., Dewey, D. W. and Gawthorne, J. M., 1975. Thiomolybdates and the copper-molybdenum-sulphur interaction in ruminant nutrition, *J. agric. Sci., Camb.* **85**: 567–8.

Diplock, A. T., 1974. The nutritional and metabolic roles of selenium and vitamin E, *Proc. Nutr. Soc.* **33**: 315–22.

Duncan, W. R. H. and Garton, G. A., 1978. Differences in the proportions of branched chain fatty acids in subcutaneous triacylglycerols of barley-fed ruminants, *Br. J. Nutr.* **40**: 29–33.

Edwin, E. E., Markson, L. M., Shreeve, J., Jackman, R. and Carroll, P. J., 1979. Diagnostic aspects of cerebrocortical necrosis, *Vet. Rec.* **104**: 4–8.

Evans, W. C., Evans, I. Antice, Humphreys, D. J., Lewin, B., Davies, W. E. J. and Axford, R. F. E., 1975. Induction of thiamine deficiency in sheep with lesions similar to those of cerebrocortical necrosis, *J. Comp. Pathol.* **85**: 253–67,

Everet, G. B., Mitchell, A. D. and Benevenga, N. J., 1979. Methionine transamination and catabolism in vitamin B-6 deficient rats, *J. Nutr.* **109**: 597–605.

Fee, J. G. and Valentine, J. S., 1977. Chemistry and physical properties of superoxide. In *Superoxide and Superoxide Dismutases* (ed. A. M. Michelson, J. M. McCord and I. Fridovich), pp. 20–60. Academic Press, New York.

Flohé, L., Gunzler, W. A. and Shock, H. H., 1973. Glutathione peroxidase: a selenoenzyme, *FEBS Lett.* **32**: 132–4.

Fraser, D. R., 1975. Advances in the knowledge of the metabolism of vitamin D, *Proc. Nutr. Soc.* **34**: 139–43.

Fridovich, I., 1972. Superoxide radical and superoxide dismutase *Acc. Chem. Res.* **5**: 321–5.

Frieden, E., 1971. Caeruloplasmin, a link between iron and copper metabolism. In *Bioinorganic Chemistry, Advances in Chemistry Series* (ed. R. F. Gould), pp. 292–321. American Chemical Society, Washington, DC.

Gast, D. R., Horst, R. L., Jorgensen, N. A. and DeLuca, H. F., 1979. Potential use of 1,25-dihydroxycholecalciferol for prevention of parturient paresis, *J. Dairy Sci.* **62**: 1009–13.

Gawthorne, J. M., 1968. The excretion of methylmalonic and formiminoglutamic acids during the induction and remission of vitamin B_{12} deficiency in sheep, *Aust. J. biol. Sci.* **21**: 789–94.

Grace, N. D. and Suttle, N. F., 1978. Some effects of sulphur intake on molybdenum metabolism in sheep, *Br. J. Nutr.* **41**: 125–36.

Hafeman, D. G., Sunde, R. A. and Hoekstra, W. G., 1974. Effect of dietary selenium on erythrocyte and liver glutathione peroxidase in the rat, *J. Nutr.* **104**: 580–7.

Henderson, L. M. and Gross, Carol J., 1979. Transport of niacin and niacinamide in perfused rat intestine, *J. Nutr.* **109**: 646–53.

Herbert, V. and Das, K. C., 1976. The role of vitamin B_{12} and folic acid in haemato-and other cell-poiesis, *Vitams Horm.* **34**: 1–30.

Hill, C. H., 1974. Reversal of selenium toxicity in chicks by mercury, copper and cadmium, *J. Nutr.* **104**. 593–8.

Hill, C. H., Starcher, B. and Matrone, G. 1964. Mercury and silver interrelationships with copper. *J. Nutr.* **83**: 107–112.

Holtzman, N. A. and Gaumnitz, B. M., 1970. Identification of an apoceruloplasmin-like substance in the plasma of copper-deficient rats, *J. biol. Chem.* **245**: 2350–3.

Hopkins, F. G., 1906. The analyst and the medical man, *Analyst, Lond.* **31**: 385–97.

Howard, L., Wagner, C. and Schender, S., 1974. Malabsorption of thiamin in folate-deficient rats, *J. Nutr.* **104**: 1024–32.

Hoyumpa, A. M., Middleton, H. M., Wilson, F. A. and Schenker, S., 1975. Thiamine transport across the rat intestine. I. Normal characteristics, *Gastroenterology* **68**: 1218–27.

Ishmael, J., Gopinath, C. and Howell. J. McC., 1971. Experimental chronic copper toxicity in sheep: histological and histochemical changes during the development of the lesions in the liver, *Res. vet. Sci.* **12**: 358–66.

Ishmael, J., Howell, J. McC., Treeby, P. J. and Bramley, P. S., 1977. Copper methionate for parenteral copper therapy in sheep, *Vet. Rec.* **101**: 410.

Johnston, R. B. and Lehmeyer, J. E., 1977. The involvement of oxygen metabolites from phagocytic cells in bactericidal activity and inflammation. In *Superoxide and Superoxide Dismutases* (ed. A. M. Michelson, J. M. McCord and I. Fridovich), pp. 291–305. Academic Press, New York.

Jones, D. I. H., 1970. Effect of cobalt applications to pasture on herbage digestibility, *Nature, Lond.* **226**: 772–3.

Kuchel, R. E. and Buckley, R. A., 1969. The provision of selenium to sheep by means of heavy pellets, *Aust. J. agric. Res.* **20**: 1099–107.

Lawrence, R. A., Parkhill, L. K. and Burk, R. F., 1978. Hepatic cytosolic non-selenium dependent glutathione peroxidase activity: its nature and the effect of selenium deficiency, *J. Nutr.* **108**: 981–7.

Lee, G. R., Ragan, H. A., Nacht, S. and Cartwright, G. E., 1969. The effect of caeruloplasmin on plasma iron in copper-deficient swine, *Clin. Res.* **17**: 152.

McCollum, E. V., 1957. *A History of Nutrition*, pp. 201–383. Riverside Press, Cambridge, Mass.

McDonald, I., Mills, C. F., Dalgarno, A. C. and Simpson, A. M., 1979. Rates of loss of hepatic copper during copper-depletion of cattle, *Proc. Nutr. Soc.* **38**: 59A (Abstr.).

McMurray, C. H. and McEldowney, P. K., 1977. A possible prophylaxis and model for nutritional degenerative myopathy in young cattle, *Br. vet. J.* **133**: 535–42.

MacPherson, A. and Moon, F. E., 1974. Effects of long term maintenance of sheep on a low-cobalt diet as assessed by clinical condition and biochemical parameters. In *Trace Element Metabolism in Animals-2* (ed.

W. G. Hoekstra, J. W. Suttie, H. E. Ganther and W. Mertz),
pp. 624–7. University Park Press, Baltimore.

MacPherson, A., Voss, R. C. and Dixon, J., 1979. The effect of copper
treatment on the performance of hypocupraemic calves, *Anim. Prod.*
29: 91–9.

Mason, J. and Cardin, C. J., 1977. The competition of molybdate and sulphate
ions for a transport system in the ovine small intestine, *Res. vet. Sci.*
22: 313–5.

Masuhara, T. and Migicovsky, B. B., 1963. Vitamin D and the intestinal
absorption of cobalt, *J. Nutr.* **80**: 322–6.

Matrone, G., 1974. Chemical parameters in trace element antagonisms. In
Trace Element Metabolism in Animals–2 (ed. W. G. Hoekstra, J. W.
Suttie, H. E. Ganther and W. Mertz), pp. 91–103. University Park
Press, Baltimore.

Mertz, W., 1974. The newer essential trace elements, chromium, tin,
vanadium, nickel and silicon, *Proc. Nutr. Soc.* **33**: 307–13.

Middleton, H. M., 1977. Uptake of pyridoxine hydrochloride by the rat
jejunal mucosa *in vivo*, *J. Nutr.* **107**: 126–31.

Middleton, H. M., 1979. Intestinal absorption of pyridoxal-5-phosphate:
disappearance from perfused segments of rat jejunum *in vivo*, *J. Nutr.*
109: 975–81.

Millar, K. R. and Lorentz, P. P., 1979. Urinary methyl malonic acid as an
indicator of the vitamin B_{12} status of grazing sheep, *N.Z. vet. J.*
27: 90–2.

Miller, J. K., Swanson, E. W., Spalding, G. E., Lyke, W. A. and Hall, R. F.,
1974. The role of the abomasum in recycling of iodine in the bovine. In
Trace Element Metabolism in Animals-2 (ed. W. G. Hoekstra, J. W.
Suttie, H. E. Ganther and W. Mertz), pp. 638–40. University Park
Press, Baltimore.

Mills, C. F., Dalgarno, A. C. and Wenham, G., 1976. Biochemical and
pathological changes in tissues of Friesian cattle during the experimental
induction of copper deficiency, *Br. J. Nutr.* **35**: 309–31.

Mistilis, S. P. and Mearrick, P. T., 1969. The absorption of ionic, biliary and
plasma radiocopper in neonatal rats, *Scand. J. Gastroenterol.* **4**: 691–6.

Morgan, K. T., 1974. Amprolium poisoning of pre-ruminant lambs. An
ultrastructural study of the cerebral malacia and the nature of the
inflammatory response, *J. Pathol.* **112**: 229–36.

Morton, R. A., 1974. The vitamin concept, *Vitams Horm.* **32**: 155–66.

Okonkwo, A. C., Ku, P. K., Miller, E. R., Keahey, K. K. and Ullrey, D. E.,
1979. Copper requirement of baby pigs fed purified diets, *J. Nutr.*
109: 939–48.

Ott, E. A., Smith, W. H., Stob, M., Parker, H. E., Harrington, R. B. and
Beeson, W. M., 1965. Zinc requirement of the growing lamb fed a
purified diet, *J. Nutr.* **87**: 459–63.

Patil, B. D., Jones, D. I. H. and Hughes, R., 1969. Wool characteristics as an
indication of nutritive attributes in herbage varieties, *Nature, Lond.*
223: 1072–3.

Patterson, D. S. P., Sweasey, D. and Herbert, C. N., 1971. Changes occurring
in the chemical composition of the central nervous system during

References

451

foetal and post-natal development of the sheep, *J. Neurochem.*
18: 2027–40.

Payne, J. M., 1963. The danger of using massive doses of vitamin D_3 in the
prevention of milk fever, *Vet. Rec.* **75**: 848–9.

Pickford, J. R., 1968. The effect of mill processing on vitamin levels in diets. In
Proc. 2nd Nutr. Conf. Feed Mfrs Univ. Nott. (ed. H. Swan and
D. Lewis), pp. 175–84. Churchill, London.

Pill, A. H., 1967. Evidence of thiamine deficiency in calves affected with
cerebrocortical necrosis, *Vet. Rec.* **81**: 178–81.

Russel, A. J. F., Whitelaw, A., Moberly, Patricia and Fawcett, A.R., 1975.
Investigation into diagnosis and treatment of cobalt deficiency in lambs,
Vet. Rec. **96**: 194–8.

Sansom, B. F., Vagg, M. J. and Taylor, P. J., 1973. The whole-body counter
as an instrument for studying the input-output relationships of mineral
elements. In *Production Disease in Farm Animals* (ed. J. M. Payne,
K. G. Hibbitt and B. F. Sansom), pp. 122–31. Baillière Tindall,
London.

Sauberlich, H. E., 1980. Interactions of thiamin, riboflavin and other B
vitamins. In *Proc. N.Y. Acad. Sci Conf. Micronutrient Interactions: Vitams
Minerals Hazardous Elements* (ed. O. Levander).

Scott, M. L., 1962. Anti-oxidants, selenium and sulphur amino acids in the
vitamin E nutrition of chicks, *Nutr. Abstr. Rev.* **32**: 1–8.

Scott, M. L., Noguchi, T. and Combs, G. F., 1974. New evidence concerning
mechanisms of action of vitamin E and selenium, *Vitams Horm.* **32**:
429–44.

Scrutton, M. C., 1971. Purification and some properties of a protein containing
manganese (avimanganin), *Biochemistry, Wash. D.C.* **10**: 3897–905.

Serfass, R. E. and Ganther, H. E., 1975. Defective microbicidal activity in
glutathione peroxidase deficient neutrophils of selenium deficient rats,
Nature, Lond. **255**: 640–1.

Shand, A. and Lewis, G., 1957. Chronic copper poisoning in young calves,
Vet. Rec. **69**: 618–21.

Smith, J. C., Brown, E. D. and Cassidy, W. A., 1977. Zinc and vitamin A:
interrelationships. In *Zinc Metabolism: Current Concepts in Health
and Disease*, pp. 29–44. Alan R. Liss, New York.

Smith, C. M., De Luca, H. F., Tanaka, Y. and Mahaffey, K. R., 1978.
Stimulation of lead absorption by vitamin D administration, *J. Nutr.*
108: 843–7.

Smith, R. M. and Marston, H. R., 1970. Some metabolic aspects of vitamin
B_{12} deficiency in sheep, *Br. J. Nutr.* **24**: 879–91.

Smith, R. M., Osborne-White, W. S. and O'Dell, B. L., 1976. Cytochromes
in brain mitochondria from lambs with enzootic ataxia, *J. Neurochem.*
26: 1145–8.

Smith, B. S. W. and Wright, H., 1980. The response of serum 25-hydroxy-
vitamin D concentrations to vitamin D intake and insolation in sheep,
Br. J. Nutr. **43**: 533–40.

Somers, M. and Gawthorne, J. M., 1969. The effect of dietary cobalt intake on
the plasma vitamin B_{12} concentration of sheep, *Aust. J. exp. Biol. med.
Sci.* **47**: 227–33.

Suttie, J. W. and Jackson, C. M., 1977. Prothrombin structure, activation and biosynthesis, *Physiol. Rev.* **57**: 1–70.

Suttle, N. F., 1977. Reducing the potential copper toxicity of concentrates to sheep by the use of molybdenum and sulphur supplements, *Anim. Feed Sci. Technol.* **2**: 235–46.

Suttle, N. F., 1978a. Determining the copper requirements of cattle by means of an intravenous repletion technique. In *Proc. 3rd int. Symp. Trace Element Metab. Man Anim.* (ed. M. Kirchgessner), pp. 473–80. Arbeit Tierernärung, Weihenstephan.

Suttle, N. F., 1978b. Effects of sulphur and molybdenum on the absorption of copper from forage crops by ruminants. In *Proc. Symp. Sulphur Forages* (ed. J. C. Brogan), pp. 197–211. An Foras Talúntais, Dublin.

Suttle, N. F., 1979a. Treatment of bovine hypocuprosis by the oral administration of cupric oxide needles, *Proc. Nutr. Soc.* **38**: 135A (Abstr.).

Suttle, N. F., 1979b. Copper, iron, manganese and zinc concentrations in the carcases of lambs and calves and the relationships to trace element requirements for growth, *Br. J. Nutr.* **42**: 89–96.

Suttle, N. F., Field, A. C., Nicolson, T. B., Mathieson, A. O., Prescott, J. H. D., Scott, N. and Johnson, W. S., 1980. Some problems in assessing the physiological and economic significance of hypocupraemia in beef suckler herds, *Vet. Rec.* **105**: 302–5.

Suttle, N. F. and Grace, N. D., 1978. A demonstration of marked recycling of molybdenum via the gastrointestinal tract of sheep at low sulphur intakes, *Proc. Nutr. Soc.* **37**: 68A (Abstr.).

Thafvelin, B. and Oksanen, H. E., 1966. Vitamin E and linoleic acid content of hay as related to different conditions, *J. Dairy Sci.* **49**: 282–6.

Ullrey, D. E., 1974. The selenium deficiency problem in animal agriculture. In *Trace Element Metabolism in Animals-2* (ed. W. G. Hoekstra, J. W. Suttie, H. E. Ganther and W. Mertz), pp. 275–93. University Park Press, Baltimore.

Underwood, E. J., 1977. Introduction. In *Trace Elements in Human and Animal Nutrition*, 4th edn, pp. 1–12. Academic Press, New York.

Vallee, B. L., 1964. Zinc and the active centre of carboxypeptidase A. In *Proc. 6th int. Congr. Nutr. Edinb.* (ed. D. P. Cuthbertson, C. F. Mills and R. Passmore), pp. 270–88. Livingstone, Edinburgh.

Vallee, B. L., 1974. The entatic properties of cobalt carboxypeptidase and cobalt pro-carboxypeptidase. In *Trace Element Metabolism in Animals-2* (ed. W. G. Hoekstra, J. W. Suttie, H. E. Ganther and W. Mertz), pp. 5–17. University Park Press, Baltimore.

Weigand, E. and Kirchgessner, M., 1978. Homeostatic adjustments in zinc digestion to widely varying dietary zinc intake, *Nutr. Metab.* **22**: 101–12.

Whitelaw, A., Armstrong, R. H., Evans, C. C. and Fawcett, A. R., 1979. A study of the effects of copper deficiency in Scottish Blackface lambs on improved hill pasture, *Vet. Rec.* **104**: 455–60.

Wiener, G. and Field, A. C., 1970. Genetic variation in copper metabolism of sheep. In *Proc. 1st int. Symp. Trace Element Metab. Anim.* (ed. C. F. Mills), pp. 92–102. Livingstone, Edinburgh.

Yasumoto, K., Iwami, K. and Yoshida, M., 1979. Vitamin B_6 dependence of seleno-methionine and selenite utilisation for glutathione peroxidase in the rat, *J. Nutr.* **109**: 760–6.

Section 3

DIET AND ANIMAL PERFORMANCE

11 FOOD CHARACTERISTICS THAT LIMIT VOLUNTARY INTAKE

R. C. Campling and I. J. Lean

In many production systems large intakes of food are required to ensure high outputs of animal products and, by reducing the proportion of total energy intake used for maintenance, efficient conversion of food into product. Also, it may be financially worthwhile to substitute bulky foods of low digestibility for highly digestible foods in diets for ruminants, and to a more limited extent in those for pigs and poultry. Ruminants, poultry and piglets are often offered food *ad libitum* but, because of the propensity of the weaned pig to deposit fat, food is restricted in most intensive pig-rearing systems.

The view is widely held that animals regulate their energy balance, the intake of food being adjusted to maintain energy equilibrium, although the size of the energy store of the body varies with the physiological state of the animal (Hervey, 1975). Farm animals tend to show this type of regulation provided that the characteristics of the food allow the animal to consume sufficient energy. However, limitations to food intake arising from the characteristics of the food are a common feature of many production systems. The aims of this chapter are to describe and discuss these limitations and to indicate ways of overcoming them.

The voluntary intake of food by a farm animal is, of course, influenced by many factors other than those associated with the food; these include factors arising from the climatic, physical and social environments of the animal as well as its physiological state. Body size, pregnancy, lactation and fatness each affect food intake, and changes in the animal due to any one of these factors may mask food characteristics limiting intake. A most potent factor is lactation: cows, ewes and sows eat considerably more when lactating than when dry. In the cow and ewe food intake increases daily from a low level at parturition to a maximum some weeks after peak milk production is reached (Forbes, 1970; Foot and Tessier, 1978; Bines, 1979), and similar changes have been observed in the sow (Friend, 1971). The amount of food eaten during lactation varies directly with milk output and with the body condition of the lactating animal. Intake is inversely related to the amount of body tissue gained during gestation: fat animals eat less than thin animals (Friend, 1971; Bines 1979; Foot and Russel, 1979). Also, fatness affects food intake in the non-lactating animal. Whether male animals eat more food than castrated males or females is uncertain. In some experiments, but not in others, bulls have shown larger intakes than castrated male cattle and young females (Kay and Houseman, 1975); castrated male pigs eat slightly more than females (Agricultural Research Council, 1967). Lastly, relative to body weight, young animals often have higher intakes than older, heavier animals. Growing animals will exhibit very high intakes per unit of body weight during compensatory growth following a period of restricted feeding (Wilson and Osbourn, 1960; Owen, Ridgman and Wyllie, 1971).

There are two main categories of food, concentrates and forages. Most concentrates are cereal and legumes seeds or residues of their processing, and they contain high levels of reserve carbohydrate (mainly starch) together with proteins and lipids. Some concentrates are also derived from oil seeds, e.g. oilseed meals and oil products, and a small number are of animal origin, e.g. fish meals, meat and bone meal, and milk. The oilseed and animal products include materials rich in protein (for the animal products, protein of high biological value) and materials having a high lipid, and thus digestible energy, content. The forages include herbages, conserved green crops and cereal straws. They are fibrous foods, the components of the fibre being the cell wall constituents, cellulose, hemicellulose, lignin and silica (see Butler and Bailey, 1973).

Plant cell contents, starch, sugars, organic acids, non-protein nitrogen (NPN) compounds, soluble protein and pectin, can be almost completely digested by ruminants and non-ruminants alike provided that the microbial and digestive enzymes can penetrate into the cells. Some form of processing is generally necessary with cereal grains to allow the entry of the digestive enzymes (Hutton and Armstrong, 1976). Plant cell wall constituents on the other hand are only susceptible to microbial digestion, as in the rumen or caecum, and are poorly digested in most simple-stomached animals. Concentrates have a high ratio of cell contents to cell walls, whilst in forages the ratio is much lower. Moreover, in forages, the proportion of cell wall and the degree of lignification of the wall varies with the type of plant, and in all cases increases as the plant matures through the flowering and seed formation stage so that the forage becomes increasingly more resistant to digestion, even in the ruminant gut.

The chemical composition and nutritive value of British foods, and of American and Canadian foods, were described by the ARC (1976) and the National Academy of Sciences (1971), respectively. Shorter lists of foods used in Britain were published by the Ministry of Agriculture, Fisheries and Food, Department of Agriculture and Fisheries for Scotland, and Department of Agriculture for Northern Ireland (1975), and by McDonald, Edwards and Greenhalgh (1981). Foods used for pigs were considered by Whittemore and Elsley (1976), and those used for poultry by Scott, Neshiem and Young (1976), Feltwell and Fox (1978), and McDonald *et al.* (1981). Foods of tropical origin were described botanically and chemically by Göhl (1975).

The characteristics of foods that limit voluntary intake are attributes of the physical and chemical composition of the foods, and vary with the different animal species and with the age of the animal. Voluntary intake is a function of both the food and the type of digestive system the animal possesses. Whilst ruminants are well equipped to eat and digest bulky forages containing a high proportion of structural carbohydrate, non-ruminants have much smaller stomachs and a limited ability to digest cellulose (Pond and Maner, 1974). Neonates have undeveloped digestive systems and calves (Roy, 1980), lambs (Large, 1965) and piglets (Kidder and Manners, 1978) will only consume nutrients in liquid form. Development of the full complement of digestive enzymes and/or a functional reticulo-rumen confers much greater ability on the animals to eat and digest a wide range of foods.

Attributes of food that are considered here are: bulk, including physical form; content of digestible energy; content of protein and protein degradation products; acidity and alkalinity; associativity with supplementary starchy concentrates; flavour; and content of toxic substances. Separate consideration is given to grazed forage, in which the spatial distribution of the forage affects intake, and, finally, methods of predicting voluntary food intake are discussed.

BULK

This property is determined by the air and water spaces in the food and by the content of structural carbohydrates. Bulk operates through distension of the gut in limiting intake, and its limiting effect can be altered by reducing the particle size of a food by grinding or by compressing the food to reduce air and water contents, as in pelleting and drying. With forages it has been established that the content of cell wall and its resistance to breakdown in the reticulo-rumen largely determine the extent to which the food is eaten by ruminants. Van Soest (1975) has expounded the concept that the structural volume of a forage in the rumen – its filling effect – is due primarily to the cell wall content; intracellular spaces in the forage may be filled with air and/or water. Intake is governed largely by the rate of reduction in particle size of the units of structural carbohydrates, and the rate of removal of the undigested and partially digested particles from the reticulo-rumen. Thus the more susceptible the cell wall of a forage is to comminution within the rumen, the greater will be its voluntary intake. The susceptibility will depend on the chemical composition of the cell walls and the effects of microbial digestion and chewing, particularly during rumination (Van Soest, 1973 and 1975; Osbourn, Terry, Outen and Cammell, 1974). A comparison of lucerne and grass can be used as an example. Both in its leaves and stem, lucerne has, on average, a lower content of cell walls than is found in the corresponding tissues in grass, and thus lucerne tends to be more rapidly digested than grass in the rumen. Consistent with this, sheep eat a greater quantity of lucerne than of grass harvested at a corresponding stage of growth (Demarquilly and Jarrige, 1974; Van Soest, 1975).

Reducing the structural volume or bulk of a forage by grinding it into small particles using a hammermill will often improve its intake, and, since milled foods can be dusty, intake may be further improved through pelleting. The more resistant the forage to comminution during chewing and to microbial attack in the rumen, the greater will be the effects of physical processing on intake; benefits from grinding and pelleting foods which are rapidly broken down in the rumen are small (van der Honing, 1975). Similarly, since superficial water on a food can rapidly be lost from the rumen, extracellular water does not have a lasting effect on rumen distension. Even with wet immature herbages there was no correlation between DM content and voluntary intake by sheep (Wilson, 1978), although there may be a critical content of plant DM below which voluntary intake is limited. Wilson (1978) suggested this critical level may be approximately 125 to 145 g DM per kg, which is likely to occur only with immature herbage in the spring. A direct association has usually been observed in cattle between the amount of DM eaten and the DM content of silages. However, this is probably not a causal relationship (Ekern and Vik-Mo, 1979). Calves offered concentrates *ad libitum* in wet (850 g water per kg) and air-dry forms ate similar amounts of DM (Fitzgerald and Kay, 1974).

Roots and tubers are types of food containing a large proportion of water; swedes, mangels and turnips may have 880 g water per kg or more, and potatoes and fodder beet contain 780 to 800 g/kg. There is evidence that beef cattle weighing 250 kg, and given diets composed of less than half as rolled barley and the remainder as swedes, were unable to eat sufficient to achieve live-weight gains as high as similar cattle given a diet containing a higher proportion of barley (Kay,

Macdearmid and Innes, 1977). When the cattle had been on the diet for approximately 10 weeks, their intake of roots began to improve. Similar experiments with cattle offered potatoes and fodder beet did not show any restriction in voluntary intake due to the roots. Lambs were unable to eat sufficient DM as swedes and potatoes to equal their voluntary DM intake of a barley concentrate diet (Ørskov, Andrews and Gill, 1969).

The only other food in which water is a major constituent is milk. Each species of mammalian farm animal produces milk of characteristic composition, differing widely in DM content. Milk from cows contains 125 g DM per kg, from ewes 184 g/kg and from sows 160 g/kg. Artificial rearing, using liquid diets based on reconstituted skim milk powder and added fat, is frequently used for young animals. It seems that the calf and lamb can tolerate a wide range in concentration of DM in the liquid diet (Large, 1965; Ternouth, Stobo and Roy, 1978). A concentration as low as 80 g DM per kg did not appear to impair the calf's ability to take in milk. However, in veal calves of 7 to 16 weeks of age there was evidence that distension of the abomasum limited intake of liquid diets when the concentration of DM was 140 g/kg. With this diet the calves were unable to drink sufficient to satisfy their requirements for maximum growth (Stobo, Roy and Ganderton, 1979).

Physical form

Certain foods are prepared by processing before feeding to various classes of farm animals. This is done to ensure efficient digestion. Cereal grains are normally rolled or milled before being given to cattle, and it is also possible to process them chemically by treatment with sodium hydroxide (Ørskov and Greenhalgh, 1977). The changes in physical form may affect voluntary intake. It is not usual to offer grain *ad libitum* to cattle, except for those kept in some intensive beef systems. Food consumption by these cattle may be reduced if the grain is too finely milled and digestive upsets may occur if insufficient coarse material is given. The inclusion of a small amount of forage with concentrate foods offered *ad libitum* will maintain rumen function and often stabilize the voluntary intake of concentrates (Preston and Willis, 1974).

In the tropics, where cattle production may be largely dependent on sugar cane and its derivatives (e.g. molasses) and not on cereal grains, it is particularly important to provide cattle with long roughage which ensures maximum intake and utilization of foods rich in sugar. Also, with molasses-based diets, urea is supplied to provide a source of nitrogen for the rumen microflora, and a high-quality protein supplement relatively resistant to rumen degradation (fish meal) given to ensure that amino acid supply in the intestine is not limiting. The physical properties of the pith of the stalks of sugar cane (derinded sugar cane) are not adequate to maintain normal rumen function, and inclusion of roughage is beneficial (Preston and Willis, 1974).

Alteration in the physical form of roughages may occur as a result of conservation processes. For example, grass is chopped before ensiling to enable air to be excluded from the ensiled herbage and ensure good preservation. However, the particle size of the chopped material may influence voluntary intake. Marsh (1978) concluded that intake of silages by sheep increased markedly with increasing fineness of chop, and that there were probably similar, although smaller, responses by growing and adult cattle. It was not possible to specify an optimum size of particle for sheep but for cattle there was little evidence to support chopping to less than 25 mm.

With artificially dried green crops it is usual to process the food to increase the bulk density of the product and thus reduce transport costs. A variety of methods of packaging such dried crops is possible, each leaving the product with a different particle size and bulk density (Shepperson, Marchant, Wilkins and Raymond, 1972). Large cobs and wafers may slow down the rate of eating by cows (Campling and Milne, 1972) but it seems unlikely that the particle size of the milled dried forage will limit intake (Tetlow and Wilkins, 1974).

With piglets from 11 to 56 days of age the physical form of a maize-based concentrate diet did not affect food intake; as much food was eaten when the diet was given as pellets as when it was offered as a coarsely milled mixture (Wu and Fuller, 1974). In older pigs, comparisons have shown larger intakes of ground rolled barley than whole grain but little difference between the processed forms of grain (Hutton and Armstrong, 1976); digestibility of whole grain was considerably lower than that of rolled grain. A wet-feeding system is often used in piggeries with meal suspended in water and pumped to the pens of pigs, using a ratio of water to dry food of approximately 3:1.

Food for poultry is offered as dry mash (meal), wet mash, pellets, crumbs (coarsely broken pellets) and as whole cereal grain. Slightly reduced intakes were found with very finely ground, dusty food (ARC, 1975). To ensure maximum intake, food must be offered *ad libitum* throughout the day with a supply of drinking water (Feltwell and Fox, 1978). If water is limited then a wet mash can be used to improve intake, but the mash rapidly becomes mouldy and unacceptable if left in the hoppers. Pellets of 3.2 to 4.7 mm diameter are eaten by birds (broilers) in probably the greatest quantity; intake is some 60 to 80 g/kg more than when the food is given in mash form (ARC, 1975; Scott *et al.*, 1976).

DIGESTIBLE ENERGY

With diets in which bulk, physical form and essential nutrients are not limiting, cattle, sheep, pigs and poultry regulate their intakes of food to maintain a constant digestible-energy (DE) intake. They consume the same amount of DE irrespective of the concentration of DE in the diet. Thus with diets of low digestibility more food will be eaten than with highly-digestible diets. There is much evidence in support of this conclusion from studies with lambs and cattle offered concentrate diets diluted with ground fibrous material (Baumgardt, 1974). Pigs behaved in a similar manner when offered diets diluted with sawdust or oat food, or when given a diet in which the concentration of DE was increased by the inclusion of fats (ARC, 1967; O'Grady, 1978). With such diets the amount of food eaten is determined by the ability of the tissues to metabolize the digested energy. Changes in energy requirement due to normal physiological factors (e.g. lactation) would be expected to lead to increased food intake, but cows in early lactation do not eat sufficient to meet their requirements for energy (Bines, 1979). Also, young pigs and lambs may not be able to compensate as successfully as older, larger animals for the inclusion of large amounts of diluent in the diet (Owen and Ridgman, 1968; Owen, Davies and Ridgman, 1969). Morris (1968) summarized many reports on the voluntary intake of egg-laying hens and concluded that, provided that the diets contained about 11.3 MJ metabolizable energy (ME) per kg, the birds adjusted their intake of food to keep ME intake constant. The adjustment of food intake was not accurate if the ME concentration of the diet differed appreciably from 11.3 MJ/kg. Also, large birds and birds with a high rate of egg laying did not compensate as successfully as strains of birds with lower food intakes (see ARC, 1975). Further information on food intake regulation in poultry has been given by Boorman and Freeman (1979).

PROTEIN AND PROTEIN DEGRADATION PRODUCTS

In laboratory mammals there is much evidence of poor voluntary intake with low protein diets. Especially low intakes are seen if the diet contains an excessive amount of one amino acid (Harper, 1974). Similarly, in the pig and chicken intakes may be low with very low protein diets, and with those with a marked amino acid imbalance or an excessive amount of protein (Rérat, 1972; Robinson, Holmes and Bayley, 1974; ARC, 1975).

Foods with a low protein content are eaten by ruminants in small amounts and supplementary protein or NPN will often improve voluntary intake. One main class of low-protein foods is formed by the crop residues, e.g. straws and maize stover, and herbages when mature;

these foods are also bulky and of low digestibility. Limitations on intake are common in ruminants grazing mature forage grown in range areas, which frequently suffer from drought. Provision of urea, by spraying it on the standing forage or including it in a molasses lick, may improve intake and reduce loss in live weight and mortality (Loosli and McDonald, 1968). Similarly, cattle offered barley straw *ad libitum* increased their straw intake by 25% when given supplements including soya bean meal (Lyons, Caffrey and O'Connell, 1970). These improvements in intake of low protein fodders when NPN or protein are given are probably due partly to improved cellulolysis and increased rate of breakdown of cell walls in the reticulo-rumen, and partly to effects on metabolism in the body tissues (Weston, 1967). Protein supplements are likely to lead to an increased weight of rumen digesta as well as to a faster rate of breakdown of straw in the rumen. The latter comes about because several of the most important species of cellulolytic bacteria in the rumen require ammonia as their main nitrogen source (Hungate, 1966; Bryant, 1973), and unless the fodder contains 80 to 100 g crude protein per kg DM their nitrogen requirements are not met. It is also important that the source of nitrogen is susceptible to microbial degradation in the reticulo-rumen and for this reason urea is sometimes used.

The other class of food low in nitrogen is that based on sugar cane. Intake by cattle of molasses and of the pith of the stalks of sugar cane can be improved by the provision of both urea to supply ammonia in the rumen and a protected protein to increase the supply of amino acids in the small intestine (Preston and Willis, 1974).

Small amounts of supplementary groundnut meal will increase the voluntary intake by milking cows of well preserved grass silages containing 140 g crude protein per kg DM and of high digestibility (0.65 kg digestible organic matter per kg DM (DOMD)) (Thomas and Castle, 1979). These silages cannot be classed as low-protein foods and the reason for the improvement in intake is still uncertain, although the protein supplements have been shown to increase the digestibility of silage cell-wall constituents.

Substances produced by the degradation of herbage proteins during the ensiling process have been implicated in limiting the intake by ruminants of this class of food (Vetter and Von Glan, 1978). Statistical surveys have indicated that the intake of silages by sheep is negatively correlated with the ammonia-nitrogen content of the silages, expressed as a proportion of the total nitrogen content (Wilkins, Hutchinson, Wilson and Harris, 1971), and infusion of ammonium salts into the rumen of goats has depressed food intake and altered eating behaviour (Conrad, Baile and Mayer, 1977). However, this does not necessarily imply an important involvement of ammonia in the regulation of silage intake. Silages with good intake potential certainly have ammonia-nitrogen contents of less than 100 g/kg of the total nitrogen, but high ammonia-nitrogen figures are a reflexion of an adverse silage fermentation. In these situations, there is extensive degradation of forage proteins (and other constituents) in the silo with formation of a wide range of products which might influence silage intake, and with possible effects on the supply of amino acids to the small intestine in animals given the silages. With some silages, supplementation of the diet with proteins protected from ruminal attack, or with methionine given as a parenteral injection, increases silage intake (see Wilkinson, Wilson and Barry, 1976).

The potential detrimental effects on intake associated with high ammonia levels can be prevented by wilting the crop prior to ensiling and further improved by the use of an additive such as formic acid (Wilkinson *et al.*, 1976; Waldo, 1977). Indeed, it is possible not only to restrict the breakdown of protein in the silo but also its degradation by rumen microorganisms by treating the herbage with formaldehyde before ensiling. Protection of protein from microbial attack within the rumen may lead to a shortage of degradable protein, and an NPN supplement will ensure adequate rumen function and voluntary food intake. With high DM silages (400 g DM per kg), overheating of protein may occur, which will depress protein solubility and reduce protein digestibility. These effects reduce nitrogen utilization by cattle and lead to low intakes which can be improved by supplementary protein (Waldo, 1977). Histamine, tyramine and serotonin, which are present in low DM silages, have many physiological effects, including a lowering of blood pressure, and have been suggested as causes of low intakes. But there is little to indicate that these substances are normally important in intake control.

ACIDITY AND ALKALINITY

The voluntary intake by ruminants of well-preserved silages has sometimes been shown to be limited by their low pH and high contents of lactic and acetic acids (Wilkins *et al.*, 1971; Ekern and Vik-Mo, 1979). Partial neutralization of grass and maize silages with sodium bicarbonate has led to increased intake, although this has not been a consistent finding (Farhan and Thomas, 1978). Wilting the herbage before ensiling will also reduce the amount of organic acids in the silage and there is evidence that voluntary intake increased with increasing content of DM in silages (Ekern and Vik-Mo, 1979).

Few foods are alkaline; the only one that need be mentioned is alkali-treated straw. Cereal straws or other lignified, cellulose-rich materials (e.g. the mature maize rachis) are physically and chemically processed to improve feeding value: the fibrous materials are ground, treated with sodium hydroxide to disrupt the bond between lignin and cellulose, and the products pelleted (Jackson, 1977). Treated straw has a pH value of approximately 10.6 unless the residual alkali is neutralized; commonly, the pH is adjusted to 7.3. Treated straw which has not been neutralized has been fed to dry cows in large amounts without any clinical signs of alkalosis (Rexen, Stigsen and Kristensen, 1976).

SUPPLEMENTARY STARCHY CONCENTRATES

Ruminants are often offered forage *ad libitum* and given restricted amounts of concentrates, usually cereal grain, to increase the total intake of digestible energy. Small amounts (10 to 20% of total DM intake (DMI)) of supplementary grain and protein-rich concentrate will be completely additive and increase total DMI by the amount of concentrate DM given. With low-protein fodders intake of forage may even be enhanced (Crabtree and Williams, 1971), as already described above. Larger amounts of cereal grain are likely to lead to the animal decreasing its voluntary intake of forage and thus the supplement ceases to be completely additive, and substitution of concentrate for forage occurs (Blaxter and Wilson, 1963; Campling and Murdoch, 1966). The extent to which the supplement is additive and improves the digestibility of the whole diet will depend on the chemical composition and digestibility of the supplement and of the forage. Readily digested starchy supplements, e.g. rolled barley, depress forage intake more than the same amounts of a cellulose-rich supplement, e.g. a pelleted, milled, artificially dried grass or legume (Tayler and Wilkins, 1976; Bines, 1979).

For a given amount of supplementary cereal grain, the greatest depression in forage intake occurs with forages of high digestibility. Leaver (1973) found the increase in total intake of DM by calves given 1 kg DM concentrate supplement was approximately 0.3 kg DM with maize silage (0.69 DOMD) and 0.7 kg DM with barley straw (0.42 DOMD). In the milking cow, forage intakes increase as lactation advances, and thus for animals given a constant quantity of concentrate the substitution ratio improves (Østergaard, 1979). It is essential to recognize that partial substitution rather than complete additivity will occur when many medium- to high-digestibility forages are supplemented with more than small amounts of concentrates, and this may mean the substitution of a cheap food by a costly one. The detailed mechanism through which the supplement depresses forage intake is not fully known although concentrates depress the rate and extent of cellulose breakdown of the forage component of the diet in the rumen, and reduce the rate of removal of digesta (Campling, 1966).

FLAVOUR

Although it is commonly believed that flavour of a food is an important factor affecting its voluntary intake there is little evidence in support of this. That farm animals can discriminate between salt, sweet, bitter and acid solutions has been demonstrated in electrophysiological and behavioural studies (Arnold and Hill, 1972; Kare and Beauchamp, 1977). Also, there are many reports of selection between foods in cafeteria-choice situations but it is not possible to relate quantitatively such discriminatory responses to the animal's maximum intake of a food (Arnold and Dudzinski, 1978). In many farming situations the animal is not presented with a choice between foods but more often, as in indoor feeding, with only one food. Only in the grazing situation is there much opportunity for food selection. How the senses of smell and taste influence grazing behaviour and selection of plants is not known, but impairing the senses of sheep by surgery markedly altered the acceptability of plants (Arnold, 1966). A discussion of the relationship between chemical components in plants and acceptability is given by Arnold and Dudzinski (1978). As these authors point out, the signals that activate receptors of the sense organs are molecules which react chemically, and it is not possible for the animal to recognize, with the senses of taste or smell, the protein, energy or crude-fibre components of plants.

Sugar is important in determining ruminant food preferences and molasses can sometimes be used to encourage the eating of foods which cattle may be reluctant to consume normally. Similarly, sugar is used in diets for piglets to promote the eating of creep food (Whittemore and Elsley, 1976). It has not been possible to find a flavour that enhances food intake in the bird (Feltwell and Fox, 1978).

TOXIC SUBSTANCES

Several foods contain naturally occurring toxic substances and some of these may limit the extent to which the food can be eaten or included in the diet. One of the first signs of ill health is a reduction in food intake, but here discussion is restricted to a few important examples in which the toxic substances depress intake and directly restrict the use of the food. A wide variety of endogenous toxic substances are found, many of them particularly associated with oilseeds: haemagglutinins, goitrogens, cyanogens, saponins, plant oestrogens, gossypol, tannins, and substances that interfere with mineral and vitamin uptake and metabolism

(Liener, 1969). Some forages also have 'anti-quality' factors (Burns, 1978): saponins, alkaloids and flavonoids. One substance widespread in brassica crops is the haemolytic toxin which in ruminants causes loss of appetite, haemoglobinuria, jaundice and anaemia (Smith and Greenhalgh, 1977). Non-ruminants are not affected. In a herd or flock fed mainly or exclusively on kale, it is common to find a small number of clinically affected animals and several others with subclinical disease. The primary toxin is S-methylcysteine sulphoxide which is acted upon by rumen microorganisms to produce dimethyldisulphide. Administration to ruminants of this latter substance produces clinical signs characteristic of kale poisoning (Smith and Greenhalgh, 1977; Smith, 1980). In the diets of sheep and cattle brassica crops should be restricted to not more than one-third of the total DMI, for at this level kale poisoning is unlikely to occur.

One main limitation to the use by grazing ruminants of forage legumes (e.g. lucerne) is their tendency to induce bloat. This disorder is characterized by excessive foaming of the digesta in the reticulo–rumen with increased intraruminal pressure and distension of this organ. Some animals may stop eating and reduce intake while others may show severe distension and death. The exact cause of the excessive foaming of rumen contents is unknown, although the soluble plant proteins, saponins and pectins, have been strongly implicated and microbial factors may be important (Clarke and Reid, 1970). There is considerable variation between cattle in their susceptibility to bloat and it is not known if voluntary intake is depressed in subclinically affected animals. Wilted and conserved legumes do not induce bloat. Prevention of bloat has been through the use of anti-foaming agents such as poloxalene or the spraying of pastures with oils. To be effective chemical preventive measures must be taken continuously.

In the pig it is known that a haemagglutinin in raw soya beans acts as an appetite depressant or anti-palatability factor (Pond and Maner, 1974). This does not normally restrict the use of this food in pig diets since heating the beans destroys the activity of the substance. The potato is another food in which cooking before feeding to pigs improves utilization and acceptability by destroying a chymotrypsin inhibitor (Whittemore, Moffat and Taylor, 1975)

GRAZED FORAGE

In the grazing situation, in addition to the effects of chemical composition which have already been discussed, the yield of herbage and its spatial distribution are important determinants of voluntary food intake. Intake by grazing cattle and sheep will be reduced on sparse pasture, but it is not possible to predict accurately the yield below which intake will be affected since this depends on the height of the sward and the amount allowed per animal (Hodgson, 1977). Another factor of major importance is the extent to which the animal alters its grazing pattern and increases the time spent grazing. In addition, the growth habit of the herbage plant will influence grazing behaviour. The ease with which the animal can prehend the plant, or part of it, is a determining factor of bite size and number of bites. There are large differences in the spatial distribution of herbage within swards of temperate and tropical grasses, and legumes. Cattle tend to reduce their rate of intake of herbage and the proportion of leaf as they progressively defoliate the sward towards the ground (Chacon and Stobbs, 1976; Arnold and Dudzinski, 1978); only in the later stages of grazing is much stem removed. The rate of ingesting herbage is likely to be influenced by the weight and density of the grazed material. Allowing the animal more herbage, for example by altering the area of sward, will influence the extent to which the animal is forced to graze down through the grazing horizons towards the soil. Unless the animal compensates for changes in rate of intake by increasing grazing time, daily intake of herbage will be reduced as the animal is forced to graze closer to the soil. Tropical grasses are often taller, less dense and less digestible than temperate grasses. Stobbs (1974) found, with Jersey cows, that the mean size of bites during grazing varied from 0.05 to 0.50 g DM per bite on tropical pastures and from 0.31 to 0.71 g DM on the temperate pastures. He suggested that despite there being adequate DM available there was a critical level of bite size (0.3 g DM) below which a 400-kg grazing animal could not gather sufficient food.

PREDICTION OF FOOD INTAKE

It is essential to have some means of accurately predicting food intake so that diets can be formulated that are within the food intake capacity of the animals under consideration. Possible limits to the daily intake of DE in pigs were suggested to be 20 MJ at 27 kg live weight rising to 60 MJ at 100 kg live weight (Whittemore and Elsley, 1976) but, for pigs, maximum voluntary intake is seldom a constraint on diet formulation, because in most intensive systems of production feeding is restricted to ensure the carcass is not over-fat. Equations are available for predicting the intake of food by broiler chickens (ARC, 1975) and there are similar equations for laying hens based on body weight, average egg weight, rate of lay and change in body weight (McDonald, 1978).

For ruminants many relationships have been proposed as a means of estimating food intake, varying from simple expressions of intake of DM or indigestible organic matter (IOM) per unit of body weight to complex partial regression equations taking account of body weight, milk production, stage of lactation and body weight change. Maximum intake per unit of body weight is greatest in the young animal and declines as it gets older and heavier. For example, maximum intakes suggested for beef cattle kept in a semi-intensive system were 3.0 kg DM at 100 kg live weight and 10.7 kg DM at 500 kg live weight (MAFF, 1979) or, expressed in preferred terms, were 0.6 kg IOM and 3.0 kg IOM, respectively. Maximum DM intakes for sheep were suggested to be 26 g/kg of body weight calculated for a diet of an assumed digestibility of 0.59 (MAFF, 1979). For the milking cow, MAFF *et al.* (1975) proposed that the DM intake of cows in mid- and late-lactation could be estimated from the equation: DM intake (kg/day) = 0.025 M + 0.1 Y, where M = live weight (kg) and Y = milk yield (kg/day); they suggested that the estimate of intake should be reduced by 2 or 3 kg DM per day in the initial 6 weeks of lactation. Some of the equations proposed predict the intake of groups of animals quite well: with groups of 20 cows intake of DM may be predicted within 1.1 kg/day; the equations are less accurate for the prediction of intakes in individual animals (see Bines, 1979; Vadiveloo and Holmes, 1979). All the equations are also subject to uncertainties and inaccuracies due to the problems of allowing for the particular characteristics of an individual foodstuff or diet, arising from its palatability, acidity, chemical composition, method of conservation and processing, etc. The effects of these factors are at present difficult to quantify satisfactorily and there is a need for further research, especially with cattle. Because of the high cost of using cattle, data on the intake characteristics of foods have often been collected using castrated male sheep but it has now been established that sheep and milking cows do not always react alike in response to the characteristics of foods that limit voluntary intake (Marsh, 1978).

REFERENCES

Agricultural Research Council, 1967. *The Nutrient Requirements of Farm Livestock. No. 3, Pigs.* Agricultural Research Council, London.
Agricultural Research Council, 1975. *The Nutrient Requirements of Farm Livestock. No. 1, Poultry.* Agricultural Research Council, London.
Agricultural Research Council, 1976. *The Nutrient Requirements of Farm*

Livestock. No. 4, Composition of British Feedingstuffs. Agricultural Research Council, London.

Arnold, G. W., 1966. The special senses in grazing animals. II. Smell, taste and touch and dietary habits in sheep, *Aust. J. agric. Res.* **17**: 531–42.

Arnold, G. W. and Dudzinski, M. L., 1978. *Ethology of Free-ranging Domestic Animals.* Elsevier, Amsterdam

Arnold, G. W. and Hill, J. C., 1972. Chemical factors affecting selection of food plants by ruminants. In *Phytochemical Ecology* (ed. J. B. Harborne), pp. 72–101. Academic Press, London.

Baumgardt, B. R., 1974. Food intake, energy balance and homeostasis. In *The Control of Metabolism* (ed. J. D. Sink), pp. 88–112. Pennsylvania State University Press, University Park.

Bines, J. A., 1979. Voluntary food intake. In *Feeding Strategy for the High Yielding Dairy Cow* (ed. W. H. Broster and H. Swan), pp. 23–48. Granada Publishing, London.

Blaxter, K. L. and Wilson, R. S., 1963. The assessment of a crop husbandry technique in terms of animal production, *Anim. Prod.* **5**: 27–42.

Boorman, K. N. and Freeman, B. H. 1979. *Food Intake Regulation in Poultry.* British Poultry Science Ltd, Edinburgh.

Bryant, M. P., 1973. Nutritional requirements of the predominant rumen cellulolytic bacteria, *Fedn Proc. Fedn Am. Socs exp. Biol.* **32**: 1809–13.

Burns, J. C., 1978. Antiquality factors as related to forage quality, *J. Dairy Sci.* **61**: 1809–20.

Butler, G. W. and Bailey, R. W., 1973. *Chemistry and Biochemistry of Herbage,* Vol. 1. Academic Press, London.

Campling, R. C., 1966. The effect of concentrates on the rate of disappearance of digesta from the alimentary tract of cows given hay, *J. Dairy Res.* **33**: 13–23.

Campling, R. C. and Milne, J. A., 1972. The nutritive value of processed roughages for milking cattle, *Proc. Br. Soc. Anim. Prod.*, pp. 53–60.

Campling, R. C. and Murdoch, J. C., 1966. The effects of concentrates on the voluntary intake of roughages by cows, *J. Dairy Res.* **33**: 1–11.

Chacon, E. and Stobbs, T. H., 1976. Influence of progressive defoliation of a grass sward on the eating behaviour of cattle, *Aust. J. agric. Res.* **27**: 709–27.

Clarke, R. T. J. and Reid, C. S. W., 1970. Legume bloat. In *Physiology of Digestion and Metabolism in the Ruminant* (ed. A. T. Phillipson), pp. 599–606. Oriel Press, Newcastle upon Tyne.

Conrad, H. R., Baile, C. A. and Mayer, J., 1977. Changing meal patterns and suppression of feed intake with increasing amounts of dietary nonprotein nitrogen in ruminants, *J. Dairy Sci.* **60**: 1725–33.

Crabtree, J. R. and Williams, G. L., 1971. The voluntary intake and utilization of roughage–concentrate diets by sheep. 1. Concentrate supplements for hay and straw, *Anim. Prod.* **13**: 71–82.

Demarquilly, C. and Jarrige, R., 1974. The comparative nutritive value of grasses and legumes, *Växtodling* **28**: 33–41.

Ekern, A. and Vik-Mo, L., 1979. Conserved forages as feeds for dairy cows. In *Feeding Strategy for the High Yielding Dairy Cow* (ed. W. H. Broster and H. Swan), pp. 322–73. Granada Publishing, London.

Farhan, S. M. A. and Thomas, P. C., 1978. The effect of partial neutralization of formic acid silages with sodium bicarbonate on their voluntary intake by cattle and sheep, *J. Br. Grassld Soc.* **33**: 151–8.

Feltwell, R. and Fox, S., 1978. *Practical Poultry Feeding*. Faber and Faber, London.

Fitzgerald, J. J. and Kay, M., 1974. Studies on the intake and utilization of wet feed by calves, *Anim. Prod.* **19**: 149–56.

Foot, Janet Z. and Russel, A. J. F., 1979. The relationship in ewes between voluntary food intake during pregnancy and forage intake during lactation and after weaning, *Anim. Prod.* **28**: 25–39.

Foot, Janet Z. and Tessier, M., 1978. Voluntary intake of feed by lactating ewes. In *Milk Production in the Ewe* (ed. J. G. Boyazoglu, and T. T. Treacher), *Eur. Ass. Anim. Prod. Publ. No. 23*, pp. 66–73.

Forbes, J. M., 1970. The voluntary food intake of pregnant and lactating ruminants: a review, *Br. vet. J.* **126**: 1–11.

Friend, D. W., 1971. Self-selection of feeds and water by swine during pregnancy and lactation, *J. Anim. Sci.* **32**: 658–66.

Göhl, B., 1975. *Tropical Feeds*. Food and Agriculture Organization, Rome.

Harper, A. E., 1974. Control mechanisms in amino acid metabolism. In *The Control of Metabolism* (ed. J. D. Sink), pp 49–74. Pennsylvania State University Press, University Park.

Hervey, G. R., 1975. The problem of energy balance in the light of control theory. In *Neural Integration of Physiological Mechanisms and Behaviour* (ed. G. J. Mogenson, and F. R. Calaresu), pp. 109–27 Toronto University Press, Toronto.

Hodgson, J., 1977. Factors limiting herbage intake by the grazing animal. In *Proc. Int. Meet. Anim. Prod. from Temperate Grassld, Dublin* (ed. B. Gilsenan), pp. 70–5. Irish Grassland Animal Production Association/An Foras Talúntais, Dublin.

Hungate, R. E., 1966. *The Rumen and its Microbes*. Academic Press, New York.

Hutton, K. and Armstrong, D. G., 1976. Cereal processing. In *Feed Energy Sources for Livestock* (ed. H. Swan and D. Lewis), pp. 47–63. Butterworth, London.

Jackson, M. G., 1977. Review article: the alkali treatment of straws, *Anim. Feed Sci. & Technol.* **2**: 105–30.

Kare, M. R. and Beauchamp, G. K., 1977. Taste, smell and hearing. In *Duke's Physiology of Domestic Animals* (ed. M. J. Swenson), 9th edn, pp. 713–30. Cornell University Press, Ithaca.

Kay, M. and Houseman, R., 1975. The influence of sex on meat production. In *Meat* (ed. D. J. A. Cole and R. A. Lawrie), pp. 85–108. Butterworth, London.

Kay, M., Macdearmid, A., and Innes, G. M., 1977. The utilization of Brassicae by feed cattle. In *Brassica Fodder Crops* (ed. J. F. D. Greenhalgh, I. H. McNaughton and R. F. Thow), pp. 106–10. Scottish Agricultural Development Committee, Scottish Plant Breeding Station, Roslin, Midlothian.

Kidder, D. E. and Manners, M. J., 1978. *Digestion in the Pig*. Scientechnica, Bristol.

Large, R. V., 1965. The artificial rearing of lambs, *J. agric. Sci., Camb.* **65**: 101–8.

Leaver, J. D., 1973. Rearing of dairy cattle. 4. Effect of concentrate supplementation on the live-weight gain and feed intake of calves offered roughages *ad libitum*, Anim. Prod. **17**: 43–52.

Liener, I. E., 1969. *Toxic Constituents of Plant Foodstuffs*. Academic Press, New York.

Loosli, J. K. and McDonald, I. W., 1968. *Nonprotein nitrogen in the nutrition of ruminants. Agric. Stud., No. 75*. Food and Agriculture Organization, Rome.

Lyons, T., Caffrey, P. J. and O'Connell, W. J., 1970. The effect of energy, protein and vitamin supplementation on the performance and voluntary intake of barley straw by cattle, *Anim. Prod.* **12**: 323–34.

McDonald, M. N., 1978. Feed intake of laying hens, *Wld's Poult. Sci. J.* **34**: 209–21.

McDonald, P., Edwards, R. A. and Greenhalgh, J. F. D., 1981. *Animal Nutrition*. 3rd edn. Longman, London.

Marsh, R., 1978. A review of the effects of mechanical treatment of forages on fermentation in the silo and on the feeding value of silages, *N.Z. J. Exp. Agric.* **6**: 271–8.

Ministry of Agriculture, Fisheries and Food, 1979. Nutrient allowances and composition of feedingstuffs for ruminants. LGR 21, amended edn. Ministry of Agriculture, Fisheries and Food, Pinner, Middlesex.

Ministry of Agriculture, Fisheries and Food, Department of Agriculture and Fisheries for Scotland, and Department of Agriculture for Northern Ireland, 1975. *Energy Allowances and Feeding Systems for Ruminants, Tech. Bull. No. 33*. Her Majesty's Stationery Office, London.

Morris, T. R., 1968. The effect of dietary level on the voluntary calorie intake of laying birds, *Br. Poult. Sci.* **9**: 285–95.

National Academy of Sciences, 1971. *Atlas of Nutritional Data on United States and Canadian Feeds*. National Academy of Sciences, Washington, DC.

O'Grady, J. F., 1978. The response of pigs weaned at 5 weeks of age to digestible energy and lysine concentrations in the diet, *Anim. Prod.* **26**: 287–91.

Ørskov, E. R., Andrews, R. P. and Gill, J. C., 1969. Effect of replacing rolled barley with swedes or potatoes on the intake and rumen volatile fatty acid composition of lambs, *Anim. Prod.* **11**: 187–94.

Ørskov, E. R. and Greenhalgh, J. F. D., 1977. Alkali treatment as a method of processing whole grain for cattle, *J. agric Sci., Camb.* **89**: 253–5.

Osbourn, D. F., Terry, R. A., Outen, G. E. and Cammell, S. B., 1974. The significance of a determination of cell walls as the rational basis for the nutritive evaluation of forages. In *Proc. 12th int. Grassld Congr., Moscow*, pp. 514–9.

Østergaard, V., 1979. Optimum feeding strategy during lactation. In *Feeding Strategy for the High Yielding Dairy Cow* (ed. W. H. Broster and H. Swan), pp. 171–94. Granada Publishing, London.

Owen, J. B., Davies, D. A. R. and Ridgman, W. J., 1969. The control of voluntary food intake in ruminants, *Anim. Prod.* **11**: 511–20.

Owen, J. B. and Ridgman, W. J., 1968. Further studies on the effect of dietary energy content on the voluntary intake of pigs, *Anim. Prod.* **10**: 85–91.

Owen, J. B., Ridgman, W. J. and Wyllie, D., 1971. The effect of food restriction on subsequent voluntary intake of pigs, *Anim. Prod.* **13**: 537–46.

Pond, W. G. and Maner, J. H., 1974. *Swine Production in Temperate and Tropical Environments.* Freeman, San Francisco.

Preston, T. R. and Willis, M. B., 1974. *Intensive Beef Production.* 2nd edn. Pergamon Press, Oxford.

Rérat, A., 1972, Protein nutrition and metabolism in the growing pig, *Nutr. Abstr. Rev.* **42**: 13–39.

Rexen, F., Stigsen, P. and Kristensen, V. F., 1976. The effect of a new alkali technique on the nutritive value of straws. In *Feed Energy Sources for Livestock* (ed. H. Swan and D. Lewis), pp. 65–82. Butterworth, London.

Robinson, D. W., Holmes, J. H. G. and Bayley, H. S., 1974. Food intake regulation in pigs. I. The relationship between dietary protein concentration, food intake and plasma amino acids, *Br. vet. J.* **130**: 361–5.

Roy, J. H. B., 1980. *The Calf,* 4th edn. Butterworth, London.

Scott, M. L., Neshiem, M. C. and Young, R. J., 1976. *Nutrition of the Chicken.* M. L. Scott, Ithaca, NY.

Shepperson, G., Marchant, W. T. B., Wilkins, and Raymond, W. F., 1972. The techniques and technical problems associated with the processing of naturally and artificially dried forages, *Proc. Br. Soc. Anim. Prod.,* pp. 41–51.

Smith, R. H. 1980. Kale poisoning: the brassica anaemia factor, *Vet. Rec.* **107**: 12–5.

Smith, R. H., Greenhalgh, J. F. D., 1977. Haemolytic toxin of the Brassicae and its practical significance. In *Brassica Forage Crops* (ed. J. F. D. Greenhalgh, I. H. McNaughton and R. F. Thow), pp. 96–101. Scottish Agricultural Development Committee, Scottish Plant Breeding Station, Roslin, Midlothian.

Stobbs, T. H., 1974. Components of grazing behaviour of dairy cows on some tropical and temperate pastures, *Proc. Aust. Soc. Anim. Prod.* **10**: 299–302.

Stobo, I. J. F., Roy, J. H. B. and Ganderton, P., 1979. The effect of changes in concentrations of dry matter, and of fat and protein in milk substitute diets for veal calves, *J. agric. Sci., Camb.* **93**: 95–110.

Tayler, J. C. and Wilkins, R. J., 1976. Conserved forage – complement or competitor to concentrate, In *Principles of Cattle Production* (ed. H. Swan and W. H. Broster) pp. 343–64. Butterworth, London.

Ternouth, J. H., Stobo, I. J. F. and Roy, J. H. B., 1978. The effect of dry matter concentration on milk substitute intake by the calf, *Proc. Nutr. Soc.* **37**: 57A (Abstr.).

Tetlow, R. M. and Wilkins, R. J., 1974. The effects of method of processing on the intake and digestibility by lambs of dried perennial rye-grass and tall fescue, *Anim. Prod.* **19**: 193–200.

Thomas, P. C. and Castle, M. E., 1979. The work of the Nutrition and Metabolism and Dairy Husbandry Sections of the Applied Studies Department, *Rep. Hannah Res. Inst.*, 1978, pp. 108–17.

Vadiveloo, J. and Holmes, W., 1979. The prediction of the voluntary feed intake of dairy cows, *J. agric Sci., Camb.* **93**: 553–62.

van der Honing, Y., 1975. Intake and utilization of energy of rations with pelleted forages for dairy cows, *Versl. Landbouwk. Onderz. Ned., No. 836.*

Van Soest, P. J., 1973. The uniformity and nutritive availability of cellulose, *Fedn Proc. Fedn Am. Socs exp. Biol.* **32**: 1804–8.

Van Soest, P. J., 1975. Physico-chemical aspects of fibre digestion. In *Proc. 4th int. Symp. Ruminant Physiol.* (ed. I. W. McDonald and A. C. I. Warner), pp. 351–65. University of New England Publishing Unit, Armidale.

Vetter, R. L. and Von Glan, K. N., 1978. Abnormal silages and silage related disease problems. In *Fermentation of Silage–a Review* (ed. M. E. McCullough), pp. 281–332. National Feed Ingredients Association, West Des Moines, Ia.

Waldo, D. R., 1977. Potential of chemical preservation and improvement of forages, *J. Dairy Sci.* **60**: 306–26.

Weston, R. H., 1967. Factors limiting the intake of feed by sheep. II. Studies with wheaten hay, *Aust. J. agric. Res.* **18**: 983–1002.

Whittemore, C. T. and Elsley, F. W. H., 1976. *Practical Pig Nutrition*. Farming Press, Ipswich.

Whittemore, C. T., Moffat, I. W. and Taylor, A. G., 1975. Influence of cooking upon the nutritive value of potato and maize in diets for growing pigs, *J. Sci. Fd Agric.* **26**: 1567–76.

Wilkins, R. J., Hutchinson, K. J., Wilson, R. F. and Harris, C. E., 1971. The voluntary intake of silage by sheep. I. Interrelationships between silage composition and intake, *J. agric. Sci., Camb.* **77**: 531–7.

Wilkinson, J. M., Wilson, R. F. and Barry, T N., 1976. Factors affecting the nutritive value of silage, *Outl. Agric.* **9**: 3–8.

Wilson, G. F., 1978. Effect of water content of Tama ryegrass on voluntary intake of sheep, *N.Z. J. Exp. Agric.* **6**: 53–4.

Wilson, P. N. and Osbourn, D. F., 1960. Compensatory growth after under nutrition in mammals and birds, *Biol. Rev.* **35**: 324–64.

Wu, J. F. and Fuller, M. F., 1974. A note on the performance of young pigs given maize-based diets in different physical forms, *Anim. Prod.* **18**: 317–20.
growing pigs, *J. Sci. FdAgric.* **26**: 1567–76.

12 MEAT PRODUCTION

D. Lister, B. N. Perry and J. D. Wood

The eating of meat has been questioned on moral grounds but for most communities meat is, and is likely to remain, an important component of the diet. However, the protein and energy available to man from the direct consumption of grain is ten times that available after the conversion of the grain to broiler chicken or pig meat, and the continuing increase in world population and the world shortage of basic foodstuffs raises the question as to whether there should be meat production from animals that compete directly with man for food. Herbivores do not necessarily compete as they can utilize forages grown where the climate is inclement or the terrain unsuitable for crop production, and in those areas they offer a means whereby the land may be used for the production of high-quality food.

Meat does not make a unique contribution to the diet but it is a useful source of several essential nutrients and is rich in protein. The composition of meat, however, influences its nutritional value and likewise its consumer appeal. Traditionally, the animal that was outstanding to the stockman's eye was assumed to satisfy the requirements of the consumer, but it is by no means uncommon to find that animals that figure prominently in on-the-hoof classes at premier fat stock shows are unplaced in carcass competitions and achieve moderate quality scores when assessed by objective scientific methods.

In 1978 the number of animals slaughtered for meat in the United Kingdom was approximately 4×10^6 cattle and calves, 11.5×10^6 sheep and lambs, 13.75×10^6 pigs and 433×10^6 poultry. This gave a home production of red meat of 2.037 Mt, which included 1.022 Mt of beef, 6 kt of veal, 0.228 Mt of mutton and lamb, 0.634 Mt of pork and 0.148 Mt of offal, and a total of 0.726 Mt of poultry meat. This chapter considers various aspects of animal production in relation to carcass and meat quality, and the extent to which the animal's diet has an important influence on the production of red meat.

COMPOSITION OF MEAT

Meat is a good source of protein of high biological value and its energy content lies between that of bread, and milk and vegetables (Tables 12.1 and 12.2). It is a rich source of B vitamins (especially B_1), iron and other essential minerals, but not calcium. The presence of fatty tissue enhances considerably the energy value of meat and also serves as a store for the fat-soluble vitamins A, D, E and K. (Tables 12.3 and 12.4). Unlike the chemical composition of lean tissue, which varies little from one species to another, that of adipose tissue, which is composed mainly of neutral fats, varies with species and with diet. The composition of the adipose tissue triglycerides influences the hardness or softness of the fat which in turn affects the firmness of cuts of meat, the appearance and hence the appeal to the would-be purchaser. Pork lard, although the composition varies with diet, in general contains more than 500 g unsaturated fatty acids per kg, of which oleic acid predominates. Palmitic and stearic acids account for a further 200 and 100 g/kg of the total respectively. Ruminant fat is less variable in its composition, less easy to modify by change of diet because of the extensive hydrogenation of dietary unsaturated fatty acids by rumen microorganisms, and contains more saturated fatty acids (approximately 300 g palmitic and 200 g stearic per kg) and fewer essential fatty acids (Table 12.5). Although the saturation of beef fat can be reduced by feeding diets containing unsaturated lipids, for the effect to be substantial the unsaturated lipid has to be chemically protected in order to pass through the rumen intact and be absorbed in the intestines (Scott, Cook and Mills, 1971). The major differences in the properties of lard and tallow (e.g. softness, melting point and susceptibility to oxidative rancidity) are due to the different concentrations of linoleic acid.

In all species the internal fat is more highly saturated than that in the peripheral depots but the composition of all body fats is influenced by the chemical nature and form of the fats and oils contained in the diet.

CARCASS AND MEAT QUALITY

Because the ultimate objective of raising animals for meat is to eat them, the consumer becomes not only the judge of product quality but also a major influence on the success of the enterprise for, if the meat is unattractive, less will be sold and fewer animals will need to be raised. The marginal satisfaction of the consumer and the extent of his influence depends, however, on whether meat is eaten for nutrition or

Table 12.1   Approximate composition of lean meat and some other foods (g/kg fresh weight) (from Rogowski, 1980)

	Water	Crude protein	Lipids	Carbohydrates	Minerals	Energy per kg (MJ)
Meat	~750	~200	~30	<10	>10	~ 5.0
Milk	~870	>30	~40	>50	<10	~ 2.9
Cheese (cheddar)	<400	>300	>300	Trace	~30	~16.7
Bread (rye)	~400	~60	~10	~520	>10	~10.5
Cauliflower	~920	<30	<10	~40	~10	~ 1.2

Table 12.2 Approximate essential amino acid content of beef protein and some other food proteins (g/16 g N)(from Rogowski, 1980)

	Ile[†]	Leu	Lys	Met	Phe	Thr	Trp	Val	Sum
Beef	5.0	8.1	7.6	2.7	4.3	4.8	2.0	5.3	39.8
Egg	7.1	8.5	5.3	5.3	5.8	4.0	1.4	8.1	45.5
Milk	6.4	9.9	7.7	2.5	4.8	4.5	1.4	7.0	44.2
Soya	5.3	8.4	5.6	1.7	5.8	4.4	1.3	5.2	37.7
Potato	5.5	6.0	5.0	1.7	4.3	4.1	1.4	5.0	33.0
Zein	7.3	22.3	0.1	2.1	6.4	2.7	0.1	2.6	43.6
Collagen	1.7	3.7	4.5	1.0	2.1	1.5	0.1	2.1	16.7
Human requirement	0.7	1.1	0.8	1.1	1.1	0.5	0.25	0.8	6.4
Human allowance	1.4	2.2	1.6	2.2	2.2	1.0	0.5	1.6	12.8

[†] Ile, Isoleucine; Leu, leucine; Lys, lysine; Met, methionine; Phe, phenylalanine; Thr threonine; Trp, tryptophan; Val, valine.

Table 12.3 Vitamin content of some organs and meat (mg/kg fresh weight)(from Rogowski, 1980)

	B_1	B_2	Niacin	B_6	Pantothenic acid	Folic acid	B_{12}	C	A	D
Liver	2.5	34.0	130	5.5	73	0.80	0.400	290	110	0.02
Kidney	3.1	20.0	69	5.0	36	0.40	0.300	130	15	–
Brain	1.4	2.5	39	1.5	26	0.12	0.050	180	–	–
Meat										
Pork	8.0	2.0	45	5.0	10	0.07	0.010	20	0.2	0.01
Mutton	2.0	2.0	50	3.0	6	0.09	0.025	10	0.1	–

Table 12.4 Approximate composition of fatty tissue ('extracellular fat') attached to meat, and of adipose tissue (lard) of some animals (g/kg) (from Rogowski, 1980)

	Water	Crude protein	Fat	Minerals	Energy per kg (MJ)
'Extracellular fat'					
Beef	< 200	< 50	> 700	< 5	>27.2
Mutton	~ 160	< 60	> 750	< 5	>29.3
Pork	~ 170	< 50	> 750	< 5	>29.3
Adipose tissue					
Beef	< 50	< 20	> 900	< 5	~37.7
Pork	< 70	< 20	> 900	< 5	~37.7

for enjoyment and whether there are alternatives on offer. In developed countries the demand for meat is elastic, for meat does not provide a food of unique importance and there are many alternatives from which the consumer may choose. As with other foods with which meat competes, quality has increasingly become an issue but there is debate about which aspects of quality are most important and about how they can best be assessed. The eating quality of meat cannot as yet be predicted with certainty from a knowledge of the animal or the carcass from which the meat came, and the cook is probably often blamed for the consequences of the inability of the butcher to predict meat quality. Even so, values can be ascribed to the carcass and to fresh meat which, in general, reflect eating quality and they can be used as the basis for pricing structures. Thus the producer is paid according to a notional estimate of the composition of the carcass, and the retailer from the differential pricing of the various cuts and joints, which reflects their composition (proportions of lean, fat and bone) and appearance (colour, texture and freedom from drip). All of these attributes depend on an animal's genotype and on environmental influences during growth, at slaughter or *post mortem*. The impact of nutrition can only be satisfactorily identified after the contribution of these other factors has been considered.

The effects of growth

The growth of an animal entails changes in its size, composition and form. Size is so important in relation to the form an animal adopts that being the 'right size' is an important tenet in biology (Haldane, 1929). Dean Swift realized that if Gulliver was 12 times the stature of the

Table 12.5 Fatty acid composition of fats from several animals and from plants (oil seeds)(g/kg)(from Rogowski, 1980)

	Saturated fatty acids			Unsaturated fatty acids			
	Short- and medium-chain acids	Palmitic acid	Stearic acid	Others	Monoenic acids	Linoleic acid	Arachidonic acid	Others
Pork	20	210	130	50	420	90	80	Trace
Horse	–	240	50	–	300	60	110	130
Chicken	10	240	70	40	380	200	40	20
Beef	–	280	190	60	440	20	10	Trace
Mutton	–	290	250	60	360	30	Trace	10
Butter	100	230	120	70	400	80	–	–
Olive oil	–	30	–	110	790	60	–	10
Soya oil	–	10	100	180	130	510	–	70
Palm kernel fat	580	100	20	130	140	30	–	–
Palm oil	–	480	50	–	360	110	–	Trace

Lilliputians he would be 12^3 times their weight, but he did not see the physical implications. To be 18 m tall, a giant must weigh 80 to 90 t. But such a weight is quite unsupportable by human bone which has increased its cross sectional area only *pro rata*. In fact the skeleton increases its weight by 1.13 for a unitary increase in body weight (Kayser and Heusner, 1964).

The amounts of muscle and fat change dramatically as animals grow, but the overall proportions of fat, muscle and bone in the carcass alter in a predictable way (see Lister, 1980). This is why for a given species the weight of the body alone provides the best single indicator of its composition. Analysis of the relatively small residual variation in the composition of groups of animals of the same weight which results from differences in nutrition and tissue growth requires the application of rather sophisticated techniques. Nevertheless, these differences have important commercial implications. Kempster (1979) and Kempster and Harrington (1979) have calculated that the annual production of waste fat in sheep and cattle is approximately 75 kt if the efficiency of transformation of feed energy to lean meat production at different levels of fatness (Andersen, 1975; Frood, 1976) is taken into account. Such waste could be eliminated if it were possible to identify easily the stage in an animal's growth when the energy cost of the edible meat production is at the minimum. Unfortunately, there is no practical way of deciding when a ruminant reaches this point other than its weight and 'finish' as judged by hand and eye, or occasionally by instruments such as those employing ultrasonic scanning techniques.

Pigs show a greater uniformity of type especially in the proportion of subcutaneous backfat so that, despite the rigidly defined slaughter weights, the yield of edible meat is reasonably predictable. Moreover, the effects of differences in slaughter weight can be identified more readily. Fowler (1976) has argued that a simple procedure, such as reducing the slaughter weight of bacon pigs by 10%, would improve the efficiency of lean meat production by an amount which would require many generations if it were to be achieved by breeding and selection. This is because there is a higher proportion of lean to fat in bacon pigs at 80 kg than at 90 kg live weight, and the proportion of lean in the carcass is even greater at 65 kg. This is primarily a function of the way food is partitioned between muscle, fat and bone which, in turn, depends on the timing of the development of individual tissues.

Animal appraisal

It is recognized that the amount of body fat affects the analysis of the apparent proportional development of the 'fat-free body' (Elsley,

1976). Moreover, striking differences in the physical form of animals of the same body weight, seemingly attributable to fat, may not be evident in chemical composition (Reid, Bensadoun, Bull, Burton, Gleeson, Han, Joo, Johnson, McManus, Paladines, Stroud, Tyrell, Van Niekerk and Wellington, 1968; Stant, Martin, Judge and Harrington, 1968).

The subjective assessment of muscularity or of fatness in animals is frequently confounded. 'Conformation' and 'finish' of beef cattle are, for instance, largely attributable to the amount and distribution of fat, for the differences between beef, dairy and even 'unimproved' cattle in the relative amounts and distribution of muscle are not so great as was once thought (Berg and Butterfield, 1976).

Barton (1967) reviewed the literature concerning conformation of live cattle and the composition of their carcasses, and was unable to establish any firm relationships. Traditional beef animals may be smaller and more compact than modern strains but there are no indications that the proportion of lean in their carcasses or its distribution has been changed by selection and breeding. There is, furthermore, no evidence that such carcasses are superior to those of dairy breeds in cutability or eating quality. Fatness confuses all comparisons of conformation, and the shape not attributable to fatness is a function predominantly of skeletal geometry. The component which matters most, lean tissue development, is largely independent of conformation, and recognition of this has provided the stimulus to incorporate into beef production those breeds and types of cattle which grow rapidly, although possibly less shapely, to a large mature body size. The recent and growing use of the large exotic breeds of cattle for beef production in the UK and elsewhere is an illustration of this.

Acknowledging that an animal's shape during life is not a good indication of the merit of its carcass, however, is not particularly helpful to the producer. He still wishes to know whether his animals are of an appropriate type, whether his feeding system is the right one, when he should slaughter and on what criteria he will be paid.. Systems for classifying carcasses have therefore been designed to answer some of these questions and to provide quasi-objective measures of animal merit.

Carcass appraisal

Inspection of the throughput of any abattoir will reveal a wide range of weights, shapes and fatness of the carcasses. This is not, in itself, a problem for there is always an equivalent variation in the requirements of retailers and processors due to local and regional variations in demand for particular cuts of meat or meat products. What is difficult is finding a description of carcasses which allows purchasers to consistently obtain meat of the quality they require and to differentiate between those carcasses which generate profit for their business and those which do not. The resulting price differentials form a basis for market intelligence which serves both producer and retailer alike. Traditionally, such information depended on national grading schemes whereby somewhat arbitrary notions of quality were ascribed to carcasses, which were then designated good, medium, poor or some similar description. Time and place alter views of carcass quality and a grading nomenclature involving words such as prime or choice tends to set objectives for a producer which may ultimately diverge from the market demand.

Carcass classification schemes have been designed to overcome such limitations by providing descriptions that have the minimum of subjective overtones. To be effective the information is confined to weight, sex, fatness and conformation of carcasses. Descriptions, reported by an independent body, are based as far as possible on objective measurements or, where 'this is not possible, on subjective estimates by trained individuals. In the UK the Meat and Livestock Commission has introduced such schemes for cattle, sheep and pigs, and schemes which will allow comparisons of carcasses within all European Economic Community countries are under consideration (Harrington, 1978).

Beef carcass classification

In the MLC scheme, carcasses are described by weight, sex, assessment of fatness and conformation. Fatness is described on a scale from 1 (leanest) to 5 (fattest); Z is used to describe a grossly overfat carcass. More than half of all carcasses fall into class 3 and this is subdivided into 3L (leaner) and 3H (fatter). Unusual patterns of fat distribution are denoted by: K – excessive kidney knob and channel fat; P – patchy fat; and U – excessive udder fat. Conformation is also described on a scale of 1 to 5, and Z is again used for carcasses with very poor conformation. In the reported description a carcass might thus be designated 2 4, which indicates that it is leaner than average and above average in conformation.

The composition of carcasses classified according to this system is given in Table 12.6

Typical carcass classifications for steers of several breeds and crosses on different production systems are given in Fig. 12.1.

Sheep carcass classification

As with cattle carcasses the classification for sheep is based on weight, fatness, conformation and an indication of type of animal –

Table 12.6   Composition of steer carcasses (with kidney knob and
channel fat removed) shown in relation to the Meat
and Livestock Commission beef classification
system (g/kg)

MLC fat classes	1	2	3L	3H	4	5
Saleable meat						
Lean	680	640	610	590	560	520
Fat	70	90	100	110	130	140
Total saleable	750	730	710	700	690	660
Carcass residue						
Bone and waste	180	180	170	160	150	140
Fat trim	70	90	120	140	160	200

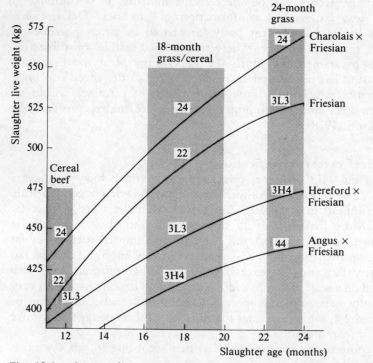

Fig. 12.1.   Average live weight and age at slaughter for steers of several breeds
and crosses on different production systems. Typical carcass classifications are indicated.

lamb, hogget or sheep. Fatness is determined by visual appraisal of
external fat development, and ranges from 1 (very lean) to 5 (very fat).
K is used to identify carcasses with excessive kidney knob and channel
fat development. Conformation is categorized into *extra* for fat classes 2

to 4 (2E, 3E, 4E) only; *average* (identified only by their fat-class numbers 1 to 5); and *poor* and *very poor* identified only as C and Z. The weight categories are agreed by organizations representing the meat industry.

Pig carcass classification

The scheme for pigs is by far the most objective and relies on the carcasses having approximately 60% of their total fat deposited in the subcutaneous fat depot. An accurate measure of the thickness of this fat permits the estimation of total fatness, and thus the correlated amount of lean, sufficiently accurately for commercial purposes. Backfat thickness was, for many years, measured along the mid-line of split carcasses at the shoulder, mid-back and loin. This was easily done for carcasses for the Wiltshire bacon trade, where it is customary to cure half carcasses, but less easily for pork carcasses, which are not usually split. The development of an optical probe, which can be pushed through the skin and fat to the underlying muscle, made it possible for the fat depth to be read directly on intact carcasses. Measurements were not limited to the mid-line, and other positions were discovered and adopted which permitted more accurate predictions of carcass fatness.

The position of the backfat measurements taken with the optical probe over the eye muscle at the level of the last rib is shown in Fig. 12.2.

The measurements designated as P_1, P_2 and P_3 are not all taken on all carcasses. There are essentially two systems of measuring, one used mainly for porkers, cutters and heavy hogs, and the second mainly for bacon pigs. In the first the measurements P_1 and P_3 are taken at 45 and

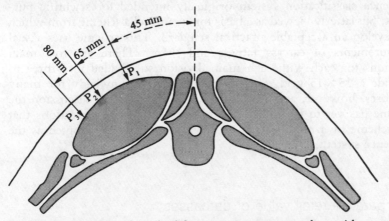

Fig. 12.2. Position where backfat measurements are taken with an optical probe (intrascope) at the level of the head of the last rib. P_1 and P_3 apply to split or unsplit carcasses (method 1) and P_2 to split carcasses (method 2).

80 mm respectively from the mid-line of the carcass, added together and the total inscribed in a triangle stamped on the trotter. In the second, the backfat thickness at the shoulder and loin are measured together with the P_2 measurement 65 mm from the mid-line. The P_2 measurement is recorded in a triangle stamped on the belly or foreleg.

Measurements of backfat thickness are reported together with the cold carcass weight. Major defects in the carcass, for example those leading to partial condemnation, deformations, soft fat or pale muscle, are classed as 'Z' or, if less badly affected, as 'C'. The length and conformation of the carcass are reported only if that information is sought by the trader; neither are now considered to be important indicators of the proportions of lean in pig carcasses.

Carcass classification in Europe

Trade in carcasses within the EEC requires a calibration standard, against which carcasses classified by national systems may be compared for price reporting as well as quality comparisons. This is particularly important for cattle carcasses where, because of the use of different breeds, sexes, carcass weights and trading needs, no national scheme is applicable for all member states. Great Britain and Ireland, for example, choose to differentiate largely on fatness, whereas Germany and France require greater differentiation amongst lean carcasses on account of the widespread use of large, lean, often double-muscled, breeds of animal and of bulls for meat. Conformation is also therefore of concern, especially in France. The European Association for Animal Production has attempted to resolve this situation by proposing a reference classification system originally intended for scientific purposes, but latterly viewed as a basis for an umbrella scheme from which to develop an acceptable practical standard. This scheme uses visual measurements of carcass fatness and shape. There are five main divisions for each with each main division subdivided into three to provide a 15×15 grid. Such a classification is unwieldy for many purposes, however, and after a decade of research and discussion the scheme has yet to be introduced, although there are indications that the scheme or a modification of it will ultimately be adopted as the reference system.

Comparative retail value of carcasses

The prediction of the composition of carcasses for commercial purposes presents no serious problems. There are good objective measurements for evaluating pig carcasses, and even the visual assessment by trained personnel of the fat cover of beef and lamb carcasses can be surprisingly accurate (see Preston and Willis, 1970). Traditionally, however, the commercial criteria for judging carcasses, especially those of ruminants, have been based not only on their apparent composition but also on conformation, since that supposedly indicates the proportions of lean and bone or of high- and low-priced joints.

Conformation is limited in its precision as an indicator by the overriding complication of fatness (Williams, 1972) and there are additional problems. The parts of a carcass do not easily divide into those of high and low value and the ratios of high- to low-value joints are determined by weight, which does not take account of composition in terms of lean, fat and bone. In practice, the retail value of a carcass will be based on a spectrum of unit prices, which may be modified appreciably by trading practices such as fat trimming. To overcome these problems, Harries, Williams and Pomeroy (1975) constructed an index of retail value for cattle carcasses to accommodate a range of prices for all the separate parts and the relative compositions of each. Using this (Harries *et al.*, 1975; Harries, Williams and Pomeroy, 1976), they showed that the index was not well correlated with the conventional ratio of high- to low-priced joints, but was highly correlated with the total proportion of carcass lean. The validity of this conclusion was extended when carcasses from different breeds of cattle were compared. In the final analysis, it was the proportions of lean, bone and fat in a carcass that determined overwhelmingly its retail value, irrespective of whether the differences in carcass composition were due to 'breed' effects or not.

Thus, as is the case for the conformation of the live animal, there is little scientific justification for the long-held view that the conformation of a carcass provides a reliable indication of its retail worth as meat. Neither, it seems, are there important hereditary differences between animals in their ability to produce carcasses with higher proportions of more valuable cuts of meat. Even so, the apparent small anatomical differences found amongst carcasses may be of commercial importance.

Fresh-meat quality

Traditionally the quality of fresh meat has been considered to be determined by the way in which an animal is slaughtered, but it is now clear that this supposition is only partly true. There is, for instance, considerable evidence that, even when animals are treated in the most humane fashion before and during slaughter, some die before they are intended to and others produce meat of undesirable commercial quality, in terms of its appearance and freedom from drip or exudate.

These problems have been of particular concern to pig producers in continental Europe and in the USA (Cassens, Giesler and Kolb, 1972), but there is no reason to suppose that animals are handled in a significantly more inhumane fashion there than in the UK. Premature death and meat quality defects are also prevalent amongst animals with desirable carcass attributes; the association is most apparent in pigs but is by no means confined to that species.

All variations in fresh-meat quality are, however, attributable to the ways in which meat acidifies in the period shortly after slaughter and the conditions under which that occurs (Bendall, 1973). There are two main categories of quality defect: those relating to the rate, and those associated with the extent of acidification in muscle, *post mortem*.

Post-mortem changes in muscle

When an animal is slaughtered, the cessation of blood-flow effectively prevents the transport of oxygen and substrates such as glucose and fatty acids around the body, and aerobiosis ceases. All metabolic processes do not stop at slaughter, however. The heart, for instance, may continue to beat, albeit ineffectually, for several minutes after an animal is stuck. Even in the absence of oxygen, excised samples of muscle can be stimulated to contract by the passage of electric current several hours after removal from a carcass. Metabolic activity is sustained by the anaerobic production of ATP. Anaerobic glycolysis, though only approximately 5% as efficient as aerobic glycolysis, may continue to produce ATP for as long as the stores of muscle glycogen permit, or until the glycolytic cycle has been blocked by the accumulation of lactate and hydrogen ions. When ATP is no longer synthesized or present in adequate amounts, *rigor mortis,* the stiffening of muscle, begins. During this period the pH of muscle falls from approximately 7.3 *in vivo* to a final value, the so-called ultimate pH, of approximately 5.4 to 5.8. In exceptional cases the pH of muscle may fall by only 0.5 units, or less.

The time for these changes to occur varies both within and between species. Pigs develop full acidity within 10 h of death, sheep within 8 to 12 h and cattle within 12 to >24 h. Pigs, on occasion, may complete rigor within a few minutes of slaughter. When this occurs, serious quality defects are found in the meat. The extreme condition is referred to as pale, soft, exudative (PSE) pigmeat (Briskey, 1964). Typically, such meat takes on a greyish/pink appearance, has a loose structure and has substantial amounts (50 to >100 g/kg) of free exudate associated with it. These effects are entirely attributable to the interaction of pH and temperature in the meat. At high temperature (>30 °C) and lowered pH (<6.3) extensive denaturation of both structural and soluble muscle proteins occurs. Their ability to bind water is lost and the precipitated proteins modify the optical properties of the surface layers of the muscle. Fluid exudes from cut surfaces, which then reflect more incident light to give the pale appearance.

Because problems of meat quality stem from the interaction between the development of acidity and the temperature at which it occurs, it is important to identify the contributions of inherent characteristics of the animals themselves, the treatments imposed on them during slaughter and the cooling of the carcasses thereafter. Poor refrigeration after slaughter may be just as damaging to meat quality as rapidity of acidification. Recommended codes of practice for refrigeration are, however, easily devised to cope with the normal variations in the rate of attainment of rigor. For those carcasses in which rapid acidification is a problem, solutions are not so easily achieved.

Bendall (1966), using Large White pigs, showed that muscle acidification post slaughter could be slowed significantly by anaesthetizing and curarizing animals to prevent neuromuscular stimulation prior to slaughter. The traditional practice of ensuring that animals are rested and unstressed at slaughter if the best quality meat is to result thus seems to be supported. However, those breeds of pig such as the Piétrain, and some strains of Landrace in which PSE is commonly found, do not show the usual slowing of muscle acidification in response to pre-slaughter treatment (Lister, Scopes and Bendall, 1969). In practice, therefore, there will always be animals which will not respond significantly in terms of improved meat quality even to extreme and quite impractical measures to avoid stress at the time of slaughter.

The explanation for these findings has not, as yet, been provided. Hypersensitivity in muscle may be a consequence of an animal's metabolic type, which also accounts for its particular somatotype and growth characteristics (Lister, Lucke and Hall, 1976). A key feature is possibly a sympathetic nervous system with a low threshold of sensitivity (Gregory and Lister, 1981). The mechanisms which induce sensitivity of the muscle to stimulation and rapidity of post-mortem change also appear to involve the autonomic nervous system (Lucke, Hall and Lister, 1979).

The second major category of quality attributes controlled by the acidification of muscle relate to an unsatisfactory degree of pH change. Typically, the fall in muscle pH may be as little as 0.1 to 0.2 pH units but problems may occur with reductions of as much as 1 pH unit. At such pH values (6.1 to 7.2) the meat of all three farm species is darker and drier than usually found. In cattle, in which the effect occurs classically in the loin and rump, it is known as the dark cutting condition. The cut surfaces of such meat are frequently of a purplish hue and tacky to the touch, and there is a high incidence of taints and off flavours in the meat. Affected pig carcasses are described as dark, firm and dry (DFD), and the condition is usually confined to the muscles of the shoulder and ham.

Dark cutting meat, although recognized long ago, has become a more significant problem in recent years because of new cutting and distribution techniques. The growing importance of supermarket sales has meant that more carcasses are cut at the abattoir or at central depots, and 'primal joints' distributed in vacuum packages. After storage for 2 weeks or so at refrigeration temperatures, the meat and exudate contained within the pack may take on a greenish appearance and may release ammonia and other offensive odours. Such occurrences pose serious problems to what is, in prospect, a most useful marketing approach.

The dark appearance of the meat is a function of the physical and chemical properties of muscle as influenced by pH. The greening of meat and the formation of exudates results from the reduction of haem pigments by the metabolic products of spoilage bacteria. The off-flavours were originally thought to be due to the pH-dependent growth patterns of spoilage organisms (pH optima 6.5 to 7.0). Recent evidence, however, suggests that there is another component of spoilage (Newton and Gill, 1978). Muscle which at slaughter contains inadequate quantities of glycogen for satisfactory anaerobic glycolysis to continue will not only fail to acidify to the usual value, but will not provide carbohydrate as the 'preferred' energy substrate for bacteria. In this event, bacteria may continue to grow by metabolizing the amino acids of muscle, the products of which produce the odours and discoloration.

The traditional explanation for this condition was that it was the consequence of profound chronic stress prior to slaughter, which caused the depletion of glycogen in muscle. This cannot be the sole explanation, however, for it is quite common to see in adjacent muscles in a carcass one which is PSE (supposedly an effect of acute stimulation) and the other DFD. The two conditions can also be seen in different portions of the same muscle. DFD is, moreover, found most commonly in particular types of animals, in stress-sensitive pigs, and also in bulls (especially Friesian) raised for beef (Duchesne, 1978).

There are no clear indications of the mechanism involved in the development of DFD. Lister (1979) suggested that it is related to substrate use at different levels of muscle stimulation. Glycogen utilization occurs when the usual substrates, FFA, tissue lipid and glucose, become depleted. This is a common, temporary occurrence in experimental animals and man during short periods of heavy exercise when aerobiosis is curtailed (Havell, 1970; Issekutz, 1970; Pernow and Saltin, 1971). Dark cutting meat is, however, a difficult condition to induce experimentally, for neither fasting, exercise, nor a combination of the two will readily produce it (Howard and Lawrie, 1956; Lawrie, 1958 and 1966). On the other hand, behavioural reactions will induce the condition: dark cutting beef often results when young bulls from different groups are mixed, even for a short period, prior to slaughter (Duchesne, 1978).

There are indications that the sympathetic nervous system and catecholamines are centrally involved, as they are in the PSE syndrome (Lister *et al.*, 1976; Lucke *et al.*, 1979). The range of meat quality from PSE to DFD or 'dark cutting' is usually attributed to the varying effects of acute or chronic stress. Recent work (Lister and Spencer, 1982) suggests that it may be more properly ascribed to the balance of α- and β- adrenergic stimulation. Acute stress will produce α-adrenergic response of the sympathetic nervous system, muscle metabolism will be stimulated, but there will be little loss of glycogen as aerobic metabolism is maintained. The consequence of this may be the initiation of the PSE condition (Lister, 1974) or the malignant hyperthermia (MH) syndrome (Lister *et al.*, 1976), to which it is closely related. In contrast to the α- mediated effects of acute stress, prolonged or severe stress induces a proportionately greater β-adrenergic response via the adrenal medulla. The characteristic metabolic reactions to this are increasing anaerobiosis, acidosis and a fall in circulating FFA levels (see Hall, Lucke, Lovell and Lister, 1980). When this occurs, muscle metabolism becomes increasingly reliant on glycogen, of muscle and liver, leading ultimately to the depletion of both reserves, and high muscle pH after rigor.

The usual range of meat quality can thus be accounted for. Why some animals should be more prone than others to meat-quality problems is not known but there is evidence of differences in thresholds of sympathetic nervous sensitivity (Gregory and Lister, 1981) which may explain the discrepancies. The nutrition of an animal, contrary to what was traditionally believed, plays only a minor part, if any, in these effects.

Eating quality

As an animal grows, its size increases; its physical characteristics and chemical composition change and it ages. These factors affect the economics of production and the acceptability of the carcass, and have general implications for meat quality. The meat from young animals tends to be pale and almost devoid of fat. Although it may lack flavour, it is tender to eat, and there has always been a market for meat from young animals such as veal calves or, indeed, sucking pigs. Older animals produce meat of darker hue due to the increased concentration of myoglobin and the development of the cytochrome system in muscle (Lawrie, 1952). There is more fat both within and between the muscles, and there is a gradual decrease in tenderness, which is not striking in pigs and lambs which are slaughtered relatively young, but can be appreciable in cattle by 1.5 years of age, at which time it stabilizes (Patterson, 1975). The change in tenderness is due mainly to an alteration in the chemical constitution of connective tissue present in muscle. As an animal ages its collagen becomes increasingly cross-linked, heat stable and insoluble (Bailey, 1974) – all factors that contribute to the toughness of the cooked meat.

The traditional notion of 'finish' as related to carcasses embodies the belief that fat endows meat with desirable eating quality. There is certainly some contribution to eating quality by the fat associated with muscle (Jeremiah, Carpenter, Smith and Butler, 1970), but the required level is appreciably lower than is commonly considered necessary (Rhodes, 1976).

Fat is important in the development of flavour. Indeed, muscle from lamb, beef or pork cooked without its own fat cannot easily be identified (Wasserman and Talley, 1968). The flavour of meat stems from flavour volatiles that are produced during cooking from the interaction of fat, protein and minor constituents of muscle (Yueh and Strong, 1960; Patterson, 1975). Since these increase during growth, the flavour of the meat from older animals is usually stronger.

All of the characteristics described above blend to provide the basic quality attributes of the meat of cattle, sheep or pigs, and combine to make meat attractive or, in certain circumstances, unacceptable. The unpopularity of lamb in the USA, for example, is largely attributable to consumers' dislike of the particular odours emanating from the fat during cooking. Tenderness is probably one of the most important properties of meat, but the toughness of old animals cannot be of the greatest consequence or beef derived from discarded dairy cows would be unsaleable. It can be concluded that differences in the age or composition of animals at slaughter cannot account satisfactorily for the range in eating quality of beef, pork or lamb which consumers normally experience.

The effects of the handling of carcasses after slaughter

The importance of interactions between temperature and the acidification of muscle in regard to fresh meat quality has already been mentioned; there are effects also on eating quality.

A good example is provided by the experience suffered first by the New Zealand meat packing industry when, to facilitate the further processing and more rapid distribution of lamb carcasses, the rate at which they were chilled to the usual holding temperatures of approximately + 2°C was increased. There was a dramatic decrease in the tenderness of the meat as a result of 'cold shortening', which occurs when muscles are allowed to develop *rigor mortis* at temperatures below 10 °C (Locker and Hagyard, 1963). In this condition the contractile units of muscle, the sarcomeres, may be shortened, commonly by 30% of their resting length, become fixed in the contracted state and make the meat tough.

The normal pattern of acidification of the muscle and the development of rigor in lambs occurs over a period exceeding 8 h and involves a fall in muscle pH from approximately 7.0 at death to between 5.6 and 5.9. During this time it is quite easy, with the refrigeration equipment currently available, to freeze the carcass, and thus cold shortening is a considerable risk in modern practice. There is also risk of inducing cold shortening in the surface musculature of beef carcasses, despite their bulk, because of the delayed onset of *rigor mortis* in this species.

The rate of acidification of muscle of a particular species is rather characteristic but, as already mentioned, is subject to individual variation. Knowledge of the acidification rate allows an appropriate chilling regime to be calculated to avoid toughness due to cold shortening. Alternatively, it is possible to identify an appropriate rate of acidification and reproduce it in carcasses to cope safely with a desired refrigeration practice. One way of achieving this, which was introduced first into industrial practice for lambs but is now available for beef carcasses (Bendall, 1980), involves the electrical stimulation of the carcass at the time of slaughter. This accelerates to a desired degree the rate of fall in pH in muscle and allows rapid chilling to proceed without risk (Chrystall and Hagyard, 1976; Davey, Gilbert and Carse, 1976).

Conclusion

This section has shown how the growth of an animal is responsible for conferring quality attributes on its carcass and meat, but has indicated that desired characteristics can probably be achieved by almost all types of animals. The technology of slaughter and the subsequent processing of the carcass has also been shown to be important in preserving the inherent quality features attributable to the animal. There is evidence of genotype/environment interaction, and that animals that tend to produce the leanest carcasses are also prone to develop adverse responses in terms of their meat quality during pre- and post-slaughter handling. The physiological mechanisms that confer particular carcass and performance characteristics on animals may also increase their sensitivity to stress. None of these issues appears to be affected to an important degree by the diet of an animal and, in the final analysis, the major concern for the nutritionist appears to be the efficient production of lean meat. This is considered in the following sections.

CONTROL OF CARCASS COMPOSITION

A major aim of animal scientists in recent years has been to increase the lean content of the carcasses of all three species of red meat-producing animals. There are two reasons for this. First, lean tissue is produced at about one-fifth of the energy cost of fat tissue during growth, so lean animals have a higher food conversion ratio. Secondly, consumers prefer lean to fat meat, partly because of an aversion to eating fat, particularly amongst young people, and partly because of an increased awareness of the possible health risks associated with excessive consumption of animal fat.

The effect of body weight on composition

As body weight increases from birth to slaughter, the most marked changes in composition are a decrease in the proportion of bone and an increase in the proportion of depot fat. Changes from 0.4 to 20 months of age are illustrated in Table 12.7 for cattle reared on a complete pelleted diet. Within the slaughter weight range, changes in composition are also marked. In Table 12.8 some recent results are given for sheep where variation in carcass weight accounted for 73.6% of variation in the weight of lean. Therefore, weight itself is a major determinant of composition, as has been shown in many studies (e.g. Burton and Reid, 1969).

The effects of breed, sex and mature weight on composition

In the sheep described in Table 12.8, four breeds were evenly represented. Fitting separate regression lines for each breed increased the proportion of overall variation in lean weight accounted for by carcass weight alone from 73.6% to 76.5%. The fattest breed, Clun Forest, had the lightest mature weight of the four breeds (73 kg for an adult ewe according to MLC figures), and one of the leanest breeds, Suffolk (the other was Colbred), had the heaviest mature weight (91 kg). Thus there was an association between mature weight and composition in the results, and similar associations have been found by other workers. In general, when fed under the same conditions, breeds with heavy mature weights are less mature, and therefore leaner, than breeds with light mature weights when both are at the same immature weight. Comparisons made at the same age cause a narrowing of breed dif-

Table 12.7 Carcass composition (g of dissected tissue per kg in side) in British Friesian steers

	Age (months)					s.e. of difference
	0.4	3	6	12	18	
Number	8	9	24	26	25	
Live weight (kg)	41.3	70.1	149.6	314.3	461.7	15.02
Kidney knob and channel fat	9	11	18	42	63	5.2
Lean	600	639	664	632	603	11.7
Bone	271	253	197	161	140	11.2
Subcutaneous fat	11	6	17	50	71	4.7
Intermuscular fat	40	40	56	101	133	7.4

From B. W. Butler-Hogg (unpublished results).

Table 12.8 Carcass composition (g of dissected tissue per kg in side) in 361 lambs in the commercial carcass weight range

	Carcass weight (kg)				s.e. of difference
	15	17	19	21	
Kidney knob and channel fat	31	37	38	41	1.7
Lean	577	568	553	550	4.5
Bone	138	124	123	117	2.1
Intermuscular fat	173	172	176	173	2.5
Subcutaneous fat	111	135	147	160	3.9

From Wood, MacFie, Pomeroy and Twinn (1980): four pure breeds (Clun Forest, Colbred, Suffolk and Hampshire) and two sexes (castrated male and female) evenly represented.

ferences in carcass composition (Table 12.9), although differences in weight remain. Empirical relationships suggest that breeds with large mature weights take longer to reach each stage of maturity (Taylor, 1968).

Differences in mature weight are probably not solely responsible for differences in composition between breeds. In one study with four breeds reared under similar conditions, McClelland, Bonaiti and Taylor (1976) found that Soay sheep consistently contained less fat (g/kg of side weight) than Finnish Landrace, Southdown or Oxford Down sheep at the same stage of maturity, defined in terms of the proportion of mature weight. In another study (Wood *et al.*, 1980) (Table 12.8), two breeds (Colbred and Suffolk) were the leanest of four examined, containing 572 g of lean per kg in the side at the mean carcass weight of

Table 12.9   Carcass composition (g of dissected tissue per kg in side) in Gloucester Old Spot (GOS) and Large White (LW) pigs given the same diet on a rationing scale based on age, and slaughtered at either the same age or weight

| | Basis for comparison | | | | | |
| | Age | | | Weight | | |
	GOS	LW	Significance of difference	GOS	LW	Significance of difference
Live weight (kg)	59.6	65.8	*	64.9	65.3	−
Days on test	55	55	−	63	54	*
Lean	511	521	NS	493	546	**
Bone	91	97	NS	87	96	NS
Total fat	355	340	NS	372	321	*

From Lodge, Lister, Wood and Wolynetz (1978): 8 castrated males and 8 females per breed × treatment group; all pigs initially 12 weeks old.

18 kg. Published mature weights (MLC, 1975) are Suffolks, 91 kg and Colbreds, 77 kg: Colbreds were thus leaner than would be indicated by published estimates of their mature weight. In recent work at the Meat Research Institute, Truscott (1980) found that 15 British Friesian and 15 Hereford steers were equally mature (i.e. had equal proportions of mature skeletal development predicted from a curve calculated for each animal) at 20 months of age following the consumption *ad libitum* of a complete pelleted diet. However, the Herefords were fatter than the Friesians (309 *v*. 285 g of dissectible fat per kg in empty body) and were also fatter when allowance was made for estimated differences in mature weight.

Differences in mature weight between males and females explain some of the difference in composition attributable to sex. Male and female sheep had a similar composition at equal stages of maturity expressed as g/kg of mature weight (McClelland *et al.*, 1976). Similarly boars, which were leaner than gilts of the same live weight, had longer carcasses and legs than gilts, suggesting a larger size and heavier weight at maturity (Wood, Lodge and Lister, 1979). On the other hand, Dutch workers found that boar, castrated male, and female Landrace pigs reached approximately the same mature live weight (approximately 330 kg), and that boars were leaner at all stages of growth.

Several authors have pointed out the difficulty in assigning probable mature weights to growing experimental animals except when mature animals have been reared and kept under the same conditions as used in the experiment.

The effects of voluntary food intake and maintenance requirement on body composition and food conversion efficiency

Under *ad libitum* feeding conditions, voluntary food intake and maintenance requirement (the amount of food needed to maintain zero energy balance) depend on body weight and the rate of growth. Breeds with heavy mature weights have larger voluntary food intakes and maintenance requirements per unit of live weight than lighter breeds when compared at the same weight. The ratio of intake to maintenance requirement is similar for light and heavy breeds at corresponding stages of maturity, and voluntary food intake and maintenance requirement are probably ultimately related to the weight and rate of deposition of body protein (Webster, 1980).

Stage of maturity influences body composition, voluntary food intake, maintenance requirement and food conversion efficiency (food intake per unit weight gain). Webster (1980) has shown that conversion efficiency remains fairly constant for approximately 30% of the weight interval from weaning to maturity and then begins to decline. This is due to a gradual convergence, in response to an altered voluntary food intake, of energy intake and heat production, and to an increasing energy cost of tissue deposition as fat makes up a higher proportion of the weight gain. Lipid is no more costly to produce than protein (both require approximately 53 MJ/kg synthesized), but lipid is stored in hydrophobic adipose tissue whereas protein is deposited, along with four times its weight of water, in muscle.

There is scope, of course, for some divergence from these general relationships and, if individual breeds or strains have unusually small voluntary food intakes or high maintenance requirements per unit of body weight, fat deposition must be reduced, resulting in a lean carcass. Such effects might explain genetic differences in body composition not accounted for by differences in stage of maturity.

Piétrain pigs have a lower mature weight than most other breeds yet, at slaughter weight after *ad libitum* feeding, they are leaner. This is apparently largely because of their low voluntary food intake. Under *ad libitum* feeding conditions, Piétrains consistently consume 20% less than Large Whites of the same live weight. To test the importance of this, J. D. Wood and B. N. Perry (unpublished results) fed eight Piétrain and eight Large White pigs the same weight of food per day over a growth period from 12 to 30 weeks of age. Daily food intake for each Large White was made equal to the average daily intake of the Piétrain group during the previous week, the Piétrains being allowed access to food for two 1-h periods each day. The food was a commercial pelleted ration containing 165 g crude protein per kg. The results (Table 12.10) showed that Piétrains had a lower live weight gain than

Table 12.10   Growth and carcass composition in Piétrain and Large White
pigs (results for four gilts and four castrated males of each
breed initially 12 weeks of age; all pigs given 229 kg food
during a 122-day growth period)

	Piétrain	Large White	s.e. of difference
Initial live weight (kg)	25.2	38.8	2.14***
Final live weight (kg)	92.9	111.6	3.80***
Live weight gain (kg)	67.7	72.8	3.11NS
Average daily gain (g)	551	592	25.3NS
Food efficiency (kg food/kg gain)	3.39	3.16	0.132NS
Lean†	598	623	9.5*
Subcutaneous plus internal fat†	250	208	11.8**
Bone†	101	121	2.7***
Leg length (mm)	568	651	11.4***
Carcass length (mm)	753	894	17.1***

From J. D. Wood and B. N. Perry (unpublished results).
† g of dissected tissue per kg in side.

Large Whites, and in these terms were less efficient because they
deposited more body fat and less lean. Estimated lean growth per day
was 123 g in Piétrains and 144 g in Large Whites. The Piétrains had
shorter legs and carcasses, indicating that they would have a smaller
body size and weight at maturity. Therefore, the normal expression of
'early maturity' as a higher proportion of body fat at a particular live
weight is offset in Piétrains by their exceptionally low voluntary food
intake. There is no evidence that the maintenance requirement of
Piétrains differs from that of other breeds (Fuller, Webster, MacPherson and Smith, 1976).

Evidence that the relationships between food intake, maintenance
requirement and protein deposition can be altered is also provided by
the results of selection experiments. At the University of Newcastle,
selection of breeding pigs has been based on high growth rate,
efficient food utilization and low backfat thickness (selection line), and a
control line has been mated randomly to maintain constant values for
these characteristics. Some results from the 6 to 8th generation of
selection (3 to 5th for control line) are given in Table 12.11. The
selected boars grew at a slightly slower rate than the controls, but had a
lower food intake and converted food into live-weight gain more
efficiently. Selected pigs deposited lean at a faster rate than the controls
and also possibly had a higher maintenance requirement (Henderson,
Whittemore, Ellis, Smith and Laird, 1980), but the marked reduction in
fat deposition resulted largely from the low food intake.

In cattle, the Limousin breed appears to possess characteristics similar to the Piétrain pig. The mature weight of this breed is not as high as

Table 12.11 Performance and carcass characteristics in 77 selection line and 80 control line boars fed *ad libitum* from 27- to 87-kg live weight

	Selection	Control	s.e. of difference
Average daily gain (g)	905	923	14.4
Food efficiency (kg food per kg gain)	2.77	2.94	0.02
Average daily food intake (kg)[†]	2.51	2.71	
Carcass length (mm)	820	805	3.1
Backfat thickness over eye muscle (mm)	14.1	18.7	0.61

From Wood, Enser, MacFie, Smith, Chadwick, Ellis and Laird (1978).
[†] Estimated from average daily gain × food efficiency.

that of other lean cattle breeds, e.g. Charolais, Simmental and South Devon, but the Limousin is especially lean (Koch, Dikeman, Allen, May, Crouse and Campion, 1976; Smith, Laster, Cundiff and Gregory, 1976).

The effects of breed, sex and mature weight on tissue distribution

Just as the major tissues grow at different relative rates between birth and slaughter, leading to changes in body composition, so do parts or units within each tissue. Some values for the growth coefficients (b) describing relative growth in Friesian steers, results for which are reported in Table 12.7, are given in Table 12.12. Values above 1.0 indicate that the contribution of a particular part increased as the whole increased. Thus, the proportions of the abdominal organs, liver, heart, lungs and trachea decreased as live weight increased between 0.4 and 18 months of age, whereas the proportion of intra-abdominal fat increased markedly, more so than for carcass fat (subcutaneous and intermuscular fat). The growth coefficient for subcutaneous fat alone was 2.02(s.e. 0.047). In a study with sheep in the carcass weight range 15 to 21 kg, the internal fat depots had growth coefficients higher than intermuscular fat and only slightly lower than subcutaneous fat (Wood *et al.*, 1980). Within the muscle mass, also, the various parts develop at different rates, the relative proportions of each part of the body varying with the weight of the total tissue present and with the animal's stage of maturity (i.e. the proportion of mature weight). In a study of the male

Table 12.12   Relative growth (growth coefficients, *b*) within the carcass, whole body and subcutaneous fat depot in British Friesian steers between 0.4 and 18 months of age; growth for each component has been described by an equation of form $\log_{10} y = a + b \log_{10} x$

x	*y*	*b*	
	Within carcass	Mean	s.e.
Dissected tissue	Lean	0.99	0.005
in side	Bone	0.72	0.009
	Subcutaneous fat	1.97	0.034
	Intermuscular fat	1.54	0.019
	Within body		
Live weight	Carcass fat	1.70	0.031
	Intra-abdominal fat[†]	1.94	0.028
	Liver	0.84	0.015
	Heart	0.76	0.017
	Lungs and trachea	0.78	0.018
	Within subcutaneous fat		
Subcutaneous fat	Shin	0.83	0.031
	Neck and clod	1.05	0.028
	Brisket	1.18	0.022
	Crop	1.30	0.018
	Leg	0.75	0.018
	Round	0.96	0.010
	Loin	1.08	0.023
	Flank	0.94	0.028

From B. W. Butler-Hogg (unpublished results).
[†] Kidney knob and channel fat, omental fat and mesenteric fat.

progeny of eight sire breeds of cattle, Berg, Andersen and Liboriussen (1978) found that, at a mean muscle weight of 87.5 kg, Hereford progeny had 38.7 kg of muscle in the high value 'pistol' cut (round and loin and hind shank) and Chianina progeny had 41.3 kg. Chianinas, being of heavier mature weight, had a less mature muscle mass and a higher proportion of total muscle in areas of low relative growth; Herefords, with the more mature muscle mass, had higher proportions in areas of high relative growth, e.g. the fore-rib and neck. There are, however, other sire breed differences in muscle weight distribution that cannot be explained by differences in stage of maturity although their commercial significance, even in breeds with obviously different conformation, is uncertain. In cattle and sheep, although not pigs, there are clear breed differences in the distribution of body fat, especially between the carcass (subcutaneous and intermuscular) and intra-abdominal (kidney knob and channel fat, omental fat and mesenteric fat) depots It is possible to separate cattle breeds into 'dairy' and 'beef' types, and sheep breeds into 'ewe' and 'ram' types, according to their use in practice and pattern of fat partitioning; the 'dairy' and 'ewe' breeds have a higher proportion of body fat in the intra-abdominal depots. Truscott (1980) found that in 20-month-old Hereford and British Friesian steers, 380 and 240 g/kg respectively of the total dissectible body fat was in the carcass following *ad libitum* consumption of a pelleted diet (11.3 MJ ME per kg DM) over a period from 6 to 20 months of age. Therefore, Herefords showed the classical 'beef' and Friesians the classical 'dairy' breed characteristics. Similarly, Clun Forest sheep (a 'ewe' breed) had a higher proportion of their body fat as intra-abdominal fat than Suffolks or Hampshires ('ram' breeds) (Wood *et al.*, 1980) although prediction of carcass lean from fat thickness at the last rib was not breed dependent, implying that breed differences in tissue distribution within the carcass were small (Wood and MacFie, 1980).

Bulls and boars appear to have a more pronounced development of forequarter muscles, particularly in the shoulder region, than corresponding females or castrated males. In bulls this is a specific effect of androgens on muscles of the neck, and is not due to differences in the stage of maturity (Brannang, 1971). However, the differences between boar and castrate pigs are extremely small when the effects attributable to differences in mature body weight and composition are allowed for.

Physiological explanations for genetic differences in body composition

Cellular basis for growth of lean and fat

In both muscle and fat tissue, the adult number of cells is probably present at birth or soon after. In pigs, muscle cells, with several nuclei, were clearly visible at birth and their number remained constant up to 200 days of age, growth being achieved by large increases in fibre size (Stickland, Widdowson and Goldspink, 1975). Fat cells, however, are not easily identified histologically until they have accumulated lipid, and the misleading conclusion can be reached that new cell formation occurs throughout growth to slaughter weight. In fact, the cell nuclei (one per cell) are present at birth but all the cells do not begin to accumulate lipid simultaneously. Some cells are clearly visible but some, the pre-adipocytes, remain quiescent until activated in some, as yet unknown, way.

In the shoulder region of pigs, the number of recognizable subcutaneous fat cells increased markedly during the period from 87 to 188 days of age (26 to 109 kg live weight) (Table 12.13). Cell size increased also and the average size at 188 days was correlated quite closely with the proportion of carcass fat ($r = 0.7$). This suggested that, in pigs

Table 12.13 Number and size of fat cells in shoulder subcutaneous fat of 12 castrated Large White pigs fed *ad libitum* from 87 to 188 days of age

| | Age of pigs (days) | | | | | |
| | 87 | | 145 | | 188 | |
	Mean	s.d.	Mean	s.d.	Mean	s.d.
Live weight (kg)	26.5	3.7	69.7	6.8	109.2	9.2
Fat cell diameter (μm)[†]	69.8	4.5	98.8	4.4	117.4	5.8
Fat cell number ($\times 10^{-3}$)[‡]	62.6	13.7	76.9	14.8	114.2	24.2

From Wood, Enser and Restall (1978).

[†] Measurements made through depth of tissue taken by biopsy or at slaughter at 188 days.

[‡] Relative number, i.e. number in a cylinder of fat whose volume was depth $\times$ area/area at 87 days.

having the same mature weight, fatness is related to fat cell size and the factors which increase fat cell size: it can be assumed that the total number of cells will be greatest in the animals with the heaviest mature weights. Recent work has shown that the pattern of activation of pre-adipocytes is similar in the subcutaneous fat of Hereford and British Friesian steers between 6 and 20 months of age (Truscott, Wood and Denny, 1980), being particularly marked after 17 months when growth of subcutaneous fat becomes most rapid. In the same study, kidney knob and channel fat (perirenal fat) had a relative growth rate similar to that of subcutaneous fat but a different pattern of development; growth in the abdominal depots occurred mainly through enlargement of the cells already observed at 6 months. The main breed difference was that Herefords had more subcutaneous fat cells than Friesians in the three subcutaneous sites studied although both breeds had similar numbers of perirenal fat cells per kilogram fat-free body weight (Table 12.14). The larger number of subcutaneous fat cells in Herefords may explain the greater fatness of the breed and the characteristic pattern of fat partitioning.

Table 12.14 Numbers of fat cells per kg fat-free body weight in 15 Friesian and 15 Hereford steers aged 20 months ($\times 10^6$)

| | Hereford | | Friesian | | |
Site	Mean	s.e.	Mean	s.e.	Significance of breed difference
Subcutaneous					
Rump	3.2	0.3	1.2	0.2	***
Midloin	1.5	0.1	0.7	0.1	***
12th rib	3.7	0.3	2.2	0.2	***
Perirenal	13.6	1.2	15.1	0.6	NS

From Truscott (1980).

Metabolism in fat cells

Several studies have been conducted to determine whether genetic differences in lipid synthesis or catabolism (fat deposition being the net result of the two processes), measured *in vitro* in fat cell preparations or adipose tissue slices, could explain differences in body fat content. In general, the results show that the rate of metabolism depends on the surface area of the fat cells present and that, at constant fat cell number, lipogenesis and lipolysis are greater in large than small cells (Smith, 1971; Zinder and Shapiro, 1971). Thus, the finding that fat cells from genetically obese rats have a greater rate of lipogenesis than those from lean rats does not provide an explanation for the greater fat content of the obese: it is simply a reflexion of their larger cell size (Kissebah, Clarke, Vydelingum, Hope Gill, Tulloch and Fraser, 1975). Similarly, Hood and Allen (1973), in an examination of activity of lipogenic enzymes in tissue slices from Hormel Miniature, Minnesota crossbred and Hampshire × Yorkshire pigs (breeds listed in order of body fat content), found that enzyme activity was greatest in the fattest animals when expressed per cell. However, when activity was expressed per unit weight of tissue slice, the fattest animals, whose fat contained larger but fewer cells, had the lowest activity. Finally, Standal, Vold, Trygstad and Foss (1973) found differences in hormone-induced lipolytic activity in fat slices between pigs from different selection lines. Activity, measured as FFA release per mg tissue, was greatest in a line selected for rapid, efficient growth and low backfat thickness, and least in a line selected for slow, inefficient growth and high backfat thickness. The authors speculated that the low fat content of the lean line might be due to a high sensitivity to lipolytic hormones. Fat cellularity measurements were not made but it is conceivable that there were more, smaller cells in tissue slices from the lean group, and that activity differences between the lines would have been reduced if corrected to the same number and size of cells. Differences in metabolic activity of adipose tissue between lean and fat genotypes appear, therefore, to be an effect rather than the cause of fatness. This conclusion is supported by results of transplantation studies, which show that it is the new environment into which the fat cells are placed, rather than the source or character of the cells themselves, which is the important determinant of future growth (Ashwell, Meade, Medawar and Sowter, 1977).

Hormones controlling tissue deposition

The two major hormones controlling body composition appear to be insulin, secreted from the pancreas, and growth hormone, from the anterior pituitary. Insulin concentrations in blood plasma increase as body fat content rises with age (Trenkle and Topel, 1978), and in some studies there have been high correlations between insulin concentration and body fat content (Wood, Gregory, Hall and Lister, 1977). There is debate as to whether high insulin concentrations are the cause of high levels of body fat through the action of insulin in stimulating lipogenesis and inhibiting lipolysis, or reflect the relative insensitivity to insulin of large as compared with small fat cells (Smith, 1971). Insulin also promotes food intake when given exogenously and is secreted from the pancreas in response to the ingestion of food.

Several studies with pigs (e.g. Gregory, Lovell, Wood and Lister, 1977; Wood et al., 1977) have demonstrated positive associations between body fat content and plasma insulin concentrations, as well as showing diurnal variations in concentration associated with the pattern of food intake. Piétrains, which were leaner than Large White pigs of the same live weight following *ad libitum* feeding, had lower insulin concentrations and lower responses in insulin secretion to tolbutamide, indicating an important, possibly causative, rôle for insulin in fat deposition. However, studies with lines of Large White pigs selected for leanness or fatness failed to demonstrate any difference in plasma insulin concentration between the lines despite significant differences in fat cell size, although only small differences in body composition (Gregory, Wood, Enser, Smith and Ellis, 1980).

Subsequent work with ruminants has also produced results which question the importance of insulin in causing body fat differences between breeds (Truscott, 1980). Plasma insulin concentrations and the secretory responses to tolbutamide were measured in British Friesian and Hereford steers, fed *ad libitum* on a complete pelleted diet, at 12 and 20 months of age. Although the Herefords were fatter than the Friesians at both ages, there was no significant difference between the breeds in plasma insulin concentration and, indeed, the Friesians had the greater secretory response to tolbutamide (Figure 12.3). For each breed, the insulin secretory response was greater at 20 than 12 months, suggesting a positive relationship with fat content within breed.

Growth hormone and insulin concentrations in blood plasma vary inversely with each other during the course of the day (Trenkle and Topel, 1978), and in some of their activities the hormones have opposing effects. Growth hormone restricts fat deposition by increasing the rate of lipolysis in fat cells and increases muscle deposition by stimulating protein synthesis from amino acids. The concentration of growth hormone in plasma falls as fattening proceeds whereas that of insulin increases (Trenkle and Topel, 1978), and growth hormone concentration tends to be negatively correlated with body fat content (e.g. Chappel and Dunkin, 1975). However, the correlation is not a very strong one, and it seems unlikely that growth hormone alone has an important rôle in determining genetic differences in fat deposition.

Some workers have suggested that the ratio of insulin to growth hormone is critical in the regulation of lipid metabolism (e.g. Mendel,

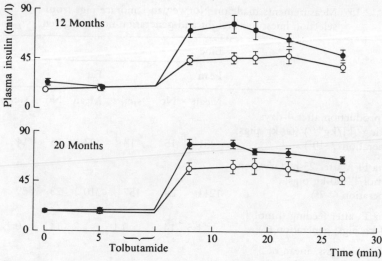

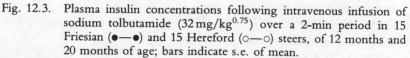

Fig. 12.3. Plasma insulin concentrations following intravenous infusion of sodium tolbutamide ($32\,mg/kg^{0.75}$) over a 2-min period in 15 Friesian (●—●) and 15 Hereford (○—○) steers, of 12 months and 20 months of age; bars indicate s.e. of mean.

1980) and, since both hormones influence the release of FFA from the fat cell, measures of this might act as an index of the balance between lipolysis and lipogenesis, which regulates fat deposition. In experiments with Piétrain and Large White pigs, there was an indication that high rates of lipolysis, caused by low ratios of insulin to growth hormone, were linked with differences in fat deposition between the breeds. Piétrains had higher circulating levels of FFA during feeding and fasting, and a greater lipolytic response to noradrenalin, infused when the pigs were under general anaesthesia (Wood *et al.*, 1977). Subsequent studies with Large White pigs showed that, between animals selected for nine generations for fast efficient growth of lean and their relatively fat controls, there were small differences in plasma FFA concentration after feeding but pronounced differences following an overnight fast (Gregory *et al.*, 1980). Similar results were also obtained with Norwegian Landrace pigs by Bakke (1975) who found that, after a 25-h period of fasting, plasma FFA concentrations were four times higher in animals from a lean- than from a fat-breeding line (Table 12.15).

High concentrations of plasma FFA during fasting could reflect a fat mobilization to meet the energy requirements for fast lean growth in animals growing to a heavy mature weight, but might also reflect an active mechanism for the regulation of body composition. The latter is consistent with the fact that the hormonal changes associated with

Table 12.15   Measurements made on Norwegian Landrace pigs from two selection lines; live weight and generation number given

	Line					
	Lean			Fat		
	Mean	No.	s.e.	Mean	No.	s.e.
Heat production after 4-days fasting (kJ/kg$^{0.75}$) (60-kg pigs; generation 7–10[†])	451	15	18	402	15	14
Plasma FFA after 25-h starvation (μmol/l) (90-kg pigs; generation 6–7[‡])	1211	24	157	310	23	39
Serum T_3 after feeding (nmol/l) (60-kg pigs; generation 6[§])	1.5	14	0.1	1.2	14	0.1
Backfat thickness, mean of 3 measurement positions (mm) (90-kg pigs; generation 8[†])	21.8			42.2		
Average daily gain from weaning at 6 weeks to 90 kg live weight (g) (generation 8[†])	594			531		

[†] Sundstøl, Standal and Vangen (1979).
[‡] Bakke (1975).
[§] Bakke and Tveit (1977).

a high lean content all tend to cause fat mobilization. For example, tri-iodothyronine (T_3) levels were higher in serum of lean pigs (Table 12.15) and thyroid hormones have lipolytic activity as well as regulating metabolic rate.

The role of FFA in the regulation of body composition in cattle breeds was investigated by Truscott (1980). He reported that the levels of plasma FFA and their rate of increase during a prolonged period without food were similar in British Friesian and Hereford steers, both at 12 and 20 months of age, despite significant breed differences in empty body composition and fat partitioning (Fig. 12.4). As indicated earlier, however, Herefords have a greater number of subcutaneous fat cells than Friesians and it is possible that this increases their potential for fat deposition irrespective of the relative hormonal status of the two breeds.

Conclusions

Carcass composition is influenced to a large extent by body weight but there are still important variations with breed, sex, selection line,

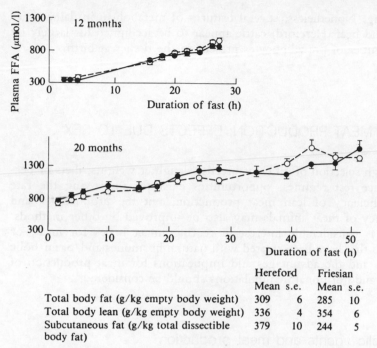

	Hereford		Friesian	
	Mean	s.e.	Mean	s.e.
Total body fat (g/kg empty body weight)	309	6	285	10
Total body lean (g/kg empty body weight)	336	4	354	6
Subcutaneous fat (g/kg total dissectible body fat)	379	10	244	5

Fig. 12.4. Plasma free fatty acid (FFA) concentrations during fasting in 15 Friesian (●—●) and 15 Hereford (○—○) steers, and body composition results at 20 months of age. Standard meals were given prior to fasting to minimize individual differences in nutritional status. Bars indicate s.e. of mean.

maintenance requirement and feeding of the animal, especially in fat deposition. Where food is given *ad libitum*, differences between animals may also be related to characteristic differences in voluntary food intake. Satisfactory comparisons can only be made, however, when the relative maturity of animals is taken into account. Breeds with light mature weight are more mature and therefore fatter than breeds of heavy mature weight when comparisons are made at a particular fixed weight. To explain the residual variations in body composition remaining between genotypes when these more obvious contributory factors have been considered, and to explain how carcass composition is controlled, measurements of cell number, cell metabolism and circulating hormone concentrations have been made. These have provided useful indices of body composition in some instances and clues about its regulation, although cause and effect are difficult to separate. Differences in fat cell metabolism between lean and fat genotypes, for example, seem mainly to reflect differences in the number and size of cells present rather than inherent differences in metabolism due to breeding. Nonetheless, several features of metabolism in dairy (Friesian) and beef (Hereford) cattle appear to be accounted for largely by the number of pre-adipocytes present in the tissues at birth.

LEAN MEAT PRODUCTION: EFFECTS DUE TO SEX

Through selection of different breeds, slaughter weights, diets or performance test regimes, opportunities exist for improving the rate and efficiency of lean meat production, but the productivity and efficiency of meat animals may also be improved by other methods. There is considerable interest in rearing intact males for meat, or animals that have been treated with natural hormones and/or anabolic agents, and the advantages and implications for meat production of sexual and hormonal manipulations should be considered.

Anabolic agents and meat production

There is widespread acceptance and use of anabolic agents in meat production because farmers are aware of the preference of most consumers for lean meat and they have recognised that, in general, lean animals use less food to grow to a particular live weight, and hence costs of production are minimized. Use of anabolic agents has been further stimulated by the problem of producing lean females at commercially acceptable slaughter weights and by the paradoxical antipathy to the use of entire males shown by some sections of the meat trade, who also impose financial penalties on producers of fat carcasses from castrated males. There is a voluminous bibliography on the use of anabolic agents in meat animals but many questions concerning their efficacy, toxicological properties, and hormonal, physiological and metabolic modes of action remain unanswered.

Undoubtedly, the major use of anabolic agents in meat production is with cattle, in veal and beef production. Their effect on sheep production is similar but less than in cattle, and probably at present insufficient to justify the cost of treatment. One proprietary product is available for use in pigs, and other combinations of androgenic and oestrogenic hormones have been investigated and reported to produce favourable effects on growth rate, food conversion, nitrogen retention and carcass fatness (Elliot and Fowler, 1973; Van Weerden and Grandadam, 1976); but, again, effects are not as marked as in cattle.

Steers have been most commonly used for investigating responses to anabolic agents. A variety of substances (diethylstilboestrol (DES), hexoestrol, zeranol and trenbolone) increase daily live-weight gain, food conversion efficiency and the economic gross margin of production (Table 12.16). Carcass composition is also improved, treated carcasses containing more edible meat and less fat. A combination of anabolic agents may act additively to improve performance and this implies that, particularly in the case of natural or synthetic oestrogens and substituted androgens, individual modes of action differ. Heitzman (1976 and 1978) has proposed that steers require a mixture of oestrogen and androgen for maximum response, whereas heifers require a predominance of androgen (trenbolone).

Table 12.16 Effects of anabolic agents on live-weight gain in steers and on profitability[†]

Treatment regime	Mean live-weight gain per day (g)	Improvement in growth rate (increase over controls, %)	Increase in gross margin, less cost of treatment (£)
Untreated	790		
Zeranol (36 mg)	910	14	8.2
Hexoestrol (60 mg)	990	25	15.9
Trenbolone acetate (300 mg)	860	8	3.8
Hexoestrol (45 mg) + trenbolone acetate (300 mg)	1050	32	19.0

[†] Evaluations were made over a 120-day period during fattening in 1557 steers, 18 to 24 months of age at slaughter, reared at 13 farms (Anonymous, 1976).

The situation is complex however, and age clearly influences responses. Young veal bulls respond in carcass gain and nitrogen retention to combined treatments (Lu and Rendel, 1976), but in fattening bulls, in which the testis is capable of synthesizing and secreting testosterone, exogenous supplemental oestrogens have little beneficial effect and may increase carcass fatness (Hedrick, Thompson and Krause, 1969; Williams, Vetter, Burroughs and Topel, 1975). These observations suggest a need to investigate the extent to which treatment with anabolic agents during early, sensitive stages of growth might improve the efficiency of meat production or carcass composition much later. However, there is an even greater need for studies comparing the performance and carcass characteristics of steers treated with anabolic agents, singly and in combination, with those of bulls.

There are no data from comparisons between bulls, steers and hormone-treated steers which allow calculation of the precise energetic efficiency of the conversion dietary nutrients to body protein (lean) and lipid (fat).

Fowler, Adeyanju, Burroughs and Kline (1970) studied the growth and compositional characteristics of steers which were untreated or implanted with DES and fed *ad libitum* for the same period of time on one of three diets. Their results, as recalculated by Trenkle (1976), are given in Table 12.17. The data show that, whereas treated steers consumed more food, gained more body weight and were considerably more efficient in converting dietary protein to tissue protein, DES-treatment caused approximately 10% reduction in the efficiency of conversion of gross energy or ME into body energy gain. Qualitatively, these results are similar to those obtained by Preston, MacDearmid, Aitken, MacLeod and Philip (1968) for bulls and steers slaughtered at the same age and fed a high concentrate diet *ad libitum*. In this instance (Table 12.18) bulls grew more rapidly and converted food energy into body weight gain more efficiently, but they also contained much less lipid in a sample joint, implying that they too were energetically less efficient than steers in converting dietary energy to body energy. Webster, Smith and Mollison (1977) have found that the predicted basal metabolism in bulls fed at levels close to *ad libitum* is approximately 20% higher than that of steers.

Griffiths (1980), on the other hand, conducted an experiment with both bulls and steers given the same amount of food at each of two levels of food intake. As in previous studies, the bulls had a greater efficiency of utilization of ME for live-weight gain than the steers (Table 12.19), but in this instance there was no difference between bulls and steers in the efficiency of energy deposition in carcass meat and fatty tissue, despite the fact that at each level of feeding the steers consistently contained a higher proportion of fat in their tissues. The steers gained weight more slowly than the bulls, however, taking 30 to 40 days longer to reach slaughter weight (Table 12.19), and the additional energy required for maintenance during this period may have been sufficient to obscure potential differences in energetic efficiency between the two groups of animals.

There is a need for more information on this question, and it is of fundamental importance to know whether the effects of exogenous oestrogen on dietary energy transformations in the steer are the same as those exerted by the testes in the bull. Some of the effect of oestrogen treatment of steers on the efficiency of energy deposition, and of the testes in bulls, undoubtedly occurs as a direct consequence of changes in net energy balance arising from hormone-induced changes in rates of lean and fat deposition, but the nature and mechanism of the additional growth response of hexoestrol-treated steers to the anabolic steroid

Table 12.17 Dietary energy and protein utilization for body weight gain by steers treated with diethylstilboestrol (DES) (20 mg/day) and fed *ad libitum*

	Diet					
	Corn-grain		High-moisture corn silage		Low-moisture corn silage	
Treatment	0	DES	0	DES	0	DES
Animals per group	9	9	10	10	10	10
Days fed	121	121	168	168	170	170
Daily DM intake (kg)	8.96	9.49	8.26	8.71	8.51	9.16
Food conversion ratio	7.3	6.4	9.4	7.9	9.4	8.3
Empty body gain (kg)	156	181	144	176	142	171
Composition of empty body gain (g/kg)						
Water	247	309	209	316	225	297
Protein	95	117	82	121	86	111
Lipid	634	544	687	533	667	563
Efficiency of						
Protein deposition (g/kg protein consumed)	113	150	77	133	79	115
Energy deposition						
(mJ/J gross energy)	335	296	347	300	322	302
(mJ/J ME)	470	415	533	461	486	456

From Trenkle (1976) and Fowler *et al.* (1970)

Table 12.18 The growth, food conversion and chemical composition of the 10th rib cut of bulls and steers slaughtered at the same age or live weight and fed *ad libitum* (from Preston *et al.*, 1968)

	Slaughtered at					
	Same age			Same live weight		
	Bulls	Steers	Significance	Bulls	Steers	Significance
No. of twin-pairs	8			7		
Age at slaughter (days)	381	381	–	401	444	***
Slaughter live weight (kg)	433	400	***	414	411	NS
Daily gain (kg)	1.06	0.97	***	0.98	0.88	**
Food conversion (MJ ME/kg gain)	59.8	64.9	**	59.4	67.4	***
Cold carcass weight (kg)	246	228	***	229	237	*
High-priced cuts (g/kg of side weight)	467	454	**	473	450	*
Chemical composition of 10th rib cut (g/kg) Water	551	482	***	567	466	***
Protein	176	158	***	175	161	*
Lipid	227	317	***	206	327	***

Table 12.19 Food utilization and meat production by pair-fed bulls and steers (from Griffiths, 1980)

	Bulls		Steers		Significance of difference due to	
	Level of feeding				Sex	Feeding level
	Medium	High	Medium	High		
Days of trial	283	236	313	277	–	–
DM intake (kg/day)	4.99	5.68	5.09	5.82	–	**
ME intake (MJ/day)	53.9	61.9	54.2	61.6	NS	**
Growth rate (kg/day)	0.91	1.10	0.79	0.92	***	***
Energy gain (MJ/day)†	5.01	6.79	4.95	6.29	NS	**
Efficiency of energy deposition (kJ/MJ ME)†	93	110	91	102	NS	NS
Efficiency of protein deposition (g/kg CP)†	121	128	96	102	**	NS
Efficiency of carcass meat deposition (g/MJ ME)†	8.0	8.5	7.0	6.8	**	NS

† In the carcass meat and fatty tissues.

trenbolone acetate (see Table 12.16) is less certain. In these animals, food conversion efficiency is superior to that of animals treated with trenbolone acetate only (Heitzman, 1976) and growth rate is superior to that of animals treated with hexoestrol alone (Anonymous, 1976). Heitzman (1976) has commented that 'the steers implanted with the combined implant were simply larger', implying they were neither leaner nor fatter and, in studies in which the rate of growth and efficiency of food utilization of female rats were manipulated endocrinologically, changes in body composition were less marked than changes in size (Perry, McCracken, Furr and MacFie, 1979).

Neither castrated nor intact male rats show a positive growth response to testosterone therapy after weaning (Vernon and Buttery, 1976) and it seems that male growth is predominantly controlled by early perinatal events regulating sexual differentiation of the brain (Perry *et al.*, 1979; Van der Schoot, 1980). Furthermore, only the androgenic anabolic agent, trenbolone acetate, consistently and significantly promotes growth and improves food utilization in female rats. Testosterone (or testosterone propionate) is ineffective (Rodway and Galbraith, 1979).

The reason for this is unknown, although trenbolone is effective and testosterone ineffective in stimulating growth in both ovariectomized rats and female rats auto-immunized against luteinizing hormone-releasing hormone (B. N. Perry and A. Toong, unpublished results). Therefore, it appears that trenbolone does not act peripherally as an anti-oestrogen but may influence growth through central neural mechanisms. Whether the same brain regions as those implicated in the characteristic perinatal male sexual differentiation of gonadotropin secretion, or defeminization of female sexual behaviour, are involved in this response has not been established.

In cattle and pigs, castration exerts profound effects on growth, food utilization and carcass composition, and trenbolone is effective in castrates as well as females (Lu and Rendel, 1976). Cattle and pigs also show a positive response in growth to oestrogens, whereas oestrogens inhibit growth in rats. These varying responses may reflect the fact that in farm species, in contrast to rats, the neural centres regulating growth remain 'open' and are therefore more sensitive to exogenous or endogenous hormonal manipulation in later life. There is no evidence that treatment of female cattle with trenbolone alone improves growth rate, food conversion, carcass composition or dietary energy utilization sufficiently to approach the performances achieved by bulls. Nevertheless, Heitzman (1976) reported that the greatest proportional response of cattle in average daily live-weight gain and food conversion ratio was obtained in heifers receiving trenbolone acetate alone, rather than in steers receiving trenbolone acetate alone or in combination with 17β-oestradiol (Table 12.20).

Table 12.20 The comparative responses to anabolic agents in live-weight gain and food conversion of steers and heifers

	Days on trial	Gain (kg/day)	Improvement (% increase over control)	Food conversion ratio	Improvement (% increase over control)
1. *Heifers approximately 370 kg at start of test[‡]*					
Control	56	0.65	–	13.9	–
TA (300 mg)	56	1.11	70.8	8.5	38.8
2. *Steers 290–310 kg at start of test[†]*					
Control	63	0.86	–	10.2	–
TA (300 mg)	63	1.02	18.6	9.2	9.8
TA + O (140 + 20 mg)	63	1.23	43.0	7.4	27.5
3. *Steers 350–360 kg at start of test[‡]*					
Control	64	0.84	–		
TA (300 mg)	64	0.91	8.3		
Hex (36 mg)	64	0.94	11.9		
TA + H (300 + 36 mg)	64	1.17	39.3		

TA, trenbolone acetate; O, oestradiol; H, hexoestrol.
[†] From Heitzman (1976).
[‡] From Heitzman (1978).

Treatments were imposed in the different sex groups at markedly different live weights, however, and the heifers were considerably heavier and, therefore, presumably older and fatter than the steers at the start of the experiment. Even with this qualification, however, the treatment of heifers appears to offer great scope for improving carcass composition and the efficiency of meat production, and it is surprising that the approach has not been subject to further investigation.

Trenbolone, or a similar yet undeveloped product, may also be important in improving the production characteristics of bulls. There is a recent report (North of Scotland College of Agriculture, 1979) that Friesian bulls implanted with trenbolone acetate and hexoestrol gained significantly more live weight (20 kg) than untreated controls, and although the treated bulls ate 14 kg more dry matter, food conversion ratios over the 90-day trial period were 6.06 and 7.45 in treated and untreated bulls, respectively. In contrast to this, the stilbene derivatives (DES and hexoestrol) alone often have zero or negative effects on performance and/or carcass characteristics in fattening bulls (Bailey, Probert and Bowman, 1966; Hedrick *et al.*, 1969; Laflamme and Burgess, 1973; Levy, Holzer and Folman, 1976), the details of the response varying with the dose rate (Table 12.21). DES-treated bulls

Table 12.21   Effect of DES on growth rate, food utilization, carcass fatness and testes weight in relation to dose rate in Holstein bulls

	DES implant level (total mg)			
	None (0)	Low (90)	Medium (150)	High (240)
Bulls per group	17	16	18	18
Daily gain (kg)[†]	1.36	1.38	1.35	1.39
Food intake (kg/day)	8.49	8.77	8.47	9.11
Food conversion ratio (kg food per kg gain)	5.98	6.22	6.04	6.41
US Department of Agriculture carcass grade[†]	8.9	9.3	10.1	9.8
Marbling score[†]	2.5	2.0	2.8	2.8
Backfat thickness (mm)[†]	38	30	38	46
Ether extract in side[‡] (g/kg)	184	–	197	204
Testes weight (g)	584	455	411	307
Testes weight (g)[†]	567	417	418	263

From Williams *et al.* (1975) and Trenkle (1976).
[†] Traits regressed to 291.5 kg hot carcass weight.
[‡] Values for three randomly selected animals per group regressed to 293.2 kg carcass weight.

also show appreciable changes in tests weight, however, which suggests disruption in the hypothalamic–pituitary–gonadal mechanism controlling testis growth. A linear relationship between testes weight and the level of DES implantation was reported by Trenkle (1976) but, as shown in Table 12.21, when results were expressed in relation to a standardized carcass weight the relationship was more complex and low doses of DES were shown to have a marked repressive activity.

Further studies of the effects of stilbenes at low dose levels in combination with trenbolone acetate are needed before potential production responses in bulls can be satisfactorily identified, and such studies could, incidentally, provide a basis for investigating the mode of action of trenbolone acetate in cattle. For example, reductions in testes weight and plasma testosterone and gonadotropin levels with trenbolone/DES treatment would indicate that trenbolone was acting as a substitute for testes androgen. Conversely, normal testes weight and testosterone and gonadotropin levels would be more consistent with trenbolone acting centrally to restore masculine neuroendocrine function and possible somatic development. In view of the high levels of growth hormone found in the pituitaries and blood plasma of steers treated with DES (Trenkle, 1976) and in the plasma of bulls as compared with steers (Galbraith, Dempster and Miller, 1978), and the low plasma thyroid hormone levels in steers treated with trenbolone and oestradiol (Heitzman, 1976), it is tempting to speculate that the anabolic effects of trenbolone and DES in bulls may be exerted through growth and thyroid hormones. Also, it may be these hormones rather than the steroids themselves that are responsible for the observed changes in muscle protein turnover (particularly catabolism) in trenbolone-treated rats (Vernon and Buttery, 1976; Buttery, Vernon and Pearson, 1978; D. J. Millward, personal communication).

Biological determinants of sex effects on meat

Although there are demonstrable commercial advantages in terms of growth rate, food conversion efficiency and carcass leanness in using entire males for meat production, and benefits from treating castrated males and females with natural steroid hormones and/or anabolic agents, most information on carcass composition relates to animals at commercial slaughter weights. There is only limited information on the nature of interrelationships between tissues during development and on the courses of changes in proportions or distribution of tissues. Also, little is known about the physiological and biochemical mechanisms controlled by anabolic hormones and agents or about the way in which the regulation of nutrient utilization, growth and body composition is achieved.

Puberty and the biological and economic costs of lean meat production

In a study conducted at the Meat Research Institute, sheep of defined breeds were reared on the same diet, slaughtered at different ages and anatomically dissected. At each slaughter age, rams were larger and proportionally leaner than ewe lambs. Thus the greater leanness of male compared with female sheep at commercial slaughter weights can be considered not only as a direct consequence of their propensity to grow to a larger adult mature size but also as a reflexion of biological differences in maturation rate between the sexes. However, rate of fattening is not constant when considered in relation to the development of the lean body. Data for intact male and female Hampshire Down lambs show that fattening is characteristically biphasic in both sexes (Fig. 12.5), and this seems to be a general phenomenon (Berg, Jones, Price, Fukuhara, Butterfield and Hardin, 1979), although it is not clear whether it should be considered as a sex effect or as a non-sexual characteristic.

It can be seen from Fig. 12.5 that the acceleration of the rate of fattening occurred in males at a heavier muscle plus bone weight than

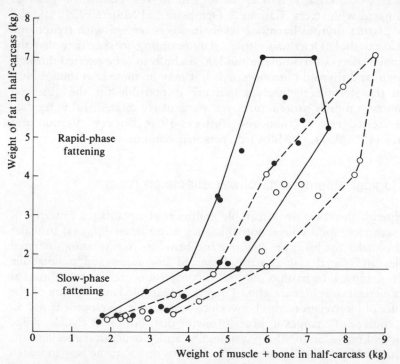

Fig. 12.5.   Effects of sex on the deposition of fat in relation to lean-body development in Hampshire Down sheep (○, males; ●, females).

in females. The studies of McClelland *et al.* (1976) suggest that the mechanism underlying the acceleration is related to the attainment of a certain proportion of adult size; ewe and ram lambs slaughtered at different proportions of adult live weight differed little in carcass composition. However, changes in fattening rate occurred at a stage of development in both ram and ewe lambs when they had apparently accumulated a similar quantity of dissectible carcass fat, which, because rams grew more rapidly, was at a similar age in rams and ewes. Berg *et al.* (1979) have reported corresponding findings for carcass fatness in heifers, steers and bulls.

In a recent study, Friesian bulls, steers and heifers were reared under defined nutritional conditions (Frood, 1976) and each category was slaughtered at various live weights. Using the results of this study, A. J. Kempster and G. Harrington (personal communication) have computed the energy costs of producing lean meat, assuming a constant energy cost for calf production. Their results, shown graphically in Fig. 12.6, indicate that the energetics of lean meat production differ consistently and appreciably between heifers, steers and bulls. In all cases, the minimum energy costs of lean meat production were attained at slaughter weights below those currently acceptable commercially for Friesian cattle.

On the other hand, if the results for steers are related to other independent data for cattle of the same breed and sex (Fig. 12.7) it may

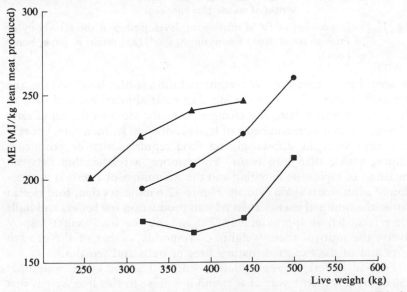

Fig. 12.6. The metabolizable energy costs of lean meat production in Friesian heifers, bulls and steers in relation to live weight at slaughter (from Frood, 1976) (■, bull; ▲, heifer; ●, steer).

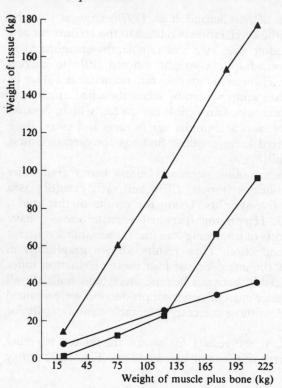

Fig. 12.7.   Deposition of fat in relation to development of the lean-body of
Friesian steers (from Anonymous, 1966) (▲, muscle; ■, fat; ●, bone).
bone).

be seen that, in terms of live weight and muscle plus bone weight, the
minimal energy cost of producing lean meat approximates closely to
the point at which fattening changes from the slow to the rapid rate.
The subsequent increasing cost of lean production is, therefore, entirely
consistent with the known greater food requirements for producing
adipose rather than lean tissue. Futhermore, a relationship between
initiation of rapid-rate fattening and the attainment of a certain proportion of adult size is again evident. Figure 12.6 indicates that, for Friesian
cattle, the minimal energy costs of lean production for heifers and bulls
were recorded at approximately 250 and 375 kg live weight respectively; the ratio of these weights corresponds to that of the growth
rates and of the expected mature sizes of bulls and females.

Friesian heifers, if appropriately fed, will attain a live weight of
250 kg by less than 1 year of age, and it is close to this live weight that
such heifers attain sexual maturity (R. J. Heitzman and I. Reynolds,
personal communication). Thus the process of rapid-rate fattening,
which apparently follows the accumulation of a given quantity of fat,

appears to be closely linked to the physiological events controlling the attainment of sexual maturity.

The concept that puberty may have important implications for the nutritional efficiency of lean meat production is a new development in animal science. Although puberty is not an easily defined event in pigs, the arguments of Fowler (1976), favouring a reduction in commercial slaughter weights as a means of significantly reducing costs of production, may depend on it. The onset of rapid fattening occurs in pigs at approximately 62 to 70 kg live weight, a weight at which ovulation can be induced (G. R. Foxcroft, personal communication); and Kempster (1980) has shown that close to this carcass weight the economic production cost per unit of carcass of a constant lean : fat ratio of 5:1 is at a minimum. Similarly, in cattle and sheep it is likely that puberty is the major determinant of the changes observed in the composition of live-weight gain during development.

In commercially reared female breeding animals, puberty may be delayed by the tendency to restrict fattening by nutritional means and to aim for a slower rate of growth. In dairy cattle the rate of growth may be particularly important since lactational performance appears to depend on a 'critical period' of udder development during the growing period. Heifers treated with trenbolone acetate show delayed puberty but puberty is attained at greater live weights, increased in direct proportion to the effects of treatment on growth rate and food utilization (R. J. Heitzman and I. Reynolds, personal communication).

It is tempting to speculate that, in heifers, anabolic agents may increase the energetic efficiency of lean meat production in direct proportion to the extent to which they delay the onset of the rapid fattening stage of growth, but there is no direct evidence in support of this idea. On the other hand, the substantial changes in the ME cost of lean meat production (Fig. 12.6) and in the pattern of fattening (Berg *et al.*, 1979) which arise from the castration of bulls, illustrate the importance of endogenous sex hormones and it is possible that such changes can be reversed by synthetic analogues. The maintenance by steers of growth rates and patterns of fattening that do not revert completely to that of the female type (Berg *et al.*, 1979) indicates, however, that regulation of the change in fattening rate is probably not simply dependent on the sex hormones alone.

Regulation of foetal neural development and postnatal neuroendocrine function

Perinatal androgenization of female rats with a single dose of testosterone propionate can induce long-term improvements in growth rate and food utilization by affecting mechanisms additional to those regulated by the secretion of gonadal steroids after puberty (Perry *et al.*, 1979), and this illustrates the ability of sex steroids to programme developmental processes early in life when animals are reproductively quiescent. Such early beneficial effects of sex steriods (or possibly other substances) on patterns of growth and development might in the future have important implications for animal production; Mainwaring (1979) has pointed out that much less is known about this rôle of sex steroids than about their ability to influence metabolic processes in tissues at later stages of growth.

The exposure of foetal female sheep to androgens will induce changes in the development of the genitalia, in sex-related patterns of behaviour and in the characteristic sex-related central neuroendocrine response to oestrogen stimulation (Short, 1974). Similar neuroendocrine effects can also be induced by direct treatment of foetal pigs *in utero* with androgen (Ellendorf, Parvizi, Elsaesser, MacLeod and Reinhardt, 1979), and the effects of foetal exposure to androgens on the rate, efficiency and patterns of tissue development are currently being investigated at the Meat Research Institute. From these and other studies conducted with rats and mice, it is now clear that one of the major early organizational rôles of sex steroids is to effect the initiation of sexually differentiated neuronal circuits within the brain (Dyer, MacLeod and Ellendorf, 1976; Toran-Allerand, 1976 and 1978).

This rôle for the brain in sex steroid responses has only recently been demonstrated, but the activities of the hypothalamus and pituitary in growth regulation have long been recognized. Even so, data are not yet available which satisfactorily explain how sexual differentiation of neuronal circuits within the brain of the male brings about increased growth and better food utilization, although the more rapid growth of males and of androgenized females is well known (Harris and Levine, 1962).

The results of Perry *et al.* (1979) suggest that sexual differences in growth rate and nutritional efficiency are induced by mechanisms which do not depend on the direct effects of sex steroids on appetite or on the partition of dietary nutrients between lean tissue and fat, although the endocrinological determinants of these processes are unknown. Some workers have suggested that the masculinized hypothalamus becomes refractory to oestrogenic influences, and there is evidence of a lack of positive oestrogen feedback on gonadotropin secretion in androgenized female and male rats, sheep and pigs. There is also now a generally accepted model to explain the action of steroid hormones on genetic expression which involves uptake of the steroid onto specific hormone receptors, activation of the hormone-receptor complex and translocation into the nucleus, where binding to chromatin acceptor-sites then brings about transcription of RNA. Using this model, Perry and Lopez (1978) have demonstrated that hypothalamic nuclear chromatin from naturally androgenized male and normal female sheep possesses comparable potential for binding of oestrogen and progesterone receptor-complexes to acceptor sites. Also, the rate of translocation of oestrogen receptor into purified hypothalamic nuclei *in vivo* has recently been shown to be similar in male rats and in female rats treated with oestrogen. This latter observation is consistent with data that show that oestradiol benzoate or the anti-oestrogen tamoxifen reduce growth; anti-oestrogens are also translocated into hypothalamic nuclei (Roy, 1978).

Briefly, therefore, these results suggest that either the sexually differentiated male brain is not a major site of dimorphism in oestrogen action in the control of growth, or that there is some unidentified sex-related mechanism acting within the hypothalamus beyond the point of interaction of receptor-complexes with chromatin, which effects differential control of pituitary hormone secretion and/or other neuronal pathways involved in growth regulation. Additionally, inter-hormonal control mechanisms may be important since some steroid hormone receptor systems are controlled by oestrogens (e.g. progesterone and androgen) (Hsueh, Peck and Clark, 1976; Leavitt, Chen, Allen and Johnston, 1977; MacLusky and McEwen, 1978; Tokarz, Harrison and Seaver, 1979), and oestrogen-receptor replenishment is affected by androgens and progesterone (Charreau and Denti, 1975; Hsueh *et al.*, 1976). Precise relationships are, however, tissue-specific (MacLusky and McEwen, 1980) and the possibility exists that, even in anatomically specialized tissues such as the hypothalamus, sexually differentiated neuronal circuits may allow steroids to elicit a variety of responses. Current biochemical analyses may not be sufficiently discriminating to detect these subtle effects. Moreover, it is becoming evident that inter-hormonal control is not restricted to structurally-related classes of hormones (e.g. steroids, amines, peptides); steroids, for example, have been shown to exert powerful influences on non-steroidal hormone receptors in the brain and other tissues. Castration and testosterone-replacement therapy have profound effects on opiate receptors (Hahn and Fishman, 1979), and catechol-oestrogens can modify the activity of dopamine receptors (Schaeffer and Hsueh, 1979) and influence pituitary hormone secretion in rats and pigs (Ellendorf *et al.*, 1979; Martucci and Fishman, 1979; Fishman, Norton and Hahn, 1980). This implies that sexual as well as neural control of the autonomic system may be important, and raises the possibility that central sex-related mechanisms may be involved in the regulation of biochemical developmental processes in peripheral organs and tissues. Perry *et al.* (1979) have also shown that auto-immunity to luteinizing hormone-releasing hormone can be used to improve growth rate and food utilization in female rats, but further studies are required to assess whether similar or alternative antigens can be used to induce beneficial effects in meat species. The sex-related accumulation of androstenone (boar taint) in the fat of pigs can also be controlled using auto-immunity (E. Diane Williamson, unpublished results), and the approach therefore has direct implications for meat quality. Equally important, however, is that boar growth rate and efficiency of food utilization are unaffected because the selectivity of the procedure achieves a separation of the hormonal determinants of anabolism and taint that cannot be attained by other means (Rhodes and Patterson, 1971).

Conclusions

Recent studies in steroid biochemistry have shown that gonadal hormones influence metabolism in many tissues and organs and only a few such studies have been considered here. Unfortunately, little is yet known about the extent to which steroid-induced anabolic responses may be the consequence of changes induced in the central nervous system. Anabolic responses induced by perinatal or foetal gonadal-steroid programming, in which the mechanisms underlying sexual differentiation of the brain are strongly implicated, could nevertheless depend on the effects of gonadal steroids acting at the periphery; and equally, the effects of administered gonadal or anabolic steroids on growth and development could primarily be mediated via central mechanisms. Dissociating the central from peripheral effects of sex hormones and anabolic agents on energy metabolism and growth is as difficult as defining the nature of the relationship between sex hormones and other endocrine and neuro-endocrine systems in the regulation of growth and metabolism. Better definition of the nature of endocrinological regulation of sites of action of hormones might provide a clearer insight into more effective means of attaining beneficial manipulations in animal production.

Reductions in circulating levels of the thyroid hormone T_4 in cattle (Heitzman, 1976) and T_3 in rats (D. J. Millward, personal communication) following treatment of the animals with trenbolone acetate could imply that the sex hormone-induced effects on the energetic efficiency of nutrient conservation, and the sex-related differences in growth rate and efficiency of food utilization, lead consequentially to the associated effects on body composition (Perry *et al.*, 1979). But the extent and precise mechanisms by which thyroid hormones act to control growth and energy metabolism are still much debated. Also, the subcellular interhormonal control mechanisms are subtle in nature, and circulating levels of hormones may not be an adequate basis for describing hormonal activity.

Analogous problems of interpretation exist with respect to the effects of sex steroids on systems controlling catecholaminergic or pep- tidergic neurotransmission in the central nervous system, and of their involvement in non-steroidal peripheral hormone action in sexual somatic development. Nevertheless, some advances have been made by endocrinologists studying the pubertal control of reproduction in females, and biogenic amines and peptide hormones in the central nervous system have been shown to be important in the feed-back regulation of gonadal oestrogen (Ojeda, Advis and Andrews, 1980). It is possible, therefore, that effects on neuronal development and/or subcellular organization, permanently induced by gonadal steroids in the critical period of brain sexual differentiation, may be manifest in changes in the functional integration of biogenic amine metabolism in the brain. Similarly, any steroid-induced effects on the relationship between the brain and autonomic nervous system might also have wide-ranging implications for the development of sexually dimorphic functions in peripheral organs and tissues. Moreover, the possibility has not yet been ruled out that some responses in growth and metabolism of animals to natural or synthetic anabolic steroids are mediated by metabolites, such as the catechol derivatives of oestrogens, which possess catecholaminergic properties affecting biogenic-amine recep- tors in some tissues (Schaeffer and Hsueh, 1979) and pituitary hormone secretion (Ellendorf *et al.*, 1979; Martucci and Fishman, 1979; Fishman *et al.*, 1980). There is a need too for greater knowledge of the rôle of neural (opiate) peptides in sexuality, growth and nutrient utilization for it is known that testosterone influences opiate receptors (Hahn and Fishman, 1979) and opiates regulate steroid metabolizing enzymes (Fishman *et al.*, 1980).

For the most part, there is still ignorance about the way in which gonadal steroids and anabolic agents influence genetic expression, particularly with regard to the control of growth and metabolism in non-reproductive tissues. Research with domestic meat species will need to consider much more carefully the nature of sex-related mecha- nisms that allow males, or animals showing male growth characteristics, to conserve not only more dietary nutrients as lean tissue but also a greater proportion of their food intake as carcass energy.

The performance and carcass characteristics of DES-treated steers do not satisfy both of these criteria, although data are not yet available to allow calculations to be made for steers treated with oestrogens (DES, hexoestrol, zeranol or oestradiol) in combination with the androgenic steroid trenbolone. In cattle, the additive effects of trenbolone on growth rate and food conversion efficiency, when combined with oestrogens, linked with its effects on circulating thyroid hormones (T_4 and T_3), that have traditionally been considered to be important determinants of metabolic rate, could reflect changes in the energetics

Table 12.22   Energy balance in castrated male pigs measured 13 to 17 days after implantation with trenbolone acetate plus 17β-oestradiol at 55 kg live weight (six pigs per group) (from Van Weerden and Grandadam, 1976)

| | Energy intake (MJ ME/day) | Energy balance (MJ/day) | | |
		Protein	Lipid	Total	Total (as proportion of intake)
Control (placebo)	28.56	2.36	11.52	13.89	0.486
Implant (140 mg trenbolone acetate + 20 mg oestradiol)	29.36	3.69	9.76	13.45	0.458

of metabolism. However, calorimetric experiments with castrated pigs treated with trenbolone acetate and oestradiol (Van Weerden and Grandadam, 1976) failed to demonstrate effects on the efficiency of utilization of metabolizable energy (Table 12.22), although, as expected, the treatment increased protein and decreased fat deposition. In another experiment in which boars and gilts were given the same total amount of ME between the start of the experiment, at 25 kg live weight, and its completion (G. A. Lodge, personal communication), boars ate less per day than gilts and took 5 days longer to consume their total allowance. However, the boars were leaner than the gilts and at least as efficient in conserving food energy, apparently partly as a result of a lower maintenance energy requirement per unit of metabolic body weight (Table 12.23). There are no corresponding data for sex comparisons in cattle that allow similar calculations to be made.

Table 12.23   Energy utilization by boars and gilts fed *ad libitum* the same total amount of food from 25 kg live weight (from G. A. Lodge, personal communication)

	Boars	Gilts
Food allowance (kg)	608	608
Mean no. of days on test	81	76
Mean weight on test (kg)	60	55.7
Mean energy retention (GJ)	1.12	1.11
Mean energy expenditure (GJ)	1.43	1.43
Energy expenditure (kJ/kg$^{0.75}$ per day)	816	925
Energy for maintenance (kJ/kg$^{0.75}$ per day)	531	632

[†] Calculated by difference from energy costs of fat and protein deposition, assuming a factor of 50 MJ/kg tissue.

Another basic requirement in relation to diet, animal performance and meat production is to determine whether differences in food and energy utilization between the sexes, or anabolic agent-treated and untreated animals, become negligible when animals are slaughtered at the same proportion of their mature weight. The sex-related differences in the carcass composition of sheep became unimportant when males and females were compared on this basis (McClelland *et al.*, 1976), but in pigs differences in carcass composition are maintained through to maturity, at which point body weights are similar for both sexes. Comprehensive information on the growth rate, food conversion efficiency and efficiency of utilization of dietary energy for breeds, types and sexes would greatly assist rational judgements on the suitability of individual groups of animals for use in particular production systems. Moreover, use of the biological effects of the interactions between breed and sex could lead to a more planned and profitable production of carcasses of desired size and desired composition, and would facilitate the application of modern and novel butchery and meat processing techniques.

REFERENCES

Andersen, H. R., 1975. The influence of slaughter weight and feeding level on the growth, feed conversion, carcass composition and conformation of bulls. *Beretn. St. Husdyrbrugs fors., No. 430.*

Anonymous, 1966. A comparison of the growth of different types of cattle for beef production. *Major Beef Research Project.* Royal Smithfield Club, London.

Anonymous, 1976. *Newsl. Meat Livest. Commn Beef Improv. Servs, No. 28.* Meat and Livestock Commission, Bletchley, Milton Keynes.

Ashwell, Margaret, Meade, C. J., Medawar, Sir Peter and Sowter, C., 1977. Adipose tissue: contributions of nature and nurture to the obesity of an obese mutant mouse (*ob/ob*), *Proc. R. Soc. Ser. B* **195**: 343–54.

Bailey, A. J., 1974. Tissue and species specificity in the crosslinking of collagen, *Path. Biol., Paris* **22**: 675–80.

Bailey, C. M., Probert, C. L. and Bowman, V. R., 1966. Growth rate, feed utilization and body composition of young bulls and steers, *J. Anim. Sci.* **25**: 132–7.

Bakke, H., 1975. Serum levels of non-esterified fatty acids and glucose in lines of pigs selected for rate of gain and thickness of backfat, *Acta Agric. scand.* **25**: 113–6.

Bakke, H. and Tveit, B., 1977. Serum levels of thyroid hormones in lines of pigs selected for rate of gain and thickness of backfat, *Acta Agric. scand.* **27**: 41–4.

Barton, R. A., 1967. The relation between live animal conformation and the carcass of cattle, *Anim. Breed. Abstr.* **35**: 1–22.

Bendall, J. R., 1966. The effect of pre-treatment of pigs with curare on the post-mortem rate of pH fall and onset of rigor mortis in the musculature, *J. Sci. Fd Agric.* **17**: 333–8.

Bendall, J. R., 1973. In *Structure and Function of Muscle,* Vol. II, 2nd edn (ed. G. H. Bourne), pp. 244–306. Academic Press, New York.

Bendall, J. R., 1980. The electrical stimulation of carcasses of meat animals, *Dev. Meat Sci.* **1**: 37–59.

Berg, R. T., Andersen, B. B. and Liboriussen, T., 1978. Growth of bovine tissues. 2. Genetic influences on muscle growth and distribution in young bulls, *Anim. Prod.* **27**: 51–61.

Berg, R. T. and Butterfield, R. M., 1976. *New Concepts of Cattle Growth.* Sydney University Press, Sydney.

Berg, R. T., Jones, S. D. M., Price, M. A., Fukuhara, R., Butterfield, R. M. and Hardin, R. T., 1979. Patterns of carcass fat deposition in heifers, steers and bulls, *Can. J. Anim. Sci.* **59**: 359–66.

Brannang, E., 1971. Studies on monozygous cattle twins. 23. The effect of castrates and age of castration on the development of single muscles, bones and special sex characters, *Swed. J. Agric. Res.* **1**: 69–78.

Briskey, E. J., 1964. Etiological status and associated studies of P.S.E. musculature, *Adv. Fd Res.* **13**: 89–178.

Burton, J. H. and Reid, J. T., 1969. Interrelationships among energy input, body composition of sheep, *J. Nutr.* **97**: 517–24.

Buttery, P. J., Vernon, B. G. and Pearson, J. T., 1978. Anabolic agents-some thoughts on their mode of action, *Proc. Nutr. Soc.* **37**: 311–5.

Cassens, R. G., Giesler, F. J. and Kolb, Q. E., 1972. *Proc. Pork Qual. Symp., Univ. Wis.*

Chappel, R.J. and Dunkin, A. C., 1975. Relation of concentration of growth hormone in blood plasma to growth rate and carcass characteristics in the pig, *Anim. Prod.* **20**: 51–61.

Charreau, E. H. and Denti, A., 1975. Characteristics of the hypothalamic and hypophyseal cytoplasmic oestradiol binding substances: effects of neonatal castration and testosterone administration, *Acta physiol. latinoam.* **25**: 279–87.

Chrystall, B. B. and Hagyard, C. J., 1976. Electrical stimulation and lamb tenderness, *N.Z. Jl agric. Res.* **19**: 7–11.

Davey, C. L., Gilbert, K. V. and Carse, W. A., 1976. Carcass electrical stimulation to avoid cold shortening toughness in beef, *N.Z. Jl agric. Res.* **19**: 13–8.

Duchesne, H., 1978. The aetiology of dark cutting beef. *Ph. D. Thesis, Univ. Bristol.*

Dyer, R. G., MacLeod, N. K. and Ellendorf, F., 1976. Electrophysiological evidence for sexual dimorphism and synaptic convergence in the preoptic and anterior hypothalamic areas of the rat, *Proc. R. Soc. Ser. B* **193**: 421–40.

Ellendorf, F., Parvizi, N., Elsaesser, F., MacLeod, N. and Reinhardt, W., 1979. Functional and organizational aspects of gonadal steroids in the pig brain, *J. Steroid Biochem.* **11**: 839–44.

Elliot, K. M. and Fowler, V. R., 1973. The response of growing castrated male pigs to various hormones of possible anabolic potential, *Proc. Nutr. Soc.* **32**: 103–4A.

Elsley, F. W. H., 1976. Limitations to the manipulation of growth, *Proc. Nutr. Soc.* **35**: 323–37.

Fishman, J., Norton, B. I. and Hahn, E. F., 1980. Opiate regulation of oestradiol-2-hydroxylase in brains of male rats: mechanism for control of pituitary hormone secretion, *Proc. natn Acad. Sci. U.S.A.* **77**: 2574–6.

Fowler, V. R., 1976. Some aspects of energy utilization for the production of lean tissue in the pig, *Proc. Nutr. Soc.* **35**: 75–9.

Fowler, M. A., Adeyanju, S. A., Burroughs, W. and Kline, E. A., 1970. Net energy evaluations of beef cattle rations with and without stilbestrol, *J. Anim. Sci.* **30**: 291–6.

Frood, I. J. M., 1976. An investigation into the effect of sex and plane of nutrition on the growth performance and carcass quality of British Friesian cattle for beef production. *Ph. D. Thesis, Univ. Reading.*

Fuller, M. F., Webster, A. J. F., MacPherson, R. M. and Smith, J. S., 1976. Comparative aspects of the energy metabolism of Pietrain and Large White × Landrace pigs during growth, *Proc. 7th Symp. Energy Metab. Fm Anim., Vichy* (ed. M. Vermorel), pp. 177–80.

Galbraith, H., Dempster, D. G. and Miller, T. B. 1978., A note on the effect of castration on the growth performance and concentrations of some blood metabolites and hormones in British Friesian male cattle, *Anim. Prod.* **26**: 339–42.

Gregory, N. G. and Lister, D., 1981. Sympathetic responsiveness in relation to fatness in pigs, *Proc. Nutr. Soc.* **40**: 11A (Abstr.).

Gregory, N. G., Lovell, R. D., Wood, J. D. and Lister, D., 1977. Insulin-secreting ability in Pietrain and Large White pigs, *J. agric. Sci., Camb.* **89**: 407–13.

Gregory, N. G., Wood, J. D., Enser, M. B., Smith, W. C. and Ellis, M., 1980. Fat mobilization in Large White pigs selected for low backfat thickness, *J. Sci. Fd Agric.* **31**: 567–72.

Griffiths, T. W., 1980. The relative efficiency of food utilization of British Friesian entire male and castrated male cattle at two levels of feeding, *Anim. Prod.* **30**: 53–9.

Hahn, E. F. and Fishman, J., 1979. Changes in rat brain opiate receptor content upon castration and testosterone replacement, *Biochem. biophys. Res. Commun.* **90**: 819–23.

Haldane, J. B. S., 1929. *Possible Worlds and Other Essays*. Chatto and Windus, London.

Hall, G. M., Lucke, J. N., Lovell, R. D. L. and Lister, D., 1980. Porcine hyperthermia. VII. Hepatic metabolism, *Br. J. Anaesth.* **52**: 11–7.

Harries, J. M., Williams, D. R. and Pomeroy, R. W., 1975. Prediction of comparative retail value of beef carcases, *Anim. Prod.* **21**: 127–37.

Harries, J. M., Williams, D. R. and Pomeroy, R. W., 1976. Comparative retail value of beef carcasses from different groups of animals, *Anim. Prod.* **23**: 349–56.

Harrington, G., 1978. Problems in devising a European beef carcass classification system. *Eur. Congr. Improved Beef Productivity, Paris*. Meat and Livestock Commission, Bletchley, Milton Keynes (Mimeograph).

Harris, G. W. and Levine, S., 1962. Sexual differentiation of the brain and its experimental control, *J. Physiol., Lond.* **63**: 42P (Abstr.).

Havell, R. J., 1970. Lipid as an energy source. In *The Physiology and Biochemistry of Muscle as a Food: 2* (ed. E. J. Briskey, R. G. Cassens and B. B. Marsh), pp. 609–21. University of Wisconsin Press, Madison,Wis.

Hedrick, H. B., Thompson, G. B. and Krause, G. F., 1969. Comparison of feedlot performance and carcass characteristics of half-sib bulls, steers and heifers, *J. Anim. Sci.* **29**: 687–94.

Heitzman, R. J., 1976. The effectiveness of anabolic agents in increasing the rate of growth in farm animals: report of experiments in cattle. In *Anabolic Agents in Animal Production* (ed. F. C. Lu and J. Rendel), pp. 89–98. Georg Thieme, Stuttgart.

Heitzman, R. J., 1978. The use of hormones to regulate the utilization of nutrients in farm animals: current farm practices, *Proc. Nutr. Soc.* **37**: 289–93.

Henderson, Ruth, Whittemore, C. T., Ellis, M., Smith, W. C. and Laird, R., 1980. Comparison of the Newcastle Large White control and selection line pigs on a fixed feed, fixed time trial, *Anim. Prod.* **30**: 464(Abstr.).

Hood, R. L. and Allen, C. E., 1973. Lipogenic enzyme activity in adipose tissue during the growth of swine with different propensitites to fatten, *J. Nutr.* **103**: 353–62.

Howard, A. and Lawrie, R. A., 1956. *Spec. Rep. Fd Invest. Bd D.S.I.R., No. 63.*

Hsueh, A. J. W., Peck, E. J. and Clark, J. H., 1976. Control of uterine oestrogen receptor levels by progesterone, *Endocrinology* **98**: 438–44.

Issekutz, B., Jr, 1970. Interrelationships of free fatty acids, lactic acid and glucose in muscle metabolism. In *The Physiology and Biochemistry of Muscle as a Food: 2* (ed. E. J. Briskey, R. G., Cassens and B. B. Marsh), pp. 623–43. University of Wisconsin Press, Madison, Wis.

Jeremiah, L. E., Carpenter, Z. L., Smith, G. C. and Butler, O. D., 1970. *Tech. Rep. Tex. agric. Exp. Stn, No. 22.*

Kayser, C. and Heusner, A., 1964. Comparative study of energy metabolism in various animals, *J. Physiol., Paris* **56**: 489.

Kempster, A. J., 1979. Variation in the carcass characteristics of commercial British sheep with particular reference to overfatness, *Meat Sci.* **3**: 199–208.

Kempster, A. J., 1980. Entire males for meat: how far has the industry come? *Meat* **53**: 13–8.

Kempster, A. J. and Harrington, G., 1979. Variation in carcass characteristics of commercial British cattle, *Meat Sci.* **3**: 53–62.

Kissebah, A. H., Clarke, P. V., Vydelingum, N., Hope Gill, H. F., Tulloch, B. R. and Fraser, T. R., 1975. Mechanism of insulin resistance associated with obesity. In *Recent Advances in Obesity Research* (ed. A. Howard) Newman, London.

Koch, R. M., Dikeman, M. E., Allen, D. M., May, M., Crouse, J. D. and Campion, D. R., 1976. Characterization of biological types of cattle 3. Carcass composition, quality and palatability, *J. Anim. Sci.* **43**: 48–62.

Laflamme, L. F. and Burgess, T. D., 1973. Effect of castration ration and hormone implants on the performance of finishing cattle, *J. Anim. Sci.* **36**: 762–7.

Lawrie, R. A., 1952. Biochemical differences between red and white muscle, *Nature, Lond.* **170**: 122–3.

Lawrie, R. A., 1958. Physiological stress in relation to dark-cutting beef, *J. Sci. Fd Agric.* **9**: 721–7.

Lawrie, R. A., 1966. *Meat Science*. Pergamon Press, Oxford.

Leavitt, W. W., Chen, T. J., Allen, T. C. and Johnston, J. O. N., 1977. Regulation of progesterone receptor formation by oestrogen action, *Ann. N.Y. Acad. Sci.* **286**: 210.

Levy, D., Holzer, Z. and Folman, Y., 1976. Effects of plane of nutrition, diethylstilboestrol implantation and slaughter weight on performance of Israeli-Friesian intact male cattle, *Anim. Prod.* **22**: 55–9.

Lister, D., 1974. The stress syndrome and meat quality: physiology. *Rapporteurs' Pap. 20th Eur. Meet. Meat Res. Wkrs*, pp. 17–27. An Foras Talúntais, Dublin.

Lister, D., 1979. Some physiological aspects of the stress cycle in relation to muscle function and meat quality, *Acta. Agric. scand., Suppl. 21*, pp. 281–8.

Lister, D., 1980. Hormones, metabolism and growth, *Reprod. Nutr. Develop.* **20**(1B): 225–33.

Lister, D., Lucke, J. N. and Hall, G. M., 1976. Pale, soft, exudative (PSE) meat, stress susceptibility and MHS in pigs: endocrinological and general physiological aspects. In *Proc. 3rd int. Conf. Prod. Dis. Fm Anim.*, pp. 144–50. Pudoc, Wageningen.

Lister, D., Scopes, R. K. and Bendall, J. R., 1969. Some properties of the muscle of Pietrain pigs, *Anim. Prod.* **11**: 288(Abstr.).

Lister, D. and Spencer, G. S. G., 1982. *Meat Sci.* In press.

Locker, R. H. and Hagyard, C. J., 1963. A cold shortening effect in beef muscles, *J. Sci. Fd Agric.* **14**: 787–93.

Lodge, G. A., Lister, D., Wood, J. D. and Wolynetz, M. S., 1978. Age, weight or total feed intake as bases for the performance testing of growing pigs, *Anim. Prod.* **27**: 345–54.

Lu, F. C. and Rendel, J., 1976. *Anabolic Agents in Animal Production*. Georg Thieme, Stuttgart.

Lucke, J. N., Hall, G. M. and Lister, D., 1979. Malignant hyperthermia in the pig and the role of stress, *Ann. N.Y. Acad. Sci.* **317**: 326–37.

McClelland, T. H., Bonaiti, B. and Taylor, St C. S., 1976. Breed differences in body composition of equally mature sheep, *Anim. Prod.* **23**: 281–93.

MacLusky, N. J. and McEwen, B.S., 1978. Oestrogen modulates progestin receptor concentrations in some brain regions but not in others, *Nature, Lond.* **274**: 276–8.

McLusky, N. J. and McEwen, B. S., 1980. Progestin receptors in rat brain: distribution and properties of cytoplasmic progestin-binding sites, *Endocrinology* **106**: 192–202.

Mainwaring, W. I. P., 1979. Androgen receptors and biologic responses: a survey. In *Receptors and Hormone Action* (ed. B. W. O'Malley and L. Birnbaumer), pp. 105–120. Academic Press, New York.

Martucci, C. P. and Fishman, J., 1979. Impact of continuously administered catechol oestrogens on uterine growth and luteinizing hormone secretion, *Endocrinology* **105**: 1288–92.

Meat and Livestock Commission, 1975. *Planned Crossbreeding and Lamb Carcase Weights*. Revised edn. Meat and Livestock Commission, Bletchley, Milton Keynes.

Mendel, V. E., 1980. Influence of the insulin-to-growth hormone ratio on body composition of mice, *Am. J. Physiol.* **238**: E231–4.

Newton, K. G. and Gill, C. O., 1978. Storage quality of dark, firm, dry meat, *Appl. & Environ. Microbiol.* **36**: 375–6.

North of Scotland College of Agriculture, 1979. Response of growing Friesian bulls to treatment with trenbolone acetate and hexoestrol, *Research Investigations and Field Trials, 1977–78*, pp. 35–37.

Ojeda, S. R., Advis, J. P. and Andrews, W. W., 1980. Neuroendocrine control of the onset of puberty in the rat, *Fedn Proc. Fedn Am. Socs exp. Biol.* **39**: 2365–71.

Patterson, R. L. S., 1975. The flavour of meat. In *Meat* (cd. D. J. A. Cole and R. A. Lawrie), pp. 359–79. Butterworth, London.

Pernow, B. and Saltin, B., 1971. *Muscle Metabolism During Exercise*. Plenum Press New York.

Perry, B. N. and Lopez, A., 1978. The binding of ^{3}H-labelled oestradiol- and progesterone-receptor complexes to hypothalamic chromatin of male and female sheep, *Biochem. J.* **176**: 873–83.

Perry, B. N., McCracken, A., Furr, B. J. A. and MacFie, H. J., 1979. Separate roles of androgen and oestrogen in the manipulation of growth and efficiency of food utilization in female rats, *J. Endocr.* **81**: 35–48.

Preston, T. R., MacDearmid, A., Aitken, J. N., MacLeod, N. A. and Philip, E. B., 1968. The effect of castration on growth, feed conversion and carcass quality of Friesian cattle given all-concentration diets, *Rev. Cubana Cienc. Agr.* **2**: 183–90.

Preston, T. R. and Willis, M. B., 1970. *Intensive Beef Production*. Pergamon Press, Oxford.

Reid, J. T., Bensadoun, A., Bull, L. S., Burton, J. H., Gleeson, P. A., Han, I. K., Joo, Y. D., Johnson, D. E., McManus, W. R., Paladines, O. L., Stroud, J. W., Tyrell, H. F., Van Niekerk, B. D. H. and Wellington, G. H., 1968. Some peculiarities in the body composition of animals. In *Body Composition in Animals and Man, Publs natn. Acad. Sci., Wash., No. 1958,* pp. 19–44.

Rhodes, D. N., 1976. What do we want in a carcass? In *Meat Animals: Growth and Productivity* (ed. D. Lister, D. N. Rhodes, V. R. Fowler and M. F. Fuller), pp. 9–24. Plenum Press, New York.

Rhodes, D. N. and Patterson, R. L. S., 1971. Effects of partial castration on growth and the incidence of boar taint in the pig, *J. Sci. Fd Agric.* **22**: 320–4.

Rodway, R. G. and Galbraith, H., 1979. Effects of anabolic steroids on hepatic enzymes of amino acid catabolism, *Hormone Metab. Res.* **11**: 489–90.

Rogowski, B., 1980. Meat in human nutrition, *Wld Rev. Nutr. Diet.* **34**: 46–101.

Roy. E. J., 1978. Anti-oestrogens and nuclear oestrogen receptors in the brain, *Curr. Stud. Hypothalamic Funct.* **1**: 204–13.

Schaeffer, J. M. and Hsueh, A. J. W., 1979. 2-Hydroxyestradiol interaction with dopamine receptor binding in rat anterior pituitary, *J. biol. Chem.* **254**: 5606–8.

Scott, T. W., Cook, L. J. and Mills, S. C., 1971. Protection of dietary polyunsaturated fatty acids against microbial hydrogenation in ruminants, *J. Am. Oil Chem. Soc.* **48**: 358–64.

Short, R., 1974. Sexual differentiation of the brain of the sheep. In *Sexual Endocrinology of the Perinatal Period* (ed. M. G. Forest and J. Bertrand), pp. 121–42. INSERM, Paris.

Smith, U., 1971. Effect of cell size in lipid synthesis by human adipose tissue in vitro, *J. Lipid Res.* **12**: 65–70.

Smith, G. M., Laster, D. B., Cundiff, L. V. and Gregory, K. E., 1976. Characterization of biological types of cattle. 2. Post-weaning growth and feed efficiency of steers, *J. Anim. Sci.* **43**: 37–47.

Standal, N., Vold, E., Trygstad, O. and Foss, I., 1973. Lipid mobilization in pigs selected for leanness or fatness, *Anim. Prod.* **16**: 37–42.

Stant, E. G., Martin, T. G., Judge, M. D. and Harrington, R. B., 1968. Physical separation and chemical analysis of the porcine carcass at 23, 46, 68 and 91 kg liveweight, *J. Anim. Sci.* **27**: 636–44.

Stickland, N. C., Widdowson, E. M. and Goldspink, G., 1975. Effects of severe energy and protein deficiencies on the fibres and nuclei in skeletal muscles of pigs, *Br. J. Nutr.* **34**: 421–8.

Sundstøl. F., Standal, N. and Vangen, O., 1979. Energy metabolism in lines of pigs selected for thickness of backfat and rate of gain, *Acta Agric. scand.* **29**: 337–45.

Taylor, St C. S., 1968. Time taken to mature in relation to mature weight for sexes, strains and species of domesticated mammals and birds, *Anim. Prod.* **10**: 157–69.

Tokarz, R. R., Harrison, R. W. and Seaver, S.S., 1979. Mechanism of androgen and estrogen synergism in chick oviduct; estrogen modulated changes in cytoplasmic androgen receptor concentrations, *J. biol. Chem.* **254**: 9178–84.

Toran-Allerand, C. D., 1976. Sex steroids and the development of the newborn mouse hypothalamus and preoptic area in vitro: implications for sexual differentiation. *Brain Res.* **106**: 407–12.

Toran-Allerand, C. D., 1978. Gonadal hormones and brain development: cellular aspects of sexual differentiation. *Am. Zool.* **18**: 553–65.

Trenkle, A., 1976. The anabolic effects of oestrogens on nitrogen metabolism of growing and finishing cattle and sheep. In *Anabolic Agents in Animal Production* (ed. F. C. Lu and J. Rendel), pp. 79–88. Georg Thieme, Stuttgart.

Trenkle, A. and Topel, D. G., 1978. Relationships of some endocrine measurements to growth and carcass composition of cattle, *J. Anim. Sci.* **46**: 1604–9.

Truscott, T. G., 1980. A study of relationships between fat partition and metabolism in Hereford and Friesian steers. *Ph. D. Thesis, Univ. Bristol.*

Truscott, T. G., Wood, J .D. and Denny, H. R., 1980. Growth and cellularity of fat depots in British Friesian and Hereford cattle. *Proc. 26th Eur. Meet. Meat Res. Wkrs, Colorado Springs, Col.,* p. A-2(Abstr.).

Van der Schoot, P., 1980. Effects of dihydrotestosterone and oestradiol on sexual differentiation in male rats, *J. Endocr.* **84**: 397–407.

Van Weerden, E. J. and Grandadam, J. A., 1976. The effect of an anabolic agent on N-deposition growth and slaughter quality in growing castrated male pigs. In *Anabolic Agents in Animal Production* (ed. F. C. Lu and J. Rendel), pp. 115–122. Georg Thieme, Stuttgart.

Vernon, B. G. and Buttery, P. J., 1976. Protein turnover in rats treated with trienbolone acetate, *Br. J. Nutr.* **36**: 575–9.

Vernon, B. G. and Buttery, P. J., 1978. Protein metabolism of rats treated with trienbolone acetate, *Anim. Prod.* **26**: 1–9.

Wasserman, A. E. and Talley, Florence, 1968. Organoleptic identification of roasted beef, veal, lamb and pork as affected by fat, *J. Fd Sci.* **33**: 219–23.

Webster, A. J. F., 1980. The energetic efficiency of growth, *Livestock Prod. Sci.* **7**: 243–52

Webster, A. J. F., Smith, J. S. and Mollison, G. S., 1977. Prediction of the energy requirements for growth in beef cattle. 3. Body weight and heat production in Hereford × British Friesian bulls and steers, *Anim. Prod.* **24**: 237–44.

Williams, D. R., 1972. Visual assessment of beef and lamb, *Wld Rev. Anim. Prod.* **8**: 87–96.

Williams, D. B., Vetter, R. L., Burroughs, W. and Topel, D. G., 1975. Dairy beef production as influenced by sex protein level and diethylstilboestrol, *J. Anim. Sci.* **41**: 1532–41.

Wood, J. D., Enser, M. B., MacFie, H. J. H., Smith, W. C., Chadwick, J. A. Ellis, M. and Laird, R., 1978. Fatty acid composition of backfat in Large White pigs selected for low backfat thickness. *Meat Sci.* **2**: 289–300.

Wood, J. D., Enser, M. B. and Restall, D. J., 1978. The cellularity of backfat in growing pigs and its relationship with carcass composition, *Anim. Prod.* **27**: 1–10.

Wood, J. D., Gregory, N. G., Hall, G. M. and Lister, D., 1977. Fat mobilization in Pietrain and Large White pigs. *Br. J. Nutr.* **37**: 167–86.

Wood, J. D., Lodge, F. A. and Lister, D., 1979. Response to different rates of energy intake by Gloucester Old Spot and Large White boars and gilts given the same total feed allowance, *Anim. Prod.* **28**: 371–80.

Wood, J. D. and MacFie, H. J. H., 1980. The significance of breed in the prediction of lamb carcass composition from fat thickness measurements, *Anim. Prod.* **31**: 315–9.

Wood, J. D., MacFie, H. J. H., Pomeroy, R. W. and Twinn, D. J., 1980. Carcass composition in four sheep breeds: the importance of type of breed and stage of maturity, *Anim. Prod.* **30**: 135–52.

Yueh, M. H. and Strong, F. M., 1960. Some volatile constituents of cooked beef, *J. agric. Fd Chem.* **8**: 491–4.

Zinder, O. and Shapiro, B., 1971. Effect of cell size on epinephrine- and ACTH-induced fatty acid release from isolated fat cells, *J. Lipid Res.* **12**: 91–5.

13 DIET AND WOOL GROWTH

P. C. Thomas and J. A. F. Rook

In the middle ages Britain was a major world exporter of wool, especially to the European centres of textile manufacturing. Nowadays,
however, whilst remaining amongst the top 10 wool-producing
countries, Britain's contribution to world wool production is modest.
Approximately 34×10^6 kg of wool are produced annually in the
United Kingdom, accounting for less than 1% of the total income from
livestock and livestock products. The wool is derived almost entirely
from enterprises whose primary concern is the production of sheep
meat; there is little specialized wool production, and in the selection,
breeding and management of sheep the yield and quality of the fleece
has tended to be a secondary consideration. Nonetheless, income from
wool is important in British sheep farming, and it can make a significant contribution to maintaining the viability of farms in marginal
and upland areas. Most of the British breeds of sheep produce wool of
the coarser quality types, unsuitable for fine cloth but with good
manufacturing properties for tweeds and carpet wool; wool from some
of the longwool breeds is especially good for these purposes and is
sought after on both the domestic and world markets (Ryder and
Stephenson, 1968).

Australia is the main wool-producing country in the world and in
Australia, in contrast to Britain, there has been specialization in wool
production. The Merino breed of sheep has become dominant and its
capacity for producing a high yield of fine-quality wool, suitable for
making worsted cloth, has been exploited.

THE STRUCTURE OF WOOL

Wool is the fibrous growth from the skin follicles of the sheep. It is
composed of three main kinds of fibre – true wool fibres, hair fibres

and kemp – which differ in coarseness, structural detail and period of growth. The fibres consist of a cuticle surrounding a cortex and, in fibres more than approximately 40 μm in diameter, a medulla consisting of a central core of highly vacuolated cells. Microscopic investigations (Fig. 13.1) have shown that the cuticle is formed by flattened overlapping cells producing a scale-like pattern. Each cell has an inner

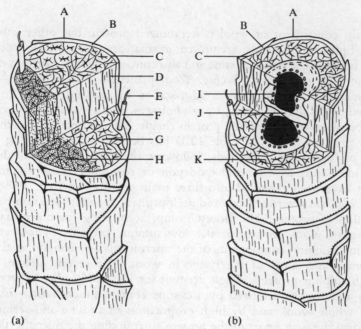

(a)   (b)

Fig. 13.1. Diagrammatic representation of the ultrastructure of (a) a non-medullated wool fibre and (b) a fibre with a medulla one cell wide (after Chapman and Ward, 1979: A – epicuticle; B – exocuticle; C – endocuticle; D – cortical cell; E – microfibril; F – macrofibril; G – orthocortex; H – paracortex; I – medullary cell; J – medullary space; and K – nuclear remnants.

layer, the endocuticle, and an outer layer, the exocuticle, which is covered with a thin, resistant membrane, the epicuticle. The cortex is formed by elongated cells, approximately 100 μm long, held together by a cell membrane complex. The cortical cells consist of filamentous bundles, macrofibrils, and the remnants of cell nuclei and organelles. Within the macrofibrils, embedded in a matrix of amorphous protein, are filaments of fibrous protein called microfibrils. These are thought to consist of groups of 11 protofibrils each containing 2 or 3 α-helical polypeptide chains (see Chapman and Ward, 1979). Various segments of cortex have been distinguished. The two most widely observed are the orthocortex and paracortex; in well-crimped fine-wool fibres these two segments are arranged bilaterally with the othocortex on the outside curvature of the fibre crimp.

THE COMPOSITION OF WOOL

The main constituent of wool is keratinized protein but other substances, lipids and minerals, are present in small amounts. Whole wool protein is especially rich in cystine and also contains high proportions of glutamic acid, serine and glycine. Wool protein is not, however, a single molecular species but an aggregation of proteins bound and stabilized by disulphide bonds, by salt linkages, and by weak hydrogen bonds between and within the protein chains. The composition of the various proteins in wool (Table 13.1) has been investigated using a variety of fractionation methods, following the initial cleavage of the disulphide bonds by chemical oxidation or reduction. The proteins isolated have been classified into three main groups (see Reis, 1979), each of which is heterogeneous and itself probably consists of a number of families of protein. The largest group, accounting for more than 600 g/kg of wool protein, is the low-sulphur proteins. These are the main structural components of the microfibrils and contain all the methionine and most of the lysine in wool. The second group is the high-sulphur proteins. These account for 180 to 350 g/kg of wool protein and are characterized by a cystine content much higher than that of whole wool, and by high proportions of proline and serine. They form the major part of the protein surrounding the microfibrils. The final group is the high-tyrosine proteins, which are rich in tyrosine and glycine. These occur in proportions varying from 10 to 120 g/kg of wool protein and are found mainly in the matrix of the fibre cortex.

WOOL SYNTHESIS

Skin follicles are of two main types called primary and secondary follicles (Fig. 13.2). The types differ histologically in that primary follicles possess a sweat gland, a sebaceous gland and an *arrector pili* muscle, whilst secondary follicles may have a sebaceous gland but are without the other accessory structures. Both primary and secondary follicles are formed in the foetus. Primary follicles are initiated after approximately 60 days gestation and by 100 days are producing an

Table 13.1   Typical amino acid analysis (mmol/mol total amino acids) of wool and some wool proteins (from Reis, 1979)

Amino acid	Whole wool	Low-sulphur proteins	High-sulphur proteins		High-tyrosine proteins	
			High	Ultra high	Type 1	Type 2
Alanine	52	77	29	20	31	0
Arginine	62	78	62	69	35	47
Aspartic acid	59	96	23	6	19	22
Cystine (half)[†]	131	60	221	299	64	102
Glutamic acid	111	169	79	79	0	0
Glycine	86	52	62	42	265	388
Histidine	8	6	7	13	0	0
Isoleucine	30	38	26	17	0	0
Leucine	72	102	34	14	35	64
Lysine	27	41	6	9	0	0
Methionine	5	6	0	0	0	0
Phenylalanine	25	20	16	5	96	27
Proline	66	33	126	128	67	17
Serine	108	81	132	127	126	124
Threonine	65	48	102	111	34	0
Tyrosine	38	27	21	18	180	208
Valine	57	64	53	43	47	0

† Cysteine plus half-cystine in original keratin.

emergent fibre. Secondary follicles are initiated after approximately 90 days gestation and mature in two waves, one just before birth and a second 4 to 18 weeks *post partum*, depending on the breed.

From a functional standpoint, the skin follicle may be considered to contain five zones. At the base of the follicle is the bulb, which is the mitotically active area of the follicle and gives rise to cells which form the cuticle, cortex and medulla of the wool fibre, the inner root sheath and the portion of the outer root sheath that surrounds the bulb. Above this is the keratogenous zone where proteins of the fibre and inner root sheath are progressively synthesized and where hardening of the fibre begins. There follows the zone of final hardening, where degradation of the inner root sheath and resorption of cell contents occurs. This process is continued into the zone of sloughing, where inner root sheath cells are shed and pass into the pilary canal which extends past the sebaceous and sweat gland ducts to the skin surface.

Intact ribonuclease-sensitive polyribosomes, keratin specific mRNA, tRNA and a complement of enzymes necessary for keratin biosynthesis have all been isolated from wool follicles (see Chapman and Ward,

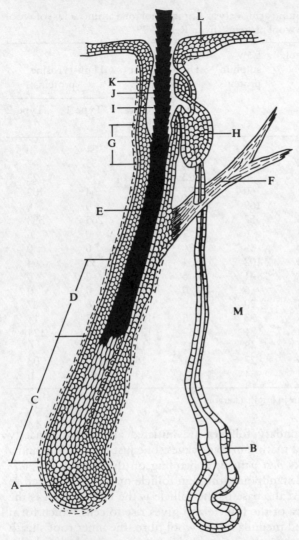

Fig. 13.2.   Diagrammatic representation of the anatomy of a primary wool
follicle with a non-medullated wool fibre (after Chapman and
Ward, 1979: A – bulb; B – sweat gland; C – keratogenous zone;
D – zone of final hardening; E – inner root sheath; F – *arrector pili*
muscle; G – zone of sloughing; H – sebaceous gland; I – wool
fibre cuticle; J – wool fibre cortex; K – pilary canal; L – epidermis;
and M – dermis.

1979), and there is no doubt that wool keratin synthesis occurs by the mechanism of protein synthesis common to other animal tissues. The microfibril-matrix complex of the wool keratins has been envisaged to be assembled by a two-stage process, involving the synthesis of the low-sulphur proteins of the microfibril low in the follicle and the subsequent synthesis of the high-sulphur matrix proteins as the fibre is formed. This idea has grown out of the observations that the sulphur content of cortex cells increases as fibres mature and that the rate of incorporation of ^{35}S-cystine into wool proteins varies between different zones of the wool follicle (see Downes, Ferguson, Gillespie and Harrap, 1966). However, a two-stage synthesis requires that the matrix proteins are formed outside the growing macrofibril and then inserted into the structure; current views are that this is unlikely, and that the fibrous and matrix proteins are synthesized concurrently. Chapman and Ward (1979) have suggested that, in contrast to the polyribosomes for the low-sulphur proteins, the polyribosomes for the high-sulphur proteins are more active when attached to a developing microfibril; the relative rates of synthesis of the two types of protein would thus vary as the macrofibril matured.

An important feature of the synthesis of keratin is the stabilization of the structure through the synthesis of disulphide bonds. These occur through the oxidation of cysteine residues present in the protein chains, but whether the oxidation is enzymic or occurs through a change in the redox potential in the cells is unknown.

^{3}H-thymidine studies (Downes, Chapman, Till and Wilson, 1966) have shown that the turnover time for the population of germinal cells in the follicle bulb is approximately 20 h. Cells which differentiate to become fibre cortical cells take approximately 72 h to pass from the bulb to the keratogenous and hardening zones, where nuclear materials are catabolized and keratinization occurs. Thus, although the skin follicle is a small metabolic pool, it is highly active and has a commensurate requirement for amino acids and for the energy substrates to produce ATP to support protein synthesis. Enzymes of the glycolytic pathway, pentose phosphate pathway and tricarboxylic acid cycle have been isolated from the follicle and the evidence is that both acetate and glucose are utilized for ATP production (Leng and Stephenson, 1965; Chapman and Ward, 1979). There is little information on the oxidation of other metabolites. Chapman and Ward (1979) have argued that the high activity of the glycolytic and pentose phosphate pathways in the follicle indicates their special rôle in follicle metabolism, in the case of the pentose phosphate pathway possibly through the provision of NADPH, but as yet there is no clear evidence in support of the proposal.

The supply of amino acids and energy substrates for wool synthesis varies with the arterial concentration of the substrates, and with blood flow in the vessels surrounding the lower part of the follicle and dermal papilla. Increased blood flow resulting from vasodilation induced experimentally by cutting the nerves leading to one side of the sheep has increased wool growth (Ferguson, 1949); and skin cooling, which would be expected to reduce blood flow, has reduced wool growth (Slee and Ryder, 1967; Lyne, Jolly and Hollis, 1970). However, no clear relationship between wool growth and blood flow has been established in normal physiological conditions in unclipped sheep.

Little is known of the uptake of nutrients by the follicle but the transfer of cyst(e)ine to wool is highly efficient: some 30% of a dose administered intravenously or intraperitoneally was taken up into wool over a subsequent 2-week period (Downes, Reis, Sharry and Tunks, 1970). On the basis of analyses of the specific activities of wool and plasma cystine, and the time curves for the proportions of ^{35}S in skin and follicles, Downes (1961 and 1965) proposed that part of the cyst(e)ine passed through an intermediate pool or pools in the non-follicular part of the skin, and that the skin may act as a nutrient reservoir facilitating the balancing of nutrients for wool growth. The reservoir could consist of peptide-bound cysteine in extravascular plasma proteins in the skin or half-cystine residues bound to those proteins by disulphide bonds. Intradermal administration of ^{35}S as half-cystine residues bound to plasma proteins has shown that the sulphur can be released to some extent in the skin, possibly through thiodisulphide exchange reactions, and can enter the pool of amino acid precursors available to the follicle (Downes, Sharry and Till, 1964). The quantitative importance of this reaction is, however, unknown.

MEASUREMENT OF WOOL GROWTH

Technically, there are major difficulties in the measurement of the rate of growth of wool over the whole surface of a sheep. Three separate methods have been devised for routine measurement of selected areas under experimental conditions.

Repeated clipping

The usual method has been the clipping of wool from a defined area, or areas, of skin at regular intervals. There are three main sources of error. First, there is the technical difficulty of clipping precisely the same area to exactly the same height above the surface of the skin.

Secondly, removal of the wool subjects the exposed skin to a lower temperature and reduces the rate of lengthening of fibres (Downes and Hutchinson, 1969). Thirdly, there are errors due to the time taken for newly-keratinized fibres, which may be modified in diameter by an experimental treatment and in that way have a marked effect on the mass of wool produced, to emerge to the point where they can be removed by clipping.

The average emergence time for fibres can be determined by the intravenous administration of [^{35}S]-cystine and the measurement of radioactivity in the wool subsequently removed from clipped areas until the maximum specific activity is recorded (Downes and Sharry, 1971). Emergence times can vary widely, from 5 to 10 days, and are affected by the rate of growth of a fibre. The accuracy of the clipping method can be improved if it is used in conjunction with the auto-radiographic assessment of time of emergence to indicate the critical period for measurement of wool growth.

Dye-banding

Fibres in a set of staples on a sheep's mid flank are dyed at skin level at intervals of a few weeks and subsequently the weights of the staple segments defined by the dye are used to determine the fleece weight associated with each period of growth. The method is more rapid than repeated clipping and less demanding of effort and equipment. The time taken to detect the emergence of newly-formed fibre is less and, since during the course of an experiment there is no removal of fleece, there are no adverse climatic effects. The method is, however, unsuitable for fleeces that are coarse, open, strongly medullated or subject to fibre shedding (Wheeler, Hedges and Mulcahy, 1977).

Autoradiography

When [^{35}S]cystine is injected intraperitoneally or intravenously into sheep, within a few minutes radioactivity is detectable just above the bulb of the follicle and some hours later in the fully keratinized fibre. Assuming the rate and position of entry of radioactivity is constant, repeated injections at known intervals may be used to measure growth by autoradiography. The technique allows the measurement of the growth of individual wool fibres with good accuracy over short periods, of the order of a few days, without the need to remove the fibre from the sheep (Downes and Lyne, 1959).

NUTRITION AND WOOL GROWTH

Maximum wool production by a sheep is ultimately determined genetically through limits on the number of wool follicles and the growth of wool fibres. However, under normal husbandry conditions, wool growth does not achieve its maximum and varies with a number of factors. Generally, the effects are expressed through changes in the length and diameter of individual wool fibres but severe undernutrition may cause a shedding of fibres and a suppression of follicle activity which is only slowly reversed (Allden, 1970 and 1979a). The number of secondary follicles developing in the foetus and lamb may also be reduced, by adverse conditions *in utero* associated with the presence of more than one foetus, or by undernutrition during the prenatal or postnatal period, and these effects may depress wool production temporarily or permanently (Allden, 1979b). Following maturation of the follicles in the young animal, the growth of wool fibres is cyclical, with alternating periods of growth and rest. A proportion of the wool fibres may be shed each season but, in breeds such as the Merino, the growth of individual wool fibres probably extends over several seasons. Conditions of climatic environment can affect wool growth (Bottomley, 1979) but the seasonal changes in growth are probably linked with changes in daylength (Nagorcka, 1979) and are under hormonal control. Thyroxine promotes wool growth and the adrenal glucocorticoids inhibit it, and these actions are modulated by the corresponding hormones of the pituitary, thyroid stimulating hormone (TSH) and adrenocorticotrophic hormone (ACTH) respectively. Growth hormone also stimulates wool growth through the release of somatomedins from the liver and kidneys (Wallace, 1979). Wool growth is reduced in growing, pregnant and lactating animals, but these effects appear to relate less to changes in hormonal status than to the competition for nutrients within the animal's tissues (Oddy and Annison, 1979) and must be dependent on the major factor influencing wool growth under many husbandry conditions, the animal's nutrition.

Food intake

Positive relationships between wool growth and food intake have been reported by a large number of workers but there is no close agreement on the precise form of the response curves (Allden, 1979a). This is perhaps not surprising since the relationship between diet amount and composition, and the supply of nutrients to the follicle, is complex because of the microbial metabolism of food materials in the rumen, and the effect of diet on mobilization and deposition of body tissues generally. Furthermore, the full effect of a change in feeding on wool growth may take as long as 3 to 4 weeks to become established and the period for which it can be maintained is uncertain: there is often opportunity for poorly understood interactions between effects due to food intake and those due to non-nutritional, environmental factors.

There has been considerable discussion about the relative importance of dietary energy and protein supplies on wool synthesis. Marston (1955) attributed the response in wool growth to an improved food intake and to the increased supply of amino acids to the tissues but Ferguson (1962) has presented evidence supporting a relation between wool growth and metabolic rate. The response to a change in food intakes is, however, affected by the dietary protein concentration. With a low protein diet, raising energy intake has caused a depression in wool growth. Conversely, high wool-growth rates can be obtained with moderate energy intakes, providing sufficient good-quality protein is available to provide an appropriate mixture of amino acids to the wool follicle (Reis, 1969). Black, Robards and Thomas (1973) observed alterations in wool growth with variations in energy supply when the protein intake was low (20 g/day) or high (100 g/day), whereas at intermediate levels only minor effects were noted. It appears that for most diets the supply of amino acids will be limiting for wool growth and that any effect of dietary energy will be exerted primarily through its influence on amino acid supply.

Amino acid supply

Although a supply of all its constituent amino acids is required for wool synthesis, it is the supply of sulphur-containing amino acids that usually limits wool growth. Under these conditions, the uptake from the gut of cyst(e)ine and of methionine, which can be converted to cysteine and cystine through transulphuration in liver, kidney and other tissues (Radcliffe and Egan, 1974), and possibly in the skin or wool follicle (Downes *et al.*, 1964) (Fig. 13.3), is of crucial importance. Marked increases in wool growth have been observed in sheep given intra-abomasal, intraperitoneal or intravenous administrations of L-cysteine, L-cystine, L-methionine or DL-methionine (D-methionine is converted to L-methionine in the tissues) (see Reis, 1979). The extent of the response is, however, affected by the genetic potential for wool growth (Williams, Robards and Saville, 1972), although possibly not at low levels of feeding (Downes, Reis and Hemsley, 1976), and by the diet. With methionine, for example, a greater response was observed to abomasal infusions with sheep receiving a high-quality forage diet of

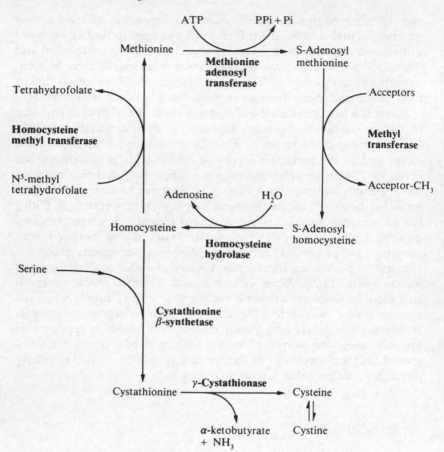

Fig. 13.3. Pathways for the metabolic interconversion of methionine to cysteine and cystine.

lucerne chaff than with sheep receiving a low-quality forage diet of wheaten hay (Dove and Robards, 1974), no response was obtained to an intraperitoneal infusion in sheep receiving a pelleted diet of wheat grain (3 parts) and wheaten hay (1 part) (Ferguson, 1975), and a negative response was obtained to an intra-abomasal infusion in sheep receiving a diet solely of wheat grain (Reis and Tunks, 1974). Responses to the administration of cystine or cysteine appear to be similar to (Reis, Tunks and Downes, 1973) or slightly less than (Williams *et al.*, 1972) those obtained with methionine, and there is no evidence to suggest that there are differences in response between the abomasal and intravenous routes of administration (Barger, Southcott and Williams, 1973; Reis *et al.*, 1973).

Under most nutritional circumstances, the supply of amino acids that do not contain sulphur is unlikely to be limiting for wool growth and, consistent with this, various non-sulphur amino acids (glycine, glutamic acid, arginine, lysine and threonine), when given as abomasal supplements to sheep receiving forage diets, had no effect on wool growth (Reis, 1970). Whole proteins, such as casein or whole-egg proteins, that contain a full complement of essential amino acids, when given abomasally stimulate growth (Colebrook and Reis, 1969), but proteins such as gelatin (even when supplemented with sulphur-containing amino acids) or zein, which are lacking not only in sulphur-containing amino acids but also in some of the other essential amino acids, have little effect or may depress growth (Reis and Schinckel, 1964; Reis and Colebrook, 1972)

Wool quality

The ratio of length to diameter of wool fibres varies between individual sheep, within the range of 9 to 22, and is little affected by wool growth rate as modified by a change of food intake (Downes, 1971). The ratio is similarly little affected when growth is promoted by abomasal supplements of casein (Reis and Downes, 1971) or parenteral infusions of sulphur-containing amino acids (Downes *et al.*, 1970). Abomasal infusions of methionine, when given to sheep receiving a diet of wheat grain only, depress wool growth with a reduction in fibre diameter (Reis and Tunks, 1974). Impairment of growth by abomasal infusion of zein (which is deficient in lysine, leucine and tryptophan) also produces weak fibres: the length of the fibre is increased but the diameter is reduced. The effect is offset by lysine supplementation alone, and a similar condition is induced by an infusion of a mixture of amino acids deficient in lysine. An endocrine mechanism could be involved as thyroxine promotes an increase in fibre length with little change in diameter, whereas cortisol depresses length and diameter proportionately (Downes and Wallace, 1965).

The sulphur content of wool is increased by infusion of casein, cysteine and methionine, due to an increase in the synthesis of sulphur-rich components of the high-sulphur proteins (Gillespie and Reis, 1966; Gillespie, Broad and Reis, 1969). Some of the cystine-rich proteins are synthesized only when there is an adequate supply of sulphur amino acids and may be absent from some wools. There is no clear indication whether such changes alter the physical properties and textile characteristics of the wool. Breeding and selection for high efficiency in wool production are associated with a reduction in sulphur content and, if this affects wool quality, it could be offset by supplementation of the diet with sulphur-containing amino acids.

The concentration of high-tyrosine proteins in wool is also affected by the supply of amino acids. It was depressed by abomasal infusion of zein or an equivalent amino acid mixture, or maize or wheat gluten (Frenkel, Gillespie and Reis, 1974). Reversal of the depression was not achieved by adding lysine, tryptophan or tyrosine to the zein and normal synthesis was not increased by supplements of tyrosine or phenylalanine. Weak wool is often characterized by a low content of high-tyrosine proteins (Frenkel, Gillespie and Reis, 1975).

The possibility exists of using the effects of amino acids on wool growth to produce a weak point in the wool fibre to facilitate harvesting. Techniques using a temporary imbalance of normal dietary amino acids have been considered but are yet to be developed. Mimosine (β-[N-(3-hydroxy-4-oxopyridyl)]-α amino propionic acid) and its analogues (which inhibit cell division in the follicle bulb, probably through effects on DNA synthesis) have, however, been used as chemical defleecing agents (Reis, 1979)

Dietary protein supply

The explanation for the diverse responses in wool growth with various diets and different levels of addition of sulphur amino acids must lie in the metabolic interactions within the rumen that affect the duodenal flow of sulphur amino acids and those within the body tissues that determine the partition of amino acid use. The requirement for amino acids for wool growth is quantitatively small, even at the maximum physiological growth rate, in relation to the needs for growth, pregnancy and lactation. Nonetheless, different balances of amino acids are required for optimal activity of the various physiological processes and the proportion of sulphur-containing amino acids needed for wool synthesis is uniquely high. Hogan, Elliot and Hughes (1979) have estimated that in sheep with high rates of wool growth cyst(e)ine deposition in wool may be as high as 2 or 3 g/day, equivalent to 500 to 800 g/kg of the total cyst(e)ine absorbed from the small intestine.

It is well recognized that the flow of total amino acids to the duodenum depends to a large degree on the extent to which dietary protein is degraded in the rumen and on the amount of dietary carbohydrate fermented to produce the ATP needed to support microbial protein synthesis. Thus, there is no simple relationship between the protein, or digestible protein, intake and the quantity of amino acids absorbed in the small intestine, and there are interactions through rumen fermentation between the intake of dietary energy and the intestinal supply of amino acids. Most food proteins are degraded in the rumen to a variable but extensive degree and the amino acid composition of the duodenal digesta tends to reflect that of microbial protein. Furthermore, neither plant nor microbial proteins are especially rich in sulphur amino acids and, whilst wool growth may respond generally to dietary changes which promote amino acid uptake in the intestine, it may be especially sensitive to an improvement in the proportion of sulphur amino acids absorbed.

Wool growth can be promoted through the dietary inclusion of proteins having a low rumen degradability or chemically 'protected' from ruminal attack through treatment with formaldehyde (Ferguson, 1975; Barry, 1976) and some attention has been given to the development of dietary supplements specifically providing sulphur amino acids. Bird and Moir (1972) suggested that since methionine itself was relatively slowly degraded in the rumen its inclusion in the diet at an appropriate level might stimulate wool growth. The approach has been tested but relatively small responses in wool growth have been obtained even with large supplements of methionine (up to 15.4 g DL-methionine per day) (Doyle and Bird, 1975; Doyle and Moir, 1979). A more promising approach may be offered through the preparation of derivatives of methionine which are resistant to ruminal attack but which are subsequently converted to the amino acid in the tissues (Salsbury and Merricks, 1972; Langar, Buttery and Lewis, 1973; Digenis, Arnes, Mitchell, Sevintosky, Yang, Schelling and Parish, 1974; Digenis, Arnes, Yang, Mitchell, Little, Sevintosky, Parish, Schelling, Dietz and Tucker, 1974). A method of encapsulating methionine with copolymers such that they resist breakdown in the rumen but disintegrate in the abomasum has been developed and under experimental conditions feeding the granules has produced an improvement in wool growth (Wheeler, Ferguson and Hinks, 1979). Feeding methionine hydroxy-analogue has increased wool growth in some experiments (Wright, 1971; Langlands, 1972) but in others has been ineffective (Carrico Cockrem, Haden and Wickham, 1970; Reis, 1970; Wickham, 1970).

Clearly, the practical problems in the use of supplements of sulphur-containing amino acids have not yet been fully overcome, and for successful application of the techniques there is a need for a much more complete knowledge of the husbandry circumstances under which the supply of sulphur-containing amino acids is not only low but also limiting for wool growth.

Dietary minerals

Suboptimal intakes of minerals are frequently accompanied by a reduced food intake and often by some impairment of digestion or metabolism in the rumen or body tissues. In these circumstances, there is likely to be an associated reduction in wool growth through effects on substrate availability. Specific effects of minerals on wool synthesis have also been described but their demonstration involves a relatively severe degree of dietary insufficiency. In a summary of the literature, Purser (1979) concluded that wool production might be affected by the dietary intake of zinc, copper, sulphur, selenium, sodium, potassium, fluorine, cobalt and phosphorus but suggested that, excepting zinc and copper, the effects of the minerals were likely to arise through their influence on food intake and ruminal metabolism. Dietary supplements of sulphur and of sodium chloride have, for example, been shown to increase the duodenal flow of protein under appropriate conditions (Hemsley, 1975; Hume and Bird, 1970).

Sheep given diets low in zinc and copper also have a reduced appetite but, additionally, the minerals appear to have specific effects on wool synthesis. Clinical signs of zinc deficiency in sheep include defects in the keratinization of hoof and horn and the occurrence of brittle wool lacking in crimp (Mills, Dalgarno, Williams and Quarterman, 1967; Underwood and Somers, 1969); wool may be shed and does not regrow without zinc supplementation. Zinc is known to have a biochemical rôle in nucleic acid metabolism and protein synthesis, and this may underlie the effects of zinc deficiency on wool growth. A deficiency in copper causes lack of pigmentation in dark-fleeced animals which is thought to occur because of the rôle of copper in tyrosinase (see Ch. 10). Additionally, copper deficiency is associated with faulty keratinization of wool and lack of crimp (Lee, 1956). Inorganic copper is known to catalyse the oxidation of thiol groups to disulphide and Marston (1949) proposed that the effects of copper deficiency on wool growth derived from impairment of the formation of disulphide linkages in keratin. A number of studies have shown that wool growth is reduced by copper deficiency occurring through either low copper intakes in the diet (Marston and Lee, 1948) or reductions in the availability of dietary copper due to interactions with sulphur and molybdenum (Wynne and McClymont, 1956). There is also evidence that copper supplements given above the level required to remedy deficiency may influence wool growth through effects on fibre diameter without change in fibre length (Palmer, 1949).

REFERENCES

Allden, W. G., 1970. The effects of nutritional deprivation on the subsequent productivity of sheep and cattle, *Nutr. Abstr. Rev.* **40**: 1167–84.

Allden, W. G., 1979a. Feed intake, diet composition and wool growth. In *Physiological and Environmental Limitations to Wool Growth* (ed. J. L. Black and P. J. Reis), pp. 61–78. University of New England Publishing Unit, Armidale.

Allden, W.G., 1979b. Undernutrition of the Merino sheep and its sequelae. V. The influence of severe growth restriction during early post-natal life on reproduction and growth in later life, *Aust. J. agric. Res.* **30**: 939–48.

Barger, I. A., Southcott, W. H. and Williams, V. J., 1973. The wool growth response of infected sheep to parenteral and duodenal cystine and cysteine supplementation, *Aust. J. exp. Agric. Anim. Husb.* **13**: 351–9.

Barry, T. N., 1976. The effectiveness of formaldehyde treatment in protecting dietary protein from rumen microbial degradation, *Proc. Nutr. Soc.* **35**: 221–9.

Bird, P. R. and Moir, R. J., 1972. Sulphur metabolism and excretion studies in ruminants. VIII. Methionine degradation and utilization in sheep when infused into the rumen or abomasum, *Aust. J. biol. Sci.* **25**: 835–48.

Black, J. L., Robards, G. E. and Thomas, R., 1973. Effects of protein and energy intakes on the wool growth of Merino wethers, *Aust. J. agric. Res.* **24**: 399–412.

Bottomley, G. A., 1979. Weather conditions and wool growth. In *Physiological and Environmental Limitations to Wool Growth* (ed. J. L. Black and P. J. Reis), pp. 115–26. University of New England Publishing Unit, Armidale.

Carrico, R. G., Cockrem, F. R. M., Haden, D. D. and Wickham, G. A., 1970. Wool growth and plasma amino acid responses of N.Z. Romney sheep to formalin-treated casein and methionine supplements, *N.Z. Jl agric. Res.* **13**: 631–40.

Chapman, R. E. and Ward, K. A., 1979. Histological and biochemical features of the wool fibre and follicle. In *Physiological and Environmental Limitations to Wool Growth* (ed. J. L. Black and P. J. Reis), pp. 193–208. University of New England Publishing Unit, Armidale.

Colebrook, W. F. and Reis, P. J., 1969. Relative value for wool growth and nitrogen retention of several proteins administered as abomasal supplements to sheep, *Aust. J. biol. Sci.* **22**: 1507–16.

Digenis, G.A., Arnes, H. E., Mitchell, G. E., Sevintosky, J. V., Yang, K., Schelling, G. T. and Parish, R. C., 1974. Methionine substitutes in ruminant nutrition. II. Stability of non-nitrogenous compounds related to methionine during *in vitro* incubation with rumen micro-organisms, *J. Pharm. Sci.* **63**: 751–4.

Digenis, G. A., Arnes, H. E., Yang, K., Mitchell, G. E., Little, C. O., Sevintosky, J. V., Parish, R. C., Schelling, G. T., Dietz, E. M. and Tucker, R. E., 1974. Methionine substitutes in ruminant nutrition. I. Stability of nitrogenous compounds related to methionine during *in vitro* incubation with rumen micro-organisms, *J. Pharm. Sci.* **63**: 745–50.

Dove, H. and Robards, G. E., 1974. Effect of abomasal infusions of methionine, casein and starch plus methionine on the wool production of Merino wethers fed on lucerne or wheaten chaff, *Aust. J. agric. Res.* **25**: 945–56.

Downes, A. M., 1961. The fate of intravenous doses of free and plasma protein-bound [^{35}S] cystine in the sheep, *Aust. J. biol. Sci.* **14**: 427–39.

Downes, A. M., 1965. A study of the incorporation of labelled cystine into growing wool fibres. In *Biology of Skin and Hair Growth* (ed. A. G. Lyne and B. F. Short), pp. 345–64. Angus and Robertson, Sydney.

Downes, A. M., 1971. Variations in wool length and diameter with sheep nutrition, *Appl. Polym. Symp.* **18**: 895–904.

Downes, A. M., Chapman, R. E., Till, A. R. and Wilson, P. A., 1966. Proliferative cycle and fate of cell nuclei in wool follicles, *Nature, Lond.* **212**: 477–9.

Downes, A. M., Ferguson, K. A., Gillespie, J. M. and Harrap, B. S., 1966. A study of the proteins of the wool follicle, *Aust. J. biol. Sci.* **19**: 319–33.

Downes, A. M. and Hutchinson, J. C. D., 1969. Effect of low skin surface temperature on wool growth, *J. agric. Sci., Camb.* **72**: 155–8.

Downes, A. M. and Lyne, A. G., 1959. Measurement of the rate of growth of wool using cystine labelled with sulphur-35, *Nature, Lond.* **184**: 1884–5.

Downes, A. M., Reis, P. J. and Hemsley, J. A., 1976. Proteins and amino acids for wool growth. In *Reviews in Rural Science, No. 2* (ed. T.M. Sutherland, J. R. McWilliam and R. A. Leng), pp. 143–8. University of New England Publishing Unit, Armidale.

Downes, A. M., Reis, P. J., Sharry, L. F. and Tunks, D. A., 1970. Metabolic fate of parenterally administered sulphur-containing amino acids in sheep and effects on growth and composition of wool, *Aust. J. biol. Sci.* **23**: 1077–88.

Downes, A. M. and Sharry, L. F., 1971. Measurement of wool growth and its response to nutritional change, *Aust. J. biol. Sci.* **24**: 117–30.

Downes, A. M., Sharry, L. F. and Till, A. R., 1964. The fate of intradermal doses of labelled amino acids in sheep, *Aust. J. biol. Sci.* **17**: 945–59.

Downes, A. M. and Wallace, A. L. C., 1965. Local effects on wool growth of intradermal injections of hormones. In *Biology of Skin and Hair Growth* (ed. A. G. Lyne and B. F. Short), pp. 679–704. Angus and Robertson, Sydney.

Doyle, P. T. and Bird, P. R., 1975. The influence of dietary supplements of DL-methionine on the growth rate of wool, *Aust. J. agric. Res.* **26**: 337–42.

Doyle, P. T. and Moir, R. J., 1979. Sulphur and methionine metabolism in sheep. III. Excretion and retention of dietary and supplemented sulphur, and production responses to intraruminal infusions of DL-methionine, *Aust. J. agric. Res.* **30**: 1185–96.

Ferguson, K. A., 1949. The effect of sympathectomy on wool growth, *Aust. J. scient. Res. Ser. B.* **2**: 438–43.

Ferguson, K. A., 1962. The relation between the responses of wool growth and body weight to changes in feed intake, *Aust. J. biol. Sci.* **15**: 720–31.

Ferguson, K. A., 1975. Protection of dietary proteins in the rumen. In *Digestion and Metabolism in the Ruminant* (ed. I. W. McDonald and A. C. I. Warner), pp. 449–64. University of New England Publishing Unit, Armidale.

Frenkel, M. J., Gillespie, J. M. and Reis, P. J., 1974. Factors influencing the biosynthesis of the tyrosine-rich proteins of wool, *Aust. J. biol. Sci* **27**: 31–8.

Frenkel, M. J., Gillespie, J. M. and Reis, P. J., 1975. Studies on the inhibition of synthesis of the tyrosine-rich proteins of wool, *Aust. J. biol. Sci.* **28**: 331–8.

Gillespie, J. M., Broad, Andrea and Reis, P. J., 1969. A further study on the dietary-regulated biosynthesis of high-sulphur wool proteins, *Biochem. J.* **112**: 41–9.

Gillespie, J. M. and Reis, P. J., 1966. The dietary-regulated biosynthesis of high-sulphur wool proteins, *Biochem. J.* **98**: 669–77.

Hemsley, J. A., 1975. Effect of high intakes of sodium chloride on the utilization of a protein concentrate by sheep. 1. Wool growth, *Aust. J. agric. Res.* **26**: 709–14.

Hogan, J. P., Elliot, N. M. and Hughes, A. D., 1979. Maximum wool growth rates expected from Australian merino genotypes. In *Physiological and Environmental Limitations to Wool Growth* (ed. J. L. Black and P. J. Reis), pp. 43–60. University of New England Publishing Unit, Armidale.

Hume, I. D. and Bird, P. R., 1970. Synthesis of microbial proteins in the rumen. IV. The influence of level and form of dietary sulphur, *Aust. J. agric. Res.* **21**: 315–22.

Langar, P. N., Buttery, P. J. and Lewis, D., 1973. N-steroyl-DL-methionine— a new form of protected methionine for ruminant feeds, *Proc. Nutr. Soc.* **32**: 86–7A (Abstr.).

Langlands, J. P., 1972. Methionine hydroxy analogue as a dietary supplement for sheep, *Proc. Aust. Soc. Anim. Prod.* **9**: 321–5.

Lee, H. J., 1956. The influence of copper deficiency on the fleeces of British breeds of sheep, *J. agric. Sci., Camb.* **47**: 218–24.

Leng, R. A. and Stephenson, S. K., 1965. Glucose and acetate metabolism by isolated sheep wool follicles, *Archs Biochem. Biophys.* **110**: 8–15.

Lyne, A. G., Jolly, M., and Hollis, D. E., 1970. Effects of experimentally produced local subdermal temperature changes on skin temperature and wool growth in the sheep, *J. agric. Sci., Camb.* **74**: 83–90.

Marston, H. R., 1949. The organization and work of the Division of Biochemistry and General Nutrition of C.S.I.R. *Proc. R. Soc. Ser. A.* **199**: 273–94.

Marston, H. R., 1955. Wool growth. In *Progress in the Physiology of Farm Animals* (ed. J. Hammond), Vol. 2, pp. 543–81. Butterworth, London.

Marston, H. R. and Lee, H. J., 1948. Nutritional factors involved in wool production by merino sheep. II. The influence of copper deficiency on the rate of wool growth and on the nature of the fleece, *Aust. J. scient. Res. Ser. B.* **1**: 376–87.

Mills, C. F., Dalgarno, A. C., Williams, R. B. and Quarterman, J., 1967. Zinc deficiency and the zinc requirements of calves and lambs, *Br. J. Nutr.* **21**: 751–68.

Nagorcka, B. N., 1979. The effect of photoperiod on wool growth. In *Physiological and Environmental Limitations to Wool Growth* (ed. J. L. Black and P. J. Reis), pp. 127–38. University of New England Publishing Unit, Armidale.

556   *Diet and wool growth*

Oddy, V. H. and Annison, E. F., 1979. Possible mechanisms by which physiological state influences the rate of wool growth. In *Physiological and Environmental Limitations to Wool Growth* (ed. J. L. Black and P. J. Reis), pp. 295–310. University of New England Publishing Unit, Armidale.

Palmer, R. C., 1949. Some properties of the wool from copper-starved Merino sheep, *J. agric. Sci., Camb.* **39**: 265–73.

Purser, D. B. 1979. Effects of minerals upon wool growth. In *Physiological and Environmental Limitations to Wool Growth* (ed. J. L. Black and P. J. Reis), pp. 243–56. University of New England Publishing Unit, Armidale.

Radcliffe, B. C. and Egan, A. R., 1974. A survey of methionine adenosyltransferase and cystathionine γ-lyase activities in ruminant tissues, *Aust. J. biol. Sci.* **27**: 465–71.

Reis, P. J., 1969. The growth and composition of wool. V. Stimulation of wool growth by the abomasal administration of varying amounts of casein, *Aust. J. biol. Sci.* **22**: 745–59.

Reis, P. J., 1970. The influence of abomasal supplements of some amino acids and sulphur-containing compounds on wool growth rate, *Aust. J. biol. Sci.* **23**: 441–6.

Reis, P. J., 1979. Effects of amino acids on the growth and properties of wool. In *Physiological and Environmental Limitations to Wool Growth* (ed. J. L. Black and P. J. Reis), pp. 223–42. University of New England Publishing Unit, Armidale.

Reis, P. J. and Colebrook, W. F., 1972. The utilization of abomasal supplements of proteins and amino acids by sheep with special reference to wool growth, *Aust. J. biol. Sci.* **25**: 1057–72.

Reis, P. J. and Downes, A. M., 1971. The rate of response of wool growth to abomasal supplements of casein, *J. agric. Sci., Camb.* **76**: 173–6.

Reis, P. J. and Schinckel, P. G., 1964. The growth and composition of wool. II. The effect of casein, gelatin and sulphur-containing amino acids given per abomasum, *Aust. J. biol. Sci.* **17**: 532–47.

Reis, P. J. and Tunks, D. A., 1974. The influence of abomasal supplements of methionine on wool growth of wheat-fed sheep, *Aust. J. agric. Res.* **25**: 919–29.

Reis, P. J., Tunks, D. A. and Downes, A. M., 1973. The influence of abomasal and intravenous supplements of sulphur-containing amino acids on wool growth rate, *Aust. J. biol. Sci.* **26**: 249–58.

Ryder, M. L. and Stephenson, S. K., 1968. World survey of sheep breeds, farming systems and wool production. A. The British Isles. In *Wool Growth*, pp. 25–84. Academic Press, London.

Salsbury, R. L. and Merricks, D. L., 1972. Susceptibility of methionine analogs to dethiomethylation by rumen micro-organisms *in vitro*, *J. Dairy Sci.* **55**: 710–1.

Slee, J. and Ryder, M. L., 1967. The effect of acute cold exposure on wool growth in Scottish Blackface and Merino × Cheviot sheep, *J. agric. Sci., Camb.* **58**: 309–26.

Underwood, E. J. and Somers, M., 1969. Studies of zinc nutrition in sheep. 1. The relation of zinc to growth, testicular development and spermatogenesis in young rams, *Aust. J. agric. Res.* **20**: 889–97.

Wallace, A. L. C., 1979. The effect of hormones on wool growth. In *Physiological and Environmental Limitations to Wool Growth* (ed. J. L. Black and P. J. Reis), pp. 257–68. University of New England Publishing Unit, Armidale.

Wheeler, J. L., Ferguson, K. A. and Hinks, W. T., 1979. Effect of nutrition, genotype, lactation and wool cover on response by grazing sheep to methionine esters and polymer-encapsulated methionine, *Aust. J. agric. Res.* **30**: 711–23.

Wheeler, J. L., Hedges, D. A. and Mulcahy, C., 1977. The use of dye-banding for measuring wool production and fleece tip wear in rugged and unrugged sheep, *Aust. J. agric. Res.* **28**: 721–35.

Wickham, G. A., 1970. Wool growth in relation to sulphur-containing amino acid administration to sheep, *Proc. N.Z. Soc. Anim. Prod.* **30**: 209–15.

Williams, A. J., Robards, G. E. and Saville, D. G., 1972. Metabolism of cystine by Merino sheep genetically different in wool production. II. The responses in wool growth to abomasal infusions of L-cystine or DL-methionine, *Aust. J. biol. Sci.* **25**: 1269–76

Wright, P. L., 1971. Body weight gain and wool growth response to formaldehyde treated casein and sulfur amino acids, *J. Anim. Sci.* **33**: 137–41.

Wynne, K. N. and McClymont, G. L., 1956. Copper-molybdenum-sulphate interactions in induction of ovine hypocupraemia and hypocuprosis, *Aust. J. agric. Res.* **7**: 45–57.

14 MILK PRODUCTION

P. C. Thomas and J. A. F. Rook

Milk production from the dairy cow is a major sector of the United Kingdom agricultural industry accounting financially for approximately 23% of the total agricultural output. Because of the rôle of milk in the nutrition of young animals, however, milk production is also important in the production of beef, from suckler-cow herds, lamb and pigmeat. Additionally, some milk for human.consumption is obtained from dairy goats kept mainly, although not entirely, by smallholders.

Because of its commercial importance and the better availability of detailed information, in this chapter attention will be concentrated mainly on milk production in the dairy cow, but many of the matters discussed have a general relevance and some specific reference will be made to milk production in other farm animals.

MILK PRODUCTION IN THE DAIRY COW

Milk production in the UK has increased progressively since the Second World War due to a continuous increase in the average yield of dairy cows and to a less regular increase in cow numbers; cow numbers reached a maximum in 1973 and have since declined (Federation of United Kingdom Milk Marketing Boards, 1979). In 1978 the average annual yield of milk was 4590 l per cow and the number of cows was 3 279 000.

The daily sales of milk off farms reach a peak during the spring, and are at a minimum during the autumn and early winter, due to the combined effects of the national calving pattern (a greater proportion of cows calve in the autumn) and the stimulus to milk production of grazing fresh pastures in the spring. The range in milk production is not extreme, however, and on average milk production for April to September is approximately 5% greater than for October to March.

Much greater seasonal variations are found in countries such as Eire and New Zealand where milk is produced mainly from grassland farming systems, and where calving is phased to make maximum use of grassland.

Legal presumptive minimum standards for milk composition of 30 g fat and 85 g solids-not-fat per kg (determined as the difference between total solids content (i.e. dry matter) and fat content) were introduced into the UK in 1901 but payment schemes based on milk composition were not adopted until the 1960s. The details of the schemes vary between the individual marketing boards. There are three boards in Scotland, one in Northern Ireland and the largest, which deals with more than 80% of the national milk production, in England and Wales. Initially, all payment schemes were related primarily to milk total solids content but the Milk Marketing Board of England and Wales introduced in 1980 a scheme of payment based on the milk contents of fat and solids-not-fat, with prices adjusted to allow for the market value of each component. The principle embodied in this scheme seems certain to form the basis for milk marketing in the future and more comprehensive schemes may well be introduced. Payment schemes based on fat, protein and lactose contents have already been discussed, and ultimately there could be quality payments taking account of milk fatty acid composition or other compositional features. Such schemes require skilled animal management by the dairy farmer if maximum financial returns are to be obtained but they ensure that milk production is sensitive to changes in the markets for milk. For many years milk marketing in the UK was dominated by sales of milk for liquid consumption but the proportion of milk used for manufacture (where milk composition is of crucial importance to the yield and quality of the product) increased from approximately 25% in the early 1950s to more than 50% in 1979.

The annual average fat and solids-not-fat contents of bulk milk supplies in England and Wales have remained rather constant since the 1950s; in 1978/79 the values were 38.6 and 87.4g/kg respectively. There are, however, significant seasonal variations in bulk milk composition: fat contents are low in the April to June grazing period, and solids-not-fat contents (both the protein and sometimes lactose portions) are low during the January to April period when conserved foods are given indoors.

The national dairy herd in the UK is now dominated by cattle of the British Friesian breed although there is a substantial proportion of Ayrshire cows in some parts of the country; Ayrshire cows account for 3.7% of the herd in England and Wales, but approximately 37% in Scotland. There are also small proportions of Guernsey, Jersey, Dairy Shorthorn, Red Poll and South Devon cows. The British Friesian has been favoured because of its 'dual purpose' character, the calves produced from the dairy cows being well suited for beef production, but recently there has been some introduction of Holstein Friesian cattle from abroad and these animals have predominantly dairying characteristics.

A wide range of management systems is used for dairy cows in commercial practice but the systems have some common features. Young stock selected for the dairy herd are allowed to grow to a stage of partial maturity before mating so that the first generation of offspring is produced when the parent animals are 2 to 2.5 years old. For this to be satisfactorily achieved, the parent should attain an appropriate body size before mating and before calving. With Friesian cows, which reach a mature live weight of 600 to 650 kg at approximately 4 years of age, typical weights of 325 kg at first mating and 500 kg at first calving are aimed for. Variations in the level of feeding and growth rate, and in the age at first mating, affect subsequent lactation performance, poor nutrition and early mating, leading to a reduced milk yield (Amir, Kali and Volcani, 1969; Kay, 1976).

Following calving, cows commence a repeating cycle of management designed to give optimum performance for the herd as a whole. The current view is that this is best achieved when cows have a calving interval close to 52 weeks, which is a common management objective. Thus, cows are mated within 12 weeks of calving and for a large part of the time are simultaneously lactating and pregnant, and, in young animals, growing also. Some cows are more persistent in lactation than others but, irrespective of this, lactation is usually curtailed at approximately 44 weeks and involution of the mammary gland is induced by cessation of milking. The animals are then given a period of 6 to 8 weeks during which they do not lactate ('dry period') before their next calving. With a dry period of inadequate length milk production in the subsequent lactation is reduced through an effect on the number (Paape and Tucker, 1969) or synthetic capacity (Swanson, Pardue and Longmire, 1967) of the secretory cells which develop in the refurbishing mammary gland. Information on this process is incomplete and somewhat contradictory, however, much of it being derived from experiments with laboratory animals which may be inadequate as a model for the dairy cow (see Baldwin, 1967).

The yield and composition of milk secreted by a cow is ultimately determined by the animal's genetic potential for milk secretion, and by limitations on the realization of that potential imposed by the hormonal regulation of the development of the mammary gland, of the initiation and establishment of lactation, and of the persistence of lactation into the next breeding cycle. In addition to these inherent factors, there are also external factors which include disease (particularly disease of the gland, referred to as mastitis), the frequency and completeness of milk removal from the gland, climatic conditions, and diet and feeding management. These external factors not only affect milk secretion directly but interact with each other and with the inherent factors, making it difficult to isolate satisfactorily one factor from another. For convenience, non-nutritional factors and those related predominantly to nutrition will be discussed separately.

Non-nutritional factors affecting milk yield and composition

Breed, strain and individuality

Although breed of cow has a distinct general effect on milk yield and composition, within a breed there is a wide range of yield and composition for the milks of individual herds, and of individual cows within the herd. Recorded differences are only partly genetic in origin as they reflect also environmental differences including diet, and analytical and sampling errors in the assessment of the lactation average. Estimates of heritability, the proportion of variation accounted for by genetic factors, range from 0.25 to 0.90 for milk yield, 0.32 to 0.75 for fat content, 0.45 to 0.75 for protein (total nitrogen × 6.38) content and 0.36 to 0.70 for lactose content (Robertson, Waite and White, 1956; Brumby, 1958; Rook, 1961a).

Breed comparisons have necessarily been made with selected populations of cows but mean values are reported in the literature for large groups of animals under commercial or near commercial conditions, and representative values for animals of the British Friesian, Ayrshire, Jersey, Guernsey and Shorthorn breeds are given in Table 14.1.

Stage of lactation

Milk yield rises quickly following calving to reach a peak after 4 to 8 weeks, and there are accompanying changes in live weight and,

Table 14.1 Typical 'average' values for the yield and composition of milk of cattle of the British Friesian, Ayrshire, Jersey, Guernsey and Shorthorn breeds

Breed	Composition (g/kg)				
	Fat	Solids-not-fat	Protein (total N × 6.38)	Lactose	Ash
British Friesian	37	87	33	45	7.5
Ayrshire	38	88	34	46	7.4
Jersey	49	92	37	46	7.7
Guernsey	45	91	36	46	7.7
Shorthorn	35	87	33	45	7.6

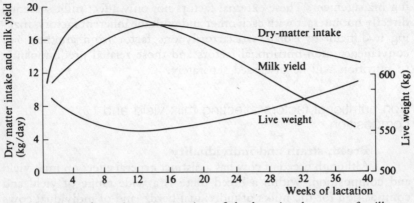

Fig. 14.1   A schematic representation of the lactational curves of milk yield, live weight and voluntary food intake of cows.

although lagging behind those in milk yield, in voluntary food intake (Fig. 14.1). Associated with the changes in yield, there are characteristic changes in milk composition throughout lactation, although in detail the shapes of the lactation curves for both yield and composition vary from cow to cow, with age, with the period between calving and subsequent conception, and with the nutrition in the pregnancy and lactation periods. Mean yield and compositional values for cows in their first lactation, given a constant amount of a diet of hay and concentrates (Rook and Campling, 1965), are shown in Fig. 14.2. Colostrum, the first secretion removed from the udder at the beginning of lactation, has a high content of fat and protein, and a low content of lactose; the contents of all protein fractions are high but there is an exceptionally high proportion of globulins, mainly immunoglobulins, which persists for 1 or 2 days only. As lactation progresses and milk yield increases, there is a rapid reduction in fat and protein contents and an increase in lactose content, changes which continue up to or beyond the peak in yield. Maximum values for lactose content may be achieved by approximately 4 weeks of lactation but minimum values for fat and protein may not be reached until a few weeks later. During the post-peak period, milk yield initially declines at a more or less constant rate of about 2 to 2.5% per week and there is a slight reversal of the previous changes in milk composition. This becomes more marked as the milk yield decline is accelerated towards the end of lactation, the point of change in the slopes of the yield and composition curves being influenced by the stage of pregnancy.

The fatty acid composition of milk fat also changes throughout lactation. The fat of colostrum removed at first milking has a lower proportion of short-chain fatty acids, especially butyric acid, and a higher proportion of palmitic acid than the fat of milk removed at

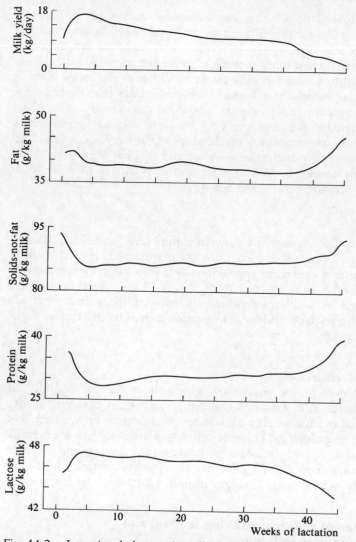

Fig. 14.2. Lactational changes in milk yield and composition in dairy cows. (Adapted from Rook and Campling, 1965.)

subsequent milkings throughout the 1st week of lactation. The relative proportions of short-chain fatty acids, possibly excepting butyric acid, increase throughout the first 8 to 10 weeks of lactation, that of palmitic acid is fairly constant, and the proportions of stearic and octadecanoic acids tend to decrease. Subsequent changes associated directly with stage of lactation are small.

The constancy of the general shape of the lactation curves for milk yield and composition has encouraged their description mathematically.

Wood (1976) has shown that the lactational curves for milk yield, for fat content and for protein content can be described by one family of equations of the type $y_n = an^b e^{cn}$, where a, b and c define the curve of production of character y at week n. In the equations, e is the base of natural logarithms, a is a scaling factor to allow for the actual yield or compositional values, and b and c are coefficients that describe the pre-peak curvature and post-peak curvature respectively. The equations, converted to the form $\log_e(y_n) = \log_e a + b \log_e n + cn$ (where the sign of b and c vary depending on the shape of the curve), can be solved relatively simply by regression analysis and this has been done using results from cows sampled as part of the National Milk Records Scheme to provide generalized equations.

Age

Analysis of results for cows in commercial herds has indicated that there are progressive reductions in fat and solids-not-fat (mainly lactose) contents averaging approximately 2.0 to 4.0 g/kg respectively over the first five lactations (see Rook, 1961a). These effects may in part be explained by a selective culling of low-yielding animals but are probably also related to udder deterioration caused by mastitis or slight physical damage.

Udder disease

Infection of the mammary gland alters the permeability of secretory tissue and impairs its secretory activity. Characteristically, there is a fall in milk yield, and in lactose and potassium contents, and an increase in sodium and chloride contents. Casein content is generally reduced but there are increases in globulin, serum albumin and proteose peptone contents so that the effect on total protein content varies with the severity of infection. Changes in milk fat content are irregular.

Stage of milking, milking interval and incomplete milking

Because of the retention of fat within the fine ducts of the mammary gland, the fat content of milk increases progressively throughout a milking; the first drawn milk contains approximately 10 g fat per kg whereas that removed at the end of a milking – the strippings – may contain 100 g/kg. Only a proportion, approximately 90%, of the milk initially present in the udder is removed with normal milking and that which is left, the residual milk, is exceptionally rich in fat. The residual milk can be obtained, and the gland milked out, with the assistance of an injection of oxytocin but the dose level must be chosen with care since oxytocin itself has effects on milk yield and composition.

When milking intervals of different lengths follow each other, the amount of milk and especially of milk fat removed from the udder is greater than the true rate of secretion after a short interval but less than the true rate of secretion after a long interval. Changes in the milk content of non-fat constituents are confounded by the diluent effect of the varying amounts of fat but the amounts of milk constituents secreted are curvilinearly related to the length of the interval between milkings. Wheelock, Rook, Dodd and Griffin (1966) found that the rate of secretion of milk and milk constituents (after a previous standardized 12-h milking interval) was virtually linear for periods of 12 h but by 18 h had started to decline. Long milking intervals were associated with reductions in the milk contents of lactose and solids-not-fat, and increases in the contents of sodium, chloride, non-casein nitrogen and fat. The milking interval at which effects on milk secretion begin to occur will however vary with the animal's daily milk yield. Accumulation of milk within the gland has a local effect on milk secretion when the hydrostatic pressure measured at the teat tip reaches approximately 4 kPa (Fleet and Peaker, 1978).

Local inhibitory effects also probably explain the effects of incomplete milking on milk yield and composition. In cows for which only 50% of the milk was removed from the gland at four successive milkings, the yields of milk and of milk constituents were subsequently depressed (Wheelock, Rook and Dodd, 1965). Excepting lactose, there were increases in the concentrations of all milk constituents, fat being especially affected.

Environmental temperature

Although cows are efficient in dissipating the heat produced by their metabolism they begin to suffer from heat stress at environmental termperatures above approximately 25 °C. The yield of milk and of milk constituents, especially fat, is reduced, possibly in part through effects on the secretion of regulatory hormones, e.g. thyroxine, growth hormone and insulin (Webster, 1976). Milk yield is also reduced below −5 °C, probably due to localized cooling effects on blood flow to the mammary gland (Thompson and Thomson, 1977).

Nutritional factors affecting milk yield and composition

Because of their high metabolic rate and their requirement for milk secretion, lactating animals have a special demand for minerals and trace nutrients but both are readily provided as supplements to the diet. Thus, in practice, milk yield and composition is influenced mainly by the dietary supplies of materials providing energy and protein, and it is on the effects of these constituents that attention will be concentrated. An increase in the amount of food given to a cow typically results in an increase in the yield of milk and of milk constituents, and either an increase in live-weight gain or a decrease in live-weight loss. The relationship with food intake is curvilinear, the response in milk yield diminishing and that in live-weight change increasing with each successive increment of food (Fig. 14.3). As discussed below, corresponding curves can be derived to describe the separate responses in

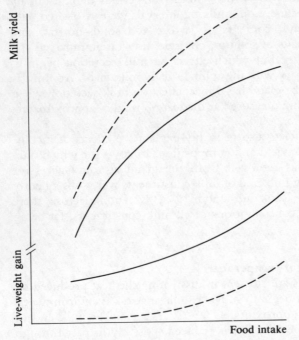

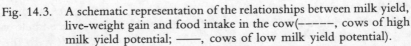

Fig. 14.3.   A schematic representation of the relationships between milk yield, live-weight gain and food intake in the cow(-----, cows of high milk yield potential; ———, cows of low milk yield potential).

milk secretion to increases in dietary energy or protein supply but, in practice, variations in energy intake are most often achieved through offering additional concentrate foods and the effects of energy intake *per se* are generally confounded with those due to the changes in the composition of the ration.

In reporting results of experiments on milk production, it has become conventional to assess responses in terms of *milk yield* (the change of volume or weight of secretion) and *milk composition* (the change of composition from that of the control milk), and to attribute a change of composition to separate treatment effects on the secretion of individual milk constituents. This approach is in line with the concept that the nutrient requirements for milk synthesis include a supply of energy-yielding materials essential for the synthesis of all milk constituents and a supply of specific precursors for each individual constituent. There is no evidence, however, that the curvilinear relationships between the supply of energy-yielding materials and rate of synthesis are identical for all milk constituents and, whilst the arbitrary separation of responses into yield and composition effects is useful for the characterization of production responses, it may mislead in any attempt to understand the causal relationships involved.

Utilization of dietary energy and protein

Conventionally, the utilization of energy in ruminants is assessed through measurement of the ME intake in the diet (where ME intake = gross energy intake − faecal energy loss − methane energy loss − urine energy loss), and the partial efficiencies of utilization of ME for maintenance and for productive processes. The situation in the lactating animal is complicated because the productive process of lactation may occur together with tissue synthesis or with tissue degradation, and energy balance may be positive or negative. The partial efficiency of utilization of ME for lactation has, however, been determined through simultaneous measurements of milk energy yield and tissue energy change under conditions where they vary relative to each other. The results of such studies have been analysed using partial regression methods, the data being fitted to a model of the type: ME intake $= a + b_1$ (body weight$^{0.75}$) $+ b_2$ (milk energy yield) $+ b_3$ (positive tissue energy balance) $+ b_4$ (negative tissue energy balance). The body weight term in this equation gives an estimate of the energy used for maintenance whilst the regression coefficients b_2, b_3 and b_4 indicate the efficiency with which energy is used for the productive processes. The efficiency of utilization of ME for lactation at zero tissue energy change (k_{l_0}) is given by $1/b_2$ and the corresponding efficiency for tissue synthesis (k_f) by $1/b_3$. The efficiency of utilization of tissue energy for milk synthesis is b_4/b_2, since b_4 reflects the amount of dietary ME spared by one unit of tissue loss, and dividing by b_2 gives the milk energy produced by that quantity of ME.

In a summary of results from a large number of experiments with cows given mixed forage and concentrate diets adequate in protein, Van Es (1976) concluded that k_{l_0} varied with diet over a narrow range from approximately 0.60 to 0.67 J/J, the value decreasing by some 0.004 for each 0.01 reduction in the metabolizability of the diet, i.e. the proportion of ME in the dietary gross energy (J/J). These results are typical of those obtained by other workers although there is evidence that efficiencies as low as 0.54 may be obtained with high-forage diets (see Flatt, Moe, Moore, Breirem and Ekern, 1972). Whereas the efficiency of tissue synthesis (k_f) varies widely with diet in growing and fattening animals, in lactating animals it is relatively constant and similar in value to k_{l_0}. Mobilized body tissue is used for milk secretion with an efficiency of 0.80 to 0.85, so that dietary energy deposited in the tissues and subsequently mobilized is used with an overall efficiency of approximately 0.50.

As a result of the similarity and constancy of the values of k_{l_0} and k_f, energy metabolism experiments have consistently demonstrated a linear relationship between ME intake and the total energy balance measured as milk plus body tissue. But this relationship hides important variations in the partitioning of energy use between milk secretion and tissue deposition. As ME intake is raised the incremental response in milk energy output, which is dependent primarily on the increase in milk yield, becomes smaller, and a greater proportion of the ME is directed towards body tissue deposition. The responsiveness of milk yield varies with the genetic merit of the cow (Fig. 14.3) and with the stage of lactation, the cow of greater genetic potential for milk secretion and earlier stage of lactation giving a greater response in milk yield and a lower response in tissue gain for a given increment of ME. Changes in energy partition may also occur in response to alterations in the composition of the diet or in feeding management. The best described effects are those observed with diets containing a high proportion of starchy concentrates and a low proportion of fibrous forages (Table 14.2), which operate mainly through a reduction in the yield of milk fat (see below). However, most changes in diet or management which enhance milk output without a concomitant increase in energy intake probably reflect a repartitioning in energy use, rather than a change in efficiency of energy utilization.

Description of the utilization of dietary energy in calorimetric terms has allowed the development of the Metabolizable Energy System for rationing dairy cows (Agricultural Research Council, 1965) and its subsequent adaptation to provide the standards for energy allowances used in Great Britain (Ministry of Agriculture, Fisheries and Food, Department of Agriculture and Fisheries for Scotland, and Department of Agriculture for Northern Ireland, 1975). In calculation of the latter, the efficiencies of utilization of ME for maintenance, lactation and tissue synthesis are assumed to be constants with values of 0.72, 0.62 and 0.62 respectively, and a value of 0.82 is adopted for the efficiency of conversion of tissue energy to milk energy. Dietary ME allowances are thus computed taking account of the cow's live weight (for maintenance requirements), the yield and energy content (calculated from milk composition) of milk, and live-weight gain or loss. It

Table 14.2 The effect of the proportions of alfalfa hay and concentrates in the diet on the partition of dietary energy (MJ/day) between milk secretion and body tissue deposition in cows in early-, mid-, or late-lactation (from Flatt, Moe, Munson and Cooper, 1969)

Dietary proportions of hay: concentrate (g/kg)	Stage of lactation	Metabolizable energy intake	Energy secreted in milk	Energy deposited in tissue	Heat production
600:400	Early	149	94	−42	97
	Mid	158	53	0	105
	Late	147	29	17	101
	Diet mean	153	58	−8	101
400:600	Early	153	80	−30	103
	Mid	164	54	7	109
	Late	141	28	16	97
	Diet mean	152	55	−2	99
200:800	Early	138	60	−15	92
	Mid	145	39	8	96
	Late	155	30	29	97
	Diet mean	146	44	7	95

is fundamental, however, that ME intake relates to the total energy balance of milk plus tissue, and one of these components must be measured before the other can be predicted.

Although the dietary crude protein (nitrogen × 6.25) intake influences milk yield and the yield of milk constituents, there is little response to additional protein in animals receiving diets providing the Woodman (1957) standard of 340 g digestible crude protein for maintenance and 60 g digestible crude protein per kg milk for production. Broster (1972) concluded that, with basal diets adequate in protein according to the standard, the yield of milk (corrected to a standard fat content of 40 g/kg) increased on average by only 0.6 kg/kg of additional digestible crude protein. On the other hand, with basal diets providing less protein than the standard, milk yield increased by an average of 4.4 kg/kg digestible crude protein, although the responses varied widely between experiments from −1 kg to +8.5 kg. Factors influencing the utilization of dietary nitrogen are discussed below but it should be noted at this stage that the utilization of nitrogen and energy are interdependent (Fig. 14.4(a)), and that the use of absorbed nitrogen is partitioned between milk secretion and tissue synthesis (Fig. 14.4 (b)). Consequently, changes in the dietary intake of crude protein or of energy, even in the absence of an effect on milk production, may have an important impact on the deposition of protein in the tissues.

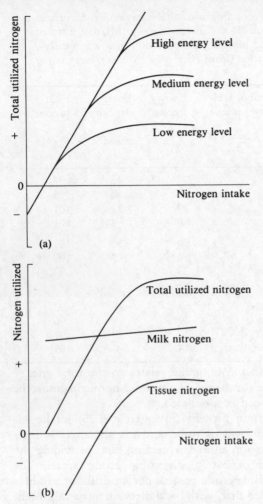

Fig. 14.4.　(a) A diagrammatic representation of the relationship between the total utilized nitrogen (nitrogen secreted in milk plus nitrogen deposited in body tissues) and the dietary nitrogen intake at various levels of energy intake (see Balch, 1967). (b) A diagrammatic representation of the relationship between the total utilized nitrogen, the nitrogen secreted in milk and the nitrogen deposited in tissue, and the dietary nitrogen intake at a fixed level of energy intake. (Based on Balch and Campling, 1965.)

Diet and the products of digestion

Assessment of nutrient supply in terms of ME and digestible crude protein has proved convenient in the practical rationing of farm livestock and is a necessary first step in the study of the relationship between diet and milk production. All the digestible organic components of a diet, including protein, are, however, a potential source of energy, although the various dietary constituents differ in the products of their digestion that are absorbed from the gut. Additionally, dietary protein is important both as a source of nitrogen and of individual amino acids. Within the tissues, certain of the pathways for the metabolism of amino acids and other substrates are common, and both the quantitative supply of substrates and the interactions in their metabolism determine the effect of diet on milk yield and composition. Over the past 10 years, much research effort has been given to the development and application of techniques for the quantitative determination of the products of digestion in the ruminant. Considerable information is now available on the digestion of a wide range of diets in sheep, and there is more limited information for the dairy cow. Typical values for the amounts of the main products of digestion formed in the rumen, small intestine, and caecum and colon are shown in Table 14.3. The figures illustrate the dominant rôle of the rumen as a site of digestion but also highlight the wide range in composition of the mixture of products of digestion formed with diets typical of those given to dairy cows in commercial practice.

Table 14.3   Estimates of the amounts and variations in amount of products of digestion absorbed from the gastro-intestinal tract of lactating dairy cows receiving mixed forage and concentrate diets. (Values are approximations, based on information from the literature on digestion in the cow, and where necessary the sheep, and have been adjusted so that they are appropriate for a cow of 600 kg live weight with a milk yield of 25kg/day and a digestible energy intake of 215 MJ/day)

Products of digestion	Gross energy absorbed (MJ/day)	Weight absorbed (kg/day)
Short-chain fatty acids		
Total acids[†]	117–147	
Acetic acid[‡]	43–75	2.9–5.1
Propionic acid	31–57	1.5–2.7
Butyric acid	24–37	1.1–1.5
Glucose[§]	4–17	0.3–1.0
Amino acids	30–45	1.3–1.9
Long-chain fatty acids	19–54	0.5–1.4

[†] 75–90% (mean 84%) of fermentation digestion usually occurs in the rumen; the remainder is in the caecum and colon.

[‡] Based on rumen fermentation patterns containing molar proportions of acetic: propionic: butyric acids of 68:20:12 and 50:35:15, and a caecal fermentation pattern of 68:20:12.

[§] Estimates include diets containing ground maize.

[‖] Estimates based on diets containing 130 to 150 g protein/kg.

[¶] Estimates assume fatty acid intake of 300 to 1000 gday.

Work is in progress on computer models for the prediction of the end-products of digestion from a knowledge of nutrient intake (Baldwin and Koong, 1980) and some attention has been given to models of substrate metabolism in the tissues (Smith, Baldwin and Sharp, 1980). However, at the present time the complexity of the relationship between diet and the products of digestion, and the uncertainties about the rôle of nutrient supply in the regulation of milk secretion (see Ch. 8), make it impossible to summarize satisfactorily in quantitative terms the links between diet, substrate supply to the tissues, and milk yield and composition. Several superficial relationships have been established, however, and these are considered below.

Conduct of lactation experiments

In the majority of nutritional experiments, animal management and climatic and other aspects of the environment are standardized as far as possible to remove any confounding of differences between dietary treatments but it should be recognized that such experiments take no account of nutritional-management or nutritional-environmental interactions, and for the dairy cow these may be quite important.

Many of the early experiments with dairy cows took little account of the effects of udder infection but nowadays strict hygiene procedures are normally imposed to minimize infections, routine bacteriological examinations are undertaken to monitor udder health and antibiotic therapy is adopted to eliminate clinical mastitis. Nonetheless, the effects of the inevitable subclinical infections and of the damage to the secretory tissue incurred through a previous mastitis infection are rarely allowed for. A system of milking individual udder quarters so that results from infected or damaged quarters may be excluded has been proposed (Waite, Abbot and Blackburn, 1963) but it is time-consuming and has not gained widespread acceptance.

The design of nutritional experiments with lactating animals presents special problems. The most relevant comparisons practically are those conducted over the whole of one or more lactations but such experiments require large groups of animals to overcome the statistical problems arising from the substantial between-animal differences in milk yield and composition. The scale and time-span of the experiments and the quantities of uniform foods (e.g. forages) required makes the studies logistically difficult, and often impossible to undertake within the constraints of available research facilities. Smaller groups of animals can be used successfully in shorter-term experiments where between-animal differences are allowed for statistically, through the use of an analysis of variance procedure, by subjecting each animal to each of the treatments to be compared. Responses in milk yield and composition to a change in diet are not immediate, however, they may not be evident for 1 to 2 weeks and may not be fully expressed for a much longer period. Assessments of dietary effects thus take some time, and experiments must be designed so that the responses to diet are not confounded by changes in milk yield and composition, which occur naturally as lactation advances. This can be done by undertaking experiments in the mid-lactation period. Experiments have been conducted from shortly after the lactational peak in milk yield over the following 15 to 20 weeks when, if nutrition is approaching the recommended standards (see below), milk yield declines slowly and more or less constantly. Under these conditions, with an appropriate choice of experimental design, the selection of a group of cows matched as closely as possible for breed, age, yield and stage of lactation, and the adoption of standardized feeding and milking procedures, a reliable indication of treatment effects can usually be obtained with treatment periods of 3 to 4 weeks and with 4 to 8 individual observations per treatment. Such short-term trials have proved of great value in establishing the general principles underlying effects of diet on milk production. However, early and late in lactation, when the yield and composition of milk produced, and the partition of nutrients between body tissue and milk secretion are changing rapidly under hormonal influences, the amount and the type of diet may not only affect milk production directly but may modify hormonal regulation, and enhance or reduce, to some extent irreversibly, the normal lactational trends in milk yield and composition. Dietary effects on milk production in early and late lactation may thus differ not only quantitatively but also qualitatively from those in mid-lactation.

Mid-lactation effects of diet on milk yield: dietary carbohydrate

The major products of the digestion of soluble and insoluble carbohydrates are the short-chain fatty acids, acetic, propionic and butyric, but small quantities of higher fatty acids are also produced. The passage of starch to the small intestine, and its subsequent digestion and absorption as glucose, is a major route of digestion only when the diet contains a large amount of starch and the source is one, such as ground maize, where the granules have a natural resistance to amylase penetration unless ruptured by moist heat-processing.

Cows given continuous intraruminal infusions of dilute solutions of short-chain fatty acids in quantities providing 500 to 2000 g acid per day have shown a slow response in milk yield with acetic but not with other acids (Fig. 14.5). Occasional but not consistent responses in milk yield have also been obtained with post-ruminal infusions of glucose (Clark, 1975; Vik-Mo, Emery and Huber, 1975; Frobish and Davis, 1977). A

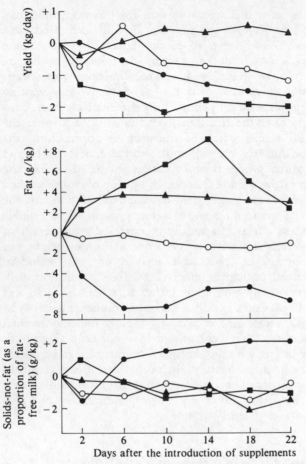

Fig. 14.5. Mean changes with time in milk yield, and fat and solids–not–fat contents, in cows following the introduction of intraruminal supplements of acetic, propionic and butyric acids (o, no supplement; ▲, acetic acid; ●, propionic acid; ■, butyric acid). On average, 98% of the response in solids–not–fat with propionic acid supplementation was accounted for by an increase in milk protein content. (After Rook and Balch, 1961.)

specific effect of acetate on the tótal yield of milk is in accordance with the rôle of acetate oxidation in the provision of ATP in the mammary gland and glucose might be anticipated to have a more specific effect in circumstances where the basal diet provides inadequate glucogenic materials to maintain glucose supply (see Ch. 8). Recent experiments have demonstrated that there can be substantial differences in milk yield between cows given isocaloric diets differing in carbohydrate composition but no consistent relationships between milk yield and the amounts

Table 14.4 The digestion of some dietary constituents, and milk yield and composition, in cannulated and intact cows given diets containing hay and concentrates of rolled barley or ground maize in various proportions (Sutton, Oldham and Hart, 1980)

| | Proportion of dietary hay:concentrate | | | |
| | 40:60 | | 10:90 | |
	Barley	Maize	Barley	Maize
Cannulated cows				
Gross energy intake (MJ/day)	$232^{a\dagger}$	227^{ab}	220^b	217^b
Proportion digested				
In whole tract	0.696^b	0.693^b	0.730^a	0.686^b
In rumen	0.515	0.482	0.522	0.429
Starch intake (kg/day)	4.10^a	4.33^a	5.75^b	6.37^c
Proportion digested				
In whole tract	0.99^a	0.92^b	0.99^a	0.89^c
In rumen	0.89^a	0.72^b	0.90^a	0.67^c
Rumen short-chain fatty acid (mmol/mol)				
Acetic acid	612^a	629^a	434^c	530^b
Propionic acid	219^a	210^a	410^b	280^a
Butyric acid	119	116	92	112
Intact cows				
Gross energy intake (MJ/day)	221	229	219	218
Milk yield (kg/day)	16.1^b	18.9^{ab}	20.6^a	15.6^b
Fat content (g/kg)	44.9^a	40.4^a	20.3^c	29.7^b
Fat yield (g/day)	725^a	761^a	419^b	461^b
Protein content (g/kg)	31.5^b	30.0^b	30.3^b	34.3^a
Protein yield (g/day)	506^b	562^{ab}	617^a	535^b
Lactose content (g/kg)	45.2	45.2	46.2	45.5
Lactose yield (g/day)	729^b	852^{ab}	954^a	714^b

$\dagger$ Means in a line that do not share the same superscript differ significantly ($P < 0.05$).

of individual short-chain fatty acids or glucose absorbed from the gut are evident (Table 14.4).

Mid-lactation effects of diet on milk yield: dietary fat

Early experiments demonstrated the need for a certain amount of dietary fat, approximately 30 to 40 g/kg of the concentrate food, for maximum milk yield and more recently this has been confirmed. An increase in milk yield of 40% was observed in cows receiving a synthetic diet when their daily intake of oil was increased from 37 to 130 g (Virtanen, 1966). Similar responses were observed in cows receiving a diet of hay and concentrates providing 81 g fat daily when 101 g of fat was substituted isocalorically for a part of the concentrate food (Banks, Clapperton, Ferrie and Wilson, 1976b); the response was greater when the substituent was soya oil or beef tallow than when it was a mixture of red palm-oil and palmitic acid.

When the basal diet contains adequate fat, responses to additional fat are small and variable, but experiments in which fats of various composition have been substituted isocalorically for a part of the concentrated food suggest that, as the chain length of the predominant fatty acid of the substituent fat increases from C_{12} and C_{14} to $C_{18:1}$, there is a corresponding change of response from a small depression to a small increase in milk yield (Fig. 14.6). *Additions* of red palm-oil and of groundnut oil, at a level of 23 g/kg of the concentrated food, have increased milk yield by 10 to 15% (Storry, Rook and Hall, 1967). Substitution in the diet of fat rich in polyunsaturated fatty acids (1 kg/day) but protected against the action of rumen microorganisms (Pan, Cook and Scott, 1972), or of cod-liver oil (0.3 kg/day) (Brumby, Storry and Sutton, 1972), has had no significant effect on milk yield. The basis of the depression of milk yield by a diet deficient in fat, or of

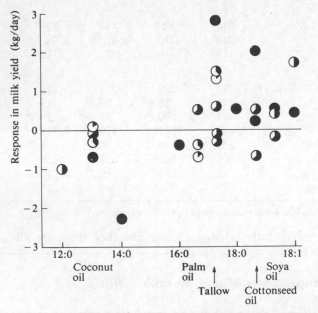

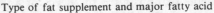

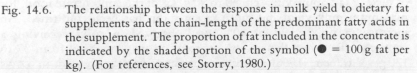

Type of fat supplement and major fatty acid

Fig. 14.6.   The relationship between the response in milk yield to dietary fat supplements and the chain-length of the predominant fatty acids in the supplement. The proportion of fat included in the concentrate is indicated by the shaded portion of the symbol (● = 100 g fat per kg). (For references, see Storry, 1980.)

the possible small differential responses to the inclusion in a normal diet of fats of different composition, is unknown.

Inclusion of large amounts of fat in the diet, in excess of approximately 100 g/kg of the concentrated food, may interfere with fermentation processes in the rumen and cause a fall in food intake and a loss of milk yield. Lauric acid has an adverse effect at lower concentration (Steele and Moore, 1968).

Mid-lactation effects of diet on milk yield: dietary protein

The interactions that are observed between dietary protein and energy in their utilization by simple-stomached animals are a consequence of the deamination and catabolism of amino acids that occurs when their supply exceeds their use for protein synthesis; synthesis may be limited by the supply of individual amino acids or of energy. In ruminants, however, there are also interactions between nitrogenous and other materials in their use for microbial synthesis in the rumen. Digestible crude protein is therefore a poor index of the amount of amino acid nitrogen derived by the ruminant animal from the diet, and is inadequate as a basis for relating dietary protein intake to milk production. More soundly based systems for the evaluation of dietary protein supply have recently been published (Journet and Verité, 1977; Kaufmann, 1977; Roy, Balch, Miller, Ørskov and Smith, 1977; Satter and Roffler, 1977) and, in the system proposed by Roy *et al.* (1977) and adopted in the UK, the uptake of total amino acids from the small intestine is computed from the amounts of undegraded dietary protein and rumen-synthesized microbial protein passing to the duodenum. The microbial protein is calculated from the dietary energy fermented in the rumen, the dietary content of rumen-degradable nitrogen having been adjusted so that the microbial growth is theoretically unrestricted by nitrogen supply. The system has well recognized limitations because, in the absence of adequate information, constant factors have been used to calculate energy digestion in the rumen, microbial protein synthesis, amino acid digestion in the small intestine, and the efficiency of utilization of absorbed amino acids for milk and tissue synthesis. Additionally, much of the information on which the system is based is derived from studies with sheep given moderate levels of feeding and may not be fully applicable to the dairy cow with its high food intake.

Whilst marked differences in rumen degradability between dietary protein sources have been observed in the sheep (Smith, 1975) there is less certainty about the range of values which may be obtained in dairy cows. Feeding experiments have generally not demonstrated clear-cut effects of dietary protein source on milk production but most studies have been with animals of moderate milk yield whose requirement for amino acids was probably met largely through the synthesis of microbial protein in the rumen. In recent work, Van Horn, Zometa, Wilcox, Marshall and Harris (1979) showed that dietary inclusions of soya bean rather than cottonseed meal improved milk yield over a range of dietary protein intakes and this, to date, is probably the most convincing demonstration of yield responses to dietary protein source. Nonetheless, as has been discussed by Oldham (1980), variations in the level and source of dietary protein have important effects on the digestibility of energy, and even in the studies of Van Horn *et al.* (1979) part of the soya bean response could be accounted for by changes in digestibility. Responses in milk yield to protein supplements of low rather than high degradability have also been reported in cows receiving diets containing grass silage (Castle and Watson, 1979) or sorghum silage (Majdoub, Lane and Aitchison, 1978), where a high proportion of the crude protein in the forage is present in non-protein form, but these observations may in part be due to effects on forage intake.

Investigations of the effects of duodenal amino acid supply on milk production have been undertaken using dietary inclusions of protein protected from ruminal attack by treatment with formaldehyde (Stobbs, Minson and McLeod, 1977; Flores, Stobbs and Minson, 1979) or intra-abomasal infusions of protein (see Clark, 1975; Schwab, Satter and Clay, 1976; Clark, Spires, Derrig and Benink, 1977; Rogers, Bryant and McLeay, 1979). Milk yield responses have been observed with protein infusions in a large number of studies and in some instances with basal diets of apparently adequate digestible crude protein content. Invariably, however, casein has been the protein supplement, and the demonstration that intra-abomasal infusions of casein increase the blood concentration of growth hormone (Oldham, Hart and Bines, 1978) raises questions about the mechanisms of the milk yield response and whether observations with casein apply to other proteins. Post-ruminal infusions of single essential amino acids have generally not produced significant effects on milk yield but in some instances there have been significant responses to mixtures containing two or more amino acids (Clark, 1975; Schwab *et al.*, 1976; Rogers *et al.*, 1979). The most extensive series of experiments conducted so far is that of Schwab *et al.* (1976) with cows given diets consisting mainly of maize grain, alfalfa hay and maize silage. In these experiments, responses in milk production to an infusion of 10 essential amino acids were similar to those obtained with an infusion of casein and, as judged from the yield of milk protein, lysine was the first and methionine was the second limiting amino acid. These experiments also demonstrated significant responses in milk yield (but not protein yield) to infusions of arginine plus histidine, suggesting that there may be differential effects of individual amino acids on the secretion of the nitrogenous and non-nitrogenous milk constituents.

Mid-lactation effects of diet on milk-fat content and composition

The complex origins of milk fat are considered in Ch. 8. The C_{18} acids used by the mammary gland for milk-fat synthesis are entirely preformed. They may be derived directly from the diet or by mobilization of fat reserves of the body; the latter contain fatty acids both of dietary origin and synthesized *de novo* at the site of fat deposition or in the liver. Dietary unsaturated C_{18} acids are, however, hydrogenated extensively in the rumen and the unsaturated acids in milk are formed in part from stearic acid which is partially desaturated in the mammary gland. The short-chain acids, C_4 to C_{12}, and to a large extent C_{14}, are synthesized *de novo* in the mammary gland from acetate and 3-hydroxybutyrate, and the supply of these materials is controlled largely by the amount and composition of the non-lipid components of the diet. The C_{16} acids used for milk-fat synthesis are derived both preformed and by the *de novo* synthesis pathway.

The supplies of both the lipid and the non-lipid components of the diet have primary effects on milk-fat secretion but these may be modified by interactions between the dietary components, by dietary effects on fat mobilization and by possible competition between individual fatty acids within the mammary gland for incorporation into milk-fat triglycerides. Understandably, because of this complexity, many partly conflicting reports have appeared on the effects of diet, and especially of its lipid composition, on milk-fat secretion and, because of the small, unexplained effects of dietary fat on milk yield, there is an even greater diversity of observations on effects on milk fat content. A clearer picture can be presented for observations on the fatty acid composition of milk fat.

Non-lipid dietary factors

In the late 1930s E. B. Powell of the Ralston Purina Company, USA, fed cows throughout the whole of their lactation on diets consisting of forage and concentrated foods, in which the forage part of the diet was either finely-ground or present in an unusually low amount, and observed a distinctive fall in milk-fat content. Numerous experiments since then have confirmed and extended his findings (see review by Sutton, 1980) and the following general relationship has emerged.

Milk fat content declines as the proportion of physically fibrous material in the diet is reduced. Initially, the fall is slight but when the proportion of long forage is reduced below approximately 400 g/kg the fall becomes more pronounced and at a long-forage content of approximately 100 g/kg a precipitous fall in fat content to less than 20 g/kg may occur, and this is frequently referred to as the 'low milk-fat syndrome'. An example of these changes is shown in Fig. 14.7.

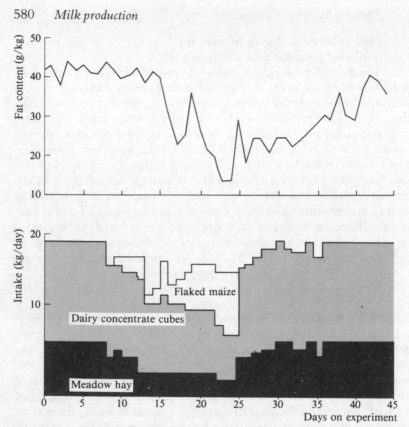

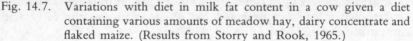

Fig. 14.7. Variations with diet in milk fat content in a cow given a diet
containing various amounts of meadow hay, dairy concentrate and
flaked maize. (Results from Storry and Rook, 1965.)

There is also a change of fat composition when milk-fat content and
yield are depressed. The proportion and sometimes the yield of
unsaturated acids is increased, and the proportion and yield of saturated
acids, especially those containing 16 carbon atoms or less, decreased.
When the fall in fat content is extreme, the proportion of $C_{18:1}$ acid
present as the *trans* isomer increases to as much as half (Storry and
Rook, 1965) and the ratio of $C_{18:1}$ to $C_{18:0}$ acids, which is usually fairly
constant, is increased (Banks, Clapperton and Ferrie, 1976a). Desaturation of $C_{18:0}$ in the mammary gland produces only the *cis* isomer and
the *trans* isomer arises from an incomplete hydrogenation of C_{18}
polyunsaturated fatty acids within the rumen; conditions in the rumen
are less reducing when diets low in fibre are offered.

Much circumstantial evidence has linked the depressed milk-fat
secretion to an alteration in the pattern of rumen fermentation,
although with some diets an enhanced passage of starch to the small intestine may also be a contributory factor. Increase in the amount of

soluble starchy foods and reduction in the amount or particle size of the fibrous forage foods in the diet causes a decrease in salivary flow into the rumen, a reduction in rumen liquor pH and dilution rate and, when the diet is offered in discrete meals, more extreme peaks and troughs in fermentation activity. The changes in dilution rate, pH, and composition and availability of substrates in combination lead to a change of microbial population typified by reduced numbers of celluloytic and fibre-digesting bacteria, and increased numbers of lactic acid- and propionic acid-producing bacteria. A specific increase in selenomonads, peptostreptococci, lactobacilli and bifidobacteria, a decrease in butyrivibrio (Latham, Sutton and Sharpe, 1974) and, in some instances, a disappearance of ciliate protozoa (Chalupa, O'Dell, Kutches and Lavker, 1967) have been reported. The microbial populations that develop, however, are unstable and there is no simple relation between the composition of the diet and that of the microbial population.

Both the products of fermentation and the flow of materials from the rumen to the intestine are altered. Typical values for the composition (mmol/mol) of the mixture of short-chain fatty acids in rumen liquor of cattle receiving high-forage diets are 650 to 740 acetic acid, 150 to 200 propionic acid and 80 to 160 butyric acid. As the fibre content of the diet is reduced progressively, the proportion of acetic acid falls and that of propionic acid rises; minimum and maximum values reported are 350 and 450 mmol/mol respectively. On some occasions, the first fall in acetic acid is associated transitorily with a rise in butyric acid and a slight fall in propionic acid but as the diet composition is altered further there is generally an abrupt increase in the proportion of propionic acid and a decrease in that of butyric acid (Storry and Rook, 1966) as a result of a switch of microbial population. The proportion of *n*-valeric acid tends to increase with that of propionic acid. Reliable estimates of the changes in the amounts of fatty acids produced are not available and, although the relative proportions of the acids reflect their rates of production, this relationship is probably not very precise. With diets containing moderate proportions of concentrates and given in frequent meals throughout the day, the molar proportions of the acids reflect closely their relative rates of production but, for animals given meals of high concentrate diets twice daily, the marked diurnal variations in rumen pH must influence the relationships between the rates of absorption of individual acids and their concentrations in the rumen, and there are major technical problems in the interpretation of isotope-dilution measurements of fatty acid production and interconversion under non-steady-state conditions (Morant, Ridley and Sutton, 1978).

Statistical relationships between the composition of the mixture of short-chain fatty acids and milk-fat content have, however, been firmly established. The proportion of acetic acid and, to a greater extent that of butyric acid, are positively related to fat content, that of propionic acid negatively. Assuming a linear relationship, at least 60% of the variation in fat content is accounted for by variation in the molar proportion of propionic acid (McCullough, 1966; Storry and Rook, 1966; Latham *et al.*, 1974). Continuous intraruminal infusions of dilute aqueous solutions of the acids into milking cows (Fig. 14.5) have confirmed those relationship. Acetic acid and butyric acid increased milk-fat secretion, butyric acid to a greater extent than acetic acid, through an increased output of fatty acids containing 16 carbon atoms or less, which was partly offset by a decreased output of C_{18} acids. Propionic acid decreased milk-fat secretion due to a decreased ouput of all acids except C_{16}. Possible mechanisms whereby those changes in products of fermentation, and associated changes in the flow of starch (Jackson, Rook and Towers, 1971) and lipid (Sutton, Storry and Nicholson, 1970) to the intestine, may cause alterations in milk-fat secretion are discussed in Ch. 8.

Because of the close relationship between milk-fat secretion and the composition of the short-chain fatty acids produced in the rumen, the influence of the non-lipid components of the diet is determined largely by their effects on fermentation pattern. Major dietary factors controlling rumen fermentation are forage : concentrate ratio, level of food intake, processing of forages and concentrates, and frequency of feeding, all of which affect fermentation rate. The chemical nature of the readily fermentable carbohydrate, in particular the relative proportions of starch and sugars, and the extent to which the starch is heat treated are also important as are feed additives designed to alter aspects of rumen environment, such as pH or redox potential, or to influence the rumen microorganisms directly, e.g. methane inhibitors, antibiotics and antiprotozoal compounds.

The general relationship between forage:concentrate ratio and milk fat content has already been described. Inclusion of an adequate amount of fibrous material in the diet is critical for the maintenance of fat content at a satisfactory level and a dietary crude fibre content of approximately 160 g/kg is often recommended. The effect of forage: concentrate ratio varies with the level of feeding, with the individual and with the breed, however; Jersey cattle are less susceptible to a depression in milk-fat content than are British Friesian or Holstein cattle. In most experiments dietary energy intake has not been held constant during the change of diet composition and the effects of forage:concentrate ratio on fat yield are less certain than those on fat content. In a recent study (I. H. L. Ormrod and P. C. Thomas, unpublished results) diets containing 200 or 400 g chopped hay per kg with concentrates were given to cows at levels providing their theoretical ME requirements for maintenance and for either 80 or 110% of milk production. At fixed levels of intake the content rumen and high and yield of milk fat both declined with the proportion of forage in the diet (Table 14.5).

Changes in level of food intake have in the majority of experiments been achieved by varying the amount of concentrated food offered and holding the amount of forage constant, and the effects on fat secretion have therefore been confounded with those of change in diet composition. Increases in the intake of a diet of constant composition cause a decrease in fat content and the effect is more pronounced when the proportion of the concentrated food in the diet is high (Table 14.5).

Table 14.5 The effect of the proportion of hay in the diet on milk yield and composition in cows with high or low energy intakes (I. H. L. Ormrod and P. C. Thomas, unpublished results)

Level of energy intake	Proportion of hay:concentrate	Milk yield (kg/day)	Fat content (g/kg)	Fat yield (g/day)
Low	40:60	16.4	39.7	650
	20:80	17.2	36.8	634
High	40:60	17.8	36.9	657
	20:80	19.1	31.0	593
s.e. of difference		0.07	2.7	17

The quality of forage of major importance for fat secretion, its physical fibrousness, is not chemically definable and has yet to be defined precisely in physical terms. Attempts have been made to characterize it in terms of the screen size used for milling, and a critical aperture size of 6.4 mm has been suggested (O'Dell, King and Cook, 1968). However, using a single screen size of 1.6 mm aperture, particle size and hence milk fat content have been altered by speed of milling (Rodrigue and Allen, 1960). Balch (1971) has proposed a biological assessment of fibrousness, based on the chewing time required per unit of dry matter consumed, which is claimed to relate closely to the milk-fat depressing effect of a diet.

Many soluble sugars, when introduced into the diet as isolated materials or as part of natural foods such as fodder beet or whey, tend to promote butyric acid production in the rumen and to maintain or increase milk-fat content (Kellog and Owen, 1969; Clark, Geerken, Preston and Zamora, 1973; Schingoethe, 1976). An apparent exception is found with young herbage, which has a high content of soluble carbohydrates but tends to depress milk-fat content (Rook, 1961b). This effect is generally ascribed to low dietary fibre content but it is notable that silages made from immature grass have quite different characteristics and tend to produce low-propionate fermentations in the milk-fat contents (Chalmers, Thomas and Belibasakis, 1978).

It is customary to process cereal grains when they are offered to cattle, which are less efficient than sheep in digesting the whole grain, and milo and maize are usually heat treated as they are less digestible than other cereals (Armstrong, 1972). Heat treatment of cereals exacerbates their depressing effect on milk-fat content, especially when the cereals are included in diets containing less than approximately 400 g of forage per kg (Coppock, 1976). Extensive processing treatments are now common; an example is the steam-flaking of maize. In general, the effect of processing is related to the effect on fermentation in the rumen: the more rapid the rate of fermentation induced, the wider the ratio of propionate to other acids and the lower the milk-fat content. A slower rate of fermentation may be achieved by selecting cereals with a high fibre content, such as oats, or those which are less fermentable, such as raw maize. Reducing the degree of processing is also effective, and Ørskov and Greenhalgh (1977) have recently developed a technique which avoids the need for physical processing through treatment of the whole grain with sodium hydroxide.

Altering the frequency of feeding of cows from the usual twice-daily feeding to between 6 and 24 times daily feeding without changing the amount of diet has increased milk-fat yield, although not invariably. In a recent study, increases in milk-fat content of up to 10 g/kg were observed in response to an increase in the frequency of feeding of cows from 2 to 6 or 24 times daily when the diet contained 900 g of concentrated food per kg but not when the diet contained only 600 g of concentrated food per kg (see Broster, Sutton and Bines, 1979). When complete diets, in which all the components are mixed together intimately, were first introduced, they were generally pelleted with the forage component finely ground, and such diets often caused a depression in milk-fat content. With the development of feeder wagons, diet components can be efficiently mixed in an unmodified form and there is then no consistent effect on milk-fat content.

When low-forage diets are offered there are inverse relationships between the molar proportion of propionic acid in the rumen, and the rumen pH and liquid clearance rate (Sutton and Johnson, 1969; Hodgson and Thomas, 1976), and attempts have been made to prevent the depression of milk-fat content by the inclusion in the diet of additives designed to increase salivary flow or to buffer rumen liquor. Plastic particles have proved ineffective, but aspen sawdust (320 g/kg) or bentonite (50 g/kg) included in the concentrate have reduced the depression in milk-fat content and the reduction in food intake and milk yield has been slight. Dietary additions of sodium and potassium bicarbonate, calcium hydroxide, magnesium carbonate and magnesium oxide, but not calcium carbonate, have reduced the depression of milk fat but often in association with a reduction in food intake and milk yield (see Sutton, 1980). The mechanism of action of magnesium oxide, however, is thought to be a stimulation of triglyceride uptake by the mammary gland and not a change in rumen fermentation. A partial recovery in milk-fat content can be achieved by addition of acetic acid to the diet or drinking water: the most practical and physiologically acceptable forms would appear to be the calcium and ammonium salts but additions of these materials to normal diets have had only a small effect on milk-fat content (Hutton, Prescott, Seeley and Armstrong, 1969; Jackson and Rook, 1970).

Dietary lipid

As the observed response in milk-fat secretion to an alteration in the amount and composition of dietary fat is the net result of several independent but interrelated processes, these will be considered separately before attempting to assess the overall effect on milk composition.

Synthesis de novo *of fatty acids in the mammary gland.* The synthesis within the mammary gland of C_4 to C_{16} fatty acids is often depressed by dietary addition of lipids, whether they are in the form of fats, oils or long-chain fatty acids, an effect which has been attributed primarily to an altered rumen fermentation causing a reduction in the plasma concentrations of acetate and 3-hydroxybutyrate (Storry, 1972). Offering the fats or oils in a 'protected' form (see p. 587) reduces substantially the influence on rumen fermentation and the depression in the synthesis *de novo* of fatty acids; the form of inclusion of unprotected oils or fats and their frequency of feeding (Banks, Clapperton, Kelly, Wilson and Crawford, 1980) also modifies the extent of the changes. Certain fatty acids, for example lauric acid, when fed as the free acid or as a component of an unprotected oil, can have a profound effect on rumen fermentation (Rindsig and Schultz, 1974). Whether or not effects on fatty acid synthesis *de novo* can be explained principally in terms of an altered rumen fermentation is, however, still unresolved (Banks *et al.*, 1976b).

Microbial synthesis of fatty acids in the rumen. A net synthesis of lipid during the fermentation of food in the rumen is frequently observed, and there is evidence that this is enhanced by diets that contain a high proportion of starchy concentrated foods (Sutton *et al.*, 1970) and depressed by dietary supplements of fats and oils (Sutton, Smith, McAllan, Storry and Corse, 1975). The constituent fatty acids of the synthesized fat are mainly stearic and palmitic but also include small amounts of acids with an odd number of carbon atoms or a branched-chain that are components of the structural lipids of bacteria.

Mammary uptake and desaturation of plasma fatty acids.   The desaturase of the mammary gland is inhibited by normal C_{18} unsaturated fatty acids (Bickerstaffe and Annison, 1970) and by cyclopropene fatty acids, such as the sterculic acid of *Sterculia* seeds, not normally present in the diet of the cow (Bauman and Davis, 1975). The cyclopropene fatty acids also inhibit mammary uptake of fatty acids from plasma triglycerides, as do the polyunsaturated fatty acids containing 20 or more carbon atoms that are found in cod-liver and other fish oils (Storry, Brumby, Hall and Tuckley, 1974b; see Ch. 8).

Transfer of individual fatty acids from the diet to milk fat.   Supplementation of the diet with lipids is usually associated with an increased transfer of component fatty acids of the supplement to milk fat but, because of the several factors that influence the metabolism and secretion of individual fatty acids, the relative efficiency of transfer of the various acids from the diet to milk is difficult to assess with certainty. In comparisons of diets containing fat in a constant amount of different composition, values of 900 g/kg have been obtained for the transfer of incremental amounts of palmitic acid and of 300 to 550 g/kg for total C_{18} acids (Banks *et al.*, 1976a). A value as low as 270 g/kg has been observed for lauric acid included in the diet as the free acid (Storry, Hall and Johnson, 1971), probably because of a change of rumen fermentation pattern causing a depression of synthesis *de novo* of fatty acids, including lauric acid. A higher efficiency of 420 g/kg for lauric acid and a value of 480 g/kg for myristic acid was found when the dietary supplement was in the form of 'protected' coconut oil (Bauman and Davis, 1975). Low efficiencies of transfer are obtained for fatty acids containing less than 12 carbon atoms as, in addition to any effect there may be on synthesis *de novo* in the mammary gland, the acids are rapidly metabolized in liver and other tissues (Guisard, Gonand, Laurent and Debry, 1970). There is also a low transfer of C_{20} and C_{22} acids, of cod-liver oil for example (Brumby *et al.*, 1972), as these are incorporated preferentially into the cholesterol ester and phospholipid fractions of the plasma lipoproteins that are not used by the mammary gland for milk fat synthesis. The efficiency of transfer of individual fatty acids is also affected by the extent of desaturation of the longer-chain fatty acids in the mammary gland and, especially, by the extensive hydrogenation of unsaturated, particularly C_{18} polyunsaturated, fatty acids in the rumen. Also of importance is the level and frequency of feeding, and the amount of fat and of individual fatty acids in the diet, which influence the partition of nutrient use between the mammary gland and other tissues and the extent of fatty acid synthesis *de novo* in the mammary gland. These modifying factors presumably account, for example, for the poor correlation between dietary intake of palmitic acid and its output in milk fat observed in

many experiments; small amounts (100 g/day) of supplementary palmitic acid, as a component of soya bean oil, included as a substituent in a fat-deficient basal diet cause a pronounced depression in the
output of C_{16} and of other short-chain acids in milk fat because
of a substantial reduction in the *de novo* synthesis of fatty acids
(Banks *et al.*, 1976b).

Net effects on the fatty acid composition of milk fat.　Storry (1980)
has quoted examples of the effects on milk fatty acid composition of
adding different amounts of red palm-oil, tallow, coconut oil or
cod-liver oil to diets of hay and concentrated foods low in fat offered
twice daily, and these are given in Table 14.6, together with similar
observations for soya bean oil. The observations selected are broadly
consistent with others obtained using basal diets containing either a
high or a low proportion of hay, or silage and cereals containing a normal or a low amount of fat (for references, see Storry, 1980).

These results demonstrate that a substantial increase in the dietary
supply of a fatty acid containing 12 to 20 carbon atoms increases the
uptake of the fatty acid by the mammary gland and the proportion of
the fatty acid in milk fat. This is true even for C_{18} polyunsaturated fatty
acids that are extensively hydrogenated in the rumen, but there is often
a lack of consistency in response when only small amounts of supplementary C_{18} polyunsaturated fatty acids are offered.

The incorporation of preformed fatty acid in the diet necessarily
causes decreased proportions of other acids in milk fat, unless the acid is
used for the formation of other fatty acids in the mammary gland or in
the rumen. When myristic, palmitic and stearic acids are given singly,
there is an increase not only in the parent acid but also in the
corresponding mono-unsaturated acids, myristoleic, palmitoleic and
oleic, respectively, due to intramammary desaturation. Hydrogenation in
the rumen of dietary linoleic and linolenic acids gives as products the *trans*
isomer of oleic acid (elaidic acid) and stearic acid, and the proportions of
these acids increase when the dietary supply of linoleic and linolenic acids
is increased.

Further reductions in the proportions of other acids can occur when
there is inhibition of mammary uptake or desaturation of fatty acids, or
depression of fatty acid synthesis *de novo*.

The observed changes in the fatty acid composition of milk fat reflect
largely those in the main triglyceride fraction but smaller changes are
observed in the composition of the phospholipids of the fat globule
membrane (Smith and Abraham, 1975).

'Protection' of dietary fat.　The ingestion of large amounts of
dietary fat interferes with rumen function and causes a loss of appetite.
Conversely, there is extensive hydrogenation in the rumen of dietary

Table 14.6 Effect of inclusion of increasing amounts of fats or oils† on the composition (g/kg) of the major fatty acids of milk fat (sources of information: Storry, 1980 and Banks et al., 1980)

Proportion of added oil or fat(g/kg)	Coconut oil			Red palm-oil			Tallow			Soya bean oil			Cod-liver oil		
	0	40	100	0	40	80	0	40	100	0	50	100	0	19	56
Fatty acid															
4:0	33	38	33	33	33	38	31	34	39	ND‡	ND	ND	19	18	18
6:0	22	21	21	25	24	24	29	26	21	28	23	18	28	28	21
8:0	13	13	12	17	16	15	18	16	11	17	12	9	17	18	12
10:0	39	36	32	42	31	29	47	37	21	34	21	16	40	36	27
12:0	59	90	132	58	44	35	56	41	22	44	28	21	50	47	42
14:0	154	171	193	153	125	111	153	130	93	120	93	73	155	154	149
14:1	22	21	24	19	16	13	27	22	14	18	13	10	14	16	19
16:0	417	387	312	394	352	368	365	318	295	400	270	240	391	374	348
16:1	33	30	29	27	30	28	33	29	34	29	27	23	17	22	35
18:0	27	27	29	35	70	66	44	75	101	76	150	190	14	19	2
18:1	126	122	138	144	207	236	149	197	281	190	310	360	199	208	243
18:2 } 18:3	7	6	4	11	9	9	15	19	14	−32	44	47	17	13	10

† The major fatty acids are: coconut oil, 10:0, 12:0, 14:0, 16:0; red palm-oil, 16:0, 18:0, 18:1, 18:2; tallow, 16:0, 18:0, 18:1, 18:2; soya bean oil 16:0, 18:1, 20:1, 20:5, 22:1, 22:6.
‡ ND, not determined.

unsaturated fatty acids, a factor that accounts for the characteristically low content of polyunsaturated fatty acids in the flesh and milk fat of ruminants. Processing methods have been devised to restrict the interaction between dietary lipids and rumen microorganisms. These methods involve coating minute droplets of lipid with protein and then treating the protein such that it resists breakdown in the rumen but is hydrolysed readily in the abomasum. Initially, extracted oils were used, mixed with casein, spray-dried and then treated with formaldehyde. Subsequently, a more economic method was developed of using crushed oil seeds to supply both the oil and much of the protein (Scott, Bready, Royal and Cook, 1972).

Feeding oils rich in linoleic acid protected in this way has produced milk fats containing 50 to 60 g linoleic acid per kg of fatty acids with preparations based on soya bean or cottonseed oil (oils containing 530 to 600 g linoleic acid per kg) and up to 350 g/kg for preparations based on safflower oil (an oil containing up to 800 g linoleic acid per kg). The value for commercial bulk milk is approximately 30 g/kg (Fogerty and Johnson, 1980). 'Protected' non-polyunsaturated fats when included in the diet give greater responses in fat yield (increases of up to 25 to 30% have been observed with normal diets) than corresponding amounts of unprotected fat, as the depression in mammary synthesis *de novo* of fatty acids is much reduced (Storry, Brumby, Hall and Johnson, 1974a). 'Protected' lipids can be used also to offset the depression in milk-fat content caused by diets lacking in physical fibrousness. By this means fatty acids can be incorporated in the diet in quantities sufficient to compensate for the increased partition of fatty acid use towards adipose tissue as well as compensating for the decreased mammary synthesis of fatty acids, without having an adverse effect on rumen fermentation (Storry *et al.*, 1974a).

Structural and physical characteristics of milk fat. The physical properties of fats are affected both by the component fatty acids and by the distribution of fatty acids in the triglyceride molecule. In spite of the complex mixture of triglycerides in milk fat, which differ substantially in molecular weight and degree of saturation, there is considerable constancy in the stereospecific distribution of the fatty acids in the triglycerides. The major source of variation in physical characteristics is probably, therefore, the relative proportions of triglycerides of different molecular weight and degree of unsaturation, and consequently the chain length and degree of unsaturation of the constituent fatty acids. The greater the contribution from low molecular weight and unsaturated triglycerides, the greater the proportion of low-melting triglycerides and the softer the milk fat. In New Zealand, milk production is largely from grass, and as the grazing season progresses the properties of milk fat change from soft in the spring to hard in the summer and softer again in the autumn. These changes have been related to a gradual, probably lactational, decline in the proportion of butyric acid in milk fat, and to increases in the proportion of C_6 to C_{16} saturated acids and decreases in $C_{18:0}$ and $C_{18:1}$ acids from spring to summer, and reverse changes in the autumn (McDowall, McGillivray and Hawke, 1961), which are probably dietary in origin. In the northern hemisphere, the dominant dietary influence on milk-fat composition is the change from winter stall feeding to spring and summer grazing; winter milk fat is harder, and has a lower proportion of $C_{18:0}$ and $C_{18:1}$ acids, and a higher proportion of $C_{16:0}$ acids, than summer milk fat (Reiter, Sorokin, Pickering and Hall, 1969).

Supplementation of normal diets with oils or fats causes the changes in physical properties of the milk fat that would be expected from the change in fatty acid composition. This is exemplified most readily by feeding 'protected' oils rich in linoleic acid, which results in a substantially increased content of the acid in milk fat (Morrison and Hawke, 1977); and by increasing the ratio of C_{18} to C_{16} acids in the diet, which increases the proportion of monounsaturated (specifically oleic) acids because of the more extensive desaturation of $C_{18:0}$ than of $C_{16:0}$ in the mammary gland of the cow. Both treatments produce a softer fat for butter production (Banks, Clapperton and Ferrie, 1974).

Mid-lactation effects of diet on milk protein content

In many feeding experiments the non-protein nitrogenous (NPN) constituents of milk have been ignored and milk protein content has been measured as total nitrogen $\times 6.38$ (the accepted average nitrogen content for milk protein has traditionally been 156.8 g/kg although modern analyses suggest a more appropriate value is 158.9 g/kg). NPN is present in milk in concentrations which range from 150 to 500 mg/kg, and the largest and most variable component is urea. Urea diffuses freely throughout body water and the concentration in milk reflects that in blood plasma. Factors that influence plasma urea concentration, such as the nitrogen content of the diet or the ingestion of large quantities of water, also affect therefore the NPN content of milk. There is no evidence of dietary effects on the composition of milk proteins in the cow, although effects of dietary protein, carbohydrate and lipid intake on milk total protein content have been observed.

Dietary protein

Experiments using conventional diets of hay and concentrate foods have demonstrated effects of dietary protein content on milk true protein content (crude protein − NPN) where there has been protein undernutrition, although effects on crude protein content reflecting changes in milk NPN occur more widely. With diets providing 80% of the digestible crude protein standards for maintenance and milk production, no effect on milk true protein content was evident (Frens and Dijkstra, 1959; Rook and Line, 1962) but, with diets providing only 60% of these standards, reductions in protein content of 1 to 2.5 g/kg were observed (Rowland, 1946; Breirem, 1949). These effects presumably reflect inadequacies in the supply of amino acids to the tissues and, in support of this, Schwab *et al.* (1976), using diets containing 107 to 115 g crude protein per kg, observed that responses in milk protein yield to postruminal infusions of essential amino acids occurred mainly through effects on milk protein content. Responses in protein content to dietary additions of proteins resistant to ruminal breakdown might therefore occur in practice in situations where, with high yielding cows or with particular diets, the demand for amino acids exceeds the supply reaching the small intestine. Unusually low values for milk protein content have been reported in some experiments with grass-silage diets (Murdoch and Rook, 1963; Castle and Watson, 1969). These diets contain adequate digestible crude protein but they are associated with low concentrations of methionine, and to a lesser extent lysine, in the mixture of proteins passing to the duodenum (Thomas, Chamberlain, Kelly and Wait, 1980). Rogers *et al.* (1979) observed that, in cows given diets solely of grass silage, intra-abomasal infusions of methionine (12 g/day) increased milk protein content by 3 g/kg, which is consistent with the idea that milk protein content is limited by methionine supply. However, in a more recent experiment with cows given diets of 700 g silage and 300 g mineralized barley per kg, intravenous infusion of methionine (8 g/day) gave a significant increase in milk fat yield but with no response in milk protein content (D. G. Chamberlain and P. C. Thomas, unpublished results).

Dietary carbohydrate

The most widely recognized effect of diet on milk protein content is that observed with a change in the 'plane of energy nutrition'. The effect is often interpreted as a simple relationship between milk protein content and dietary energy supply but it is in reality more complex. An increase in the 'plane of energy nutrition' has in most experiments been achieved through the feeding of additional starchy concentrate foods, such as flaked maize, and the effects on milk protein content are related to combined changes in the energy intake, proportion of concentrate in the diet and composition of the concentrate mixture.

'Plane of energy nutrition' effects have been observed to increase milk protein content by as much as 5 g/kg but increases are more typically 2 to 3 g/kg and in some dietary circumstances may be less than 1 g/kg (Wright, Rook and Wood, 1974). The dietary response is due in part to the change in energy intake *per se*, since animals given a diet of constant composition show a depression in milk protein content of approximately 1 g/kg when subjected to mild undernutrition (I. H. L. Ormrod and P. C. Thomas, unpublished results). However, reductions in the dietary ratio of forage to concentrate have increased milk protein content both in animals receiving an adequate energy intake and in those subjected to moderate undernutrition (Chalmers, Thomas and Kelly, 1977), and similar responses have been obtained, although not invariably, when flaked maize has been substituted for barley in the diet (Balch, Balch, Bartlett, Johnson, Rowland and Turner, 1954). Fine-grinding of the forage can enhance milk protein content too, as can the feeding of 'low-fibre' forages. Increases in milk protein content are generally observed when cattle commence grazing pasture in the spring although the response is modified by the level of feeding during the winter period (Rook, Line and Rowland, 1960).

The observed changes in milk protein content have been related to the effects of the amount and composition of the diet on the pattern of fermentation in the rumen, specifically on the ruminal production of propionic acid. Infusions of dilute aqueous solutions of propionic acid into the rumen of cows receiving hay and concentrate diets have given increases in milk protein content of the same order as those achieved by a change of diet (Rook, Balch and Johnson, 1965; Fig. 14.5), although infusions given intra-abomasally (Frobish and Davis, 1977) or intravenously (Fisher and Elliot, 1966) have not produced a similar response. With diets containing silage, prepared from grass cut at an early stage of growth, and possibly with other silages also, the amount and composition of cereals in the diet has a comparatively small effect on rumen fermentation pattern and milk composition (Chalmers *et al.*, 1978). Additionally, with these diets intraruminal infusions of propionic acid have failed to elicit a significant response in milk protein content (Chalmers, Thomas and Chamberlain, 1980), possibly because of limitations on milk secretion imposed by the supply of amino acids to the small intestine (p. 591).

Dietary fat

Depressions in milk protein content consequent upon the incorporation in the diet of fats of various composition have been reported (Steele, Noble and Moore, 1971; Macleod and Wood, 1972; Maltos and Palmquist, 1974) but the basis of the effects has yet to be explained.

Mid-lactation effects on lactose and other water-soluble constituents

The direct effect of feeding on milk lactose content is slight. Underfeeding causes a small depression, usually less than 1 g/kg (Dawson and Rook, 1972) but there are more marked changes during starvation (Smith, Howat and Ray, 1938; Robertson, Paver, Barden and Marr, 1960). The changes are linked to a fall in milk yield and appear to derive from a reduction in the contribution of lactose to the osmotic pressure of milk as secretory activity is depressed; the milk concentrations of sodium and chloride are increased.

Studies at other stages of lactation

There is an underlying cyclical pattern in the reproducing, lactating animal of a deposition of nutrients during pregnancy (in addition to those deposited in the foetal and uterine tissues and fluids) and of a mobilization of nutrients during lactation, especially in the early stages. Thus, with the usual systems of dairy cow management the course of lactation is accompanied by a progressive change from mobilization of body tissue at the beginning of lactation to deposition at the end, and in the dry period (see Fig. 14.1). The diet offered at one stage of the lactation cycle may thus influence milk production at other stages, directly through effects on the growth, development and maintenance of mammary tissue, and indirectly through effects on body condition and nutrient stores. The responses in milk production identified in mid-lactation are therefore modified at other stages of lactation by the inherent trends of the lactation cycle, and the modulation of those trends by present and previous nutrition.

Early lactation: milk yield

The daily intakes of food pre- and post-calving have pronounced, separate effects on milk yield during the early lactation period. As with feeding during lactation, responses to pre-calving feeding follow the pattern of the law of diminishing returns, and a model linking pre- and post-calving feeding in their effects on milk yield has been proposed (Fig. 14.8). There is an innate limit to milk yield above which it cannot be raised by improved feeding either pre- or post-calving and severe undernutrition at either stage may preclude the possibility of maximum yield being achieved. Between these extremes, however, the effects of feeding before and after calving are additive and complementary, but the effect of pre-calving nutrition may be restricted by the cow's ability to mobilize body tissues in support of milk secretion. In mature, high-yielding cows, the amounts of tissue mobilized can be very large, and Flatt, Coppock and Moore (1965) observed a maximum value of more than 80 MJ/day in one individual animal. The tissue mobilized is mainly adipose tissue since, although cows may go into negative nitrogen balance in early lactation (Wohlt, Clark and Blaisdell, 1978), the evidence indicates that their labile body protein reserves are limited. Coppock, Tyrell, Merrill and Reid (1968) estimated that in Holstein cows protein reserves may provide amino acids for the production of 126 kg of milk whereas fat reserves could with some cows provide energy for the production of 1000 kg.

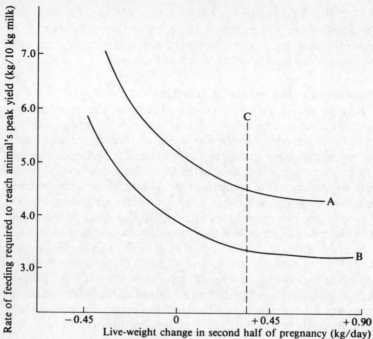

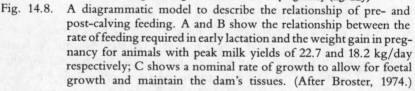

Fig. 14.8.   A diagrammatic model to describe the relationship of pre- and post-calving feeding. A and B show the relationship between the rate of feeding required in early lactation and the weight gain in pregnancy for animals with peak milk yields of 22.7 and 18.2 kg/day respectively; C shows a nominal rate of growth to allow for foetal growth and maintain the dam's tissues. (After Broster, 1974.)

The extent of utilization of body reserves in early lactation is dependent on the body condition at calving, on the animal's capacity for milk secretion, and on the amount and composition of the diet. In mid-lactation the absorption of large amounts of propionic acid from the rumen or glucose from the small intestine, as may occur with high-concentrate diets, alters the partition of energy use between milk secretion and body tissue deposition, and leads to a reduction in milk fat content (p. 579). In early lactation such diets reduce tissue mobilization (Table 14.2) and depress milk yield as well as milk fat content.

Protein undernutrition may also limit tissue mobilization under certain circumstances, although whether protein deficiency limits milk synthesis and therefore energy use by the mammary gland or influences tissue mobilization more directly has not been fully established (see below). In newly calved cows severely underfed for both energy and protein, Ørskov, Grubb and Kay (1977) demonstrated substantial responses in milk yield to the intra-abomasal infusion of casein that could only be accounted for in energetic terms by an enhanced mobilization of body tissues; the infusion of glucose was without effect. More recently, however, in cows given a low protein diet at a level of intake typical of that normally achieved by cows in the early lactation period, the effect of casein infusion was small and not significant (Oldham, Lobley, Konig, Parker and Smith, 1980). Additionally, in several other experiments conducted with cows given 'normal' levels of feeding, dietary inclusions of fish meal, a protein food with a low rumen–degradability that might be anticipated to increase the passage of amino acids to the small intestine, have given relatively small responses in milk yield and little evidence of a protein-regulated stimulation of tissue mobilization (P. C. Thomas, D. G. Chamberlain and S. Robertson, unpublished results; E. R. Ørskov, personal communication).

Early lactation: milk composition

The typical, mid-lactation responses in milk composition to feeding are modified in early lactation by the level of pre-partum feeding, by the contribution to milk secretion of nutrients from body stores, and by the early-lactational relationships between milk yield and composition. Variations in energy and protein nutrition leading to an enhanced mobilization of adipose tissue increase milk-fat content and alter its fatty acid composition towards that of body fat. Energy undernutrition pre- or immediately post-calving may also delay or prevent the attainment of peak yield and in these circumstances the lactose content fails to increase to its maximum value, which is usually more or less coincident with the peak in yield, and the lactational reduction in protein content is slowed. As a consequence, energy undernutrition may have less effect on milk-protein content in early lactation than in mid-lactation, and in the first few days of lactation protein content may actually be increased by underfeeding (Wright *et al.*, 1974). In cows given low-protein or low-protein, low-energy diets, milk protein content has been raised significantly by the intra-abomasal infusion of casein (Ørskov *et al.*, 1977; Oldham *et al.*, 1980) and corresponding, although smaller, effects on protein content have been observed, in cows given moderate-protein diets, in response to dietary additions of fish meal (P. C. Thomas, D. G. Chamberlain and S. Robertson, unpublished results).

Late lactation

In late lactation, the effects of feeding on milk yield and composition tend to be dominated by the influence of the level of energy intake on the rate of loss of secretory function. Giving additional food produces a slight reversal or retardation of the lactational trends in milk yield and composition whilst underfeeding leads to a sharp and sometimes irreversible decline in milk yield, to a decrease in lactose content, and to increases in milk-fat and protein contents (Dawson and Rook, 1972; Thomas and Kelly, 1976).

Interactions between early and later stages of lactation

As indicated earlier, the responsiveness of milk yield to changes in energy intake declines as lactation progresses and milk yield itself declines. Thus the milk yield attained in early lactation influences the yield which can be achieved in later lactation and in the lactation as a whole. The residual effects of level of early-lactation feeding on subsequent milk production have been studied by Broster and his colleagues in a number of large-scale feeding experiments with heifer cows (see Broster, 1974). These experiments have shown that underfeeding in early lactation not only depresses the current milk yield but establishes a pattern in the partition of dietary nutrients between milk secretion and body tissue deposition which persists into the mid-lactation period (Fig. 14.9). Summarizing these results, Broster (1974) suggested that, for cows underfed for 8 to 12 weeks in early lactation and subsequently given the same amount of food as their normally fed counterparts, the effect of underfeeding on the whole lactation yield is approximately four times as great as that on the yield in early lactation. The size of the residual effect, however, varies with the degree of underfeeding in early lactation (and this should be defined in terms of the amounts of nutrients available from the diet and body tissues relative to the amounts required to allow the development of the cow's full milk-yield potential) and with the scope for underfed cows to compensate for their early lactation undernutrition by increasing food intake in mid and late lactation. In several studies with cows given reduced amounts of concentrates in early lactation with silage *ad libitum*, followed by grazing in the mid-lactation period, milk yield in early lactation has been reduced but residual effects have been less pronounced and less persistent than those observed by Broster and his colleagues, and the reduction in total lactation yield has been small (see Gordon, 1977). Likewise, only small effects on total lactation yield were obtained by varying the pattern of distribution of a fixed quantity of food during the first 20 weeks of lactation, although in high-yielding cows graded rates of feeding produced higher early lactation milk yields than flat rates of feeding (Johnson, 1977).

Effects of underfeeding in early lactation on milk composition in subsequent periods of adequate feeding have been suggested in a number of studies, but the results are not clear-cut. Effects on milk-fat content vary between experiments and no consistent pattern has emerged (see Broster, Broster and Smith, 1969), and whilst effects on solids-not-fat content are more reproducible there are difficulties in their interpretation. Wright *et al.* (1974) found that underfeeding in the pre-calving and early-lactation periods led to a reduction in milk

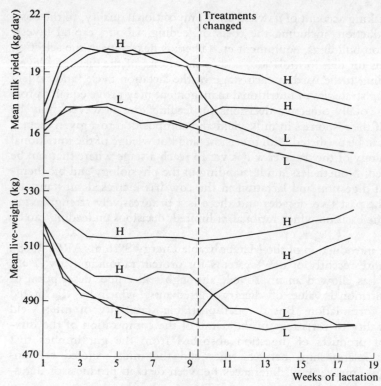

Fig. 14.9. Mean milk yields and live weights of groups of first lactation Friesian cows given one of two levels of feeding in weeks 1 to 9 of lactation followed by one of the same two levels in weeks 10 to 18 (H, high level of feeding; L, low level of feeding). (After Broster, 1974.)

solids–not–fat content in early lactation; initially, there was a distinct depression of lactose content but as lactation progressed that effect was lessened and protein content was decreased. Restoration of normal feeding in mid-lactation produced only a small improvement in milk solids–not–fat and protein contents but, when the cows were later turned out to graze, milk protein content increased substantially. These results therefore suggest that the lack of response to improved feeding in mid-lactation was a reflexion of the character of the mid-lactation diet rather than of any inherent inability of the animals to respond due to the residual effect of previous underfeeding.

Nutritional management of the dairy cow

Strategies for the nutritional management of dairy cows must ulti-mately be judged in economic terms that relate the income from milk, taking account of its yield and compositional quality, to the costs of production, including the costs of feeding, labour, capital investments on buildings, equipment etc. There is flexibility in the selection of foods for diet formulation, and in the choice of the diets and levels of feeding to be used at each stage of the lactation cycle, and widely differing strategies of nutritional management may prove equally profitable. Totally objective decisions on feeding can, however, only be made if the responses in milk yield and composition to a given dietary input can be predicted with precision, and knowledge of the nutritional physiology of the dairy cow has yet to reach a stage where that can be achieved. Nonetheless, understanding of the physiology and biochemistry of digestion and lactation in the cow has increased substantially over the past two decades and there is a progressively strengthening scientific basis on which rational, if limited, decisions on feeding can be made.

The introduction of the Metabolizable Energy System (ARC, 1965), and more recently of new systems for protein rationing (Roy *et al.*, 1977), has allowed an improved, although still crude, description of the nutritional value of dietary ingredients, which has facilitated ration formulation. But the demonstrable sensitivity of milk yield and quality to variations in the detail of the composition of the mixture of products of digestion absorbed from the gut implies that precise relationships between diet and the milk secreted are unlikely to emerge until differences between diets in products of digestion are taken into account.

Additionally, there is need to allow for the differences between individual cows, and between early and late lactation, in the partition of dietary nutrients between milk secretion and body tissue deposition, and for the residual effects of pre-calving and early-lactation feeding on later lactation performance. Some progress in these areas has been made through the development of a system for condition scoring (Lowman, Scott and Somerville, 1973) that provides an estimate of body tissue reserves, and through the use of the mathematical description of the shape of the lactation curve (p. 563) to extrapolate from one stage of lactation to another.

In practice, most current strategies of nutritional management place emphasis on adequacy of feeding in early lactation to allow the cow to achieve its full potential in terms of peak milk yield. Thereafter the diet is adjusted to meet the animal's estimated requirements for maintenance, milk production and, as appropriate, body weight gain. This approach focuses particular attention on the use of body reserves in early lactation and on the nutrient density of the diet, which must be sufficiently high to offset the effects of the post-calving restrictions on dry-matter intake (Fig. 14.1). Nutrient density is most frequently increased through the dietary inclusion of cereal concentrate foods in

replacement for forages and, understandably, there has been application in early lactation of techniques for manipulation of rumen fermentation, to avoid the development of high-propionate fermentation
patterns and associated effects on milk yield and composition. An
alternative way to increase the energy content of the diet is to use
concentrates containing protected lipid. This will improve total energy
intake although there may be reductions in the *ad libitum* intake of
forage, probably as a consequence of an incomplete protection of the
lipid and interference with rumen microbial function (see Storry,
Brumby and Dunkley, 1980). Protected supplements of soya bean/
tallow included in a hay and concentrate diet increased milk, milk
energy, fat and lactose yields with additions of up to 1 kg/day but at
higher levels the response disappeared or became negative, particularly
for lactose. The effects on protein yield were much less marked and
became negative at intakes over approximately 0.5 kg/day. Fat content
increased, protein content was reduced and responses in lactose content
were variable. There was no indication of a change in live-weight loss
due to the inclusion of the supplement but yield of total milk fat was
related positively to dietary intakes of total fatty acids and carbohydrate, and negatively to live-weight changes (Bines, Brumby, Storry,
Fulford and Braithwaite, 1978).

Dietary manipulation of milk composition

The modification of milk composition by diet offers the possibility of
manipulating by natural means the composition and characteristics of
milk and its products to meet the needs of specialist consumers, and yet
to retain the distinctive nature of a dairy product. Several possibilities
have been investigated and some products have been test-marketed.

Fat and protein contents

Diets based on ground and pelleted hay and ground or heated
corn (maize) have been used for the production of milk with a depressed fat content (Ensor, Shaw and Tellechea, 1959). A depression in
milk-fat content of greater, on average, than 50% was obtained both
with a diet of 12.7 kg ground and pelleted hay and 1.8 kg heated corn,
and with one of 2.7 kg ground and pelleted hay and 8.2 kg heated corn,
but there was a lack of consistency between cows presumably because
with low fibre, high cereal diets, fermentation pattern is variable and
unstable. There is no reason to suppose that milk of a reduced fat
content could not be produced readily under commercial conditions but
development work is required to determine the particular depression in

milk-fat content that should be sought and the certainty with which the selected fat content may be achieved.

The diets that reduce fat content also give a small increase in protein content and a further benefit is that the milk fat is richer in linoleic acid than normal milk fat; values as high as 40 to 50 g/kg of the total fatty acids have been recorded (King and Hemken, 1962; Storry and Sutton, 1969). Attempts have been made to enhance further the linoleic acid content by incorporation in the diet of 'unprotected' oil seed preparations, but so far unsuccessfully (Clapperton, Kelly, Banks and Rook, 1980). With the current medical concern about the high intake of saturated animal fats, a milk with a lower proportion of fat, rich in essential fatty acids, and of high protein content could have market potential.

Milk-fat composition

The presence within the mammary gland of a desaturase mechanism and its high specificity for the conversion of stearic to oleic acid allows the physical properties of milk fat to be manipulated by feeding free oils. Generally, if an oil is rich in C_{18} acids the milk fat will contain a high proportion of relatively low-melting material and produce a soft butter, whereas if the oil is rich in C_{16} acids the proportion of the higher-melting material will be increased and a harder butter produced.

The addition of soya oil to the diet has been used by Banks and his colleagues (Banks *et al.*, 1976a) to improve the low-temperature spreadability of butter. An effect is achieved principally because the soya oil is rich in C_{18} acids but also because a high proportion of these acids is polyunsaturated and there is a partial transfer to milk fat of the small proportion of the polyunsaturated acids that escape hydrogenation in the rumen.

A more extensive transfer of polyunsaturated fatty acids achieved by 'protecting' the oil from rumen microbial action has also been used to increase the essential fatty acid content of milk fat and to alter the physical characteristics (Scott, Cook, Ferguson, McDonald, Buchanan and Loftus-Hills, 1970). Although the feeding of 'protected' polyunsaturated oils has in some instances produced milk fats containing 200 to 300 g of linoleic acid per kg of fatty acids, the response has been variable. The proportion of dietary 'protected' linoleic acid that has ultimately appeared in milk fat has ranged from 80 to 400 g/kg, the value varying with the amount of supplement, the basal diet, the stage of lactation, and the individuality and breed of cow.

The effect of modification of milk-fat composition on the melting profile of the anhydrous fat, and on the stand-up and oiling-off properties of the butter, is shown in Fig. 14.10 and Table 14.7 in comparison with values for conventional fats. The milk fat of cows re-

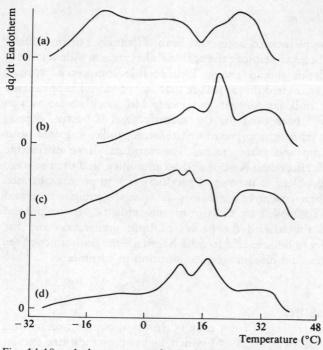

Fig. 14.10. A thermogram obtained using a differential scanning calorimeter of various anhydrous milk fats: (a) a luxury tub margarine; (b) a winter milk fat; (c) a milk fat from cows receiving a winter diet supplemented with soya bean oil; and (d) a mixture of sunflower seed oil (200 g/kg) and milk fat (800 g/kg).

Table 14.7 The stand-up and oiling-off properties of various spreads (see Rook, 1977)

Spread	Temperature (°C)	Stand-up height (proportion of original height)	Oiling off (weight of free oil) (g/kg)
Polyunsaturated butter ($120 \text{ g } C_{18:2}$ per kg)	21	0.95	8
Polyunsaturated butter ($200 \text{ g } C_{18:2}$ per kg)	21	0.71	27
Tub margarine	21	0.93	22
Conventional butter	21	0.98	2
'Winter' butter	15	1.00	1
	30	0.94	55
'Soya' butter	15	1.00	2
	30	0.57	115

ceiving a diet supplemented with soya bean oil shows a distinct melting gap, which helps to stabilize the spreadability over a wide temperature range, and this should give it considerable commercial appeal, but there is the associated disadvantage that soya bean oil supplements tend to depress milk-fat content and yield. Milks with a fat rich in linoleic acid have been used for the manufacture of butter, cheese, yoghurt, cream cheese, ice cream, pasteurized milk, cultured sour cream, cheese dip and table cream. The products have distinctive properties which affect their flavour and acceptability, and their storage life: the major problem to the use of products rich in polyunsaturated fatty acids is their oxidative instability (a special problem in liquid milk) which is controlled by the use of antioxidants. At the present time, however, the cost of the protected lipid preparation and the restricted transfer of linoleic acid to milk has made the economics of the process uncertain, and discouraged its adoption in commerce.

Heat stability

The heat stability of fresh milk is closely dependent on its urea content (Muir and Sweetsur, 1976) which, as has been indicated earlier, can be readily manipulated through changes in the level and type of nitrogenous constituents in the diet. With milks which have been concentrated during manufacturing, e.g. those containing 400 to 480 g total solids per kg, the relationship between heat stability and urea content disappears, and one dependent on the concentrations of inorganic constituents in milk becomes established. The crucial features of this relationship have still to be fully elucidated but the evidence suggests that the concentration of calcium and the partition of calcium between its soluble and colloidal phases are important. Feeding experiments have shown that milk soluble–calcium content is closely correlated with citric acid content and that both are influenced by diet. Together with milk fat content they are reduced by an increase in the proportion of cereal concentrate in the diet (Ormrod, Thomas and Wheelock, 1979) and increased by dietary inclusions of tallow (Ormrod, Thomas and Wheelock, 1980).

MILK PRODUCTION IN SUCKLING CATTLE AND SHEEP

Milk let-down in the dairy cow is readily stimulated and, excepting the residual fraction, the milk can be completely removed from the udder by hand or machine milking. The yield can be measured with accuracy and, provided that appropriate weighted mean samples from a number of milkings are taken for analysis, small effects of diet on milk composition can be determined reproducibly. In contrast, in suckling farm livestock milking is dependent on the sucking of the young, and thus on the number and appetite of the offspring in the litter; if the litter is removed, there may be difficulties in stimulating a satisfactory milk let-down. Accurate measurements of milk yield and truly representative samples of milk for analysis are therefore more difficult to obtain than from the dairy cow, and both can be affected by the completeness of removal of milk from the gland during normal sucking. In experimental studies milk yield has been measured by the gain in weight of the young during sucking, following the standardization of litter size by fostering or crossfostering, and by hand or machine milking following the removal of the young for several hours and the injection of oxytocin to promote milk let-down. Other methods of measurement based on the estimation of body water distribution (Macfarlane, Howard and Siebert, 1969) or using isotope dilution techniques (Wright and Wolff, 1976) have also been devised but they have not been widely adopted.

Udder infections are generally considered to be less of a problem in suckling animals than in those that are machine milked but infections do occur, and, since bacteriological monitoring of milks is rarely undertaken, they may not be recognized until there are advanced chemical signs of mastitis.

Needless to say, in comparison with the dairy cow, there is only limited information about the effects of diet on milk production in suckling farm livestock, and the information available reflects the restricted range of diets and production systems that have been studied. For suckler cows the limitations on information may not be too serious since much of what is known about the dairy cow is directly applicable. However, there are important differences in detail, for beef cows have lower milk yields than dairy cows and a greater propensity to partition nutrients towards tissue deposition, and this reflects differences in their circulating hormone levels (see Bines and Hart, 1978) and metabolic responses to nutrition, as well as differences in udder size. Additionally, the lactational changes in milk yield and composition in beef cows are influenced by the sucking demands of the calves; typically, the lactation curve in yield differs from that observed in the dairy cow, the peak in yield tending to be suppressed in part by the incompleteness of milking.

Milk production in the ewe

Recent experiments with Blackface, East Friesland × Blackface and Merino ewes have shown that similar, although not necessarily identical, milk yields can be obtained using the 'lamb weight' and 'oxytocin-milking' methods (Doney, Peart, Smith and Louda, 1979). It therefore seems that, with careful application, either method is satisfactory for use in nutritional studies and here no distinction is drawn between them.

Under traditional systems of management, lactation in the ewe may continue over a period of 12 to 14 weeks but the lamb begins to eat significant amounts of solid food by approximately 3 to 4 weeks of age, and after 6 weeks begins progressively to wean itself. Thus a high proportion of the total lactational milk yield, as much as 60 to 70%, may be produced during the first 6 weeks of lactation. With intensive systems of lamb production, the object is to wean the lamb rapidly so that the ewe may be returned quickly to lamb production. Under these circumstances the lamb is introduced to creep food at approximately 10 days of age and weaned abruptly at 4 weeks of age, so that lactation is curtailed.

In ewes allowed to complete a 12-week lactation, the lactational changes in milk yield and composition show many features similar to those described earlier for the cow, although the changes are accentuated because of the shortening of the lactation period, and are dependent on the size and number of lambs in the litter. As compared with ewes suckling single lambs, those with twins or triplets show higher milk yields and a much more pronounced lactational peak in yield, and there are associated differences in the composition and in the lactational changes in composition of the milk (Fig. 14.11). These differences influence the average fat, protein and lactose contents of the milk produced during the lactation (Table 14.8) and, understandably, complicate any attempt to describe the characteristic differences in composition of milk between breeds.

Energy nutrition

Estimates of the efficiency of utilization of dietary ME in the ewe given a variety of diets have indicated that the efficiency for lactation (k_{l_0}) is approximately 0.63 to 0.75 and that the efficiency of tissue synthesis has a corresponding value of approximately 0.60 to 0.71 (Graham, 1964; Maxwell, Doney, Milne, Peart, Russel, Sibbald and MacDonald, 1979). Thus, as in the cow, changes in the carbohydrate composition of the diet leading to effects on the products of digestion are likely to alter the partition of energy use between milk secretion and tissue synthesis rather than the efficiency of energy utilization. Evidence of depressions in milk-fat content in ewes given low–fibre diets has been presented by Poulton and Ashton (1972) and it seems likely that the influence of diet on milk composition is broadly similar to that described for the cow.

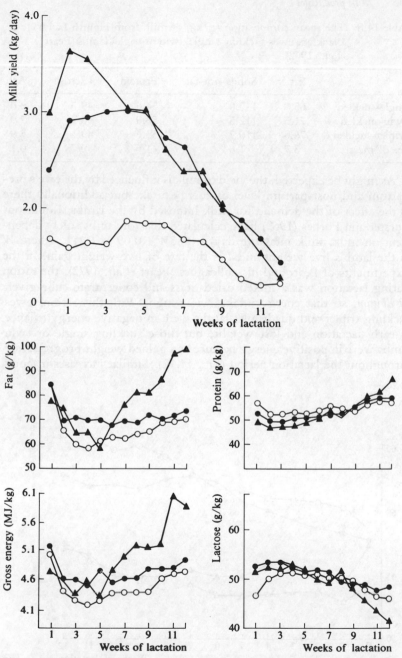

Fig. 14.11. Lactational changes in milk yield and composition in single-suckled (○), twin-suckled (●) and triplet-suckled (▲) Finnish Landrace × Blackface ewes (results taken from Peart, Edwards and Donaldson, 1972.)

Table 14.8   The mean composition (g/kg) of milk from Finnish Landrace ×
Blackface ewes suckling single, twin or triplet lambs (Peart
et al., 1972)

	Fat	Solids-not-fat	Protein	Lactose	Ash
Single-suckled	65.9	112.0	54.6	49.3	8.0
Twin-suckled	71.3	112.5	53.9	50.7	7.9
Triplet-suckled	76.8	110.7	53.6	49.1	7.9
s.e. of mean	3.7	1.6	1.6	0.7	0.1

As might be expected, the yield of milk is influenced by the ewe's pre-partum and post-partum level of energy intake but additionally there is the effect of the demand for milk imposed by the lambs; Robinson, Forster and Forbes (1969) have calculated that for lambs solely dependent on milk, milk intake $(g/day) = 38.3W + 0.09\ I^2 + 411$, where W is the lamb's live weight and I is the rate of live-weight gain. In the experiments of Peart and his colleagues (Peart *et al.*, 1972), the ration during lactation was a mixed dried grass and concentrate cube given *ad libitum*, so that energy intakes were high. With this ration, ewes suckling triplet and quadruplet lambs were in negative energy balance in early lactation and lost weight, but those suckling single or twin lambs were in positive energy balance and gained weight progressively throughout the lactation period (Fig. 14.12). Similar increases in body

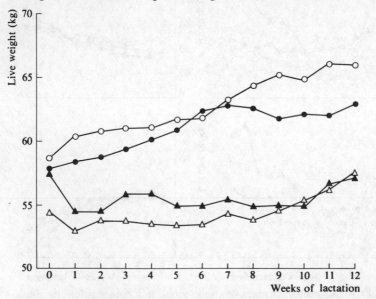

Fig. 14.12.   Lactational changes in live weight in ewes suckling single lambs
(○), twin lambs (●), triplet lambs (△) and quadruplet lambs (▲)
(results taken from Peart *et al.*, 1972.)

weight have been observed in ewes suckling single or twin lambs and grazing pasture *ad libitum* (Maxwell *et al.*, 1979) or given *ad libitum* pelleted diets (Peart, 1967), and in these studies even severe undernutrition during late pregnancy has had little or no effect on milk production. When the dietary energy intake is restricted during the lactation period, the situation, understandably, is different, milk production is reduced in parallel with the energy intake, and there are interactions between the current level of feeding, the number of lambs suckled, the body condition at lambing and the subsequent weight loss in lactation. For example, in ewes given restricted amounts of diet for the first 4 weeks, of lactation, milk production of twin-suckled ewes that were fat at parturition was significantly greater than that of twin-suckled ewes that were lean, but there was no difference in milk production between fat and lean single-suckled ewes (Peart, 1970).

Protein nutrition

The protein nutrition of the lactating ewe, and in particular the interactions between dietary protein and dietary energy supply, has been investigated in a series of experiments by Robinson and his colleagues (see Robinson, 1980). The results of their work have been summarized in a schematic form which shows that, for ewes of a given milk yield, there is a curvilinear relationship between the dietary requirement for crude protein and the dietary energy intake; low requirements for protein are associated with high intakes of energy, and *vice versa*. These relationships are an alternative form of expression of response curves of the type given in Fig. 14.4 (a) and suggest that in ewes receiving a low energy intake milk production may be especially sensitive to changes in the supply of amino acids to the small intestine. Consistent with this, ewes in negative energy balance have shown responses in milk production to dietary protein supplements of low rumen-degradability (Fig. 14.13). These effects correspond with those described for dairy cows given intra-abomasal infusions of casein (see p. 595), which have been interpreted to indicate an influence of protein supply on adipose tissue mobilization. However, the results of comparative slaughter experiments with ewes tend to suggest that protein supply influences the utilization of mobilized tissue rather than tissue mobilization itself (Cowan, Robinson and McDonald, 1980).

MILK PRODUCTION IN THE SOW

Milk production is technically more difficult to study in the sow than in the cow or ewe since the 'oxytocin-milking' technique can be used to

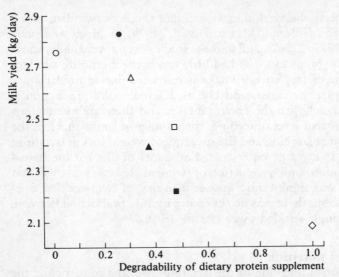

Fig. 14.13.   The relationship between milk yield and the rumen-degradability of dietary protein supplements in ewes given a basal control diet and supplements of blood meal (○), fish meal (●), linseed meal (△), meat and bone meal (▲), soya bean meal (□), groundnut meal (■) and urea (◇). (Gonzalez, Robinson, McHattie and Mehrez, 1979.)

obtain milk samples for analysis but cannot be satisfactorily employed for measurements of milk yield. A routine procedure of weighing piglets before and after suckling over a period of 12 to 24 h, with suckling intervals of not more than 1 h, has been adopted for milk yield measurements but even this procedure may be subject to serious error (Elsley, 1971).

The milk yield of the sow varies with litter size, increasing by 0.9 to 1.0 kg per pig for litters of less than eight piglets and by 0.7 to 0.8 kg per pig for litters of 9 to 12 piglets. An average yield for a typical 8-week lactation is 300 to 400 kg of milk, and there is a peak in yield usually between the 3rd and 5th weeks of lactation (Fig. 14.14). Sow's milk is more concentrated than that of the cow but trends in composition throughout lactation are similar, except for fat content, which is low early and late in lactation, and at a maximum in mid-lactation (Fig. 14.14). Day-to-day variations in composition are greater in the sow, especially for fat content, for which variations of up to 30% have been observed. The fat content is similar for milk from different teats but varies erratically throughout a milking and there is not the progressive increase observed in the cow. Colostral fat is richer in oleic and linoleic acids, and lower in palmitic and palmitoleic acids, than the milk fat and there are day-to-day variations in oleic and palmitic acids

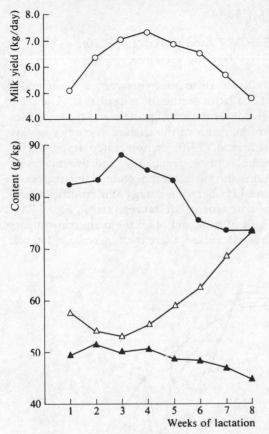

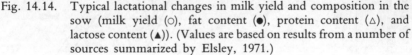

Fig. 14.14. Typical lactational changes in milk yield and composition in the sow (milk yield (○), fat content (●), protein content (△), and lactose content (▲)). (Values are based on results from a number of sources summarized by Elsley, 1971.)

of the milk fat that may reflect variations in the extent to which the fat is derived from preformed or newly-synthesized fatty acids.

Energy nutrition

A majority of the comparisons of different levels of energy nutrition have been made between groups of sows, not within animals; the errors attached to observed differences inevitably are large but consistent relationships have emerged. Elsley (1971), from a pooled (within experiment) regression analysis of the results of several studies obtained the following relationships between milk energy (kJ/day) or milk yield (kg/day) and food intake (MJ/day):

milk energy = 22.5 + 0.47 food intake (s.e. 0.10);
milk yield = 3.74 + 0.60 food intake (s.e. 0.10).

It was not possible statistically to distinguish between a linear and a curvilinear relationship but the latter seems more probable. The diets used in the studies had a high concentration of protein and the responses were attributed primarily to the result of the change of energy intake: O'Grady, Elsley and MacPherson (1970) demonstrated responses to energy intake when the feeding during pregnancy, and the intakes of protein minerals and vitamins during lactation were standardized.

The more detailed relationships between energy undernutrition and the secretion of major milk constituents are represented in Fig. 14.15: there is a decrease in the yields of milk and of all the main constituents but, whereas lactose content is decreased, there is an increase in fat, ash and usually protein contents.

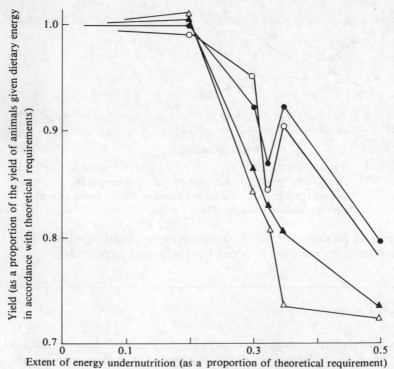

Fig. 14.15. The effect in the sow of energy undernutrition during lactation following normal feeding during pregnancy on the yields of milk protein (○), milk fat (●), lactose (△) and milk (▲). (After Rook and Witter, 1968.)

The level of energy intake in lactation also affects the overall body weight change during lactation; in the first 1 or 2 weeks of lactation there may be little change of weight, in sows receiving a low energy intake, or a gain of weight in sows receiving a higher energy intake, but subsequently the trend is towards a fall in weight, which is more rapid in underfed animals (O'Grady *et al.*, 1970). These changes are consistent with mobilization of body reserves being influenced by nutritional status (see Salmon-Legagneur, 1965). Sows subjected to a very high energy intake or a low energy intake over three successive lactations differed in body weight, and the proportion of the carcass accounted for by subcutaneous fat and skin; average values were 139.7 and 101.1 kg, and 307 and 167 g/kg, respectively (O'Grady *et al.*, 1970).

Food intake during pregnancy is also of importance. Live-weight gain during pregnancy is related inversely to live-weight loss during lactation, primarily as a consequence of an increased milk production mainly in the early part of lactation; milk-fat content is also higher (Elsley and MacPherson, 1966). The response to level of feeding during pregnancy is modified by that during lactation, being smaller the higher the level of intake during lactation; intake *ad libitum* during lactation is inversely related to level of intake during pregnancy.

Protein nutrition

Distinct effects of the amount and quality of dietary protein on milk secretion have not been observed in comparisons in which diets contained at least 140 g crude protein per kg. Diets containing only 120 g crude protein per kg would probably be satisfactory for milk production, providing their lysine content was adequate (Elsley, 1971). The lower intakes of protein may, however, increase live-weight loss during lactation. Salmon-Legagneur (1965) compared diets containing 150 and 180 g protein per kg and observed, as would be expected, a significant effect on the urea content of milk but also one on the lactalbumin content.

Amount and composition of dietary fat

Effects of the amount and type of dietary fat on the yield and composition of milk fat are firmly established. The first detailed, systematic study was made by Salmon-Legagneur (1965), and his observations have since been confirmed and extended (deMan and Bowland, 1963; Tollerz and Lindberg, 1965; Witter and Rook, 1970).

Increases in milk-fat content have been observed when, during lactation, lard has been added alone or with fish meal to, or as an isocaloric substituent for, a low-fat diet, or when tallow has been added to the diet; dietary addition of maize oil during pregnancy was without effect.

The effects on milk-fat composition reflect the fatty acid composition of the supplement but differences exist between individual fatty acids in their efficiency of transfer to milk fat. There are intermediate changes in the fatty acid composition of plasma triglycerides, and the degree of change is affected by the extent of fat digestion and of liver metabolism of individual fatty acids. Short-chain fatty acids are extensively metabolized, and there is a negligible transfer of butyric and caprylic acids from the diet to the triglycerides of the plasma. As chain length increases so the efficiency of transfer increases, to a maximum, for saturated acids, with myristic acid; at that chain length and above, digestibility of the fat, and therefore transfer of fatty acids, may be depressed, a factor unimportant for oils rich in unsaturated acids. However, erucic acid ($C_{22:1}$), present in rapeseed oil, is transferred to plasma triglycerides to only a very limited extent. The changes in milk-fat composition are, broadly, proportionately similar to those in the composition of the plasma triglycerides, except for the transfer of capric, lauric and myristic acids when present in coconut oil.

An increased content of palmitic acid in milk fat is associated also with an increased content of palmitoleic acid, due to the presence in sow mammary tissue of a desaturase system highly active towards palmitic acid (Bickerstaffe and Annison, 1970). During the feeding of cottonseed oil, the constituent sterculic and malvalic acids interfere with the desaturation mechanism. Increases in the content of stearic and palmitic acids, and decreases in palmitoleic and oleic acids in milk are observed which are independent of similar changes in the plasma triglycerides.

REFERENCES

Agricultural Research Council, 1965. *The Nutrient Requirements of Farm Livestock. No. 2, Ruminants*, pp. 193–264. Agricultural Research Council, London.

Amir, S., Kali, J. and Volcani, R., 1969. Influence of growth rate on reproduction and lactation in dairy cattle. In *Growth and Development of Mammals* (ed. G. A. Lodge and G. E. Lamming), pp. 234–56. Butterworth, London.

Armstrong, D. G., 1972. Developments in cereal processing – ruminants. In *Cereal Processing, Tech. Publ. U.S. Feed Grains Coun., Lond.*, pp. 9–37.

Balch, C. C., 1967. Problems in predicting the value of non-protein nitrogen as a substitute for protein in rations for farm ruminants, *Wld Rev. Anim. Prod.* **3**: 84–90.

Balch, C. C., 1971. Proposal to use the time spent chewing as an index of the extent to which diets for ruminants possess the physical property of fibrousness characteristic of roughages, *Br. J. Nutr.* **26**:383–92.

Balch, C. C., Balch, D. A., Bartlett, S., Johnson, V.W., Rowland, S. J. and Turner, J., 1954. Studies on the secretion of milk of low fat content by cows on diets low in hay and high in concentrates, *J. Dairy Res.* **21**:305–17.

Balch, C. C., and Campling, R. C., 1965. Utilization of urea by milking cows, *J. Dairy Res.* **28**: 157–63.

Baldwin, R. L., 1967. Enzyme activities in mammary glands of several species, *J. Dairy Sci.* **49**: 1533–42.

Baldwin, R. L. and Koong, L. J., 1980. Mathematic modelling in analysis of ruminant digestive function: philosophy, methodology and application. In *Digestive Physiology and Metabolism in Ruminants* (ed. Y. Ruckebusch and P. Thivend), pp. 251–70. MTP Press, Lancaster.

Banks, W., Clapperton, J. L. and Ferrie, Morag E., 1974. The composition of milk from cows fed on various fat-supplemented diets, *Proc. Nutr. Soc.* **33**: 82A (Abstr.).

Banks, W., Clapperton, J. L. and Ferrie, Morag E., 1976a. Effect of feeding fat to dairy cows receiving a fat-deficient basal diet. II. Fatty acid composition of the milk fat, *J. Dairy Res.* **43**: 219–27.

Banks, W., Clapperton, J. L., Ferrie, Morag E. and Wilson, Agnes G., 1976b. Effect of feeding fat to dairy cows receiving a fat-deficient diet. I. Milk yield and composition, *J. Dairy Res.* **43**:213–8.

Banks, W., Clapperton, J. L., Kelly, Morag E., Wilson, Agnes G. and Crawford, R. J. M., 1980. The yield, fatty acid composition and physical properties of milk obtained by feeding soya oil to dairy cows, *J. Sci. Fd Agric.* **31**: 368–74.

Bauman, D. E. and Davis, C. L., 1975. Regulation of lipid metabolism. In *Digestion and Metabolism in the Ruminant* (ed. I. W. McDonald and A. C. I. Warner), pp. 496–509. University of New England Publishing Unit, Armidale.

Bickerstaffe, R. and Annison, E. F., 1970. The desaturase activity of goat and sow mammary tissue, *Comp. Biochem. Physiol.* **35**:653–65.

Bines, J. A., Brumby, P. E., Storry, J. E., Fulford, Rosemary J. and Braithwaite, G. D., 1978. The effect of protected lipids on nutrient intakes, blood and rumen metabolites and milk secretion in dairy cows during early lactation, *J. agric. Sci., Camb.* **91**: 135–50.

Bines, J. A. and Hart, I. C., 1978. Hormonal regulation of the partition of energy between milk and body tissue in adult cattle, *Proc. Nutr. Soc.* **37** : 281–7.

Breirem, K., 1949. Norwegian experiments regarding the effects of the feed on the composition and quality of the milk and milk products, *Proc. 12th int. Dairy Congr., Stockholm*, Vol. 1, pp. 28–60.

Broster, W. H., 1972. Protein requirements of cows for lactation. In Handbuch der Tierernährung, Vol. II (ed. W. Lenkeit, K. Breirem and E. Crasemann), pp. 292–321. Parey, Hamburg.

Broster, W. H., 1974. Response of the dairy cow to level of feeding, Bienn. Rev. Natn. Inst. Res. Dairy., pp. 14–34.

Broster, W. H., Broster, V. J. and Smith, T., 1969. Experiments on the nutrition of the dairy heifer. VIII. Effect on milk production of level of feeding at two stages of the lactation, J. agric. Sci., Camb. 72: 229–45.

Broster, W. H., Sutton, J. D. and Bines, J. A., 1979. Concentrate:forage ratios for high yielding dairy cows. In Recent Advances in Animal Nutrition – 1978 (ed. W. Haresign and D. Lewis), pp. 99–126. Butterworth, London.

Brumby, P. J., 1958. Monozygotic twins and dairy cattle improvement, Anim. Breed. Abstr. 26: 1–12.

Brumby, P. E., Storry, J. E. and Sutton, J. D., 1972. Metabolism of cod-liver oil in relation to milk fat secretion, J. Dairy Res. 39: 167–82.

Castle, M. E. and Watson, J. N., 1969. The effect of level of protein in silage on the intake and production of dairy cows, J. Br. Grassld Soc. 24:187–93.

Castle, M. E. and Watson, J. N., 1979. Silage and milk production: a comparison between soya, groundnut and single-cell protein as silage supplements, Grass & Forage Sci. 34: 101–6.

Chalmers, J. S., Thomas, P. C. and Belibasakis, N., 1978. Rumen fermentation and milk yield and composition in cows given silage diets. In Proc. 5th Silage Conf. (ed. R. D. Harkess), pp. 18–19 (Abstr.). Hannah Research Institute, Ayr.

Chalmers, J. S., Thomas, P. C. and Chamberlain, D. G., 1980. The effect of intraruminal infusion of propionic acid on milk composition in cows given silage diets, Proc. Nutr. Soc. 39: 27A(Abstr.).

Chalmers, J. S., Thomas, P. C. and Kelly, Morag E., 1977. The effect of the level of feeding and composition of the diet on milk secretion in the Ayrshire cow, Proc. Nutr. Soc. 36: 35A(Abstr.).

Chalupa, W., O'Dell, G. D., Kutches, A. J. and Lavker, R., 1967. Changes in rumen chemical characteristics and protozoa populations of animals with depressed milk fat tests, J. Dairy Sci. 50: 1002(Abstr.).

Clapperton, J. L., Kelly, Morag E., Banks, Jean M. and Rook, J. A. F., 1980. The production of milk rich in protein and low in fat, the fat having a high polyunsaturated fatty acid content, J. Sci. Fd Agric. 31: 1295–302.

Clark, J. A., 1975. Lactational responses to postruminal administration of proteins and amino acids, J. Dairy Sci. 58: 1178–97.

Clark, J., Geerken, C. M., Preston, T. R. and Zamora, A., 1973. Molasses as a source of energy in low fibre diets for milk production, Cuban J. Agric. Sci. 7: 155–67.

Clark, J. H., Spires, H. R., Derrig, R. G. and Benink, M. R., 1977. Milk production, nitrogen utilization and glucose synthesis in lactating cows infused postruminally with sodium caseinate and glucose, J. Nutr. 107: 631–44.

Coppock, C. E., 1976. Cereal grain processing as related to diets for lactating cows, Proc. Cornell Nutr. Conf., pp. 67–71.

Coppock, C. E., Tyrell, H. F., Merrill, W. G. and Reid, J. T., 1968. The significance of protein reserve to the lactating cow, *Proc. Cornell Nutr. Conf.*, pp. 86–94.

Cowan, R. T., Robinson, J. J. and McDonald, I., 1980. The effects of diet on the body composition of lactating ewes, *Anim. Prod.* **30**: 477(Abstr.).

Dawson, R. R. and Rook, J. A. F., 1972. A note on the influence of stage of lactation on the response in lactose content in milk to a change in plane of energy nutrition in the cow, *J. Dairy Res.* **39**: 107–11.

deMan, J. M and Bowland, J. P., 1963. Fatty acid composition of sow's colostrum, milk and body fat as determined by gas-liquid chromatography, *J. Dairy Res.* **30**: 339–43.

Doney, J. M., Peart, J. N., Smith, W. F. and Louda, F., 1979. A consideration of the techniques for estimation of milk yield by suckled sheep and a comparison of estimates obtained by two methods in relation to effect of breed, level of production and stage of lactation, *J. agric. Sci., Camb.* **92**: 123–32.

Elsley, F. W. H., 1971. Nutrition and lactation in the sow. In *Lactation* (ed. I. R. Falconer), pp. 393–412. Butterworth, London.

Elsley, F. W. H. and MacPherson, R. M., 1966. Utilisation of nitrogen by lactating sow and litter, *Proc. 9th int. Congr. Anim. Prod., Edinb.*, p. 104(Abstr.).

Ensor, W. L., Shaw, J. C. and Tellechea, H. F., 1959. Special diets for the production of low fat milk and more efficient gains in body weight, *J. Dairy Sci.* **42**: 189–91.

Federation of United Kingdom Milk Marketing Boards, 1979. *United Kingdom Dairy Facts & Figures 1979*. Federation of United Kingdom Milk Marketing Boards, Thames Ditton.

Fisher, L. J. and Elliot, J. M., 1966. Effect of intravenous infusion of propionate or glucose on bovine milk composition, *J. Dairy Sci.* **49**: 826–9.

Flatt, W. D., Coppock, C. E. and Moore, L. A., 1965. Energy balance studies with lactating non-pregnant dairy cows consuming rations with varying hay: grain ratios. In *Energy Metabolism* (ed. K. L. Blaxter), pp. 121–30. Academic Press, London.

Flatt, W. P., Moe, P. W., Moore, L. A., Breirem, K. and Ekern, A., 1972. Energy requirements in lactation. In *Handbuch der Tierernährung,* Vol. II (ed. W. Lenkeit, K. Breirem and E. Crasemann), pp. 341–92. Parey, Hamburg.

Flatt, W. P., Moe, P. W., Munson, A. W. and Cooper, T., 1969. Energy utilization by high producing dairy cows. II. Summary of energy balance experiments with lactating Holstein cows. In *Energy Metabolism of Farm Animals* (ed. K. L. Blaxter, J. Kielanowski and Greta Thorbek), pp. 235–51. Oriel Press, Newcastle upon Tyne.

Fleet, I. R. and Peaker, M., 1978. Mammary function and its control at the cessation of lactation in the goat, *J. Physiol., Lond.* **279**: 491–507.

Flores, J. F., Stobbs, J. H. and Minson, D. J., 1979. The influence of the legume *Leucaena leucocephala* and formal-casein on the production and composition of milk from grazing cows, *J. agric. Sci., Camb.* **92**: 351–7.

Fogerty, A. C. and Johnson, A. R., 1980. Influence of nutritional factors on the yield and content of milk fat: protected polyunsaturated fat in the diet. In *Factors Affecting the Yields and Contents of Milk Constituents of Commercial Importance, Bull. int. Dairy Fed., Docum. 125* pp. 96–104.

Frens, A. M. and Dijkstra, N. D., 1959. Feeding trial about the desirable protein allowance in winter rations for dairy cows, *Versl. landbouwk. Onderz., Wageningen*, **65**: 1–39

Frobish, R. A. and Davis, C. L., 1977. Effects of abomasal infusions of glucose or propionate on milk yield and composition, *J. Dairy Sci.* **60**: 204–9.

Gonzalez, J. S., Robinson, J. J., McHattie, I. and Mehrez, A. Z., 1979. The use of lactating ewes in evaluating protein sources for ruminants, *Proc. Nutr. Soc.* **38**: 145A(Abstr.).

Gordon, F. J., 1977. The effect of three concentrate input levels on the performance of dairy cows calving during mid-winter, *Anim. Prod.* **25**: 373–9

Graham, N. McC., 1964. Energy exchanges of pregnant and lactating ewes, *Aust. J. agric. Res.* **15**: 127–41.

Guisard, D., Gonand, J. P., Laurent, J. and Debry, G., 1970. The plasma clearance of synthetic emulsions containing long-chain fatty acids and medium-chain fatty acids, *Eur. J. Clin. Biol. Res.* **15**: 674–8.

Hodgson, J. C. and Thomas, P. C., 1976. A relationship between the molar proportion of propionic acid and the clearance rate of the liquid phase in the rumen of the sheep, *Br. J. Nutr.* **33**: 447–56.

Hutton, K., Prescott, J. H. D., Seeley, R. C. and Armstrong, D. G., 1969. Ammonium salts of short-chain fatty acids for milk production. 2. The effect of feeding a salt containing ammonium acetate on the yield and fatty acid composition of Jersey milk fat, *Anim. Prod.* **11**: 209–18.

Jackson, P. and Rook, J. A. F., 1970. Responses in milk yield and composition to the inclusion of ammonium salts of short-chain fatty acids in the drinking water of dairy cows, *Anim. Prod.* **12**: 503–12.

Jackson, P., Rook, J. A. F. and Towers, K. G., 1971. Influence of the physical form of a barley grain and barley straw diet on nitrogen metabolism in sheep, *J. Dairy Res.* **38**: 33–42.

Johnson, C. L., 1977. The effect of the plane and pattern of concentrate feeding on milk yield and composition in dairy cows, *J. agric, Sci., Camb.* **88**: 79–94.

Journet, M. and Verité, R., 1977. Levels of energy and nitrogen intake in relation to animal protein production during lactation. In *Proc. 2nd int. Symp. Protein Metab. Nutr.* (ed. S. Tamminga), pp. 119–21. Centre for Agricultural Publishing and Documentation, Wageningen, the Netherlands.

Kaufmann, W., 1977. Calculations of the protein requirements for dairy cows according to measurements of N metabolism. In *Proc. 2nd int. Symp. Protein Metab. Nutr.* (ed. S. Tamminga), pp. 130–2. Centre for Agricultural Publishing and Documentation, Wageningen, the Netherlands.

Kay, M., 1976. Meeting the energy and protein requirements of the growing animal. In *Principles of Cattle Production* (ed. H. Swan and W. H. Broster), pp. 255–71. Butterworth, London.

Kellog, D. W. and Owen, F. G., 1969. Relation of ration sucrose level and grain content to lactation performance and rumen fermentation, *J. Dairy Sci.* **52**: 657–62.

King, R. L. and Hemken, R. W., 1962. Composition of milk produced on pelleted hay and heated corn, *J. Dairy Sci.* **45**: 1336–42.

Latham, M. T., Sutton, J. D. and Sharpe, M. E., 1974. Fermentation and micro-organisms in the rumen and the content of fat in the milk of cows given low-roughage rations, *J. Dairy Sci.* **57**: 803–10.

Lowman, B. G., Scott, N. and Somerville, S., 1973. Condition scoring in cattle, *Bull. E. Scotl. Coll. Agric., No. 6.*

McCullough, M. E., 1966. Relationship between rumen fluid volatile fatty acids and milk fat percentage and feed intake, *J. Dairy Sci.* **49**: 896–8.

McDowall, F. H., McGillivray, W. A. and Hawke, J. C., 1961. Growth of ryegrass-dominant pasture grazed by cows and properties of New Zealand butterfat, *Nature, Lond.* **191**: 303–4.

Macfarlane, W. V., Howard, Beth and Siebert, B. D., 1969. Tritiated water in the measurement of milk intake and tissue growth of ruminants in the field, *Nature, Lond.* **221**: 578–9.

Macleod, G. K. and Wood, A. S., 1972. Influence of amount and degree of saturation of dietary fat on yield and quality of milk, *J. Dairy Sci.* **55**: 439–45.

Majdoub, A., Lane, G. T. and Aitchison, T. E., 1978. Milk production response to nitrogen solubility in dairy rations, *J. Dairy Sci.* **61**: 59–65.

Maltos, W. and Palmquist, D. L., 1974. Increased polyunsaturated fatty acid yields in milk of cows fed protected fat, *J. Dairy Sci.* **57**: 1050–4.

Maxwell, T. J., Doney, J. M., Milne, J. A., Peart, J. N., Russel, A. J. F., Sibbald, A. R. and MacDonald, D., 1979. The effect of rearing type and prepartum nutrition on the intake and performance of lactating Greyface ewes at pasture, *J. agric. Sci., Camb.* **92**: 165–74.

Ministry of Agriculture, Fisheries and Food, Department of Agriculture and Fisheries for Scotland, and Department of Agriculture for Northern Ireland, 1975. Energy allowances and feeding systems for ruminants, *Tech. Bull. 33.* Her Majesty's Stationery Office, London.

Morant, S. V., Ridley, J. L. and Sutton, J. D., 1978. A model for the estimation of volatile fatty acid production in the rumen in non-steady-state conditions, *Br. J. Nutr.* **39**: 451–62.

Morrison, I. M. and Hawke, J. C., 1977. Triglyceride composition of bovine milk fat with elevated levels of linoleic acid, *Lipids* **12**: 994–1004.

Muir, D. D. and Sweetsur, A. W. M., 1976. The influence of naturally occurring levels of urea on the heat stability of bulk milk, *J. Dairy Res.* **43**: 495–9.

Murdoch, J. C. and Rook, J. A. F., 1963. A comparison of hay and silage for milk production, *J. Dairy Res.* **30**: 391–7.

O'Dell, G. D., King, W. A. and Cook, W. C., 1968. The effect of grinding, pelleting and frequency of feeding of forage on fat percentage of milk and milk production of dairy cows, *J. Dairy Sci.* **51**: 50–5.

O'Grady, J. F., Elsley, F. W. H. and MacPherson, R. M., 1970. The response of lactating sows and their litters to different energy allowances, *Anim. Prod.* **12**: 374(Abstr.).

Oldham, J. D., 1980. Protein and the high-yielding cow. In *Feeding Strategies for Dairy Cows* (ed. W. H. Broster, C. L. Johnson and J. C. Tayler), pp. 7.1–7.19. Agricultural Research Council, London.

Oldham, J. D., Hart, I. C. and Bines, J. A., 1978. Effect of abomasal infusions of casein, arginine, methionine or phenylalanine on growth hormone, insulin, prolactin, thyroxine and some metabolites in blood from lactating goats, *Proc. Nutr. Soc.* **37**: 9A(Abstr.).

Oldham, J. D., Lobley, G. E., Konig, B. A., Parker, D. S. and Smith, R. W., 1980. Amino acid metabolism in lactating dairy cows early in lactation. In *Proc. 3rd int. Symp. Protein Nutr. Metab.* (ed. H. J. Oslage and K. Rohr), Vol II, pp. 458–464. European Association for Animal Production, Braunschweig.

Ormrod, I. H. L., Thomas, P. C. and Wheelock, J. V., 1979. The effect of diet on the citric acid and soluble calcium content of cow's milk, *Proc. Nutr. Soc.* **38**: 121A(Abstr.).

Ormrod, I. H. L., Thomas, P. C. and Wheelock, J. V., 1980. The effect of dietary inclusions of tallow on the citric acid and soluble calcium content of cow's milk, *Proc. Nutr. Soc.* **39**: 33A(Abstr.).

Ørskov, E. R. and Greenhalgh, J. F. D., 1977. Alkali treatment as a method for processing whole grain for cattle, *J. agric. Sci., Camb.* **89**: 253–5.

Ørskov, E. F., Grubb, D. A. and Kay, R. N. B., 1977. The effect of postruminal protein or glucose supplementation on milk yield and composition in Friesian cows in early lactation and negative energy balance, *Br. J. Nutr.* **38**: 397–405.

Paape, M. J. and Tucker, H. A., 1969. Influence of length of dry period on subsequent lactations in the rat, *J. Dairy Sci.* **52**: 518–22.

Pan, Y. S., Cook, L. J. and Scott, T. W., 1972. Formaldehyde-treated casein-safflower oil supplement for dairy cows. 1. Effect on milk composition, *J. Dairy Res.* **39**: 203–10.

Peart, J. N., 1967. The effect of different levels of nutrition during late pregnancy on the subsequent milk production of Blackface ewes and on the growth of their lambs, *J. agric. Sci., Camb.* **68**: 365–71.

Peart, J. N., 1970. The influence of live weight and body condition on the subsequent milk production of Blackface ewes following a period of undernourishment in early lactation, *J. agric. Sci., Camb.* **75**: 459–69.

Peart, J. N., Edwards, R. A. and Donaldson, E., 1972. The yield and composition of the milk of Finnish Landrace × Blackface ewes, *J. agric. Sci., Camb.* **79**: 303–13.

Poulton, S. G. and Ashton, W. M., 1972. The effect of high cereal diets on ewes and on the yield of milk and milk constituents, *J. agric. Sci., Camb.* **78**: 203–13.

Reiter, B., Sorokin, Y., Pickering, A. and Hall, A. J., 1969. Hydrolysis of fat and protein in small cheeses made under aseptic conditions, *J. Dairy Res.* **36**: 65–76.

Rindsig, R. B. and Schultz, L. H., 1974. Effect of feeding lauric acid to lactating cows on milk composition, rumen fermentation and blood lipids, *J. Dairy Sci.* **57**: 1414–8.

Robertson, A., Paver, H., Barden, P. and Marr, T. G., 1960. Fasting metabolism in the lactating cow, *Res. vet. Sci.* **1**: 117–24.

Robertson, A., Waite, R. and White, J. C. D., 1956. Variations in the chemical composition of milk with particular reference to solids-not-fat. II. Effect of heredity, *J. Dairy Res.* **23**: 82–91.

Robinson, J. J., 1980. Energy requirements of ewes during late pregnancy and early lactation, *Vet. Rec.* **106**: 282–4.

Robinson, J. J., Forster, W. H. and Forbes, T. J., 1969. The estimation of the milk yield of the ewe from body-weight data on the suckling lamb, *J. agric. Sci., Camb.* **72**: 103–7.

Rodrigue, C. B. and Allen, N. N., 1960. The effect of fine grinding of hay on ration digestibility, rate of passage, and fat content of milk, *Can. J. Anim. Sci.* **40**: 23–9.

Rogers, G. L., Bryant, A. M., McLeay, L. M., 1979. Silage and dairy cow production. III. Abomasal infusions of casein, methionine and glucose and milk yield and composition, *N.Z. Jl agric. Res.* **22**: 533–41.

Rook, J. A. F., 1961a. Variations in the chemical composition of the milk of the cow – Part I, *Dairy Sci. Abstr.* **23**: 251–8 (references: 307–8).

Rook, J. A. F., 1961b. Variations in the chemical composition of the milk of the cow – Part II, *Dairy Sci. Abstr.* **23**: 303–8.

Rook, J. A. F., 1977. Dietary manipulation of the composition and quality of milk and milk products, *J. Soc. Dairy Technol.* **30**: 169–77.

Rook, J. A. F. and Balch, C. C., 1961. The effect of intraruminal infusion of acetic, propionic and butyric acids in the yield and composition of milk in the cow, *Br. J. Nutr.* **15**: 361–9.

Rook, J. A. F., Balch, C. C., and Johnson, V. W., 1965. Further observations on the effects of intraruminal infusions of volatile fatty acids and lactic acid on the yield and composition of the milk of the cow, *Br. J. Nutr.* **19**: 93–9.

Rook, J. A. F. and Campling, R. C., 1965. Effect of the stage and number of lactation on the yield and composition of cow's milk, *J. Dairy Sci.* **32**: 45–55.

Rook, J. A. F. and Line, C., 1962. The influence of the level of dietary protein on the yield and chemical composition of milk, *Proc. 16th int. Dairy Congr. Copenh.*, Vol. A, pp. 57–63.

Rook, J. A. F., Line, C. and Rowland, S. J., 1960. The effect of the plane of energy nutrition of the cow during the late winter-feeding period on the changes in the solids-not-fat content of milk during the spring-grazing period, *J. Dairy Res.* **27**: 427–33.

Rook, J. A. F. and Witter, R. C., 1968. Diet and milk secretion in the sow, *Proc. Nutr. Soc.* **27**: 71–6.

Rowland, S. J., 1946. The problem of low solids-not-fat, *Dairy Inds* **11**: 656–63.

Roy, J. H. B., Balch, C. C., Miller, E. L., Ørskov, E. R. and Smith, R. H., 1977. Calculation of the protein requirements for dairy cows according to measurements of nitrogen metabolism. In *Proc. 2nd int. Symp. Protein Metab. Nutr.* (ed. S. Tamminga), pp. 125–9. Centre for Agricultural Publishing and Documentation, Wageningen, the Netherlands.

Salmon-Legagneur, E., 1965. Some aspects of the nutritional relations between pregnancy and *lactation* in the sow, *Annls Zootech.* **14**: *Spec. Ser., No. 1.*

Satter, L. D. and Roffler, R. E., 1977. Calculating requirements for protein and non-protein nitrogen by rumminants. In *Proc. 2nd int. Symp. Protein Metab. Nutr.* (ed. S. Tamminga), pp. 133–6. Centre for Agricultural Publishing and Documentation, Wageningen, the Netherlands.

Schingoethe, D. J., 1976. Whey utilisation in animal feeding: a summary and evaluation, *J. Dairy Sci.* **59**: 556–70.

Schwab, C. G., Satter, L. D. and Clay, A. B., 1976. Response of lactating cows to abomasal infusion of amino acids, *J. Dairy Sci.* **59**: 1254–70.

Scott, T. W., Bready, P. J., Royal, A. J. and Cook, L. J., 1972. Oil seed supplements for the production of polyunsaturated ruminant milk fat, *Search* **3**: 170–1.

Scott, T. W., Cook, L. J., Ferguson, K. A., McDonald, I. W., Buchanan, R. A. and Loftus-Hills, G., 1970. Production of polyunsaturated milk fat in domestic ruminants, *Aust. J. Sci.* **32**: 291–3.

Smith, R. H., 1975. Nitrogen metabolism in the rumen and the composition and nutritive value of nitrogen compounds entering the duodenum. In *Digestion and Metabolism in the Ruminant* (ed. I. W. McDonald and A. C. I. Warner), pp. 399–415. University of New England Publishing Unit, Armidale.

Smith, S. and Abraham, S., 1975. The composition and biosynthesis of milk fat, *Adv. Lipid Res.* **13**: 195–239.

Smith, N. E., Baldwin, R. L. and Sharp, W. M., 1980. Models of tissue and animal metabolism. In *Energy Metabolism* (ed. L. E. Mount) pp. 193–8. Butterworth, London.

Smith, J. A. B., Howat, G. R. and Ray, S. C., 1938. The composition of the blood and milk of lactating cows during inanition, with a note on an unidentified constituent present in certain samples of abnormal milk, *J. Dairy Res.* **9**: 310–22.

Steele, W. and Moore, J. H., 1968. The effects of a series of saturated fatty acids on milk fat secretion in the cow, *J. Dairy Res.* **35**: 361–70.

Steele, W., Noble, R. C. and Moore, J. H., 1971. The effects of two methods of incorporating soybean oil into the diet on milk yield and composition in the cow, *J. Dairy Res.* **38**: 43–8.

Stobbs, T. H., Minson, D. J. and McLeod, M. N., 1977. The response of dairy cows grazing a nitrogen fertilized grass pasture to a supplement of protected casein, *J. agric. Sci., Camb.* **89**: 137–41.

Storry, J. E., 1972. Milk fat: its synthesis and composition in relation to the nutrition of the dairy cow, *J. Soc. Dairy Technol.* **25**: 40–6.

Storry, J. E., 1980. Influence of nutritional factors on the yield and content of milk fat: non-protected fat in the diet. In *Factors Affecting the Yields and Contents of Milk Constituents of Commercial Importance, Bull. int. Dairy Fed., Docum. 125*, pp. 88–95.

Storry, J. E., Brumby, P. E. and Dunkley, W. L., 1980. Influence of nutritional factors on the yield and content of milk fat: protected non-polyunsaturated fat in the diet. In *Factors Affecting the Yields and Contents of Milk Constituents of Commerical Importance, Bull. int. Dairy Fed., Docum. 125*, pp. 105–25.

Storry, J. E., Brumby, P. E., Hall, A. J. and Johnson, V. W., 1974a. Response of the cow to different methods of incorporating casein and coconut oil in the diet, *J. Dairy Sci.* **57**: 61–7.

Storry, J. E., Brumby, P. E., Hall, A. J. and Tuckley, B., 1974b. Effects of free and protected forms of codliver oil on milk fat secretion in the dairy cow, *J. Dairy Sci.* **57**: 1046–9.

Storry, J. E., Hall, A. J. and Johnson, V. W., 1971. The effects of increasing amounts of dietary coconut oil on milk fat secretion in the cow, *J. Dairy Res.* **38**: 73–7.

Storry, J. E. and Rook, J. A. F., 1965. The effects of a diet low in hay and high in flaked maize on milk fat secretion and on the concentration of certain constituents in the blood plasma of the cow, *Br. J. Nutr.* **19**: 101–9.

Storry, J. E. and Rook, J. A. F., 1966. The relationship in the cow between milk fat secretion and ruminal volatile fatty acids, *Br. J. Nutr.* **20**: 217–28.

Storry, J. E., Rook, J. A. F. and Hall, A. J., 1967. The effect of the amount and type of dietary fat on milk fat secretion in the cow, *Br. J. Nutr.* **21**: 425–38.

Storry, J. E. and Sutton, J. D., 1969. The effect of change from low-roughage to high-roughage diets on rumen fermentation, blood composition and milk fat secretion in the cow, *Br. J. Nutr.* **23**: 511–21.

Sutton, J. D., 1980. Influence of nutritional factors on the yield and content of milk fat: dietary components other than fat. In *Factors Affecting the Yields and Contents of Milk Constituents of Commercial Importance, Bull. int. Dairy Fed., Docum. 125*, pp. 126–34.

Sutton, J. D. and Johnson, V. W., 1969. Fermentation in the rumen of cows given rations containing hay and flaked maize or rolled barley in widely differing proportions, *J. agric. Sci., Camb.* **73**: 459–68.

Sutton, J. D., Oldham, J. D. and Hart, I. C., 1980. Products of digestion, hormones and energy utilization in milking cows given concentrates containing varying proportions of barley or maize. In *Energy Metabolism* (ed. L. E. Mount), pp. 303–6. Butterworth, London.

Sutton, J. D., Smith, R. H., McAllan, A. B., Storry, J. E. and Corse, D. A., 1975. Effect of variations in dietary protein and of supplements of cod-liver oil on energy digestion and microbial synthesis in the rumen of sheep fed hay and concentrates, *J. agric. Sci., Camb.* **84**: 317–26.

Sutton, J. D., Storry, J. E. and Nicholson, J. W. G., 1970. The digestion of fatty acids in the stomach and intestines of sheep given widely different rations, *J. Dairy Res.* **37**: 97–105.

Swanson, E. W., Pardue, F. E. and Longmire, D. B., 1967. Effect of gestation and dry period on deoxyribonucleic acid and alveolar characteristics in bovine mammary glands, *J. Dairy Sci.* **50**: 1288–92.

Thomas, P. C., Chamberlain, D. G., Kelly, N. C. and Wait, M. K., 1980. The nutritive value of silages. Digestion of nitrogenous constituents in sheep receiving diets of grass silage and grass silage and barley, *Br. J. Nutr.* **43**: 469–79.

Thomas, P. C. and Kelly, Morag E., 1976. The effect of frequency of feeding on milk secretion in the Ayrshire cow, *J. Dairy Res.* **43**: 1–7.

Thompson, G. E. and Thomson, E. M., 1977. Effect of cold exposure on mammary circulation, oxygen consumption and milk secretion in the goat, *J. Physiol., Lond.* **272**: 187–96.

Tollerz, G. and Lindberg, P., 1965. Influence of dietary fat and short-time starvation on the composition of sow-milk fat, *Acta vet. scand.* **6**: 118–34.

Van Es, A. J. H., 1976. Factors influencing the efficiency of energy utilization by beef and dairy cattle. In *Principles of Cattle Production* (ed. H. Swan and W. H. Broster), pp. 237–54. Butterworth, London.

Van Horn, H. H., Zometa, C. A., Wilcox, C. J., Marshall, S. P. and Harris, B., Jr, 1979. Complete rations for dairy cattle. VIII. Effect of percent and source of protein on milk yield and ration digestibility, *J. Dairy Sci.* **62**: 1086–93.

Vik-Mo, L., Emery, R. S. and Huber, J. T., 1975. Milk protein production in cows abomasally infused with casein or glucose, *J. Dairy Sci.* **57**: 869–77.

Virtanen, A. I., 1966. Milk production in cows on protein-free feed, *Science, Wash., D.C.* **153**: 1603–14.

Waite, R., Abbot, J. and Blackburn, P. S., 1963. The use of quarter samples in the assessment of the effects of feeding treatments on milk composition, *J. Dairy Res.* **30**: 209–15.

Webster, A. J. F., 1976. The influence of the climatic environment on metabolism in cattle. In *Principles of Cattle Production* (ed. H. Swan and W. H. Broster), pp. 103–20. Butterworth, London.

Wheelock, J. V., Rook, J. A. F. and Dodd, F. H., 1965. The effect of incomplete milking or of an extended milking interval on the yield and composition of cow's milk, *J. Dairy Res.* **32**: 237–48.

Wheelock, J. V., Rook, J. A. F., Dodd, F. H. and Griffin, T. K., 1966. The effect of varying the interval between milkings on milk secretion, *J. Dairy Res.* **33**: 161–76.

Witter, R. C. and Rook, J. A. F., 1970. The influence of the amount and nature of dietary fat on milk fat composition in the sow, *Br. J. Nutr.* **24**: 749–60.

Wohlt, J. E., Clark, J. H. and Blaisdell, F. S., 1978. Nutritional value of urea versus preformed protein for ruminants. II. Nitrogen utilization by dairy cows fed corn based diets containing supplemental nitrogen from urea and/or soybean meal, *J. Dairy Sci.* **61**: 916–31.

Wood, P. D. P., 1976. Algebraic models of the lactation curves for milk, fat and protein production with estimates of seasonal variations, *Anim. Prod.* **22**: 35–40.

Woodman, H. E., 1957. Rations for livestock. 11th edn. *Bull. Minist. Agric. Fish. Fd, Lond., No. 48.*

Wright, J. A., Rook, J. A. F. and Wood, P. D. P., 1974. The responses in milk solids-not-fat and protein contents to improved feeding of cows receiving winter-stall diets and underfed for varying periods, *J. Dairy Res.* **41**: 155–64.

Wright, D. E. and Wolff, J. E., 1976. Measurement of milk intake in lambs suckling grazing ewes by a double isotope dilution method, *Proc. N.Z. Soc. Anim. Prod.* **36**: 99–102.

15 EGG PRODUCTION

C. Fisher

The average production characteristics of modern laying hens vary, principally according to breed, environmental factors and the incidence of disease. Brown egg-laying strains, which now form 90% of the national flock, show the following typical results (National Poultry Tests, 1978). At hatching a chick weighs 35 g and grows to approximately 2.0(s.d. 0.3) kg at sexual maturity (first egg), reached at 160 (s.d. 8) days of age. Body weight increases rapidly just prior to sexual maturity reflecting the development of the reproductive tract and associated tissues, but after maturity the rate of growth falls and body weight reaches 2.20(s.d. 0.22) kg at 500 days. Of the total body mass, protein mass is approximately 6, 260 and 300 g and fat mass 2, 300 and 500 g at 1, 160 and 500 days respectively.

Eggs are laid on successive days in sequences, or clutches, separated typically by single 'eggless' days. Average production is 270 to 280 eggs per hen to 500 days, the s.d. being approximately 56 to 60 eggs. However, this distribution is skewed by the proportion of birds which lay very poorly, or not at all. At sexual maturity egg weight is 48 (s.d. 4) g rising to 66(s.d. 6) g at the end of lay, so that in total approximately 16 to 17 kg of egg material is produced by each bird.

The nutrients secreted in a typical egg are shown in Table 15.1. These values give some idea of the turnover of material in egg production. Thus the protein content of 1 year's egg production (17 kg) is equivalent to some eight times the total body protein, corresponding figures for fat and calcium being 5.75 and 32. In comparison with other animals these average rates of turnover of material are very high.

The values in Table 15.1 can also be considered as the net requirement of nutrients for egg production and provide a starting point for defining the relationship between diet and animal performance. By combining them with appropriate coefficients for the efficiency of nutrient utilization, and with allowances for the maintenance of body

Table 15.1   The net requirement of nutrients for egg production

	Nutrients present in a 60-g egg	(yolk:albumen:shell)	Nutrients present in a 17-kg egg§	Nutrients present in a 2-kg hen
Weight (g)	60.0	(32:57:11)	–	–
Dry matter (g)	19.9	(49:21:30)	5638	–
Energy (MJ)	0.372	(81:19:0)	105	34
Fat (g)	6.1	(99.9:0.1:0)	1728	300
†Linoleate (g)	1.2	(99.9:0.1:0)	–	–
Protein (nitrogen × 6.25) (g)	7.08	(45:52:3)	2006	260
Arginine (mg)	429	(52:45:3‡)	–	–
Histidine (mg)	158	(48:49:3‡)	–	–
Isoleucine (mg)	384	(47:50:3‡)	–	–
Leucine (mg)	604	(47:50:3‡)	–	–
Methionine (mg)	237	(38:59:3‡)	–	–
Methionine + cystine (mg)	431	(41:56:3‡)	–	–
Phenylalanine (mg)	360	(38:59:3‡)	–	–
Phenylalanine + tyrosine (mg)	649	(41:56:3‡)	–	–
Threonine (mg)	330	(49:48:3‡)	–	–
Tryptophan (mg)	134	(47:50:3‡)	–	–
Valine (mg)	459	(43:54:3‡)	–	–
Calcium (g)	2.24	(1.2:0.2:98.6)	635	20
Phosphorus (g)	0.14	(81:4:15)	40	40
Sodium (g)	0.069	(20:80:0)	20	1.8
Potassium (g)	0.079	(27:73:0)	22	4.7

Chloride (g)	0.077	(31:69:0)	20	0.5
Copper (mg)	0.3	(94:6:trace)	—	—
Iodine (mg)	0.02	(80:20:trace)	—	—
Iron (mg)	2	(95:5:trace)	—	—
Manganese (mg)	0.02	(93:7:trace)	—	—
Zinc (mg)	1.0	(99:1:0)	—	—
Magnesium (g)	0.048	(51:7:42)	14	0.5
Selenium (mg)	0.3	(75:25:0)	—	—
†Vitamin A (μg)	360	(100:0:0)	—	·
†Vitamin D$_3$ (μg)	2.5	(100:0:0)	—	—
†Vitamin E (mg)	1.0	(100:0:0)	—	—
†Thiamin (μg)	12	(100:0:0)	—	—
†Riboflavin (μg)	85	(65:35:0)	—	—
†Pyridoxine (μg)	12	(100:0:0)	—	—
†Cyanocobalamin (μg)	6	(100:0:0)	—	—
†Folic acid (μg)	46	(82:18:0)	—	—
†Nicotinic acid (μg)	40	(22:78:0)	—	—
†Biotin (μg)	9	(81:19:0)	—	—
†Pantothenic acid (μg)	200	(93:7:0)	—	—
†Choline (mg)	380	(100:0:0)	—	—

† The levels of these nutrients in the egg are influenced by dietary supply. The values given are typical for practical diets used in commercial egg production in the United Kingdom.

‡ Proportion in shell assumed to be constant for all amino acids.

§ Equivalent to 1 year's egg production.

tissues and function, the familiar *factorial* equation can be written:

Dietary nutrient requirement (mass per day)

$$= \frac{\begin{array}{l} \text{Nutrient used} \\ \text{for maintenance} \end{array} + \begin{array}{l} \text{Nutrient content} \\ \text{of products} \end{array}}{\text{Efficiency of nutrient utilization}}.$$

The nutrient concentration in the diet required to supply this level of requirement is then a simple function of food intake:

Dietary concentration required (mass per mass)

$$= \frac{\text{Nutrient requirement}}{\text{Food intake}}.$$

Since laying hens are normally fed *ad libitum*, a knowledge of food intake under different conditions is essential to the understanding of the relationship between diet and animal performance.

PROTEIN AND AMINO ACIDS

There are only minor qualitative differences in protein metabolism between domestic fowl and mammals. In so far as these occur they are associated mainly with the uricotelic mode of nitrogen excretion.

Protein digestibility is a characteristic of the diet, and with mixed foods of the type normally used it ranges from 0.80 to 0.85 (coefficient of apparent digestibility) and from 0.85 to 0.90 (true digestibility). The biological value of the protein in such foods is approximately 60. A typical N balance for a laying hen whose protein intake is just sufficient to meet requirements is as follows: ingested N, 2.88 g/day; faecal-N loss, 0.56 g/day; urinary-N loss, 1.42 g/day; N in products, 0.90 g/day, of which egg protein accounts for 0.86 g/day and tissue growth for 0.04 g/day. The N in the urine is distributed between (g/kg) uric acid (840), urea (50), ammonia (70), creatinine (5), amino acids (17) and miscellaneous minor compounds (17). N losses of endogenous origin are approximately 208 mg/day, equally divided between the urine and faeces. In the fowl, faeces and urine are excreted together and separation for analysis requires special chemical or surgical techniques.

The concept of a maintenance requirement for protein has several theoretical weaknesses. However, studies with adult 'roosters' have shown that zero N-balance can be maintained by 250 mg digestible N per kg per day (1.56 g digestible protein) and this is consistent with the value of 2 g crude protein per kg per day suggested by feeding experiments with hens. Thus the total maintenance cost, defined in this way, is approximately twice the endogenous loss. For individual amino acids the Agricultural Research Council (1975) has suggested the following maintenance requirements (mg/kg body weight per day): lysine, 60; methionine, 40; methionine + cystine, 60; and tryptophan, 10.

The utilization of amino acids for egg production cannot be measured directly and varies in a complex manner with rate of lay. However, for hens in the earlier stages of lay (up to 40 weeks of age), the efficiency coefficient appears to be relatively constant and to vary for different amino acids only between 0.80 and 0.85. These values are based on the analysis of results from feeding experiments and are defined as the ratio of amino acid in the egg to amino acid used for egg production. They lead to the reasonable assumption that, for practical purposes, the amino acid requirements for egg production can be calculated as $1.2 \times$ the amino acid content of the egg (an efficiency of 0.83).

Thus for lysine, which is present in whole egg (including shell) at a level of 7.9 g/kg, the requirement for dietary available lysine is $7.9/0.83 = 9.5$ g/kg egg. The factorial equation is then:

$$\text{Lysine requirement (mg/day)} = 9.5\,E + 60\,W,$$

where
$$E = \text{egg production (g/day)};$$
$$W = \text{body weight (kg)}.$$

Similar equations can be derived for other amino acids:

$$\text{Methionine requirement (mg/day)} = 4.2\,E + 40\,W;$$
$$\text{Tryptophan requirement (mg/day)} = 2.25\,E + 10\,W.$$

It is important to recognize the limitations of such calculated requirements. They refer only to hens laying regularly during the early stages of production; they assume that there are no major discontinuities over the period concerned; they ignore variations in egg composition; and other forms of amino acid utilization, such as tissue or feather growth, are assumed to be zero. This latter assumption is probably reasonable in mature hens as the majority of the energy retained is as fat. Finally, they can only be applied strictly to individual animals; to obtain the requirements for populations of animals both the mean values of E and W for the population, *and* the variability in these values must be taken into account.

In recent years it has been shown that simple linear factorial models can be reconciled with a non-linear response curve, by considering individuals and populations separately. The elements of this theory are given in Fig. 15.1, which shows the linear factorial model for an individual bird, and how linear models for individuals combine to give

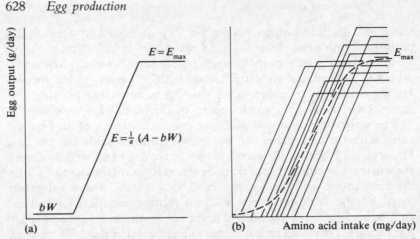

Fig. 15.1.   Diagram showing how a response based on a simple factorial
model and assumed to apply to an individual hen (a) produces a
diminishing response curve when applied to a group of hens which
exhibits variation in mean body weight and egg production (b).
The parameters of the flock curve (——) are: E = mean egg output
(g/day) (maximum = E_{max}); W = mean   body   weight   (kg);
σ_E = standard deviation of egg production; σ_W = standard deviation of body weight: ρ = correlation between E and W; a = kg
amino acid per kg E; b = mg amino acid per kg W; A = amino acid
intake (mg/day).

a non-linear model for a population if variations in E and W are taken
into account.

The biological and statistical characteristics of this simple model
have been worked out in some detail (Fisher, Morris and Jennings,
1973). If normal distributions are assumed a statement of an economically optimum requirement can be given in the following terms:

$$\text{Optimum requirement (mg/day)} = a\overline{E} + b\overline{W} + x\sqrt{a^2\sigma_E^2 + b^2\sigma^2w}$$

where a, b, $\overline{E}$, $\overline{W}$, σ_E and σ_W are as defined in Fig. 15.1, and x = the
deviate of the normal distribution corresponding to an area ak in one
tail (where k = cost per kg amino acid per value kg egg).

In practice, $\overline{E}$ and $\overline{W}$ are characteristics of a particular flock a and b
are constants, and σ_E and σ_W can be computed as $0.20 \, \overline{E}$ and $0.10 \, \overline{W}$,
respectively. The economic ratio k is calculated from 'local' data and the
normal deviate x is obtained from statistical tables. The optimum
requirement is defined as that which equates marginal returns to
increasing amino acid supply with marginal costs. Obviously, the
higher the cost in relation to the value of production the lower is the
optimal requirement.

This method of calculating requirements, which takes into account
the most important variables, has been widely used as the basis of

practical feeding recommendations. It also provides a procedure whereby the results of different experiments, carried out on stocks with differing characteristics, can be reconciled.

Such an elementary model obviously has a number of theoretical limitations and these are fully discussed in the original publications. For the present, the most important assumption is that the efficiency of utilization of amino acids for egg production, i.e. the coefficient a, is a constant. Whilst this appears to be generally true, an important qualification is that average utilization declines as the laying year progresses and the model cannot be used to calculate requirements in older birds. In simple terms, this decline in average amino acid utilization appears to result from rates of lay below 50% (i.e. less than one egg every 2 days). To lay at such a low rate birds must be cycling physiologically between the laying and non-laying states and protein synthesis for egg production is intermittent. When synthesis stops there will be no utilization of dietary amino acids for egg production and thus, over a period of time, efficiencies will range from zero, at zero egg production, to 0.80 to 0.85 at 50% egg production or above. Since, as birds age, the proportion of poor egg-layers in the flock increases, this provides a satisfactory explanation of the observed decline in the average efficiency of amino acid utilization.

With the range of foodstuffs in normal use, essential amino acid requirements are met by 17 to 19 g protein per day and non-essential amino acids or total protein are supplied in excess. It is important, however, to know the level at which the total protein supply rather than the supply of individual amino acids becomes the limiting factor. This has not been determined precisely for laying hens but estimates range from 12 to 16 g per day.

MINERAL SUPPLY AND EGG SHELL FORMATION

Calcium and phosphorus requirements

The metabolism of calcium in the hen is very intense owing to the large and rapidly fluctuating demands for egg shell formation; the Ca requirement of a laying hen is some 20 to 30 times that of a non-laying hen. The egg enters the shell-gland region of the oviduct – the uterus – 19 h prior to oviposition, with the shell membranes, two fibrous layers 70 μm thick, already formed. Some preliminary calcification has also occurred in the formation of mamillary knobs. In the uterus the process of 'plumping', due to water uptake, continues for 6 to 7 h and a further 13 to 14 h is required to complete shell formation. The completed shell weighs approximately 5 g and is 300 to 340 μm thick. Chemically, 980 g/kg of the shell mass consists of calcium carbonate, in the form of calcite, although small quantities of phosphorus and magnesium can also be detected. The remaining 20 g/kg is proteinaceous and forms the organic matrix of the shell. After 2 to 3 h of mineralization a constant rate of approximately 300 mg/h is reached, equivalent to a transfer of 155 mg Ca^{2+} per h from the blood; there is no prior storage of Ca^{2+} ions in the shell gland. The average rate of absorption of Ca from the digestive tract is 83 mg/h and the short-term demand for calcification has therefore to be met partly from labile stores in medullary bone. These labile stores are deposited in the maturing bird under the influence of ovarian oestrogens and represent 4 to 5 g Ca. Under the influence of the parathyroid hormone cortical bone may also be mobilized although, if this occurs to an excessive extent, a pathological condition known as 'cage layer fatigue' may ensue.

Over time intervals longer than those needed for the formation of a single egg, Ca balance is maintained positive. The absorption of Ca from the gut is dependent on the dietary supply, an effect which is mediated by vitamin D, but with conventional diets 0.5 to 0.6 of that ingested is absorbed. Thus, deposition of 2 g Ca per day in the egg shell requires an intake of 3.5 to 4.0 g Ca per day. This static view of the provision of Ca to the hen is a gross oversimplification of the processes involved, however, for, in view of the importance of Ca and the high rate of Ca turnover, it is not surprising that there are a number of complex mechanisms which interact to ensure the supply of Ca for egg formation.

Faced with an extreme Ca deficiency (dietary levels less than 1 g/kg) the hen stops laying completely, an effect which can be reversed by the administration of anterior-pituitary hormones. With less severe deficiencies a variety of responses are observed, including a reduction in the rate of lay, but many birds continue in production until tetany and death occur.

Under conditions of dietary adequacy the hen adjusts to its varying Ca needs by changing food intake. Thus, during 24-h periods when an egg is calcified and laid, food intake is up to 20% higher than on days when no eggs are produced. Separation of Ca from the remainder of the food diminishes this effect indicating that it is, in major part, a specific response to meet short-term Ca needs. Furthermore, when Ca is offered separately from the food, for example in the form of oyster shell, the supplement is consumed preferentially at times when it is required. A consequence is that the provision of a Ca source which is being digested at the time of shell calcification leads to a reduction in the turnover of labile Ca stores and an improvement in shell quality.

In addition to these adaptations of food intake, the efficiency of absorption of dietary Ca is almost twice as great during egg shell formation as during periods when no shell is being formed. This regulatory change, which is initiated no later than 3 h after the start of shell calcification, occurs throughout the small intestine but especially in the jejunum.

Because of the interacting factors influencing Ca metabolism, a simple factorial model, as used above for amino acids, is unsatisfactory for predicting Ca requirements, and response data from experiments must be used. An example is shown in Fig. 15.2, from which it can be seen that the requirement for maximum shell thickness is greater than that for other economic characteristics. Some experiments, unlike this one, have shown that the provision of excessive Ca can depress food intake and egg production, and thus a compromise is required. When Ca is incorporated entirely in the food this is usually to provide 3.5 to 4.0 g Ca per day, although there is an increasing move towards feeding systems which allow the hen to select the amount required. The mechanisms summarized above suggest that she will do this efficiently.

Quantitatively, the egg shell contains only small amounts of phosphorus, approximately 20 mg, compared with 120 mg in the egg contents. These needs, and those of the many metabolic functions of phosphorus, can be met at very low dietary levels. However, the hen also loses a significant amount of P in the urine during lay. This originates from the bone which is mobilized to meet the requirement for calcium, and the amount lost therefore varies with the Ca status of the

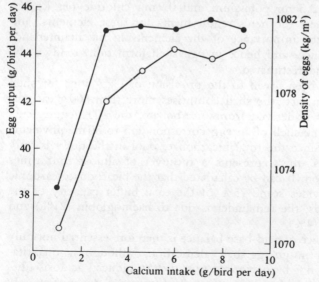

Fig. 15.2. An illustration of data on the response of laying hens to calcium intake which can be used as the basis for determining a requirement (●, egg output; ○, density). (From MacIntyre, Chancey and Gardiner, 1963.)

bird: values range from 1 g/day on a deficient diet to virtually zero when excess Ca is provided. From dose-response studies, the total P requirement of the hen is met when approximately 0.3 g/day available P is provided.

Although the P content of the shell is low there is variation in its distribution. Thus P: Ca is 0.002 for the inner layers and 0.012 for the outer layers. This difference may be associated with the inhibitory effect of phosphate ions on $CaCO_3$ precipitation, the phosphate bringing shell formation to an end. It might also provide an explanation for recent observations that excessive levels of P lead to a reduction in egg shell thickness.

A considerable proportion of the P in poultry foods is present as phytate and is usually considered to be completely unavailable, as high levels of Ca inhibit any exogenous phytase activity. Since Ca and other phytates are very insoluble, mineral requirements are increased by the presence of phytate.

Sodium, potassium and chloride; the maintenance of acid-base balance

For practical purposes, it can be simply stated that diets containing 1.0 mg sodium, 2.5 mg potassium and 0.9 mg chloride per kg are satisfactory to meet the hen's requirements for these elements, and because of this the importance of the elements in the maintenance of acid-base balance, and hence in egg shell formation, tends to be overlooked or underestimated.

Emphasis has been given to the provision of Ca^{2+} ions for shell formation but, in fact, the shell comprises more than 600 g carbonate per kg. This is derived from bicarbonate, the 100 mequivalents of carbonate in the shell of an egg corresponding to 50 mequivalents of bicarbonate. Since the total bicarbonate pool in the body is only 13.5 mequivalents, this represents a turnover of almost four times during calcification. It can be calculated that the bicarbonate-carbonic acid system provides some 75% of the total buffer capacity of the extracellular fluids; the remainder is due to haemoglobin (21%) and plasma proteins (4%).

The maintenance of acid-base balance is therefore essential not only for life but for optimum egg shell calcification. Although the quantitative details have not been worked out, dietary-induced acidosis (disadvantageous) or alkalosis (generally advantageous) depends mainly on the balance between sodium, potassium and chloride. Under some conditions the substitution of sodium bicarbonate for chloride has led to an improvement in egg shell quality.

Trace minerals

Provided that overt deficiencies are avoided, the provision of trace minerals to the hen presents few problems. As foods for laying hens contain high levels of Ca and phytate, both of which can reduce the availability of trace minerals, especially manganese and zinc, it is normal practice to ensure that about 2 to 3 times the mineral requirement is provided in the food.

VITAMINS

Provided, of course, that minimum requirements are met, there are no special problems in supplying vitamins to the hen. Because of the low cost of synthetic vitamins it is normal practice to make relatively generous additions to the diet. Vitamins are stored in the egg at a level which depends on the dietary intake. However, this is mainly important in reproduction, as has been discussed in Ch. 6.

ESSENTIAL FATTY ACIDS

In common with other animals the essential fatty acid (EFA) requirements of the hen can be considered in terms of linoleic acid; arachidonic acid, the other important EFA, can be derived *in vivo* from linoleic acid.

The hen requires 8 to 10 g linoleic acid per kg diet to meet its needs for most production purposes but a higher intake is necessary for maximum egg size to be achieved; some studies have suggested that dietary allowances as high as 20 g/kg can be justified. However, attempts to define precisely the response to linoleic acid have led to confusing results and, on economic grounds, dietary levels are usually fixed at approximately 12 g/kg.

EGG YOLK PIGMENTATION

The desired degree of egg yolk pigmentation varies from country to country but the ability to control it is an important aspect of ration design. In the United Kingdom relatively high levels of pigmentation are required.

The carotenoid pigments involved are, generally speaking, oxidation and/or breakdown products of carotenes. Of the many substances in this class, dihydroxy- and diketo-carotenoids are good pigmentors whilst others with mono- or poly-substituted side chains are not. The chemistry of these substances is complex and the simple analyses used for 'total' carotenoids involve only the separation of chlorophyll and β-carotene fractions from the total extractable lipid. As this is still a heterogenous component a utilization factor, based on feeding experiments, is applied to the results obtained with different foodstuffs. The pigmenting power of a mixed diet is indicated approximately by the sum of lutein and zeaxanthin, commonly referred to as xanthophyll.

A deep golden-yellow yolk contains 20 to 30 mg pigment per kg yolk substance. However, the relationship between pigment content and perceived yolk colour is complex and feeding decisions are normally based on the relationship between a yolk colour score, or index, determined by comparative methods, and the dietary level of pigmenting carotenoids or xanthophylls. Synthetic pigments, both yellow (the ethyl ester of β-apo-8'-carotenoic acid) and red (canthaxanthin), are now universally used to control very precisely the degree of pigmentation in eggs.

ENERGY REQUIREMENT AND FOOD INTAKE

In the discussion up to this point attention has been paid to the provision of adequate nutrients for egg production and the response of the hen to different levels of nutrient supply. In practical feeding, food intake is a key element since this determines the amount of food in which the nutrients must be conveyed, and hence the required nutrient concentration.

In common with other animals, the hen regulates food intake to maintain energy balance and, if feeding is *ad libitum*, it can be argued that the energy consumption and the energy requirement are one and the same thing. This has led to two approaches to the quantitative assessment of energy requirements. In the first, requirements are derived from summation of the various components of energy utilization as determined by calorimetric and balance techniques. In the second, requirements are determined from the measured food intake obtained under experimental conditions with animals of defined rates and production characteristics.

For some time these two approaches did not give consistent answers: the calorimetric approach provided predictions of energy requirements which were lower than the energy intakes observed in feeding experiments. However, it is now apparent that the discrepancies between the two approaches resulted from differences in methodology rather than principle.

A typical energy balance for a 2-kg hen is: ME intake, 1530 kJ/day; energy secreted in a 50-g egg, 335 kJ/day (22% of intake); energy stored in 0.75 g body tissues, 15 kJ/day (1% of intake); and energy lost as heat, 1180 kJ/day (77% of intake).

Of the energy lost as heat, some 19% is associated with the energy cost of egg production, 0.25% with the energy cost of growth and the remainder is conventionally attributed to maintenance. The major factors influencing this last component are environmental temperature, feathering and activity; minor factors include age and breed.

There are small, but consistent, differences, between maintenance energy requirements measured in light (white egg) strains and heavy (brown egg) strains. For the former, maintenance requirements in birds adapted to 25 °C are approximately 480 kJ/kg per day and for the latter 375 kJ/kg per day. Over the range of weights observed in commercial flocks it is valid to assume that maintenance energy requirements are proportional to body weight to the power 1.0 and not to the more usual power 0.75.

The effects of temperature and feather cover on these requirements interact in a complex way. The effect of temperature is greater (up to three times in extreme cases) in unfeathered than in well-feathered birds but temperature itself can affect feather cover, which is sometimes better at high than at low temperatures. Morris and Freeman (1974) provide a detailed discussion of these effects but, for the present, it is enough to say that overall differences in feathering are of sufficient importance to require consideration in the accurate prediction of food intake in laying hens.

In normally well-feathered flocks maintenance energy requirements change with temperature by approximately 9.2 and 8.4 kJ/kg per day per °C for white- and brown-egg strains respectively. Thus for practical purposes maintenance energy requirements (MJ/day) can be calculated as follows:

$$\mathrm{ME}_m = W[480 + 9.2(25 - T)] \text{ for white birds;}$$
$$\mathrm{ME}_m = W[375 + 8.4(25 - T)] \text{ for brown birds;}$$

where W = body weight (kg) and T = environmental temperature (°C)

Corrections for subjective feathering scores can be included in such calculations.

The energy content of egg, 6.7 MJ/kg, is relatively constant unless the proportions of yolk and albumen vary widely but, because of the experimental difficulties inherent in the measurements, there is uncertainty about the efficiency with which dietary ME is utilized for egg formation. Experimental estimates vary from 0.60 to 0.86 J/J and, whilst a value of 0.8 is widely used, this must be subject to modification in the light of further evidence. Assuming $k_{p,egg} = 0.80$, the ME requirement for egg production is 8.4 MJ/kg of egg.

There is even more uncertainty about the energy associated with small changes in body weight during lay but in the prediction of total energy intakes there is little potential error from this source, except in short-term studies. Changes in body weight are largely due to fat deposition or loss, and a value of 25 kJ/g can reasonably be used.

The summation of these components of energy utilization provides estimates of food intake which correspond fairly closely with the intakes observed in practice. For improved agreement the calculations would need to take account of age, activity, microclimate, feeding system and possibly food wastage, all of which can influence the food intake of flocks of hens to a minor extent.

Responses to dietary energy level

If energy consumption were the same on all diets, with food intake varying according to dietary energy concentration, then the optimum diet would provide a unit of energy at least cost. However, the adjustment of food intake is not always precise and it is necessary to know the response that hens make to diets of differing energy content. This response appears to vary with the type of bird, being more precise in small than in large breeds. Thus, in an analysis of several experiments, it was found that small birds eating approximately 1300 kJ/day increased their energy intake by 2 to 3% for each 10% increase in dietary energy content. For larger birds, eating 1880 kJ/day, the corresponding value was 4 to 5%.

Although important in economic terms, these small differences in energy intake do not influence egg production and most of the energy consumed in 'excess' of that required for egg production is deposited as fat, leading to small differences in body weight gain during lay.

Controlled feeding of laying hens

The normal deposition of body fat in hens fed *ad libitum* can be considered wasteful, and this has raised the possibility that restricting food intake to a level below *ad libitum* might increase profitability. In other aspects of poultry production, for example in the rearing of laying hens and the feeding of female parents of meat chickens, food restriction has an effect on birds' production characteristics, which may be beneficial. However, in egg laying hens food saving is the main objective and any effects on production would need to be small so as not to offset the benefit in food costs.

Although the available experimental data are variable, the larger and longer-term experiments indicate that, under conditions prevailing in the UK, restriction in food intake below *ad libitum* leads to a reduction in egg production, and the economics of production are not improved. Similarly, there is no evidence that increasing energy intake will lead to an increase in production. When foods in meal form are pelleted, energy intake is increased by up to 10% but this tends only to increase fat deposition. Thus, the mechanism for food intake regulation is sufficiently accurate for optimum performance to be achieved with diets given *ad libitum* in meal form.

Choice or selective feeding in laying hens

Two topics already discussed in this chapter indicate a possible rôle in feeding hens for selective feeding systems, in which individual birds are allowed to choose their own diet from a range of foods of differing composition.

Firstly, in the discussion on amino acids it was shown that variation in requirements between birds contributes to the inefficiency with which amino acids are utilized when a single food is given. Secondly, it was noted that hens given an opportunity to do so would consume a separate source of Ca specifically to meet variations in their needs for this nutrient.

Both of these can, in theory at least, be exploited if hens have the ability to select from a number of foods (differing appropriately in composition) a diet which just 'supports their maximum level of production. There is some evidence that they have this capacity and attempts are now being made to develop practical feeding schemes based on this principle.

The provision of a separate Ca source is now widespread and is probably a beneficial practice. Extension of choice feeding to two or three feeds differing in Ca, protein and other nutrient contents has been tried experimentally, and can be made to work, at least on a small scale. Exploitation of the concept in practical feeding is more difficult because of the technical problems of presenting the different foods in a way which allows the hens to express their preferences.

Success in this area could lead to a situation in which each hen, and therefore each flock, receives its own unique and optimum diet, leading to improvements in efficiency over the present methods whereby a single food is used to provide the best compromise between the conflicting needs of individuals. In the meantime, however, the development of methods for the better definition of this compromise will continue.

REFERENCES

Agricultural Research Council, 1975. *The Nutrient Requirements of Farm Livestock. No. 1, Poultry.* 2nd edn. Agricultural Research Council, London.

Fisher, C., Morris, T. R. and Jennings, R. C., 1973. A model for the description and prediction of the response of laying hens to amino acid intake, *Br. Poult. Sci.* **14**: 469–84.

MacIntyre, T. M., Chancey, H. W. R. and Gardiner, E. E., 1963. Effect of dietary energy and calcium level on egg production and egg quality, *Can. J. Anim. Sci.* **43**: 337–43.

Morris, T. R. and Freeman, B. M., 1974. *Energy Requirements of Poultry.* British Poultry Science, Edinburgh.

National Poultry Tests, 1978. Final report, 12th brown egg test. *Poultry Testing, July 1978,* pp. 5–16. National Poultry Tests Ltd, Godalming.

16 NUTRITION AND THE THERMAL ENVIRONMENT

A. J. F. Webster

This chapter deals with effects of heat and cold on the metabolism by farm animals of energy and protein. Energy is the more important of these for the reason that once converted to heat it cannot be recycled. An adult dairy cow converts to heat each year an amount of chemical energy equivalent to about five times that contained in her body at any one time. The conversion by a farm animal of the food energy it eats to products that the farmer can sell depends essentially upon three things:

1. the nutritive value of the diet, usually expressed as digestible energy or ME;
2. energy retention in the body (RE) where RE is the difference between ME intake and metabolic heat production (H_p);
3. the energy content of animal products, e.g. milk or meat.

The thermal environment can affect all three of these aspects of animal production. The most important (and best understood) effects involve (2), the conversion of ME to RE where the environment can influence H_p or ME or both. These will be considered first.

HOMEOTHERMY IN FARM ANIMALS

The heat exchanges between any homeotherm and the environment over a given period of time can be described most simply by equation [1]. For a more detailed treatment, see Monteith and Mount (1974).

$$H_p \pm H_s = H_1 = H_n + H_e \qquad [1]$$

where
H_p is heat produced in metabolism (W or MJ/day);
H_s is heat storage in the body, or $\rho \, \Delta T$. W where W is body weight (kg), ΔT is change in body temperature (°C) and ρ is the specific heat of the body (*ca.* 3.5 kJ/kg);

H_l is total heat loss from the animal to the environment (W or MJ/day);
H_e is heat loss by evaporation of moisture from the skin and from the respiratory tract (2.52 MJ/kg water); and
H_n is sensible heat transfer by the pathways of conduction, convection and radiation. The subscript $_n$ is used because sensible heat transfer approximately follows Newtonian laws of cooling. This may be written, in its simplest form

$$H_n = h \cdot A(T_1 - T_2)$$ [2]

where
$(T_1 - T_2)$ is the temperature difference between two bodies (°C), A is surface area (m²) and h is the coefficient of heat transfer (W/m² per °C).

For practical purposes the resistance of an animal to H_n can be described best by the use of the expressions tissue insulation (I_t) and external insulation (I_e).

Tissue insulation describes the resistance of an animal to heat loss by convection and conduction from the sites of heat production in the body core to the surface of the skin and respiratory tract. In this case $H_p = H_n$ and I_t is described by

$$I_t = (T_r - \bar{T}_s)/H_p.$$ [3]

When T_r is rectal temperature and $\bar{T}_s$ is mean skin temperature (°C), H_p is expressed in W/m^{-2}, the units of I_t become °C/m² per W. This equation neglects the fact that the surface of the skin and that of the respiratory tract are not likely to have the same mean temperature, in order to avoid incorporating an expression for evaporative heat loss from the respiratory tract, which is difficult to measure.

External insulation (I_e) describes the resistance to sensible heat loss from the surface of the skin ($\bar{T}_s$) through the coat of hair, wool or feathers to the air (T_a)

$$I_e = (\bar{T}_s - T_a)/H_n.$$ [4]

When H_n is expressed in W/m² the units are again °C/m² per W. Most measurements of heat exchange in animals are based on the measurement of metabolic heat production (H_p) using the techniques of indirect respiration calorimetry. In equation 4, therefore, it is usual to substitute ($H_p - H_e$) for H_n (see Blaxter, 1977).

The common farm animals may be divided into two types according to the way they maintain homeothermy in a temperate climate such as that of the United Kingdom. One group, which includes pigs and poultry, maintains a constant body temperature in most environments to which they are naturally exposed by regulating metabolic heat production in order to keep warm. The second group, which includes horses and all the ruminants, except in the earliest days of life,

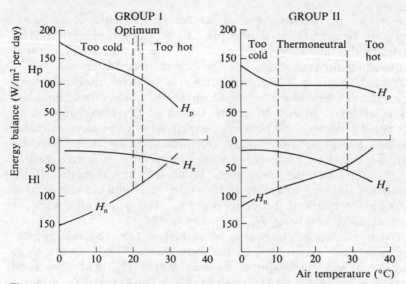

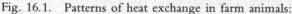

Fig. 16.1.   Patterns of heat exchange in farm animals:

    (a) *group I*, e.g. pigs and chickens, animals who maintain homeothermy primarily by regulating H_p. The vertical lines indicate the narrow zone of air temperature wherein food conversion efficiency is optimal;

    (b) *group II*, e.g. horses and ruminants, animals who maintain homeothermy primarily by regulating H_e.

    For further explanation see text.

maintains T_r in most UK environments by regulating heat emission, principally H_e, in order to keep cool. This point is illustrated in Fig. 16.1.

Pigs and chickens (group 1) have little ability to regulate evaporative heat loss, since active secretion of sweat is negligible (Ingram, 1974; Van Kampen, 1976). While they exhibit thermal panting when subjected to heat stress, the process is not very efficient. Both pigs and chickens are intolerant to heat stress experienced, for example, during transport. In the environment of the traditional farmyard, heat stress is not a problem because poultry can seek shade and pigs can wallow in mud, which provides an excellent substitute for sweat. However, for most of the year pigs and poultry in traditional farmyards utilize a significant proportion of dietary energy to keep warm. While this rarely constitutes a stress for well fed animals, it does affect their efficiency as converters of animal food to animal products. In modern intensive units for pigs and poultry, air temperature is usually regulated in order to maximize food conversion efficiency. Above the optimal temperature efficiency declines because the animal is too hot and maintains homeothermy by reducing ME intake. Below optimal temperature the environment appears to be too cold to the cost-conscious farmer if not to the pig or the chicken. Figure 16.1(a) illustrates this point in schematic form. Specific details of optimal temperatures for pigs and poultry will be discussed later.

Animals in group 2 (Fig. 16.1(b)), i.e. horses and ruminants, have very efficient mechanisms for regulation of H_e. In the case of Equidae, this is achieved mainly by active sweating. *Bos taurus* appears to partition H_e about 50:50 between cutaneous and respiratory evaporative loss. Sheep, not surprisingly, rely little upon sweating under the fleece but can sweat profusely over such temperature-sensitive areas as the scrotum. For the most part, however, they regulate H_e by ventilating the very extensive and very vascular mucous membranes covering the turbinate bones in the nose. For a general review of mechanisms of regulating H_e, see Hales (1974).

The regulation of H_e in group 2 animals is achieved at negligible metabolic cost except in extreme conditions. There is, for these animals, a wide *thermoneutral zone* in which H_p, and thus food conversion efficiency, are independent of T_a. The limits of the thermoneutral zone are called the upper and lower critical temperatures. The upper critical temperature is the point above which the animal cannot comfortably sustain homeothermy by H_e alone and so reduces H_p by reducing ME intake. At the lower critical temperature, active sweating and thermal panting cease and H_e is reduced to a minimal value associated with the obligatory loss of water from the skin and the respiratory tract. Below this point further increases in H_n enforce increases in H_p. The lower critical temperature (T_{1c}) for group 2 animals can be expressed in terms of the equations described already as follows:

$$T_{1c} = (T_r + H_{e, min.} \cdot I_e) - H_p^*(I_t + I_e)   [5]$$

H_p^* is thermoneutral heat production and $H_{e, min.}$ is minimal loss of heat by evaporation in cold environments (W/m^2). Specific examples of the effects of heat and cold on animals in group 2 and the extent of the thermoneutral zone will be discussed again later.

METABOLIC HEAT PRODUCTION

The amount of heat that an animal produces in metabolism is a function of its size and physiological state, its food intake (best expressed as ME), activity, and that which it may need to produce in order to maintain homeothermy, usually defined as cold thermogenesis.

Body size

The effect of body size is expressed most directly by basal metabolic rate, which is H_p in a fasted animal engaged in minimal activity and in a thermoneutral environment. While it is relatively easy to measure H_p, body size is a difficult concept to define precisely. It is possible to measure body weight easily and accurately, surface area with more difficulty and less accuracy (Brody, 1945) and volume (in the large, live, conscious animal) at some risk to life and limb. The relationship between surface area (A, m^2), which determines H_n, and body weight (W, kg) can be described by the formula

$$A = 0.09 \, W^{0.67}.$$ [6]

The exponent 0.67 (or 2/3) suggests that the ratio of surface area to volume is similar to that which obtains for a perfect sphere.

As a first approximation, basal metabolic rate (F), which defines the effect of size on H_p in a particular physiological state in all adult homeotherms, is related to W by the formula (see Kleiber, 1961)

$$F = 300 \, \text{kJ} \cdot \text{kg} \; W^{0.75}/\text{day}.$$ [7]

The value of $300 \, \text{kJ} \cdot \text{kg}^{0.75}/\text{day}$ is quite close to observed values for thermoneutral fasting metabolism in adult pigs and poultry. Most ruminants e.g. cattle and deer, have a fasting metabolism slightly above the interspecies mean, of approximately $350 \, \text{kJ} \cdot \text{kg}^{0.75}/\text{day}$. For sheep the value is rather lower, approximately $280 \, \text{kJ} \cdot \text{kg}^{0.75}/\text{day}$ (Blaxter, 1967; Mount, 1968).

Since H_n, which dominates heat loss in cold environments, is a function of surface area (or $W^{0.67}$), it follows that the larger the size of the adult animal the greater its basal metabolism per unit of surface area and thus, other things being equal, the greater its cold tolerance. It has conventionally been assumed that the effect of size on basal metabolism in the growing animal should be described by the same exponent. However, recent comprehensive reviews for the Agricultural Research Council of the data for ruminants (ARC, 1980) and pigs (ARC, 1982) indicate that the effect of increasing size on the basal metabolism of a growing individual is best described by an exponent not differing significantly from 0.67. Thus the increase in size of an individual during growth does not, of itself, confer any increase in cold tolerance, since the ratio of H_p to A appears to remain constant.

Food intake

The more an animal eats the more heat it produces. The resting heat production of an animal eating a maintenance ration is 25 to 40% above basal metabolism, depending on the efficiency of utilization of ME for maintenance, which is about $0.8 J/J$ in pigs and 0.63 to 0.73 in ruminants, depending on the fibrousness of the diet (Blaxter and Boyne, 1978). When an animal is consuming food to appetite its H_p is about 2.2 times basal metabolic rate (F) (Table 16.1). Thus, in growing cattle, H_p at *ad libitum* intake (A) is 800, F is 350, the ratio $A:F$ is 2.3; for lambs A is 620, F is 280 and $A:F$ is 2.2. The high heat production of the dairy cow at *ad libitum* intake is associated with a high apparent maintenance requirement (Moe and Tyrrell, 1975) of this physiologically hard-working animal. The data of Holmes and Close (1977) indicate that for the rapidly growing pig $A:F$ is above 1.8; again, basal metabolic rate per $kg^{0.75}$ exceeds that of the mature animal, reflecting the more active physiological state during growth.

Not only is there a marked similarity between species in the ratio $A:F$ but H_p at *ad libitum* intake is remarkably independent of the quality of the diet. Thus store cattle consuming a relatively fibrous diet with a high heat increment, and retaining little energy, have a maximum H_p very similar to that of 'barley beef' animals or even veal calves consuming a liquid diet with a metabolizability of 0.90. This suggests that among the many factors that influence appetite should be included the possibility that there is an upper limit to the extent to which an animal is prepared to do work in order to metabolize food. This level is lowest in the non-pregnant, non-lactating adult, higher in the growing animal and higher still under the physiological stimulus of peak lactation. However, these differences in physiological state are reflected in differences in apparent maintenance requirement or predicted basal metabolism (Webster, Brockway and Smith, 1974), so the ratio $A:F$ remains constant. In the context of this chapter, however, the most important point to emphasize is the degree to which food intake can affect H_p; in simple terms, the more an animal eats the more tolerant it will be to cold and the less tolerant to heat. This phenomenon will be expressed quantitatively for the different farm species later.

Activity

The effect of activity on H_p refers, in this context, only to those observable actions performed by the animal in relation to the external environment. In practice, the effect of activity on H_p is a function of the energy cost of each activity per unit of time and the length of time spent on each activity, when confined in a calorimeter for a conventional measurement of H_p. Excluding, for the moment, the energy cost of cold thermogenesis, the main activities of an unconstrained and unstressed farm animal are: (1) standing, (2) changing position,

Table 16.1 The metabolic heat production of different farm animals consuming food at or near to appetite

	Reference†	Body weight (kg)	Surface area (m²)	Heat production kJ/kg$^{0.75}$ per day	W/m²
Broiler chick	1	2.0	0.14	700	97
Laying hen	2	1.8	0.13	580	80
Growing pig	3	60	1.40	645	115
Growing lamb	4	35	0.97	620	106
Cattle	5				
Veal calf		100	1.97	800	148
Barley beef		450	5.40	810	170
Store cattle		250	3.64	790	158
Dairy cow (35 kg milk/day)		550	6.17	880	187

† References: 1. Siegel (1977); 2. Emmans and Charles (1977); 3. Holmes and Close (1977); 4. Webster, Smith and Brockway (1972); 5. Webster (1974).

(3) walking, and (4) eating. Table 16.2, taken from Webster (1978), illustrates the effect of activity on H_p for a 500-kg steer on range compared with that of a similar animal confined in a calorimeter. The two major elements are the energy cost of grazing out of doors (excluding the energy costs of standing and walking to graze) and the energy cost of walking, both of which, in normal circumstances, increase H_p by less than 10% above that of a confined animal, although this value can approach 25% on open range.

Cold thermogenesis

When the sum of sensible and inevitable evaporative heat loss $(H_n + H_{e, min})$ from a homeotherm exceed thermoneutral H_p (a function of its size, physiological state, food intake and activity with respect to the external environment), i.e. when it is below its lower critical temperature, it must perforce increase H_p in order to maintain homeothermy. This component of H_p is called cold thermogenesis. For adult farm animals this is probably achieved entirely by shivering or a similar mechanism involving the generation of heat by contraction of striated muscle. Newborn lambs and calves (Alexander, 1974; Alexander, Bennett and Gemmell, 1975) possess brown adipose tissue (BAT) which can produce heat *in situ* in response to sympathetic stimulation. The capacity of 1 kg of BAT to generate heat undoubtedly exceeds that of striated muscle by many orders of magnitude (Foster and Frydman, 1978), and non-shivering thermogenesis involving BAT is undoubtedly a major factor influencing the survival of newborn calves and lambs born out of doors. However, BAT appears to lose its effectiveness within the 1st week of life in these species and there is no evidence for non-shivering thermogenesis involving BAT in the newborn pig or chicken.

There has recently been a revival of interest in BAT in the adult animal, stimulated by the observation that adult rats, persuaded to overeat by being offered a variety of decadent foodstuffs, appear to show an enhanced thermogenic response in BAT to the infusion of noradrenalin (Rothwell and Stock, 1979). For the moment, however, there is no evidence to indicate that heat increment of feeding in farm animals alters as a consequence of prolonged over-eating. The bulk of the evidence suggests that (except in some neonates) non-shivering thermogenesis involving BAT plays little or no part in keeping farm animals warm in the cold, or in adjusting energy output to accommodate excessive ME input.

The four factors that contribute to H_p in a cold environment are not necessarily additive. The heat increment of feeding (HIF) is not

Table 16.2 The daily energy expenditure of a beef cow on range compared with that of a similar animal confined in a calorimeter (from Webster, 1978)

Activity	Energy cost of activity	Amount of activity		Additional cost of activity on range (kJ/day)
		Confined	On range	
Eating	35 J/kg$W$ per min	1.5 h	5–9 h	3700–7900
Standing	5.5 J/kg$W$ per min	5 h	5–15 h	1600
Changing position	55 J/kg$W$	20 actions	20–30	300
Walking	2.1 J/kg$W$ per horizontal m	Nil	1–6 km	1000–6300
	26.5 J/kg$W$ per vertical m			
Extra energy cost of outdoor activity (MJ/day)		4.7–16.1		
Heat production at maintenance in confinement (MJ/day)		49.8		
Heat production on range (MJ/day)		54.4–65.8		
Increase due to activity (%)		9–32		

constant over 24 h and peak increment may not coincide with peak heat loss in the case, for example, of a sow fed once per day at 10.00 h and exposed to a maximum intensity of cold at 06.00 h the following morning. Fig 16.2 shows that inevitable heat loss ($H_n + H_{e,min}$) exceeds H_p derived from (F + HIF) from 23.00 h until feeding time at 10.00 h. Thereafter, (F + HIF) exceeds inevitable heat loss and the animal maintains homeothermy by regulating H_e until 23.00 h when the lines once again cross over. In this case much of HIF has been wasted. Had the animal been fed so that HIF coincided better with the

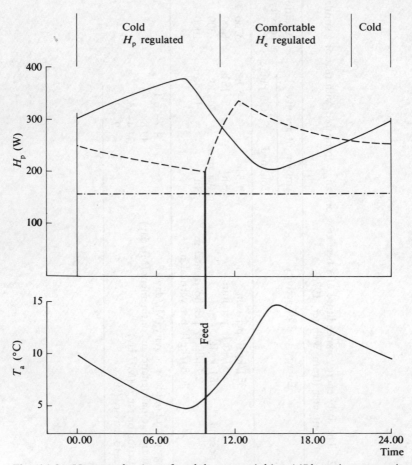

Fig. 16.2   Heat production of a adult sow weighing 165 kg, given an mainte- nance ration in one feed at 10.00 h and exposed to an air temperature fluctuating from +5 to +15°C ($\cdot-\cdot-\cdot$, indicates basal metabolism; ---, indicates the magnitude of the heat increment of feeding; ——, indicates obligatory heat loss ($H_n + H_{e,min.}$)). The metabolic heat production is indicated by the top line at any instant.

intensity of cold stress, the efficiency of utilization of the food, and thus the maintenance requirement of the animal, could have been improved. In ruminants, HIF is spread more evenly over 24 h and thus HIF substitutes more effectively for cold thermogenesis. Figure 16.3 illustrates the relationship between air temperature and H_p for individual sheep (Blaxter, 1977) and pigs (Close and Mount, 1978) in calorimeters. In the case of closely shorn sheep (Figure 16.3(a)) the effect of increasing HIF is simply to move the point of inflexion of the line (the lower critical temperature). Below this point the relationship between H_p and T_a is described by a single slope, indicating that HIF substitutes entirely, in this example, for shivering cold thermogenesis. In the case of pigs (Figure 16.3(b)), the lines relating H_p to T_a at different levels of ME intake converge as T_a falls but never meet, indicating that in this example HIF is never able to substitute entirely for cold thermogenesis.

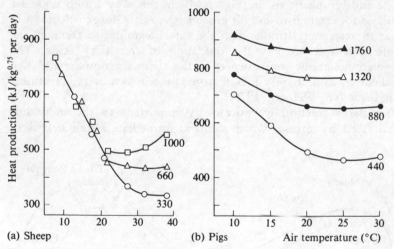

Fig. 16.3.   Interactions between the effects of air temperature and food intake on metabolic heat production in (a) sheep and (b) pigs. Units of H_p are $kJ/kg^{0.75}$ per day and the numbers to the right of each line indicate ME intake, also in $kJ/kg^{0.75}$ per day. These curves have been adapted slightly from (a) Blaxter (1977) and (b) Close and Mount (1978) to permit direct comparison.

METABOLIC RESPONSES TO THERMAL STRESS

It is important here to distinguish between three phenomena. Prolonged exposure to heat or cold involves *hormonal* and *metabolic* changes specific to each stress. Acute exposure of an animal to heat, cold, danger and distress arouses a non–specific but typical response termed by Selye (1950) the 'alarm reaction'.

Alarm reaction

Immediately following any stress, the secretion of glucocorticoid hormones from the adrenal cortex is increased. At the same time increased activity in the sympathetic nervous system is augmented by increased secretion of catecholamines from the adrenal medulla. The principal metabolic action of the catecholamines is to mobilize energy-rich substrates for catabolism. These substrates come mainly from fat but also from glycogen in liver and protein in muscle (Figure 16.4). The catecholamines also selectively inhibit glucose uptake in muscle by inhibiting insulin release and therefore spare glucose for vital tissues like the brain. They may also inhibit the release of insulin and growth hormone (Himms-Hagen, 1967). Glucocorticoids stimulate the breakdown and inhibit the synthesis of protein in major stores like skin, gut, muscle and lymphatic tissue (Fig. 16.4). In this way amino acids are mobilized for catabolism and for gluconeogenesis. Glucocorticoids also appear to act synergistically with the catecholamines to facilitate the mobilization and possibly the oxidation of free fatty acids. The immediate metabolic consequences of the alarm reaction are a loss of stored energy as heat and a loss of stored protein as urea and creatinine in the urine (see Webster, 1976).

The alarm reaction is enormously important to the individual animal faced by stresses which demand immediate action if it is to

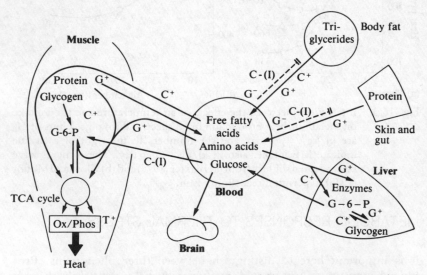

Fig. 16.4.   Probable metabolic actions of catecholamines, corticosteroids and thyroxine (C+, catecholamines stimulate; C-(I), catecholamines inhibit insulin; G+, glucocorticoids stimulate; T, thyroxine; G-6-P, glucose-6-phosphate). (From Webster, 1976.)

survive. Cold stress falls within this category since homeothermy in the cold requires increased work. Faced by acute heat stress, an animal which exhibits an alarm reaction involving an increase in H_p is obviously at a disadvantage. Indeed, the exaggerated alarm response to heat stress, seen in stress-susceptible pigs of the Piétrain and other breeds, can lead rapidly to death from hyperthermia (Sybesma and Eikelenboom, 1969).

The rôle of farm animals is anabolism rather than catabolism and each alarm reaction must reduce the efficiency of food conversion to saleable product. For this reason an environment which is designed to minimize stress in any form is likely to maximize productive efficiency. This is the basis of a strong, albeit incomplete, argument in favour of the theory that optimum productivity in farm livestock equates with optimum welfare. One exception to the 'no stress is best' theory is seen in dairy cows. Ekesbo (1966) noted that in Sweden the incidence of lactation ketosis was seven times greater in cows tethered and housed all winter in insulated barns than in those offered intermittent activity and cold stress in open-fronted yards. The stimulus to increased catabolism evoked by activity, cold and the onset of lactation are qualitatively similar. It may be that an environment which succeeds in protecting an animal from any environmental stress may leave it unprepared to meet the more demanding stress of lactation.

Cold stress

Once the initial alarm reaction has subsided the hormonal and metabolic responses of an animal alter subtly as it adapts to prolonged cold. Cold stress of constant intensity is, of course, only a figment of the controlled experiment; in practice the intensity of cold stress is inconstant and unpredictable. There is, moreover, good evidence that the nature of metabolic adaptation to cold differs markedly according to the nature of the stimulus. Héroux (1963) has listed differences in the metabolic response of rats *acclimated* to constant cold in the laboratory or *acclimatized* to the fluctuating, but severe, cold stresses of a Canadian winter. Briefly, Héroux (1963) concluded that acclimation to constant cold stimulated a general and persistent increase in all aspects of energy metabolism; both thermoneutral H_p and summit metabolism in severe cold were enhanced, but thermal insulation was unaffected. Acclimatization to winter conditions increased thermal insulation but apparently had little affect on energy metabolism. In similar experiments with sheep, Webster, Hicks and Hays (1969) obtained similar results: for example, animals adapted to constant cold of moderate intensity rather rapidly developed an increased appetite and an enhanced metabolic response to severe cold, whereas those acclimatized to the Canadian winter developed more slowly a more persistent response, which included an increase in appetite but a decreased metabolic response to severe cold. The animals appeared to *habituate* to winter conditions in the sense that their metabolic response to a standard cold stimulus was reduced rather than enhanced. In other words, they were prepared to tolerate a lower skin temperature in the interests of energy conservation. In terms of the physics of heat transfer this is equivalent to an increase in tissue insulation. It is probable that the physiological response of most farm animals to naturally occurring cold conditions involves a stoic response of this type. Unfortunately, nearly all studies on adaptation to cold have been conducted in controlled environment chambers. It is almost certain that these experiments exaggerate the metabolic response of an animal in the field but, bearing this in mind, some general conclusions may be drawn.

The increase in glucocorticoid secretion in response to cold probably does not persist unless the animal is undernourished and in chronic negative energy balance. If adequate food is available and the stress is not too severe, thyroid secretion rate increases, reaching a maximum by approximately 36 h. This increase may or may not be accompanied by an increase in metabolic rate. Catecholamine secretion rates are probably elevated throughout any period of cold exposure. Since they act synergistically with thyroid hormones their secretion during cold exposure is inversely related to the level of thyroid activity at that time. These hormonal changes appear to be initiated at air temperatures slightly (approximately 5 °C) above the lower critical temperature. In other words, metabolic consequences of changes in hormone secretion may occur without any increase in H_p. For a more complete review, see Webster (1976). In practice, this means that growth or milk production may be affected even though the energy metabolism of the animal appears to be unaltered.

The most important nutritional consequences of the physiological response of an animal to cold are as follows. Food intake is usually reduced during the alarm reaction but increases during acclimation to constant cold. As indicated above, this response is less obvious and slower to develop in field studies (Webster *et al.*, 1969). Growing cattle reduce food intake during periods of driving wind and rain but develop a large appetite for high-energy foods when exposed on feedlots to the prolonged severe cold of a north American winter (Webster, 1976). These animals (and their owners) can afford the luxury of a hedonistic or enhanced metabolic response to cold since if, in the growing animal, ME intake is increased more than H_p, then the overall efficiency of ME utilization (RE/ME) is also increased. Adult stock on poor-quality winter range do not have the opportunity to increase ME intake. In this case stresses of cold and undernutrition combine to create a chronic problem of energy shortage, and in these circumstances the stoic response involving increased tolerance to low skin temperatures and a diminished metabolic response to cold has a greater survival value. In this context it is significant that semi-domesticated ruminant species like the sheep and the red deer spontaneously reduce food intake as daylength shortens (Forbes, 1977).

The digestibility of forages by sheep and cattle is reduced when the animals are subjected to cold stress. This reduction is associated with an increase in thyroid secretion rate and an increase in rate of passage of digesta through the gut (Kennedy, Christopherson and Milligan, 1976). The ME content of the dry matter is therefore reduced. Utilization of ME depends primarily, as indicated earlier, upon the extent to which cold increases H_p, which is determined not only by the total thermal demand of the environment ($H_n + H_{e,min}$.) but also by the pattern of feeding, which affects the degree to which HIF can substitute for cold thermogenesis (Fig. 16.2).

Prolonged severe cold can also have marked effects on the way in which an animal allocates retained nutrients to different tissues. D. L. Ingram raised piglets in very cold and hot environments and observed extraordinary differences in patterns of growth (see Mount, 1968). The piglets raised in the cold not only grew more hair, which was expected, but also developed a completely different shape from those raised in the heat, even though the two groups were retaining energy at the same rate. Martha Heath and D. L. Ingram (unpublished results) have recently extended this work. Pigs in the cold were shorter in all the extremities (ears, snout, tail, legs) than pigs in the heat. Furthermore, in the cold they tended to deposit fat intra-abdominally rather than subcutaneously, which had the undesirable effect of reducing their tissue insulation. Undoubtedly some of these differences in tissue growth were simple consequences of different patterns of blood (and thus substrate) flow in the different environments, since when piglets in the cold were given a muff for one ear, that ear grew larger. There are, however, reasons for suspecting that some of the differences in growth attributable to cold, in particular the relative decrease in the ratio of protein to fat in the body gains, may have been due to a cold-induced inhibition of secretion of the major anabolic hormones, prolactin, growth hormone and insulin. The conditions in these experiments were more severe than normally occur in practice but it is reasonable to conclude that hormonal response to less severe cold stress can also affect the pattern of growth. Siegel (1977) has reviewed evidence for similar changes in the pattern of growth in poultry. Thompson and Thomson (1977) have shown that the reduced milk production of goats in cold environments can probably be attributed mainly to a reduced blood flow to the mammary gland but may also be due in part to reduced secretion of lactogenic hormones. Presumably the same applies to cattle.

Cold may therefore affect each stage of the conversion by livestock of animal food into animal products: intake, digestibility, energy and protein retention, and the distribution of retained nutrients. Thus well controlled field trials which measure the ultimate expression of all these responses in the entire animal may often provide more sensitive indicators of the practical importance of cold stress than laboratory-based experiments which measure, albeit very precisely, only certain aspects of the metabolic response and often in animals not appropriately adapted to the field environment which the experimenters wish to simulate.

Heat stress

Heat is potentially a greater commercial problem than cold because it affects first the animal that is growing fastest or producing the most milk by virtue of its high metabolic rate, and the main effect is a reduction in food intake. Thus while *Bos taurus* will usually eat more and grow faster than *Bos indicus* in a thermoneutral environment, it can seldom compete in the tropics (Colditz and Kellaway, 1972). Much of the difference between *Bos taurus* and *Bos indicus* in heat tolerance can be attributed to the superior heat dissipation mechanisms of the latter, e.g. sweating, thermal panting, reflexion of incoming solar radiation by the coat. These considerations are, however, outside the scope of this chapter and have been covered thoroughly by Bianca (1965) and Thompson (1973).

The basal metabolic rate of *Bos indicus* is lower than that of *Bos taurus*. In more practical terms, at the same body size and ME intake the physiological state of *Bos indicus* is such that it produces less heat (Frisch and Vercoe, 1977). This less active physiological state confers greater tolerance to both heat and drought, but limits the potential for growth or milk production on a high-quality diet in a thermoneutral environment.

The hormonal and metabolic changes invoked by heat stress begin with the alarm reaction. Thereafter there is a fall in the thyroid secretion rate (even if food intake is maintained by force-feeding) and in the turnover of insulin and growth hormone. Quite simply, during prolonged heat exposure both catabolic and anabolic hormone secretions are depressed and as a result the whole process of metabolism slows down (see Webster, 1976). This inevitably reduces appetite and thus performance in the growing or lactating animal. Moreover (as in the case of cold stress), the reduced secretion of anabolic hormones appears to reduce the efficiency of utilization of digested nutrients. Thus hyperthermic steers given a controlled food intake show an increased urinary excretion of urea and creatinine, indicating a diminished capacity for protein deposition in the growing body (Colditz and Kellaway, 1972). Undoubtedly, animals adapt to prolonged heat but the recovery of normal nitrogen metabolism would appear to be very slow (McDowell, 1968).

The effect of heat stress on lactation is similar. Even when food intake is maintained, milk secretion is reduced. The reduction in yield involves all the major components but milk fat appears to be the most severely depressed. Again, this is presumably due to reduced secretion of lactogenic hormones and acclimation is slow and incomplete (see Webster, 1976).

Drought

In many of the tropical areas grazed by domesticated ruminants, heat stress is compounded for long periods every year by the problem of drought. The water balance of ruminants in hot, arid environments has been studied and reviewed by McFarlane (1976). However, drought also has important nutritional consequences because the amount of food available to the animals is markedly reduced. Even if the area is not overgrazed, the standing hay on range is extremely fibrous and low in crude protein.

There has been little fundamental research on the nutritional consequences of drought for ruminants and other farm species, but it is possible to construct from first principles a satisfactory explanation of the metabolic mechanisms invoked for survival in a drought and the reasons why, for example, the west African goat and the donkey appear to thrive in conditions that are intolerable to European cattle or horses.

Excluding the extreme case where there is no food at all, the nutritional problems of drought are lack of water, lack of dietary nitrogen and low digestibility of dietary energy. Digestible energy is low because dietary fibre content is high and because degradable nitrogen content cannot sustain sufficient microbial growth in the rumen and/or hind gut to ensure optimal fermentation of potentially digestible dry matter. Thus, even though food may be available in plenty, the animal has difficulty in consuming enough ME for maintenance within the constraints of gut fill. Tropically adapted breeds, e.g. *Bos indicus*, have a lower H_p at maintenance than *Bos taurus* so are at an advantage in this respect.

Species adapted to the dry tropics, like the African goat and donkey, have a greater ability to concentrate urine than cattle (*Bos indicus* or *Bos taurus*) or horses (Schmidt-Nielsen, 1964; McFarlane, 1976). Not only does the ability to concentrate urine conserve water, it also conserves urea produced by catabolism of body protein in an animal at or below maintenance. This urea can be recycled to the rumen or hind gut and incorporated into microbial protein. Thus the animal best able to concentrate urine is best able to digest low-nitrogen, high-fibre, dry tropical grasses. The ability of ruminants to recycle the end products of catabolism of body protein through the rumen in order to generate more ME and amino acids in conditions of drought is undoubtedly of far greater evolutionary and practical significance than their much more assiduously studied ability to use dietary sources of non-protein nitrogen for productive purposes.

The other prime requirement for survival in the dry season is a large stomach to accommodate large amounts of fibrous material long enough to ensure optimal fermentation. Here again the native goat and the donkey have a conspicuous advantage over 'improved' cattle and horses.

At the end of the long, dry season in, e.g. northern Nigeria, the native Fulani cattle and (surprisingly) sheep are emaciated even on well-managed units, presumably because they have been unable to obtain sufficient energy for maintenance from the food available. The little native goats are, however, in excellent condition, due mainly to their relatively enormous stomachs and powerful kidneys.

PRACTICAL CONSEQUENCES FOR FARM SPECIES

Chickens

Most poultry are nowadays kept in strictly controlled environments and the conditions for most economic performance are known with some precision. Because respiratory disease can be controlled by selective breeding and vaccination, it is possible to stock animals at very high density and the only environmental variable which significantly interacts with nutrition is air temperture.

Broilers

For growing birds, air temperature is regulated to ensure an optimal balance between ME intake and H_p so as to achieve maximum growth rate and food conversion efficiency. Figure 16.5, which is adapted from Ota and McNally (1965), shows that in 9-week-old broilers food conversion efficiency improved with increasing T_a over the range 5 to 30 °C but that growth rate was optimal at 21 °C. The temperature requirements for growing birds are summarized by Sains-

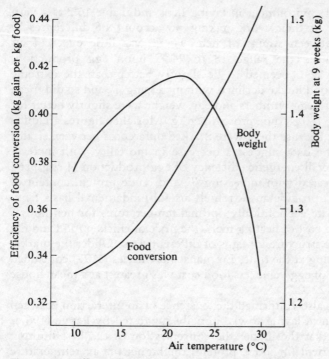

Fig. 16.5. Effect of air temperature on growth rate, expressed as weight achieved at 9 weeks, and food conversion efficiency (kg gain per kg food) in broiler chickens. (Adapted from Ota and McNally, 1965.)

bury (1978). Conventionally, 1–day-old chicks are provided with a heat source that maintains T_a in a confined area at 35 °C. This is subsequently reduced by 3 °C per week. House temperature outside the confines of the brooder is approximately 21 °C. Alternatively, blown hot air can be used to provide an initial T_a of 31 °C, falling by 0.5° per day to 21 °C by 3 weeks of age. Thereafter, 21 °C is optimal for growth, food conversion and mortality, but the increased cost of heating fuels relative to chicken food may demand a review of the economic wisdom of providing a temperature as high as this under winter conditions. For a review of the effects of heat, cold and temperature fluctuations on metabolism in growing chickens, see Siegel (1977).

Layers

Even the modern, highly selected hen does not lay more than one egg per day. In order to achieve maximum conversion of food into eggs the intensive producer uses control of air temperature to restrict the food intake of his birds. Emmans and Charles (1977) have thoroughly investigated the interactions between nutrition, egg production and the thermal environment in laying hens and Table 16.3 is a very brief summary of their work, taking no account of differences in performance between strains of hen. There was little effect of air temperature within the range 18 to 24 °C upon egg production, although 20 to 22 °C seemed to be slightly better than the extreme temperatures. Food intake declined with increasing T_a and so did mean egg weight. Both egg numbers and egg weight were slightly better for diets containing 180 g crude protein per kg. Mortality figures are difficult to interpret because there were marked differences between strains of birds, but the data suggest a decrease in mortality with increasing T_a. The overall energetic efficiency of egg production (J egg per J ME) again increased with increasing T_a and crude protein content of diet. These data provide an extremely useful fundamental basis from which to calculate economically optimal temperatures for hen houses according to the cost of heating fuels, the price of chicken food and the differential price structure for eggs of different sizes. Under the market conditions existing at the time, Emmans and Charles (1977) concluded that the margin of egg value less food cost was greatest at a mean house temperature of 22 °C.

These results also confirmed the existence of an interaction between T_a and nutrition in laying fowls, initially suggested by Payne (1967), who proposed that the higher the concentration of the first limiting non-energy nutrient (in short, protein) the higher the air temperature associated with maximum egg production. In other words, as T_a is increased so the birds' requirement for ME is decreased relative to other nutrients. This interaction will assume particular importance if, as is possible, alternative systems of husbandry to battery cages develop in response to legislation on welfare grounds or to unacceptable increases in the costs of installing and running battery units. Sainsbury (1978) has provided some evidence to show that a low-cost, well-designed straw yard system for laying hens can be economically competitive with the battery unit. The increased food requirement of birds in straw yards is not large because the birds are better feathered and on straw rather than wire, both of which combine to improve external insulation. Moreover, the increased requirement is almost entirely for energy. This means that the dietary concentration of other nutrients, e.g. amino acids and vitamins, can be much less than in a high temperature battery unit and some of these nutrients can be found by the birds themselves in deep litter. Low cost egg production has not received the scientific attention offered to the battery hen, but one can predict from first principles that adequate production might be achieved in unheated units on diets with crude protein contents as low as 120 g/kg. This would make it possible to provide a very large part of the hen's diet from cereals produced on the farm and reduce the dependence of the true chicken farmer on proprietary foodstuffs.

Table 16.3   Effect of air temperature and crude protein content of diet on productivity of laying hens in battery cages (from Emmans and Charles, 1977).

	Air temperature (°C)							
	18		20		22		24	
Crude protein (g/kg)	150	180	150	180	150	180	150	180
Eggs per hen per day	0.715	0.736	0.728	0.731	0.722	0.743†	0.712	0.724
Food intake (g/hen per day)	116	115	115	114	111	110	105	103
Mean egg weight (g)	60.4	61.1	60.0	60.8	59.6	60.4	58.6	59.0
Mortality (%)	15.4	14.9	14.3	13.6	14.7	11.2	11.2	9.6
Energetic efficiency (J egg per J ME)	0.223	0.234	0.229	0.236	0.232	0.247	0.240	0.250

† Numbers underlined indicate 'best' value for each attribute of performance.

Pigs

For practical purposes, the most important pieces of information necessary to design a system of feeding and housing pigs for optimal growth are lower critical temperature (T_{lc}) and the increase in rate of heat loss (or ME requirement) per °C fall in T_a below T_{lc}. From these one can calculate the increased food requirement to meet the demands of cold thermogenesis or, alternatively, the decrease in live-weight gain if those needs are not met. Table 16.4 provides calculated values for individually-housed growing pigs summarized from Holmes and Close (1977). The decrease in live-weight gain occasioned by cold if extra food is not provided was calculated on the assumption either that the energy for cold thermogenesis was derived (a) entirely from fat, or (b) equally from all body tissues. The difference is striking, particularly in the young animal. Effects of cold on nitrogen metabolism in growing animals have been discussed earlier. It is probable that the effect of cold on live-weight gain is close to the upper values (b) (Table 16.4) on initial exposure when the alarm reaction operates and steroid hormones stimulate nitrogen catabolism but declines towards the lower values (a) as the animal adapts.

Undoubtedly, pigs huddled in groups lose less heat than individuals. In their review, Holmes and Close (1977) suggested that this effect might be quite small but the results of Verstegen, van der Hel and Willems (1977) suggest that, at least to 50 kg live weight, the lower critical temperature of groups of, for example, nine pigs is approximately 6 °C lower than that of individuals, and the rate of increase in heat loss per °C fall in T_a only about half as great.

Table 16.4   Calculated values for lower critical temperature (T_{lc}) in growing pigs housed individually, rates of increase in heat production (H_p) per °C below T_{lc} and the equivalent weight of meal required to meet the increase or the decrease in live-weight gain expected if the increase in intake was not met (from Holmes and Close, 1977).

	Live weight (kg)			
	2	20	60	100
Lower critical temperature (°C)[†]	29	17	16	14
ΔH_p (kJ per pig per day per °C)	47	163	316	430
Extra food requirement (g per pig per day per °C)	4	14	26	36
Decrease in live-weight gain (g per pig per day per °C) (a)[‡]–		4	8	11
(b) –		29	16	19

[†] ME intake 2 to 3 times maintenance.
[‡] (a) assuming energy for cold thermogenesis derived only from fat;
   (b) assuming energy for cold thermogenesis derived equally from all tissues.

Table 16.5 Predicted values for the lower critical temperatures (°C) of growing pigs (from Bruce and Clark, 1979)

Body weight (kg)	Group size	Straw floor Food intake* $2 \times M^{\dagger}$	Food intake $3 \times M$	Concrete floor Food intake $2 \times M$	Food intake $3 \times M$
20	1	22	17	26	22
	15	17	11	21	16
40	1	19	14	23	19
	15	13	7	18	13
60	1	18	12	22	18
	15	12	5	16	11
80	1	17	11	21	17
	15	10	4	15	10

† Maintenance.

Floor type obviously affects heat loss and food requirements, particularly in the growing pig which spends so much time lying down. Bruce (1979) has measured the effects of different floor types on heat loss from simulated pigs, and Bruce and Clark (1979) have derived an elegant model to predict the lower critical temperature according to body weight, food intake, group size and floor type. Table 16.5 summarizes their conclusions. For example, at a body weight of 40 kg, T_{lc} for pigs group-housed on concrete is 13 °C, on straw it is 7 °C. Under UK winter conditions, straw bedding effectively dispenses with the need for supplementary heating for pigs over approximately 20 kg.

In many modern pig units the adult pregnant sow is held in individual stalls on concrete and fed only a maintenance ration. The three factors, isolation, high conductive heat loss and low thermoneutral H_p, combine to make the sow extremely sensitive to cold and in these circumstances her critical temperature is approximately 20 °C. Thus, in addition to the other insults to the welfare of a sow compelled to spend most of her adult life in an individual pen and on concrete, she is unnecessarily exposed to cold and her ME requirement for maintenance is elevated accordingly. There have been several descriptions of the 'thin sow syndrome', an irreversible loss of condition in adult sows being fed allegedly a maintenance ration. Straightforward cold stress is an adequate explanation of this phenomenon (Hovell, Gordon and MacPherson, 1977).

Sheep

The lower critical temperature of sheep is affected by body size, food intake and environmental conditions affecting external insulation, such as wind and rain. Values in Table 16.6 are drawn from a variety of sources, all of which are quoted in the review by Alexander (1974). The lamb at birth is obviously acutely sensitive to cold and one may conclude that in most UK conditions it is exposed to air temperatures below T_{1c} almost continually for the 1st month of life. By the time it reaches slaughter weight T_{1c} in still air has fallen to $-15\,°C$ by virtue of increased H_p and thermal insulation. The fleece of the adult sheep provides excellent insulation in dry, still air conditions ($T_{1c} = -7\,°C$) but wind and rain elevate T_{1c} markedly (Table 16.6). A starving ewe in full fleece by virtue of her low thermoneutral H_p has a T_{1c} of approximately $10\,°C$. The stress of winter for sheep kept out of doors on the hills in the UK is therefore severe only if cold is accompanied by undernutrition. Shearing elevates T_{1c} initially to approximately $+20\,°C$ in still air. This is quite a severe thermal stress for the animals, to which they adapt in part by increasing food intake (Davey and Holmes, 1977). There has been a tendency in recent years to shear ewes at housing in the winter, the logic being to increase voluntary food intake in late pregnancy and thus increase birth weight, and therefore viability, in lambs (Kneale and Bastiman, 1977). There are undeniably cases where ewes housed over winter when in full fleece are subject to mild heat stress, to which they are likely to respond by reducing food intake, and this is undoubtedly undesirable in late pregnancy. Moreover, in dry, draught-free conditions inside a sheep house no shorn ewe, adequately fed, is likely to be intolerably stressed by low air temperatures alone. However, it is likely, again from first principles of energy exchange, that the ME requirement of ewes from housing in January to lambing

Table 16.6   The lower critical temperature of sheep and lambs under different conditions of management

	Management	Lower critical temperature (°C)
Lamb, newborn	Dry, still air[†]	+28
Lamb, 1-month-old	Dry, still air	+10
Lamb, fat	Dry, still air	−15
Ewe, pregnant, full fleece	Dry, still air	−7
	Dry, draughty[‡]	+2
	Wet, draughty	+10
Ewe, starved, full fleece	Dry, still air	+10
Ewe, newly shorn	Dry, still air	+20
	Wet, draughty	+25

[†] 'Still air': wind speed = 0.18 m/s (0.65 km/h)
[‡] 'Draughty': wind speed = 1.8 m/s (6.5 km/h)

in March would be increased at least 25% by shearing. This seems to be an unacceptable increase in food costs relative to the small potential gain in lamb crop. It may be better to ensure adequate natural ventilation in the building to avoid any inappetence due to mild heat stress.

Cattle

Table 16.7, updated slightly from Webster (1974), illustrates in some detail effects of food intake and differences in thermal insulation on the lower critical temperature in still air for different classes of cattle. The most obvious point is the extreme degree of cold tolerance of all but very young calves. For practical purposes it can be said that low air temperatures, as such, have negligible effects on the metabolic rate of cattle. The combined effects of cold on metabolic rate, digestibility and utilization of nutrients for growth can, in the most severe conditions such as a western Canadian feedlot (Milligan and Christison, 1974), have small effects.

The low T_{lc} of veal calves is of particular interest, since these animals have conventionally been housed in heated buildings at air temperatures of 15° to 20 °C. Veal calves produce heat at an exceptionally high rate by virtue of their high ME intake and so are, contrary to popular opinion, more tolerant to cold and more susceptible to heat stress than conventionally raised calves (Webster, 1979).

For dairy cows T_{lc} is misleading since lactation is depressed at temperatures below approximately 0 °C, presumably, as indicated earlier, because local cooling reduces blood supply to the mammary gland.

Table 16.8 illustrates differences in cold tolerance of cattle attributable to effects of adaptation to cold in the individual, differences in wind speed, differences between beef and dairy types, and differences in body condition, itself conditioned by prior nutrition. For a detailed discussion of acclimatization to cold in cattle and of the effects of wind, rain and sun on heat exchange, see Webster (1974). Only one extreme example from Table 16.8 need be illustrated here. A beef-type suckler cow, in good condition and acclimatized to the winter environment has a still-air critical temperature of −17 °C. In a similar individual, unacclimatized to cold, T_{lc} is −2 °C. For a suckler cow of dairy type acclimatized to winter conditions but in poor condition, T_{lc} is +7 °C. Thus acclimatization, body type and body condition all markedly influence cold tolerance in cattle. The cow that enters the winter in poor condition is the first to be cold stressed. This generates a vicious circle of cold and undernutrition wherein each exacerbates the effects of the other.

Table 16.7 Critical temperature of cattle housed in conditions of very low air movement (wind velocity 0.18 m/s)

	Body weight (kg)	Coat depth (mm)	Thermal insulation (°C/m² per W)		Heat production† (W/m²)	Critical temperature (°C)
			I_t	I_e		
Calves						
Newborn	35	12	0.09	0.25	100	+9
1-month-old	50	14	0.10	0.26	120	0
Veal calf	100	12	0.12	0.25	154	−14
Beef cattle						
Young, 1 kg gain/day	150	14	0.14	0.26	139	−12
	350	14	0.19	0.26	144	−12
Young, 1.3 kg gain/day	150	14	0.13	0.26	150	−15
	350	14	0.19	0.26	155	−26
Store cattle, maintenance	250	22	0.16	0.33	123	−16
0.4 kg gain/day	250	22	0.14	0.33	158	−30
Fat stock, 0.8 kg gain/day	450	20	0.17	0.32	157	−32
1.5 kg gain/day	450	14	0.16	0.26	175	−32
Beef cow, maintenance	450	29	0.22	0.36	107	−17
Dairy cattle						
Dry, pregnant	500	16	0.21	0.29	104	−18
9 l/day	500	14	0.21	0.26	129	−17
23 l/day	500	12	0.20	0.25	154	−26
36 l/day	500	12	0.18	0.25	178	−33

† Heat production at critical temperature.

Table 16.8 Some effects of acclimatization, type and condition on the critical temperatures of cows in winter condition (from Webster, 1974)

	Condition	Heat production (W/m²)	Thermal insulation (°C/m² per W)		Critical temperature V (m/s)[†]	
			I_t	I_e	0.4	4.1
Beef cows (dry)						
Unacclimatized	Good	107	0.21	0.24	− 2	+10
Acclimatized	Good	117	0.22	0.35	−18	− 5
	Poor	97	0.15	0.35	− 1	+10
Dairy cows(dry)						
Unacclimatized	Good	107	0.17	0.22	0	+16
Acclimatized	Good	117	0.18	0.30	− 8	+ 5
	Poor	97	0.12	0.30	+ 7	+17

[†] Overcast, radiant temperature of the environment close to air temperature; V, wind speed.

Practical nutritional aids to the amelioration of cold stress in cattle involve the exploitation of the high appetite of the cold acclimatized individual and heat increment of feeding as a substitute for cold thermogenesis. For example, in western Canada, it is quite common practice to provide for beef cows on range a feed of barley straw additional to the normal maintenance requirement when air temperature drops below −18 °C. This feed is provided in the evening before the period of maximum cold. Not only are the cows prepared to eat an extra meal of forage in these circumstances, but the relatively low efficiency of utilization of the ME of barley straw (high heat increment) no longer constitutes a loss in efficiency since heat increment substitutes for cold thermogenesis at this time. In other words, the ME of barley straw is as useful as that of good hay to a cold cow.

Heat stress is, as indicated earlier, a much more serious impediment to productivity in cattle. The air temperature above which cattle lose appetite and retard growth or milk yield varies again according to type and degree of acclimatization but few animals of the class *Bos taurus* perform at their best above 25 °C (see Webster, 1976).

The effects of heat are a composite of reduced appetite and altered partition of retained nutrients between lean tissue, fat and milk, where relevant. The most useful ways of improving productivity in such climates involve modifications to the local environment for the animals and breeding for heat tolerance. The only possible nutritional aid to the amelioration of heat stress would be to feed diets of low heat increment at times of day when heat stress is least. The factors that affect the heat increment of diets for ruminants are complex and cannot be explained by any single hypothesis such as the molar ratios of glucogenic to ketogenic volatile fatty acids produced in fermentation. All that can be said for certain is that heat increment is intimately related to the fibre content of the diet (Annison and Armstrong, 1970; Webster, 1980). Unfortunately, many low-fibre diets tend to be expensive and inappropriate to tropical agriculture. Nevertheless, there is a good case to be made for investigating a selection of tropical foods and forms of physically processing those foods in order to minimize heat increment. This would not only increase the efficiency of utilization of ME in a thermoneutral environment but also increase appetite and thus productivity in areas where a major constraint on ruminant production is that of heat stress.

REFERENCES

The scope of this chapter embraces both nutrition and environmental physiology. It is not possible to provide a comprehensive list of references. Most of the references listed below are review articles. Original communications are quoted where the information is at present unreviewed or controversial.

Agricultural Research Council, 1980. *The Nutrient Requirements of Ruminant Livestock*. Commonwealth Agricultural Bureaux, Slough.

Agricultural Research Council, 1982. *The Nutrient Requirements of Farm Livestock. No. 3, Pigs*. 2nd edn. Agricultural Research Council, London.

Alexander, G., 1974. Heat loss from sheep. In *Heat Loss from Animals and Man: Assessment and Control* (ed. J. L. Monteith and L. E. Mount), pp. 173–203. Butterworth, London.

Alexander, G., Bennett, J. W. and Gemmell, R. T., 1975. Brown adipose tissue in the new-born calf (*Bos taurus*), *J. Physiol., Lond.* **244**: 223–34.

Annison, E. F. and Armstrong, D. G., 1970. Volatile fatty acid metabolism and energy supply. In *Physiology of Digestion and Metabolism in the Ruminant* (ed. A. T. Phillipson), pp. 422–37. Oriel Press, Newcastle on Tyne.

Bianca, W., 1965. Cattle in a hot environment, *J. Dairy Res.* **32**: 291–345.

Blaxter, K. L., 1967. *The Energy Metabolism of Ruminants*. 2nd edn. Hutchinson, London.

Blaxter, K. L., 1977. Environmental factors and their influence on the nutrition of farm livestock. In *Nutrition and the Climatic Environment* (ed. W. Haresign, H. Swan and D. Lewis), pp. 1–16. Butterworth, London.

Blaxter, K. L. and Boyne, A. W., 1978. The estimation of the nutritive value of feeds as energy sources for ruminants and the derivation of feeding systems, *J. agric. Sci., Camb.* **90**: 47–68.

Brody, S., 1945. *Bioenergetics and Growth*. Reinhold, New York.

Bruce, J. M., 1979. Heat loss from animals to floors, *Fm Bldg Prog., No. 55*, pp. 1–4.

Bruce, J. M. and Clark, J. J., 1979. Models of heat production and critical temperature for growing pigs, *Anim. Prod.* **28**: 353–69.

Close, W. H. and Mount, L. E., 1978. The effects of plane of nutrition and environmental temperature on the energy metabolism of the growing pig. 1. Heat loss and critical temperature, *Br. J. Nutr.* **40**: 413–21.

Colditz, P. J. and Kellaway, R. C., 1972. The effect of diet and heat stress on feed intake, growth, and nitrogen metabolism in Friesian, F_1 Brahman × Friesian, and Brahman heifers, *Aust. J. agric. Res.* **23**: 717–25.

Davey, A. W. F. and Holmes, C. W., 1977. The effects of shearing on the heat production and activity of sheep receiving dried grass or ground hay, *Anim. Prod.* **24**: 355–61.

Ekesbo, I. 1966. Disease incidence in tied and loose housed dairy cattle and causes of this incidence variation with particular reference to cowshed type, *Acta Agric. scand., Suppl. 15*.

Emmans, G. C. and Charles, D. R., 1977. Climatic environment and poultry feeding in practice. In *Nutrition and the Climatic Environment* (ed. W. Haresign, H. Swan and D. Lewis), pp. 31–49. Butterworth, London.

Forbes, J. M., 1977. Interrelationships between physical and metabolic control of voluntary food intake in fattening, pregnant and lactating mature sheep: a model, *Anim. Prod.* **24**: 91–101.

Foster, O. and Frydman, M. L., 1978. Non-shivering thermogenesis in the rat. 2. Measurements of blood flow with microspheres point to brown adipose tissue as the dominant site of the calorigenesis induced by noradrenaline, *Can. J. Physiol. Pharmac.* **56**:110–22.

Frisch, J. E. and Vercoe, J. E., 1977. Food intake, eating rate, weight gains, metabolic rate and efficiency of feed utilization in Bos taurus and Bos indicus crossbred cattle, *Anim. Prod.* **25**: 343–58.

Hales, J. R. S., 1974. Physiological responses to heat. In *MTP International Review of Science and Environmental Physiology*, Physiology Ser. 1, Vol. 7 (ed. D. Robertshaw), pp. 107–62. Butterworth, London.

Heroux, O., 1963. Patterns of morphological, physiological and endocrinological adjustments under different environmental conditions of cold, *Fedn Proc. Fedn Am Socs exp. Biol.* **22**: 789–94.

Himms-Hagen, J., 1967. Sympathetic regulation of metabolism, *Pharmac. Rev.* **19**: 367–461.

Holmes, C. W. and Close, W. H., 1977. The influence of climatic variables on energy metabolism and associated aspects of productivity in the pig. In *Nutrition and the Climatic Environment* (ed. W. Haresign, H. Swan and D. Lewis), pp. 51–73. Butterworth, London.

Hovell, F. D. DeB., Gordon, J. G. and MacPherson,, R. M., 1977. Thin sows. 2. Observations on the energy and nitrogen exchanges of thin and normal sows in environmental temperatures of 20 and 5 °C, *J. agric. Sci., Camb.* **89**: 523–33.

Ingram, D. L., 1974. Heat loss and its control in pigs. In *Heat Loss from Animals and Man: Assessment and Control* (ed. J. L. Monteith and L. E. Mount), pp. 233–54. Butterworth, London.

Kennedy, P. M., Christopherson, R. J. and Milligan, L. P., 1976. The effect of cold exposure of sheep on digestion, rumen turnover time and efficiency of microbial synthesis, *Br. J. Nutr.* **36**: 231–42.

Kleiber, M., 1961. *The Fire of Life.* Wiley, New York.

Kneale, W. A. and Bastiman, B., 1977. In wintering of ewes. Part V. The effect of shearing at housing, *Expl Husb., No. 32,* pp. 70–74.

McDowell, R. E., 1968. Climate versus man and his animals, *Nature, Lond.* **218**: 641–5.

McFarlane, M. V., 1976. Water and electrolytes in domestic animals. In *Veterinary Physiology* (ed. J. W. Phillips), pp. 461–539. Wright-Scientechnica, Bristol.

Milligan, J. D. and Christison, G. I., 1974. Effects of severe winter conditions on performance of feedlot steers, *Can. J. Anim. Sci.* **54**: 605–10.

Moe, P. W. and Tyrrell, H. F., 1975. Efficiency of conversion of digested energy to milk, *J. Dairy Sci.* **58**: 602–10.

Monteith, J. L. and Mount, L. E., 1974. *Heat Loss from Animals and Man: Assessment and Control.* Butterworth, London.

Mount, L. E., 1968. *The Climatic Physiology of the Pig.* Edward Arnold, London.

Ota, H. and McNally, E. H., 1965. Preliminary broiler heat and moisture data for designing poultry houses and ventilating systems, *Am. Soc. Agric. Engrs, Pap.* 65–411.

Payne, C. G., 1967. Environmental temperature and egg production. In *The Physiology of the Domestic Fowl* (ed. C. Horton-Smith and E. C. Amoroso), pp. 235–41. Oliver and Boyd, Edinburgh.

Rothwell, Nancy J. and Stock, M. J., 1979. A role for brown adipose tissue in diet-induced thermogenesis, *Nature, Lond.* **281**: 31–5.

Sainsbury, D. W. B., 1978. Poultry. In *The Care and Management of Farm Animals* (ed. W. N. Scott), pp. 176–215. Baillière Tindall, London.

Schmidt-Nielsen, K., 1964. *Desert Animals: Physiological Problems of Heat and Water.* Clarenden Press, Oxford.

Selye, H., 1950. *Stress.* Acta Inc., Montreal.

Siegel, H. S., 1977. Effects of temperature and light on growth. In *Growth and Poultry Meat Production* (ed. K. N. Boorman and B. J. Wilson), *Symp. Br. Poult. Sci., No. 12,* pp. 187–226.

Sybesma, W. and Eikelenboom, G., 1969. Malignant hyperthermia syndrome in pigs, *Neth. J. Vet. Sci.* **2**: 287–92.

Thompson, G. E., 1973. Climatic physiology of cattle, *J. Dairy Res.* **40**: 441–73.

Thompson, G. E. and Thomson, E. M., 1977. Effect of cold exposure on mammary circulation, oxygen consumption and milk secretion in the goat, *J. Physiol., Lond.* **272**: 187–96.

Van Kampen, M., 1976. Evaporative temperature regulation in birds. In *Progress in Biometeorology,* Div. B, Vol. 1 (ed. S. W. Tromp), pp. 158–66. Swets and Zeitlinger, Amsterdam.

Verstegen, M. W. A., van der Hel, W. and Willems, G. E. J. M., 1977. Growth depression and food requirements of fattening pigs at low environmental temperatures when housed either on concrete slats or on straw, *Anim. Prod.* **24**: 253–59.

Webster, A. J. F., 1974. Heat loss from cattle with particular emphasis on the effects of cold. In *Heat Loss from Animals and Man: Assessment and Control* (ed. J. L. Monteith and L. E. Mount), pp. 205–31. Butterworth, London.

Webster, A. J. F., 1976. The influence of the climatic environment on metabolism in cattle. In *Principles of Cattle Production*. (ed. H. Swan and W. H. Broster). pp. 103–20. Butterworth, London.

Webster, A. J. F., 1978. Prediction of the energy requirements for growth in beef cattle, *Wld Rev. Nutr. Diet.* **30**: 189–227.

Webster, A. J. F., 1979. Housing and husbandry of the veal calf, *Vet. A.* **19**: 49–53.

Webster, A. J. F., 1980. The energy cost of digestion and metabolism in the gut. In *Digestive Physiology and Metabolism in Ruminants* (ed. Y. Ruckebusch and P. Thivend), pp. 423–38. MTP Press, Lancaster.

Webster, A. J. F., Brockway, J. M. and Smith, J. S., 1974. Prediction of the energy requirements for growth in beef cattle. 1. The irrelevance of fasting metabolism, *Anim. Prod.* **19**: 127–39.

Webster, A. J. F., Hicks, A. M. and Hays, F. L., 1969. Cold climate and cold temperature induced changes in the heat production and thermal insulation of sheep, *Can. J. Physiol. Pharmac.*, **47**: 553–62.

Webster, A. J. F., Smith, J. S. and Brockway, J. M., 1972. Effects of isolation, confinement and competition for feed on the energy exchanges of growing lambs, *Anim. Prod.* **15**: 189–201.

17 NUTRITION AND GASTROINTESTINAL PARASITISM

J. H. Topps

Certain helminth parasites have a profound effect on the production of farm animals. For this reason essential features of their taxonomy, morphology and life cycles have been studied and recorded in detail in order to devise and use appropriate control measures (see Dunn, 1978). A few species which are widely occurring and particularly well known have also been the subject of intensive pathophysiological studies involving ruminant animals. These parasites are responsible for two major conditions in ruminants, namely fascioliasis and parasitic gastroenteritis. It is the intention in this chapter to consider the latter, since the effects on the nutrition of farm animals are more direct and better defined. For information on the pathogenesis of fascioliasis and related factors reference may be made to the papers of Sinclair (1967), Dargie (1975), Murray and Rushton (1975), Berry and Dargie (1976) and Dargie, Berry and Parkins (1979).

Gastrointestinal helminth parasites which have been studied in relation to physiological effects on the host animal, and their site of infection, are shown in Table 17.1. All but two belong to the family Trichostrongyloidea, the pathogenesis of which has been reviewed in detail by Fitzsimmons (1969). Although they differ appreciably in morphology and in their anatomical effects, they tend to produce similar effects on ruminant production. These effects will be reviewed before more detailed attention is given to the physiological changes caused by parasites.

EFFECTS ON ANIMAL PERFORMANCE

All the gastrointestinal helminths listed in Table 17.1 are capable of either reducing the rate of growth or causing loss of weight in ruminants. There appears to be no great difference between site of infection in this characteristic of parasites. In general, the heavier the infection the greater is the effect, but there is a level below which the

Table 17.1 Some common gastrointestinal parasites of ruminants and their site of infection.

Parasite	Common host animal	Site of infection
Chabertia ovina	Sheep	Large intestine
Haemonchus contortos	Sheep and goat	Abomasum
Oesophagostomum columbianum	Sheep and goat	Large intestine
Ostertagia circumcincta	Sheep and goat	Abomasum
Ostertagia ostertagi	Cattle	Abomasum
Trichostrongylus axei	Cattle and sheep	Abomasum
Trichostrongylus colubriformis	Sheep	Small intestine
Trichostrongylus vitrinus	Sheep	Small intestine

animal is apparently unaffected. A large part of the reduced growth rate or weight loss is due to a lower food intake. Only in one study, on sheep infected with mixed nematodes, has wool growth and weight gain been depressed without any apparent effect on food intake (Southcott, Heath and Langlands, 1967). The importance of depressed food intake has been measured by several workers (e.g. Bremner, 1961; Bawden, 1969a; Sykes and Coop, 1976 and 1977) by providing uninfected control animals with the amount of food consumed daily by infected animals, i.e. by using a pair-feeding technique. The results show that the reduction in intake accounts for approximately 40 to 90% of the differences in growth rate between infected and controls, both fed *ad libitum*. It is not clear why gut parasites reduce the food intake of the ruminant. No published study appears to have been devised to answer this particular question. Instead, results of work on parasitized calves and sheep have led to suggestions to explain the fall in intake. It seems too naïve to assume that local damage of the gut, which can be severe, could make an animal less inclined to eat. However, in some infections this may be a contributory factor, since lesions occur in locations in which there are receptors concerned with controlling gut motility, tension and content of digesta. A more important consideration is that there is a progressive fall in food intake as the infection persists and this is usually more apparent on poor-quality diets. Such an effect could be explained by the clinical condition or low metabolic status determining the level of intake; if this were the case as the condition became worse, less and less food would be eaten.

A reduced food intake in infected animals must inevitably lower the efficiency of conversion of food to weight gain, although early work by Andrews (1938) indicated there was also an increased heat production from infected lambs. Such an effect, if it occurs, may be transient. MacRae, Sharman, Smith, Easton and Coop (1979) have found recently that lambs infected with *T. colubriformis*, when compared with pair-fed controls, showed a decrease of 17% in the metabolizability of dietary energy by the 4th week of infection, but 4 weeks later the difference started to decline, and after another 4 weeks the metabolizability of energy by the two groups was identical. Energy balances followed a similar trend. However, nitrogen balances of infected lambs were considerably less than the controls by the 4th week and did not return to normal. A similar adverse effect of parasites has been seen in other studies and the reasons for it will be discussed later. Some limitation to protein deposition could lower the efficiency of conversion of food to weight gain but the effect may be too small to measure in experiments of 10 to 15 weeks duration. On the other hand, changes in body composition or carcass quality may be more apparent.

Differences in body composition of infected and worm-free sheep have been found by Reveron, Topps, MacDonald and Pratt (1974b) and by Sykes and Coop (1976 and 1977). The latter authors found that the percentage of water in infected animals was higher than normal and that the deposition of fat, protein and skeletal calcium and phosphorus was 15 to 45% lower than in worm-free controls. Reveron, Topps and Gelman (1974a) also found less calcium and phosphorus as well as less magnesium in the skeleton of infected lambs but there was some evidence that a lower content of body protein was offset by a higher content of fat. Clearly, from these studies, carcass quality can be affected adversely by parasites and this should be investigated further.

A variety of field evidence, and that derived from comparing the results of different trials, has indicated that young ruminants are more severely affected by parasites than older or mature animals. For example, in Britain, *Ostertagia ostertagi* is most commonly seen in cattle in the latter part of their first season at grass, when they are likely to be 6 months to 1 year old (Fitzsimmons, 1969). Sometimes older cattle are infected but with less marked clinical signs. Reasons for this age difference are related to the development of immunity and a lower requirement for certain nutrients by older animals. The quality of the diet of the host animal also affects the severity of infection (Gibson, 1963). As expected, a higher-quality diet offsets to a greater extent the lower utilization of nutrients but it may also affect the establishment of the parasite within the host. Such a difference has been clearly seen, with high- and low-protein diets, by Bawden (1969b). Young sheep fed on a low- protein diet (60 g/kg) had a greater susceptibility to infection with *Oesophagostomum columbianum* than those on a high-protein diet (180 g/kg). Both the number of adult worms recovered 56 days after infection and the fecundity of the female worms was greater in sheep given low levels of protein. While the quality of the host's diet has an effect on the establishment of the parasite, it appears to have less influence on established infections. If the production of worm eggs is a reliable indicator of the degree of infection, Brunsdon (1964) has found that a natural *Trichostrongylus* parasitism in lambs was not markedly affected by the host's plane of nutrition.

Since wool consists mainly of protein, it is not surprising that two groups of workers have reported an adverse effect of gastrointestinal parasites on wool production (Southcott *et al.*, 1967; Barger, Southcott and Williams, 1973). Both the diameter and length of fibres are reduced. In both reports there are indications that wool growth is affected at levels of infection which have little or no effect on body weight.

CLINICAL CHANGES CAUSED BY PARASITES

Although changes in the gastrointestinal tract are not seen until the animal is slaughtered, they are important in initiating a series of events which have serious consequences and may lead to a premature death. Invasion of the gut tissues causes lesions which arise directly from the penetration, migration and feeding habits of the parasite. For example, Armour, Jarrett and Jennings (1966) found that the larvae of *Ostertagia circumcincta*, in developing, growing and emerging onto the mucosal surface, destroyed the gastric glands of the abomasum of sheep. In contrast, it is the adult worm of *Haemonchus contortus* which mutilates the mucosa of the abomasum and causes haemorrhage. Parasites of the small intestine tend to produce atrophy and flattening of the villi (Barker, 1973), while two that invade the large intestine cause ulceration and haemorrhage (Bawden, 1969a; Herd, 1971). Recently, Angus, Coop and Sykes (1979) found that treatment of sheep with an anthelmintic, after the animals had been dosed daily with 4000 *Trichostrongylus colubriformis*, resulted in the restoration after 3 weeks of a normal mucosa of the small intestine.

Once tissue damage has been caused there is a replacement of functional by undifferentiated cells, together with hyperplasia and inflammation of the epithelium which thickens most of the parasitized surfaces of the mucosa. Such changes lead to functionally immature cells being placed in secretory and absorptive areas and a 'leak lesion' develops, which has a mucosa with a greater permeability to macromolecules (Murray, Jennings and Armour, 1970). A variety of abnormalities may follow, depending on the site of infection. For example, in the abomasum there may be changes in pH, while parasites lodged in the small intestine may induce or exacerbate deficiencies of certain brush-border enzymes.

Anaemia and changes in plasma proteins are common clinical signs of gastrointestinal parasitism. Their incidence and severity appear to be unrelated to the site of infection, and they undoubtedly affect the performance of the ruminant animal. Changes in plasma proteins are usually a decrease in albumin concentration and increases in the concentrations of globulin and total protein. In severe infections both albumin and globulin are reduced. There is a consistent pattern in the development of these changes, including that of anaemia. It is characterized by three basic stages which occur separately or together in a group of animals. The initial stage is a decrease by approximately 25% in packed cell volume and levels of serum albumin. This is followed by a second stage when levels of these blood constituents remain relatively constant but are still depressed, and a third stage during which further deterioration occurs. The pattern can be explained by changes in fractional rates of removal of red blood cells. and albumin from the circulation, and in the synthesis of haemoglobin and albumin in parasitized animals. The magnitude of both changes has been measured in lambs infected with *Haemonchus contortus* (Dargie, 1973). Increased fractional rates of removal of plasma, albumin or protein, or of all three materials, have been found by Bremner (1969) in parasitized calves and by Herd (1971), Holmes and MacLean (1971), and Barker (1973) in lambs infected with different nematodes.

Other clinical changes which result from parasitic infections are diarrhoea and oedema, depressed blood levels of certain essential minerals, and elevated activities of plasma pepsinogen and certain enzymes produced by the liver.

EFFECTS ON GUT FUNCTION, DIGESTION AND ABSORPTION

Unfortunately, little is definitely known about gut function in parasitized ruminants. Some information has been inferred from digestion and balance studies, but this has limited value since measurements have often been of apparent rather than true digestibility, and such studies do not reveal the importance of local dysfunctions. To overcome this omission more studies are required on animals fitted with cannulae in different parts of the gastrointestinal tract.

There is a little evidence that parasites alter gut motility and the rate of flow of digesta. Roseby (1977) found that, in lambs with a medium-sized burden of *Trichostrongylus colubriformis*, digesta flow from the rumen was reduced but in the small and large intestine it was enhanced. The results are a little equivocal since the sheep may have suffered from diarrhoea and the flow of solid material was not measured. Bawden (1970) showed earlier a slower rate of flow of fluid digesta through the whole gut in lambs infected with *Oesophagostomum columbianum* which did not show diarrhoea, but pair-fed animals were not used so the effect could be attributed to a lower food intake. French work, in which the electrical activity of the gut wall was measured, provides good evidence for altered gut motility and a more rapid flow of digesta through the intestine of sheep affected by diarrhoea caused by a mixed infection (Ruckebusch, 1970). It now seems that if motility and digesta flow are accelerated the change for most infections is likely to be restricted to certain sections of the gut.

Firmer evidence is available for the fact that some parasites affect the release of gastrointestinal hormones. Such an effect was intimated in work by Jennings, Armour, Lawson and Roberts (1966) on calves which were infected with *Ostertagia ostertagi* and fitted with an abomasal cannula. The calves had abomasal contents with a high pH (up to 7.5), increased concentrations of sodium and greater numbers of viable bacteria, but concentrations of potassium and chloride and pepsin activity were reduced. To explain these findings, it was suggested that there was a leakage of body fluid into the abomasum via the damaged hyperplastic epithelium. This may be the main, though possibly not the sole, causative factor. More recent work in Australia (Titchen and Anderson, 1977) with sheep infected with the abomasal parasite *Ostertagia circumcincta* has clearly indicated an increased secretion of gastrin. The sheep (and also a few calves subsequently infected with *Ostertagia ostertagi*) were prepared with separated, innervated pouches made from the region of the abomasum which secretes acid. After infection, secretory activity of parasitized mucosa was compared with that of non-parasitized mucosa by means of cannulae inserted in the abomasum and pouch. The main part of the abomasum showed a loss of its capacity to maintain acidity and the pH of the contents rose to between 5 and 7 units approximately 2 weeks after infection. Conversely, acid secretion and acidity in the pouches increased from 4 days after infection and reached a maximum approximately 12 days later when food intake was reduced, which normally causes a reduction in the volume secreted from the fundic pouches. The contrary reactions were thought on the one hand to be due to a direct suppressive effect on acid secretion of substances released locally by the parasite or injured host tissue, whereas increased secretion of the hormone, gastrin, was thought to be responsible for the stimulating effects of infection on acid secretion within the pouches. Furthermore, hypersecretion from fundic pouches failed to develop in infected sheep after total removal of the antrum, which is the major source of gastrin. Radioimmunoassay showed that blood gastrin levels of infected sheep increased to more than 10 times those of worm-free sheep; the hypergastrinaemia was reversed by anthelmintic treatment and developed again on re-infection of treated sheep. These changes provide evidence for a direct causal relationship between the presence of parasites and hypergastrinaemia.

As far as is known, the effect of hypergastrinaemia is purely homeo-static, but since gastrin increases water and electrolyte secretion by the liver, pancreas and ileum, and pentagastrin inhibits activity of the reticulorumen and abomasum, other physiological changes cannot be discounted. An equally important consideration is the possibility of parasites altering the secretion of other gastrointestinal hormones.

Since gastrointestinal parasites cause distinct pathological lesions it is not surprising that impaired digestion and absorption are considered to be major causes of a poor utilization of food by parasitized ruminants. Evidence for such a relationship is not convincing, however. The find-ings of Bremner (1969), Holmes and MacLean (1971), Parkins, Holmes and Bremner (1973) and Sykes and Coop (1976 and 1977), who used pair-fed animals, suggest some reduction in the digestion or absorp-tion of dietary nitrogen as indicated by values for apparent digest-ibility, but such measures are poor indicators of malabsorption. This is particularly so in the parasitized ruminant in which, as described in detail later, there is additional passage of endogenous nitrogen into the gut. It cannot be concluded that there is poor digestion or malabsorp-tion if the excess of a certain nutrient appearing in the faeces could be accounted for by endogenous losses. In only one reported study (Sykes and Coop, 1977) with pair-fed animals is there a strong indication of poor digestion or malabsorption. The difference between infected and control sheep in apparently digested nitrogen was initially too large (see Table 17.2) to be accounted for by leakage into the gut, but later it was reduced sufficiently for this phenomenon to have been the explanation. The authors gave considerable emphasis to the digestive disturbance caused by the parasite, *Ostertagia circumcincta*, but the correlation observed between weight gain and differences in nitrogen digestibility was low. If there is a true reduction in nitrogen absorption due to this parasite, the impact of the reduction on ruminant production appears small. It is interesting to note that Barger *et al.* (1973) found that reduced wool growth induced by trichostrongylosis could not be attributed to malabsorption of cysteine.

Two Australian researchers, working separately, have studied gut fermentation in parasitized sheep and both report a 30% reduction in production of rumen VFA by animals infected with *Trichostrongylus colubriformis* after allowing for reduced food intake (Steel, 1972; Roseby, 1977). The results of Steel (1972) also indicate that ammonia production in the rumen is decreased but that the production of VFA and ammonia in the large intestine are increased. These results, together with those in a later report (Steel, 1974), indicate that, in terms of fermentation as well as enzymic digestion, digestive activity is shifted caudally to some extent. Such changes may seriously alter the amount of amino acids and ammonia absorbed by the parasitized ruminant and for this reason merit further attention.

Table 17.2   Nitrogen balance (g/day) of parasitized animals compared with controls which were pair-fed[†]

Host and parasite	Weeks after infection	Group	Nitrogen			
			Intake	Faeces	Urine	Balance
Calves *Oesophagostomum radiatum*	4–5	Control	78.0	26.9	58.1	−7.0
		Infected	77.8	35.0	58.9	−16.1
Sheep *Ostertagia cirumcincta*	1–2	Control	2.1	1.7	3.2	−2.8
		Infected	2.2	1.6	5.1	−4.5
Sheep *Trichostrongylus colubriformis*	6–7	Control	32.9	14.1	16.5	+2.3
		Infected	33.4	14.6	18.0	+0.8
Sheep *Ostertagia circumcincta*	2–3	Control	31.1	12.6	17.6	+0.9
		Infected	32.2	18.0	17.6	−3.4
	7–8	Control	32.3	11.7	17.8	+2.8
		Infected	34.4	15.6	16.5	+2.3
	12–13	Control	29.4	9.5	17.4	+2.5
		Infected	31.3	12.0	17.2	+2.1

[†] Results of Bremner (1969), Holmes and Maclean (1971), Parkins *et al.* (1973) and Sykes and Coop (1976 and 1977).

EFFECTS ON PROTEIN METABOLISM

Gastrointestinal parasites have an adverse effect on the nitrogen balance of calves and sheep. The results of comparative work in which pair-fed animals have been used are shown in Table 17.2. In the most recent work, Sykes and Coop (1976 and 1977) confirmed the lower nitrogen balance observed in their infected animals by showing a lower content of protein in the carcass. The inferior balances are due to greater losses of faecal nitrogen or urinary nitrogen or both. The first may be explained by additional leakage of endogenous nitrogen into the gut or a lower true digestibility of nitrogen, as mentioned earlier. Greater urinary loss indicates a lower efficiency of utilization of absorbed nitrogen. Hence it would seem that disturbances of the animal's protein metabolism are the major causes of the lower protein deposition even though these disturbances are initiated by lesions in the gut.

These derangements of protein metabolism, as caused by *Trichostrongylus colubriformis* in sheep, have been summarized by Roseby (1977) and the major pathways of nitrogen transfer are outlined in Fig. 17.1. This

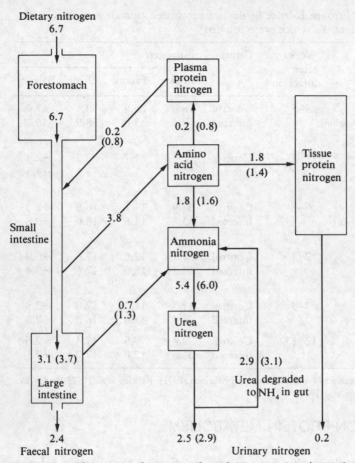

Fig. 17.1.   The rates of net transfer of nitrogen (mg/min) between body
'pools' in worm-free sheep and in sheep infected with *Trichostrongylus colubriformis* (values in parenthesis where different from the
worm-free animals).

summary, which is based on the results of Barker (1973), Roseby
(1973 and 1977), Roseby and Leng (1974) and Steel (1974), follows the
approach of Nolan and Leng (1972) but has been simplified to include
only pathways that are relevant to a comparison of worm-free and
parasitized sheep. Roseby and Leng (1974) found that parasitized sheep
had a greater plasma concentration or pool size of urea than non-
infected animals and most of the extra urinary nitrogen excreted could
be accounted for by urea. It would appear that *Trichostrongylus colubriformis* and possibly other gut parasites cause an increase in urea synthesis
which is accompanied by a greater rate of irreversible loss in the urine,
but not by more urea recycling through the gut. This means that the

extra urea excreted comes from ammonia rather than from endogenous urea, and that the ammonia probably comes from deamination of amino acids within the gut and tissues. This sequence of events follows logically from the effects of the parasite on the small intestine, which are summarized in the flow diagram (Fig. 17.1). The greater leakage of endogenous protein into the small intestine results in a reduction in the net absorption of amino acid nitrogen. The corresponding increase in microbial deamination in the large intestine causes an increase in ammonia production, but very little is used for amino acid synthesis since most of the ammonia is converted to urea and excreted. Other work reported by Dargie (1973) and by Symons and Jones (1975) has indicated changes in rates of protein synthesis in sheep infected with either *Haemonchus contortus* or *Trichostrongylus colubriformis*. These changes are compatible with the nitrogen transfers shown in Fig. 17.1 Dargie (1973) found that synthesis of albumin was increased 2.5-fold and that of haemoglobin three-fold in parasitized animals which had the same food intake as non-infected animals. Symons and Jones (1975) measured the incorporation of labelled amino acids into mixed tissue proteins, and obtained firm evidence that in sheep infected with *Trichostrongylus colubriformis* synthesis of skeletal muscle protein was reduced while that of liver protein was increased. Furthermore, the increase in hepatic synthesis in both studies was closely associated with the development of excessive leakage of plasma into the gastrointestinal tract.

Extra energy would be needed by infected animals to meet the cost of synthesis of additional blood protein. Using a recent estimate (Puller and Webster, 1977) of the energy cost of protein deposition of 53 MJ/kg, a daily loss of 150 ml of plasma would be equivalent to about 800 kJ/day. A difference of this magnitude in deposition of body energy has been found by Sykes and Coop (1976 and 1977) between infected and control sheep which were pair-fed.

EFFECTS ON MINERAL METABOLISM

Very early work, which was reviewed by Reveron and Topps (1970), suggested that sheep with heavy infections of gut nematodes suffered from mineral disorders. The classical research of Franklin, Gordon and MacGregor (1946), which showed clearly that young sheep with subclinical infections of *Trichostrongylus colubriformis* utilized calcium and phosphorus inefficiently, was the first to confirm the occurrence of such an effect. It is now known that both abomasal and intestinal infections adversely affect deposition of calcium, phosphorus and magnesium in the growing animal, which results in reductions in bone size, the density of the bone matrix and its degree of mineralization (Barger, 1973; Reveron *et al.*, 1974a; Sykes and Coop, 1976 and 1977). However, infected animals tend to maintain normal blood levels of these minerals unless *Trichostrongylus colubriformis* is the parasite, when marked decreases in concentrations of plasma phosphorus occur. A pronounced difference in plasma phosphorus has been found between worm-free and parasitized animals even when they have been pair-fed (Coop, Sykes and Angus, 1976). Attempts to elucidate the reasons for the bone disorders have produced inconsistent results even in studies on the same parasite. Barger (1973) found that the apparent absorption of calcium but not phosphorus was reduced with *Trichostrongylus colubriformis*. Reveron *et al.* (1974a) obtained an adverse effect on phosphorus but not on calcium and magnesium absorption, while Sykes and Coop (1976) showed that both calcium and phosphorus were less well absorbed. Obviously, more work is needed to resolve these differences before the mechanism of the interference can be elucidated. An important practical consequence of this work is the recognition that increasing the dietary supplies of the three minerals is unlikely to improve the performance of infected animals.

CONCLUSIONS

As a result of research over the last 10 years there is now a clearer understanding of the ways in which gastrointestinal parasites affect the nutrition and physiology of ruminant animals. More work is needed to extend the range of parasites that have been studied, to establish the causes of the depression in food intake and of the disorders in mineral metabolism, and to assess quantitatively the changes in nitrogen metabolism. It should be remembered that under field conditions changes in food intake and ingestion of parasitic larvae, and the presence of factors which induce environmental stress, may well exacerbate or occasionally ameliorate some of the effects that have been seen in controlled experiments.

REFERENCES

Andrews, J. S., 1938. Effect of infestation with the nematode *Cooperia curticei* on the nutrition of lambs, *J. agric. Res.* **57**: 349–61.
Angus, K. W., Coop, R. L. and Sykes, A. R., 1979. The rate of recovery of

intestinal morphology following anthelmintic treatment of parasitized sheep, *Res. vet. Sci.* **26**: 120–2.

Armour, J., Jarrett, W. F. H. and Jennings, F. W., 1966. Experimental *Ostertagia circumcincta* infections in sheep: development and pathogenesis of a single infection, *Am. J. vet. Res.* **27**: 1267–78.

Barger, I. A., 1973. Trichostrongylosis and wool growth. I. Feed digestibility and mineral absorption in infected sheep, *Aust. J. exp. Agric. Anim. Husb.* **13**: 42–7.

Barger, I. A., Southcott, W. H. and Williams, V. J., 1973. *Trichostrongylus* and wool growth. II. The wool growth response of infected sheep to parenteral and duodenal cystine and cysteine supplementation, *Aust. J. exp. Agric. Anim. Husb.* **13**: 351–9.

Barker, I. K., 1973. A study of the pathogenesis of *Trichostrongylus colubriformis* infection in lambs with observations on the contribution of gastrointestinal plasma loss, *Int. J. Parasitol* **3**: 743–57.

Bawden, R. J., 1969a. Relationships between *Oesophagostomum columbianum* infection and the nutritional status of sheep. I. Effects on growth and feed utilization, *Aust. J. agric. Res* **20**: 589–99.

Bawden, R. J., 1969b. The establishment and survival of *Oesophagostomum columbianum* in male and female sheep given high and low protein diets, *Aust. J. agric. Res.* **20**: 1151–9.

Bawden, R. J., 1970. The effects of nematode parasitism on the rate of passage of food residues through the alimentary tract of sheep, *Br. J. Nutr.* **24**: 291–6.

Berry, C. I. and Dargie, J. D., 1976. The role of host nutrition in the pathogenesis of ovine fascioliasis, *Vet. Parasitol.* **2**: 317–32.

Bremner, K. C., 1961. A study of pathogenetic factors in experimental bovine oesophagostomosis. I. An assessment of the importance of anorexia, *Aust. J. agric. Res.* **12**: 498–512.

Bremner, K. C., 1969. Pathogenic factors in experimental bovine ocsophagostomosis. IV. Exudative enteropathy as a cause of hypoproteinaemia, *Expl Parasit.* **25**: 382–94.

Brunsdon, R. V., 1964. The effect of nutrition on the establishment and persistence of Trichostrongyle infestation, *N.Z. vet. J.* **12**: 108–11.

Coop, R. L., Sykes, A. R. and Angus, K. W., 1976. Subclinical trichostrongylosis in growing lambs produced by continuous larval dosing. The effect on performance and certain plasma constituents, *Res. vet. Sci.* **21**: 253–8.

Dargie, J. D., 1973. Ovine haemonchosis: pathogenesis. In *Helminth Diseases of Cattle, Sheep and Horses in Europe* (ed. G. M. Urquhart and J. Armour), pp. 63–71. Robert Maclehose, University Press, Glasgow.

Dargie, J. D., 1975. Applications of radioisotope techniques to the study of red cell and plasma protein metabolism in helminth diseases of sheep. In *Pathogenic Processes in Parasitic Infections* (ed. A. E. R. Taylor and R. Muller), pp. 1–26. Blackwell, Oxford.

Dargie, J. D., Berry, C. I. and Parkins, J. J., 1979. The pathophysiology of ovine fascioliasis: studies on the feed intake and digestibility, body weight and nitrogen balance of sheep given rations of hay or hay plus a pelleted supplement, *Res. vet. Sci.* **26**: 289–95.

Dunn, A. M., 1978. *Veterinary Helminthology*. 2nd edn. Heinemann, London.

Fitzsimmons, W. M., 1969. Pathogenesis of the *Trichostrongylus, Helminth. Abstr.* **38**: 139–90.

Franklin, M. C., Gordon, H. McL. and MacGregor, C. H., 1946. A study of nutritional and biochemical effects in sheep of infestation with *Trichostrongylus colubriformis, J. Coun. scient. ind. Res. Aust.* **19**: 46–60.

Gibson, T. E., 1963. The influence of nutrition on the relationships between gastro-intestinal parasites and their hosts, *Proc. Nutr. Soc.* **22**: 15–20.

Herd, R. P., 1971. The pathogenic importance of *Chabertia ovina* (Fabricius, 1788) in experimentally infected sheep, *Int. J. Parasitol.* **1**: 251–63.

Holmes, P. H. and MacLean, J. M., 1971. The pathophysiology of ovine ostertagiasis: a study of the changes in plasma protein metabolism following single infections, *Res. vet. Sci.* **12**: 265–71.

Jennings, F. W., Armour, J., Lawson, D. D. and Roberts, R., 1966. Experimental *Ostertagia ostertagi* infections in calves: studies with abomasal cannulas, *Am. J. vet. Res.* **27**: 1249–57.

MacRae, J. C., Sharman, G. A. M., Smith, J. S., Easton, J. F. and Coop, R. L., 1979. Preliminary observations on the effects of *Trichostrongylus colubriformis* infestation on the energy and nitrogen metabolism of lambs, *Anim. Prod.* **28**: 456 (Abstr.).

Murray, M., Jennings, F. W. and Armour, J., 1970. Bovine ostertagiasis: structure, function and mode of differentation of the bovine gastric mucosa and kinetics of the worm loss, *Res. vet. Sci.* **11**: 417–27.

Murray, M. and Rushton, B., 1975. The pathology of fascioliasis with particular reference to hepatic fibrosis. In *Pathogenic Processes in Parasitic Infections* (ed. A. E. R. Taylor and R. Muller), pp. 27–41. Blackwell, Oxford.

Nolan, J. V., and Leng, R. A., 1972. Dynamic aspects of ammonia and urea metabolism in sheep, *Br. J. Nutr.* **27**: 177–94.

Parkins, J. J., Holmes, P. H. and Bremner, K. C., 1973. The pathophysiology of ovine ostertagiasis: some nitrogen balance and digestibility studies. *Res. vet. Sci.* **14**: 21–8.

Puller, J. D. and Webster, A. J. F., 1977. The energy cost of fat and protein deposition in the rat, *Br. J. Nutr.* **37**: 355–63.

Reveron, A. E. and Topps, J. H., 1970. Nutrition and gastro-intestinal parasitism in ruminants, *Outl. Agric.* **6**: 131–6.

Reveron, A. E., Topps, J. H. and Gelman, A. L., 1974a. Mineral metabolism and skeletal development of lambs affected by *Trichostrongylus colubriformis, Res. vet. Sci.* **16**: 310–9.

Reveron, A. E., Topps, J. H., MacDonald, D. C. and Pratt, G., 1974b. The intake, digestion and utilization of food and growth rate of lambs affected by *Trichostrongylus colubriformis, Res. vet. Sci.* **16**: 299–309.

Roseby, F. B., 1973. Effects of *Trichostrongylus colubriformis* (Nematoda) on the nutrition and metabolism of sheep. I. Feed intake, digestion, and utilization, *Aust. J. agric. Res.* **24**: 947–53.

Roseby, F. B., 1977. Effects of *Trichostrongylus colubriformis* (Nematoda) on the nutrition and metabolism of sheep. III. Digesta flow and fermentation, *Aust. J. agric. Res.* **28**: 155–64.

Roseby, F. B. and Leng, R. A., 1974. Effects of *Trichostrongylus colubriformis*

(Nematoda) on the nutrition and metabolism of sheep. II. Metabolism of urea, *Aust. J. agric. Res.* **28**: 363–7.

Ruckebusch, Y., 1970. The electrical activity of the digestive tract of the sheep as an indication of the mechanical events in various regions, *J. Physiol., Lond.* **210**: 857–82.

Sinclair, K. B., 1967. Pathogenesis of Fasciola and other liver-flukes, *Helminth. Abstr.* **36**: 115–34.

Southcott, W. H., Heath, D. D. and Langlands, J. P., 1967. Relationship of nematode infection to efficiency of wool production, *J. Br. Grassld Soc.* **22**: 117–20.

Steel, J. W., 1972. Effects of the intestinal nematode *Trichostrongylus colubriformis* on ruminal acetate metabolism in young sheep, *Proc. Aust. Soc. Anim. Prod.* **9**: 402–7.

Steel, J. W., 1974. Pathophysiology of gastrointestinal nematode infections in the ruminant, *Proc. Aust. Soc. Anim. Prod.* **10**: 139–47.

Sykes, A. R. and Coop, R. L., 1976. Intake and utilization of food by growing lambs with parasitic damage to the small intestine caused by daily dosing with *Trichostrongylus colubriformis* larvae, *J. agric. Sci., Camb.* **86**: 507–15.

Sykes. A. R. and Coop, R. L., 1977. Intake and utilization of food by growing sheep with abomasal damage caused by daily dosing with *Ostertagia circumcincta* larvae, *J. agric. Sci., Camb.* **88**: 671–7.

Symons, L. E. A. and Jones, W. O., 1975. Skeletal muscle, liver and wool protein synthesis by sheep infected by the nematode *Trichostrongylus colubriformis*, *Aust. J. agric. Res.* **26**: 1063–72.

Titchen, D. A. and Anderson, N., 1977. Aspects of the physic-pathology of parasitic gastritis in the sheep, *Aust. vet. J.* **53**: 369–73.

INDEX